Enkephalins and Endorphins
Stress and the Immune System

Enkephalins and Endorphins
Stress and the Immune System

Edited by

Nicholas P. Plotnikoff

Oral Roberts University
Tulsa, Oklahoma

Robert E. Faith

University of Houston
Houston, Texas

Anthony J. Murgo

West Virginia University
Morgantown, West Virginia

and

Robert A. Good

University of South Florida
St. Petersburg, Florida

PLENUM PRESS • NEW YORK AND LONDON

Library of Congress Cataloging in Publication Data

Enkephalins and endorphins.

Bibliography: p.
Includes index.
1. Enkephalins—Physiological effect. 2. Endorphins—Physiological effect. 3. Immune response—Regulation. 4. Stress (Physiology) 5. Stress (Psychology) 6. Psychoneuroimmuno-endocrinology. I. Plotnikoff, Nicholas P.
QP552.E55E55 1986   616.07'9   85-23234
ISBN 0-306-42226-3

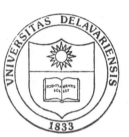

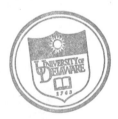

QP
552
.E55
E55
1986

© 1986 Plenum Press, New York
A Division of Plenum Publishing Corporation
233 Spring Street, New York, N.Y. 10013

Printed in the United States of America

FOREWORD

Is this a time for a sleeping giant to rise? We have known since
study of the lymphocyte and plasma cells really began in earnest in the
early 1940's that the pituitary adrenal axis under intimate control of the
hypothalamus could influence immunological functions profoundly. We have
also known for at least 20 years in my recollection that female sex hormones can maximize certain immunity functions while male sex hormones
tend to suppress many immunological reactions. The thyroid hormones
accelerate antibody production while at the same time speeding up degradation of antibodies and immunoglobulins and thyroidectomy decreases
the rate of antibody production. Further, much evidence has accumulated
indicating that the brain, yes even the mind, can influence in significant
ways susceptibility to infections, cancers and to development of a variety
of autoimmune diseases. More than 20 years ago, my colleagues and I
convinced ourselves, if no one else, that hypnosis can exert major influences on the effector limb of the classical atopic allergic reactions.
We showed with Aaron Papermaster that the Prausnitz-Kustner reaction may
be greatly inhibited, indeed largely controlled, by post-hypnotic suggestion.
And it was not even necessary for us to publish our discovery because
scientists in John Humphrey's laboratory at Mill Hill Research Center in
London had beaten us to the punch. They described hypnotic control of
both the PK reaction and delayed allergic reactions to tuberculin by
hypnosis. Although he doesn't necessarily attribute the controls to
neurological modulation, I have been convinced that the extraordinary
rhythms Franz Halberg in Minnesota has elucidated for immunological
functions that range from NK cell activity to the amount of antibody
produced and even the tempo of allograft rejection reflect neuroendocrinological interactions with the immunological systems.

Halberg's Chronoimmunologic analyses have been underway for at least
20 years and would have begun earlier and progressed even more rapidly
than they have had we immunologists been more responsive to his prodding
and that of other chronobiologists associated with him.

Why then does the present moment strike me as so propitious a moment
for a comprehensive new work considering the interaction of the major
body networks?

For me, a new and truly golden age of psychoneuroimmunoendocrinology
began when Wybran of Brussels first observed in 1979 that met-enkephalin

can talk to lymphocytes directly and its conversation with lymphocytes can be interrupted by naloxone. These rather crude beginnings have now been greatly refined and we know for sure that lymphocytes have receptors for met-enkephalin and have either surface or cytosolic receptors for a number of other hormones and neurohumoral mediators. We see in this volume and in numerous contemporary articles reaching our scientific journals that met-enkephalin, leu enkephalin and endorphins can reproducibly influence cell surface expression and functions of lymphocytes in vivo, antibody production, delayed allergic reactions and development and differentiation of lymphoid cells. We are even witnessing these days the first descriptions of responses of immunoparameters in healthy humans and patients with various kinds of immunodeficiencies including patients with AIDS and cancer. All this is happening right now and this science and this form of immunopharmacology will be rapidly developed in the years ahead.

But this is only one of many many exciting fields in psychoneuro-immunoendocrinology where incredible discoveries are turning up.

As a Visiting Professor at the University of Texas Medical Branch in Galveston last winter, I was introduced to a constellation of related studies by Blalock and his group of young colleagues. These studies established to my satisfaction that lymphocytes, like pituitary cells, can produce a molecule very like ACTH both immunologically and functionally and that like cells of the anterior pituitary, the lymphocytes have cytosolic receptors for cortisol. Through these, cortisol can suppress production of the ACTH-like molecule by these cells. As a classical cellular immunologist such a turn of events could never have entered my mind yet here it was, big as life, and it had been demonstrated by what seemed to me to be commanding and critical scientific methodology.

But these surprises are at least paralleled as surprises presented by Hall and Goldstein's (Washington) discovery that thymosin α_1 now a fully defined molecule (thymic hormone?) exerts functional and electrical influences on certain hypothalamic nuclear cells that can, in turn, exert influences on lymphoid cell function through the thymus. If these descriptions sound fanciful it is because I believe they are. Yet they and much, much more are presented in detail in this volume of collected multi-authored papers that reflect a burgeoning scientific field. Even Robert Ader and Nicholas Cohen's exciting discovery that the immune response can be regulated by taste via prior conditioning in the conditioned-aversion response after simultaneous exposure to a cytotoxic immunosuppressive chemical may before long be explained in precise immunopharmcological terms. I now would bet it will.

This field is developing more rapidly than I thought could ever be the case and I am thankful to the immunopharmacologists like Plotnikoff, Wybran, Hadden, Szentivanyi and others who have urged me to pay close attention.

Robert A. Good, M.D., Ph.D.

CONTENTS

EARLY CLINICAL TRIALS OF METHIONINE ENKEPHALIN(IN VIVO)

INTRODUCTION: YING-YANG HYPOTHESIS OF IMMUNOMODULATION

N.P. Plotnikoff, A.J. Murgo, R.E. Faith, and R.A. Good

Oral Roberts University School of Medicine
Tulsa, Oklahoma

Originally the inspiration for this book stemmed from a Symposium on Enkephalins; Endorphins: Stress and the Immune System held at the Annual meeting of the American Society of Pharmacology and Experimental Therapeutics in Philadelphia 1983. Since that meeting a significant increase in research has occurred and prompted us to compile this book. Recent research has shown that the immune system is exceedingly sensitive to the effects of enkephalins and endorphins. This sensitivity was illustrated by the immunodepressant effects of morphine on T-cells. In contrast the enkephalins and endorphins have shown to enhance T-cell function.

At the same time a major development in this field was the discovery that the adrenal glands are the source of peripheral enkephalins and endorphins. Two major prohormones have been identified in human adrenal glands, namely, Proenkephalin A as well as proopiomelanacortin hormone.

These prohormones have been shown to release various intermediate peptide fragments(Peptide E and F) as well as the final end products, methionine enkephalin, leucine enkephalin, and beta-endorphin. Since morphine is immuno-depressant and is found to have high affinity for the mu and kappa receptors, it was of great interest to find that several of the prohormone peptide fragments also has a high affinity for the same receptors, suggesting that they may also have an immuno-depressant role. In contrast the final end products methionine enkephalin and leucine enkephalin and beta-endorphin have been discovered to be immuno-stimulant and bind preferentially to the delta and epsilon receptors.

This immunomodulation by prohormone peptide fragments and enkephalin-endorphin end products led to the Ying-Yang hypothesis of immunomodulation of T-cell function. We are proposing the working opioid peptide hypothesis that various prohormone fragments are released by different stressors resulting in fluctuations of immunomodulation in concert with the steroid hormones and the catecholamines from the adrenal glands. It is possible that a number of contradictory behavioral studies reported in the literature are a result of this immunomodulation(depression and/or stimulation) as a function of differential prohormone processing and type of duration of stressors.

It is intriguing to consider the possibility that long term stress may result in "depletion or exhaustion phenomenon" of prohormone end products (enkephalins-endorphins) depending upon the state of behavioral coping.

Perhaps 'replacement therapy' with the enkephalins-endorphins would be appropriate in certain selected clinical conditions.

Finally, very recent studies indicate that methionine enkephalin stimulates the production and release of lymphokines(interferons and inter-leukins) from macrophages and T-cells. Therefore, the clinical effects of methionine enkephalin in enhancing T-cell subsets in Kaposis sarcoma, AIDS, and lung cancer patients may be of therapeutic interest(chapters at the end of the book).

We invite the reader to join us in studying the phenomenon of prohormone fragments released by stress as they impact on the immune system.

REFERENCES

Brown,S.L. and D.E. Van Epps. Beta Endorphin(BE), Met-Enkephalin(ME), and Corticotrophin(ACTH) Modulate the Production of Gamma Interferon(IFN) In Vitro. Fed. Proc. 44,4,949,1985.
Faith, R.E., N.P. Plotnikoff, and A.J. Murgo. Effects of Opiates and Neuropeptides on Immune Functions. pp. 300-311. Ed. C.W. Sharp. Mechanism of Tolerance and Dependence, NIDA Research Monograph 54,1984.
Herz, A. Multiple Endorphins as Natural Ligands of Multiple Opioid Receptors. 43-52, in Central and Peripheral Endorphins: Basic and Clinical Aspects, ed. by E.E. Muller and A.R. Genazzini. Raven Press, New York, 1984.
Kojima, K.,Kilpatrick, D.L. Stein, A.S. Jones, B.N., Udenfriend, S. 1982. Proenkephalin: a general pathway for enkephalin biosynthesis in animal tissues. Arch. Biochem. Biophys. 215:638-43.
Plotnikoff, N.P., G.C. Miller, J. Wybran, and N.F. Nimeh. Methionine enkephal: T-cell Enhancement in Kaposis's Sarcoma. Serono Symposia, Recent advances in primary and acquired immunodeficiencies(In Press). Copley Plaza Hotel, Boston, April 10,1985.
Plotnikoff, N.P., and A.J. Murgo. Enkephalins:Endorphins: Stress and the Immune System. Fed. Proc. 44,1,1.1985.
Weber, R.J. and C.B. Pert. Peptitergic Modulation of the Immune System. p. 35-42. from Central and Peripheral Endorphins: Basic and Clinical Aspects, ed. by E.E. Muller and A.R. Genazzani. Raven Press, N.Y.,1984.
Youkilis,E.; J. Chapman; E. Woods; and N.P. Plotnikoff. In Vivo immunostim-ulation and increased in vitro production of interleukin 1(IL-1) Activity by methionine enkephalin. Int. J. Immuno.Pharm. 7,3,79,1985.

CANDIDATE OPIOID PEPTIDES FOR INTERACTION WITH THE IMMUNE SYSTEM

Christopher J. Evans, Elizabeth Erdelyi, and Jack D. Barchas

Nancy Pritzker Laboratory of Behavioral Neurochemistry
Department of Psychiatry and Behavioral Sciences
Stanford University School of Medicine
Stanford, CA 94306

Endogenous opioids are a recently discovered group of peptides which have been implicated as modulators of a number of biological systems. Both opiate receptors and their peptide ligands are widely distributed throughout the CNS and are additionally located in some peripheral sites. The classical effects of opiates as analgesics have perhaps overshadowed many other important biological activities of this group of neuroactive peptides. This book provides strong indications that endogenous opioid peptides play a crucial role in the regulation of the immune system.

Many studies have shown that various stressors have dramatic affects on the functioning of the immune system. The question then becomes one of dissecting out individual components released on the stressful stimuli and determining which may be responsible for the observed changes in immunity. There is a large literature on the effects of glucocorticoids on suppression of the immune function (see Munck et al., 1984 for review). Furthermore, adrenaline has been shown to affect the immune kinetics (Depelchin and Letesson, 1981). A clue that opioids may influence immune responsiveness was indicated in early clinical studies of immuno deficiencies in heroin addicts (Brown et al., 1974). Recent work has shown that opioid peptides can modulate a number of cell types involved in the immune response, and these activities are the subject of other chapters in this book. This chapter will be concerned with the various forms of opioid peptides found in tissues actively secreting into the blood in response to a stressful stimulus, since it is these peptides that will be available for interaction with components of the immune system. Special emphasis will be placed on the opioid peptides that are present in the adrenal gland.

Opioid peptides are generated by enzymic processing of large precursors which themselves are not opiate active. Three opioid precursors have thus far been described: proopiomelanocortin (POMC or pro-ACTH-endorphin); proenkephalin (proenkephalin A), and prodynorphin (proenkephalin B or proneoendorphin/dynorphin). The cDNA representing the messenger RNA encoding the structure of all three opioid precursors has been cloned and the primary amino acid sequence deduced from the cDNA sequence (Nakanishi et al., 1979; Noda et al., 1982; Kakidani et al., 1982; Comb et al., 1982). The endogenous opioid peptides that have been isolated from various mammalian tissues all have at their N-termini an opiate core sequence: Tyr-Gly-Gly-Phe[met or leu]. The primary structure of POMC contains one opioid core sequence, proenkephalin contains seven, and prodynorphin three. The chemical and spatial integrity of certain features of this sequence are crucial for opiate activity. One essential component is the ionizable amino group at the N-terminus of the opioid core sequence in a particular spatial arrangement to the side chain of the tyrosine residue. Removal of the N-terminal positive charge by acylation of the α-amino group completely obliterates opiate-like properties of these peptides (Bradbury et al., 1977). Therefore, if the α-amino group of the opioid core sequence is engaged in a peptide linkage as in the precursor structures, or α-N-acetylated—a modification found in some tissues, the opioid core is completely inactivated. The N-terminal tyrosine residue of every opioid core sequence is preceded in the three precursors by paired basic residues and in all but one core sequence found in bovine proenkephalin this is a lysyl arginine (see Fig. 1). Cleavage of the precursor at the paired basic residues preceding the opioid core is a prerequisite for the generation of peptides with opiate-like properties. Nature has used paired basic residues as precursor processing signals for the generation of many bioactive peptides (see Steiner et al., 1974 for review). In addition, many precursors are cleaved at single arginine residues (Rehfeld, 1981; Roth et al., 1983). If all paired basics and single arginines were precursor processing sites, the opiate-active peptides would be from POMC, β-endorphin(1-27); from prodynorphin, 3 copies of leu-enkephalin; and from proenkephalin, 6 copies of met-enkephalin and one 1 copy of leu-enkephalin. However, in most tissues, complete processing does not occur such that there are whole consortium of peptides with the opioid core at the N-terminus and various C-terminal extensions. It is interesting that the extent and nature of processing can be variable between tissues, an issue addressed in detail later in this chapter. Figure 1 shows the structure of the three opioid precursors and the endogenous biologically active peptides that have been characterized in various mammalian tissues (see Weber et al., 1983b for review).

The importance of the C-terminal tails following the opioid core sequence should not be understated. The tails infer selectivity for various receptor types, provide stability against exopeptidase attack (Austen et al., 1979), and can influence both the on and off rate of receptor/effector activation. These properties may be crucial when considering an opioid peptide as a candidate for interaction with the immune system. It should, however, be remembered that all endogenous opioid peptids are pure agonists for all receptor types and the microenvironment where the peptides are released and act can be a crucial factor with regard to issues relating to the importance of receptor selectivity and ligand stability.

Identification of Precursor Products

The tissue distribution and concentration of various processing products of the three opioid precursors can be studied using specific antisera as probes. Since all endogenous opioids have a common component at the N-terminus—the opioid core sequence—these specific antisera have to be directed to the C-terminal tails of the various products. As nature would have it, rabbits will indeed direct their antigenic response to the C-terminus of short peptides when certain injection protocols are followed (Weber et al., 1982b). Consequently, antisera can be readily raised which differentiate between the processing products. Often it is possible to obtain antisera that require the C-terminal amino acid as part of the antigenic site. A good example is an antisera we raised to dynorphin(1-8) which, when

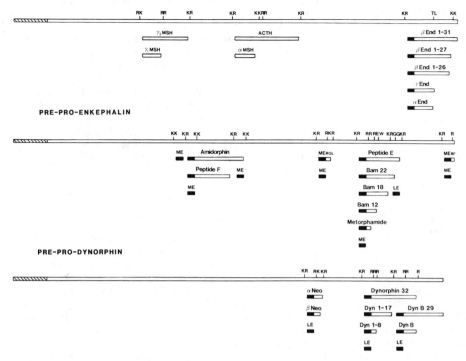

Fig. 1. A large number of endogenous bioactive peptides have been
isolated and characterized from POMC, proenkephalin, and
prodynorphin. This figure shows the molecular origin of these
peptides. The opiate active core sequences are represented by
solid bars (▬▬) and the putative signal regions of the
precursors by thatched bars (▨▨). The following abbrevia-
tions have been used: MSH, melanocyte stimulating hormone;
ACTH, adrenocorticotrophic hormone; End, endorphin; ME,
met-enkephalin; LE, leucine-enkephalin; Neo, neoendorphin; Dyn,
dynorphin; R, arginine; K, lysine; T, threonine; L, leucine; E,
Glutamic acid; W, tryptophan; G, glycine; and F, phenylalanine.
The structures are for bovine pre-pro-opiomelanocortin, bovine
pre-pro-enkephalin and porcine pre-pro dynorphin.

used in radioimmunoassay, has less than 0.1% crossreactivity with
dynorphin(1-7) or dynorphin(1-17). Radioimmunoassays using such
specific antisera have proven to be an invaluable quantitative tool in
the study of endogenous opioid peptides. These assays are quick,
sensitive and reliable, although extreme caution must be taken when
measuring in tissues such as blood and CSF where interfering substances
causing displacement can be mistaken for the presence of peptides. It
is advisable in these cases that RIAs be validated by chromatographic
analysis of the immunoreactive material. Chromatography of immunoreactive peptides can also reveal different forms containing the same
antigenic site. A common problem encountered is that most antisera
raised to β-endorphin also recognize the opiate inactive precursor
β-lipotropin. Gel filtration chromatography rapidly distinguishes
between these two immunoreactive forms. The antisera can also be used
for immunocytochemistry which provides precise localization of cells
producing a particular opiate peptide. The analysis of opioid
processing procucts by immunocytochemistry in combination with
radioimmunoasays has proved to be very powerful and enabled the

5

construction of detailed maps of the various opioid precursor products in mammalian tissues.

Opioid peptides are found in many peripheral sites that secrete into the blood stream and, consequently, could be available for activation of opiate receptors on cells concerned with the immunoresponse. The presence of β-endorphin-like immunoreactive peptides in the subpopulation of macrophages is of considerable interest in this regard (Lolait et al., 1984). If this β-endorphin-like immunoreactivity proves to be opiate active, an autocrine-like role can be postulated since opiates have been shown to stimulate the IgG mediated antibody-dependent cytotoxicity of macrophages (Foris et al., 1984). Opioid peptides are also present in high concentrations in the pituitary and adrenal glands. Both these endocrine tissues are activated during stress and warrant special attention with regard to their opioid content.

THE PITUITARY

Opioid peptides can be found in all three lobes of the pituitary gland. In the posterior lobe of many species, prodynorphin derived peptides are costored and probably coreleased with vasopressin (Martin and Voigt, 1981). In the oxytocin cells of rat there is immunocyto-chemical evidence for costorage with met-enkephalin (Martin et al., 1983). In the anterior lobe of the rat pituitary, prodynorphin derived peptides can be detected by radioimmunoassay and there is evidence that these peptides are stored in the gonadotropic hormone secreting cells. More relevant to the theme of this chapter is the β-endorphin-like peptides costored with adrenocorticotropin hormone (ACTH) in the anterior lobe. Proopiomelanocortin has within its structure both the sequence of β-endorphin and ACTH (see Fig. 1). The processing pathway in the anterior lobe of the pituitary is geared for the production of ACTH which is flanked at both the N-terminus and C-terminus by lysyl arginines. The cleavage of POMC at the C-terminus of ACTH leaves β-LPH a fragment of the precursor which contains the β-endorphin sequence yet is not opiate active. This peptide has been shown to be a major product of POMC in the anterior pituitary (Liotta et al., 1978). β-Endorphin (1-31), a very active opioid peptide in many bioassays, is also a product of POMC found in anterior pituitary extracts.

The intermediate lobe of the pituitary contains very high concentrations of POMC-derived peptides. Greater than 90% of the endorphin-like immunoreactive material in rat pituitary is present in the intermediate lobe. It has been demonstrated that certain stressors can stimulate release of the endorphin material not only from the anterior lobe of the pituitary but also the intermediate lobe (Przewlocki et al., 1982). However, the POMC products are very different in the two lobes. More complete processing of POMC occurs in the intermediate lobe than in the anterior lobe such that the major bioactive product of the ACTH portion of POMC is α-MSH--the N-terminal fragment of ACTH, acetylated at the N-terminus and amidated at the C-terminal valine. The endorphin portion of the precursor follows a similar processing pattern. The major products are extensively processed at all paired basic residues and then α-N-acetylated at the N-terminal tyrosine (see Table 1). As previously discussed, the α-N-acetylation is an important modification since it completely obliterates the opiate-like properties of this peptide (for reviews, see Eipper and Mains, 1980; O'Donohue and Dorsa, 1982). The question of why a tissue would synthesize an opioid precursor, then prior to release deactivate the opioid core remains unsolved. Perhaps the MSH portion of the precursor is the important bioactive product or else the acetylated endorphins in the pituitary have an as yet undiscovered nonopioid role.

Using an antisera we raised to α-N-acetyl-β-endorphin that did not crossreact with opiate active β-endorphin, it became possible to measure by radioimmunoassay the concentration of α-N-acetylated endorphins in tissue extracts. This assay, in conjunction with an assay that did not distinguish between the two endorphin forms (i.e., a C-terminal or middle region directed β-endorphin antisera), enabled the ratio of acetylated to nonacetylated endorphin to be assayed in various tissues (Weber et al., 1982b). In our studies, the intermediate lobe of the pituitary was found to be the only tissue where α-N-acetylation of endorphin was a prominent modification.

The human pituitary is different from other species in that it has no classical neurointermediate lobe. It is an interesting and important finding that human pituitary has no acetylated endorphins or acetylated α-MSH (Weber et al., 1982b; Evans et al., 1982). However, processing in some human pituitary cells does proceed to produce β-endorphin and α-MSH sized peptides.

OPIOID PEPTIDES IN ADRENAL GLANDS

Opioid peptides are also present in high concentrations in the adrenal glands of many species. It has been shown by immunocyto-chemistry and by RIA that the medulla portion of the gland contains the opioid peptides and that they are costored and coreleased with adrenalin (Viveros et al., 1979). Initial studies were performed on bovine adrenals since opiate activity was high and large quantities of tissue are readily available. A number of peptides containing opioid core sequences were isolated and characterized from this source including the BAM (Bovine, Adrenal, Medulla) fragments BAM 12 and BAM 22, peptide E and peptide F, and peptides containing the met-enkephalin-Arg-Phe and met-enkephalin-Arg-Gly-Leu sequence (Stern et al., 1981; Jones et al., 1982). These multiple opioid peptides subsequently were shown to be processing products of a single precursor-proenkephalin (see Fig. 1).

Recently we have identified a novel opioid processing product, BAM-18 from bovine adrenal glands (Evans et al., 1984). It is note-worthy that BAM-18 unlike BAM-12, BAM-22, peptide E and peptide F is in high concentrations in brain tissue as well as adrenal medulla. Additionally, amidorphin, a 26 amino acid opioid peptide with a C-terminal amide, has been isolated from bovine adrenal medulla (Seizinger et al., 1985). Like BAM-18, amidorphin is found in high concentrations in certain areas of brain. In general, processing of proenkephalin in brain is considerably more extensive than in bovine adrenal. For example, met-enkephalin-Arg-Gly-Leu as the heptapeptide is an abundant opioid in brain but in bovine adrenal this sequence is predominantly found as part of a 5.3 kilodalton nonopioid metabolite of proenkephalin (Jones et al., 1982; Lindberg et al., 1984). It is important to note that many of these incompletely processed fragments of proenkephalin are not opiate active, although they contain the opioid core sequence within their structure. The 5.3 and 3.6 kilodalton peptides containing respectively met-enkephalin-Arg-Gly-Leu and met-enkephalin-Arg-Phe at the C-terminus are both examples of proenkephalin processing products found in abundance in the adrenal which although not active at opiate receptors contain an opioid core embedded within their structure.

In our studies we have analyzed adrenals from a number of different species for the processing fragments of the three precursors. Specific radioimmunoassays (RIAs) to processing products have been developed and used for these studies. Table 1 illustrates a summary of the results. As a cautionary note in interpreting these data, it should be remembered

Table 1. Species Variability in Opioid Peptides In Adrenal Glands As Measured by RIA (levels in pmoles/gram)

		Human Medulla	Guinea Pig	Dog	Rabbit	Rat	Sheep
ProDyn	α-Neo-endorphin	BD	216	BD	BD	BD	BD
	Dynorphin 1-17	BD	129	BD	BD	BD	BD
	Dynorphin B	BD	113	BD	BD	BD	BD
	Leu Enkephalin	1132	209	522	85	9	150
ProEnk	Metorphamide	306	BD	33	BD	BD	7
	Met-enkephalin-RGL	957	878	28	8	6	316
	Met-enkephalin-RF	739	484	1541	136	21	200
POMC	β-Endorphin	144	BD	BD	BD	BD	BD
	α-MSH	53	BD	BD	BD	BD	BD
	ACTH	25	BD	BD	BD	BD	BD

Tissues were extracted in 5 wt vol acid/acetone and prepared for RIA using previously procedures (Weber et al., 1983b). Values were obtained from at least 5 adrenal samples for each species. The detection limit was 2-10 pmol/g depending on the assay. In many of the samples no immunoreactive material could be detected (BD). The opioid directed RIAs used above crossreact less than 0.5% with other endogenous opioids with the exception of the leu-enkephalin assay which crossreacts around 7% with met-enkephalin. The β-endorphin RIA recognizes β-LPH, β-endorphin(1-31), β-endorphin(1-27), β-endorphin (1-26) and their respective α-N-acetyl derivatives with equal crossreactivity. The α-MSH assay is C-terminally directed and does not recognize ACTH.

that the structure of the three precursors has not been characterized for all the animals investigated. Although there is considerable structural conservation of the opiate active portions of the precursors that have been sequenced from various species, mutations in certain regions affecting immunoreactivity should not be excluded. In all mammalian adrenals we analyzed, the RIAs detected peptides derived from pro-enkephalin. However, considerable differences were observed in the concentration of the various proenkephalin processing products. For example, metorphamide, an amidated opioid which has been isolated from brain (Weber et al., 1983) and pheochromocytoma (Matsuo et al., 1983) is in high concentrations in human adrenal but is undetectable in guinea pig, rabbit and rat adrenals and is in very low concentrations in dog and sheep adrenals. However, in extracts from rat and guinea pig brain, metorphamide can be detected in many regions (Sonders et al., 1984) indicating that these animals can indeed generate this processing product and that the sequence in this region of proenkephalin is probably conserved. Additional variances between species on the extent of processing have been exposed by sizing the immunoreactive material using column chromatography. Figure 2 shows the gel filtration immuno-reactivity profiles of a human adrenal extract assayed with RIAs directed to the proenkephalin processing products metorphamide, met-enkephalin-Arg-Gly-Leu and met-enkephalin-Arg-Phe. All three RIAs detected material eluting at an extrapolated molecular weight of between 0.5 and 1 kilodalton. However, analysis of a guinea pig adrenal extract (Fig. 3) shows no metorphamide and very little low molecular weight met-enkephalin-Arg-Gly-Leu or met-enkephalin-Arg-Phe immunoreactive material. The guinea pig adrenal met-enkephalin-Arg-Phe and met-enkephalin-Arg-Gly-Leu immunoreactivity may correspond to the nonopiate

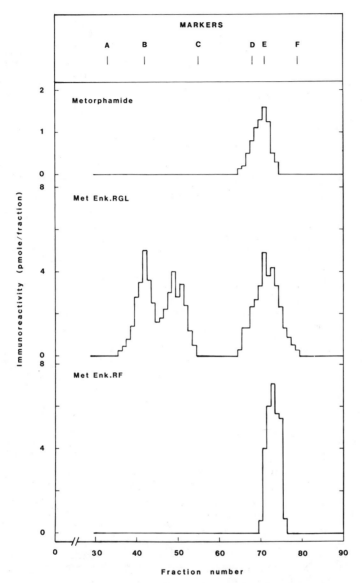

Fig. 2. Gel filtration analysis of the immunoreactive proenkephalin
peptides found in human adrenal gland. An acid/acetone extract
was loaded onto a 100 x 0.9 CM Sephadex G75 column equilibrated
and eluted with 25% acetic acid. Aliquots of the fractions
were analyzed using the metorphamide, met-enkephalin-Arg-Phe,
and met-enkephalin-Arg-Gly-Leu RIAs. The standard molecular
weight markers were A) exclusion, B) ^{125}I-lipotropin, C)
[125]I-β-endorphin(1-31), D) ^{125}I-α-MSH, E) ^{125}I-α-neo-
endorphin, and F) ^{125}I-leucine-enkephalin.

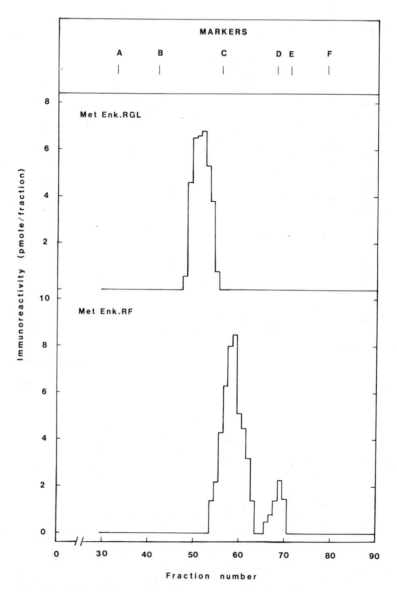

Fig. 3. Gel filtration analysis of the immunoreactive proenkephalin peptides in the guinea pig adrenal gland. The column conditions and molecular weight markers were identical to those used in Figure 3.

3.6 and 5.2 kilodalton fragments found in bovine adrenal (Stern et al., 1981; Jones et al., 1982). We must conclude that between species there is considerable heterogeneity in the stored processing products of adrenal proenkephalin.

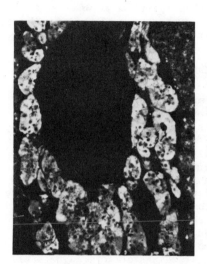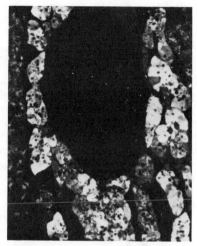

Fig. 4.   This figure shows the colocalization of the met-enkephalin-
Arg-Gly-Leu (a proenkephalin-derived peptide) and α-neo-
endorphin (a prodynorphin-derived peptide) in guinea pig
adrenal gland. Sequential 4.5 μ sections through the gland
were taken and stained alternatively with α-neo-endorphin or
met-enkephalin-Arg-Gly-Leu. The α-neo-endorphin staining
could not be blocked by 10 μM dynorphin(1-17), dynorphin B,
met-enkephalin-Arg-Phe, met-enkephalin-Arg-Gly-Leu, or
leu-enkephalin, but was blocked by α-neo-endorphin.
Met-enkephalin-Arg-Gly-Leu staining was not blocked by 10 μM
dynorphin(1-17), dynorphin B, met-enkephalin-Arg-Phe, or
α-neo-endorphin, but was blocked by met-enkephalin-Arg-Gly-
Leu. The blocking controls demonstrated that the staining was
specific and the precursor products were indeed present in the
same cells.

The guinea pig adrenal glands are somewhat unusual in that
prodynorphin-derived peptides can be detected in addition to
proenkephalin metabolites. We have analyzed the distribution of these
products by immunocytochemistry (see Fig. 4). By staining alternate
thin sections with antisera to products of pro-enkephalin and prodynorphin we have demonstrated that fragments of both precursors are
present in the same cells. Interestingly, in guinea pig adrenal almost

every medulla cell is immunoreactive with antisera directed to fragments of the proenkephalin precursor. We do not observe this is all species. Sizing chromatography of the immunoreactive material shows that the processing of prodynorphin and proenkephalin is not extensive in guinea pig adrenal medulla. The dynorphin(1-17) and dynorphin B immunoreactive material is of high molecular weight, ranging from 10 to 12 kilodaltons (Evans et al., 1985). The met-enkephalin-Arg-Gly-Leu and met-enkephalin-Arg-Phe immunoreactive material was also of high molecular weight (see Fig. 3) and consequently may not be opiate active. However, the majority of the α-neo-endorphin immunoreactive material cochromatographed with the authentic peptide on gel filtration. It is at present not clear whether there are discrete prodynorphin-containing or proenkephalin-containing granules--this awaits ongoing electron microscopy localization studies in our laboratory. If the peptides from both precursors are indeed present in the same granules, corelease would be inevitable. However, if the precursor products were stored in separate granules, there is a potential for selective release of products from one or other of the precursors.

The human adrenal medulla is extremely interesting in that processing products derived from POMC as well as proenkephalin can be demonstrated (Nakao et al., 1981; Evans et al., 1983). We have analyzed in considerable detail the processing fragments of these precursors. Since only autopsy material is available, one has to be a little cautious in conclusions drawn from these studies. However, postmortem analysis of neurosecretory peptides has demonstrated that processing patterns in general don't radically alter even a number of hours after death. Results have been consistent in the postmortem tissues we have investigated. Initial RIA shows that there is approximately half the concentration of ACTH as α-MSH. However, gel filtration analysis of the ACTH-like immunoreactivity shows only a small percentage actually chromatographing at the correct molecular weight of ACTH. Therefore ACTH is only a very minor product in these human adrenal medulla cells and α-MSH (identified as des acetyl α-MSH by reverse phase HPLC) is apparently the major product of this region of POMC (Evans et al., 1983). With regard to the endorphin region of POMC, there is processing to form β-endorphin(1-31) which is the major product. Using specific antisera for α-N-acetylated endorphin, we detected no immunoreactive material indicating that there was no α-N-acetylation in this tissue. Interesting, no β-endorphin(1-27) could be detected and less than 10% of the endorphin immunoreactivity could be attributed to lipotropin. This processing pattern is unlike the pituitary in that β-endorphin (1-31) is the major product along with des acetyl α-MSH. It appears from immunocytochemical observations that the POMC producing cells are close to the medulla-cortex interface and are different from the proenkephalin producing cells. The close proximity of POMC producing cells with the adrenal cortex may indicate a direct paracrine-like stimulatory effect on the corticotroph sensitive cells. However, the processing is not geared for ACTH, a considerably more potent cortico-troph than α-MSH, and the blood flow is generally accepted to be from the cortex to the medulla. At present it is unclear if the scattered POMC cells contain adrenaline and whether they are indeed activated during stress. With regard to the proenkephalin, the human adrenal unlike many other species fairly extensively processes this precursor to low molecular weight opioids. The met-enkephalin-Arg-Gly-Leu and met-enkephalin-Arg-Phe immunoreactive material is predominantly of low molecular weight (see Fig. 2). Furthermore, the presence of the octapeptide metorphamide would suggest that the human adrenal medulla contains an enzyme capable of cleaving at single arginine residues in addition to an amidating-like enzymic activity.

Interaction of the pituitary and the adrenal gland during a stress-ful stimuli is extremely relevant to which opiate peptides will be secreted into the blood stream. The release of corticotropic hormone releasing factor (CRF), into median eminance may be accompanied by the release of prodynorphin fragments which have been shown by immunocyto-chemistry to colocalized in the subpopulation of CRF cells (Hökfelt et al., 1983). The release of CRF in turn will induce release of ACTH and endorphins from the anterior pituitary. The ACTH stimulates the release of steroids from the adrenal cortex. The steroids have multiple actions, including primary effects on the immune system and inhibition of the continuation of ACTH secretion from the anterior pituitary. In a recent study in collaboration with Dr. James Eberwine, we have demon-strated that in guinea pig adrenal glands dexamethasone, a potent steroid agonist, can increase the proenkephalin mRNA approximately 2-fold. Interestingly, the steroid treatment did not affect the co-localized prodynorphin message levels. We found very little change in levels of the proenkephalin peptide processing products. These results could possibly be interpreted as psychological stress (generating the message) preparing the body for a physical stressor (release of opioid peptides with adrenalin). Assuming _in vivo_ opiate peptides are co-released with adrenalin from the chromaffin cells, this could be a major source of circulating opioid peptides released on stress. From our studies on the stored processing products, it would seem that the type and concentration of these opioid peptides from the adrenal would be very dependent on the species under investigation. It is perhaps the human adrenal which should be further investigated with regard to potentially useful opioid peptides that may interact with our immune system. Although in this chapter we have concentrated on the opioids in pituitary and adrenal, it should be remembered that these opioid peptides are only candidates for interaction with opioid receptors in cells involved in the immune response. It may be that other more local sources of opioids are more important factors _in vivo_.

REFERENCES

Austen, B. M., Evans, C. J., and Smyth, D.G., 1979, Susceptibility of neuroactive peptides to aminopeptidase digestion is related to molecular size, Biochem. Biophys. Res. Commun., 91:1211.

Bradbury, A. F., Smyth, D. G., Snell, C. R., Deakin, W., and Wendlandt, S., 1977, Comparison of the analgesic properties of lipotropin C-fragment and stabilized enkephalins in the rat, Biochem. Biophys. Acta, 74:748.

Brown, S. M., Stimmel, B., Taub, R. N., Kochwa, S., and Rosenfield, R. E., 1974, Immunologic dysfunction in heroin addicts, Arch Intern Med. 134:1001.

Comb, M., Seeburg, P. H., Adelman, J., Eiden, L., and Herbert, E, 1982, Primary structure of the human met- and leu-enkephalin precursor and its mRNA, Nature 295:663.

Depelchin, A., and Letesson, J. J., 1981, Adrenaline influence on the immune response. I. Accelerating or suppressor effects according to the time of application, Immunol. Lett., 3:199.

Eipper, B., and Mains, R., 1980, Structure and biosynthesis of pro-adrenocorticotropin/endorphin and related peptides, Endo. Rev., 1:1.

Evans, C. J., Erdelyi, E., Weber, E., and Barchas, J. D., 1983, Identification of pro-opiomelanocortin derived peptides in the human adrenal medulla, Science, 221:957.

Evans, C. J., Lorenz, R., Weber, E., and Barchas, J. D., 1982, Variants of alpha-melanocyte stimulating hormone in rat brain and pituitary:

evidence that acetylated α-MSH exists only in the intermediate lobe of pituitary, Biochem. Biophys. Res. Commun., 106:910.

Evans, C. J., Erdelyi, E., Makk, G., and Barchas, J. D., 1985, Identification of a novel proenkephalin derived peptide in brain and adrenal, Abstract #69, FASEB Meeting, Anaheim, CA 1985.

Foris, G., Medgyesi, G. A., Gyimesi, E., and Hauck, M., 1984, Met-enkephalin induced alterations of macrophage functions, Mol. Immuno., 21:747.

Geisow, M. J., Deakin, J. F. W., Dostrovsky, J. O., and Smyth, D. G., 1977, Analgesic activity of lipotropin C fragment depends on carboxyl terminal tetrapeptide, Nature, 269:167.

Hazum, E., Chang, K. J., and Cuatrecasas, P., 1979, Specific nonopiate receptors for beta-endorphin, Science, 205:1033.

Hökfelt, T., Fahrenkrug, J., Tatemoto, K., Mutt, V., Werner, S., Hulting, A.-L., Terenius, L., and Chang, K. J., 1983, The PHI (PHI-27)/corticotropin-releasing factor/enkephalin immunoreactive hypothalamic neuron: Possible morphological basis for integrated control of prolactin, corticotropin, and growth hormone secretion. Proc. Natl. Acad. Sci. USA, 80:895.

Jones, B. N., Shively, J. E., Kilpatrick, D. L., Kojima, K., and Udenfriend, S., 1982, Enkephalin biosynthetic pathway: A 5300-dalton adrenal polypeptide that terminates at its COOH end with the sequence [Met]enkephalin-Arg-Gly-Leu-COOH, Proc. Natl. Acad. Sci. USA, 79:1313.

Kakidani, H., Furutani, Y., Takahashi, H., Noda, M., Morimoto, Y., Hirose, T., Asai, M., Inayama, S., Nakanishi, S., and Numa, S., 1982, Cloning and sequence analysis of cDNA for porcine β-neo-endorphin/dynorphin precursor, Nature, 298:245.

Lindberg, I., Yang, H-Y. T., and Costa, E., 1983, A high molecular weight form of $Met^5Arg^6Gly^7Leu^8$ in rat brain and bovine chromaffin granules. Life Sci., 33(Suppl):5.

Liotta, A. S., Suda, T., and Krieger, D. T., 1978, β-Lipotropin is the major opioid-like peptide of human pituitary and rat pars distalis: Lack of significant β-endorphin, Proc. Natl. Acad. Sci. USA, 75:2950.

Lolait, S. J., Lim, A. T., Toh, B. H., and Funder, J. W., 1984, Immunoreactive beta-endorphin in a subpopulation of mouse spleen macrophages, J. Clin. Invest., 73:277.

Martin, R., Geis, R., Holl, R., Schaffer, M., and Voigt, K. H., 1983, Co-existence of unrelated peptides in oxytocin and vasopressin terminals of rat neurohypophyses: Immunoreactive methionine-enkephalin-, leucine-enkephalin- and cholesystokinin-like substances, Neurosci., 8:213.

Martin, R., and Voigt, K. H., 1981, Enkephalins co-exist with oxytocin and vasopressin in nerve terminals of rat neurohypophysis, Nature 289:502.

Matsuo, H., Miyata, A., and Mizuno, K., 1983, Novel C-terminally amidated opioid peptide in human phaeochromocytoma tumour, Nature 305:721.

McCain, H. W., Lamster, I. B., Bozzone, J. M., and Grbic, J. T., 1982, Beta-endorphin modulates human immune activity via non-opiate receptor mechanisms, Life Sci., 31:1619.

Munck, A., Guyre, P. M., and Holbrook, N. J., 1984, Physiological functions of glucocorticoids in stress and their relation to pharmacological actions, Endocrin. Rev., 5:25.

Nakanishi, S., Inoue, A., Kita, T., Nakamura, M., Chang, A. C. Y., Cohen, S. N., and Numa, S., 1979, Nucleotide sequence of cloned cDNA for bovine corticotropin-β-lipotropin precursor, Nature, 278:423.

Nakao, K., Yoshimasa, T., Ohtsuki, H., Oki, S., Tanaka, I., Nakai, Y., and Imura, H., 1981, β-Endorphin, ACTH and γ-MSH in human sympathoadrenal system, Presented at the Eighth International Congress of Pharmacology, Tokyo.

Noda, M., Furatani, Y., Takahashi, H., Toyosato, M., Hirose, T., Inayama, S., Nakanishi, S., and Numa, S., 1982, Cloning and sequence analysis of cDNA for bovine adrenal preproenkephalin, Nature 295:202.

O'Donohue, T. L., and Dorsa, D. M., 1982, The opiomelanotropinergic neuronal and endocrine systems, Peptides, 3:353.

Przewlocki, R., Millan, M. J., Gramsch, G. H., and Millan, M. H., 1982, The influence of selective adeno- and neurointermedio-hypophysectomy upon plasma and brain levels of β-endorphin and their response to stress in rats, Brain Res., 242:107.

Rehfeld, J. F., 1981, Four basic characteristics of the gastrin cholecystokinin system, Am. J. Physiol., 240:6255.

Roth, K. A., Evans, C. J., Lorenz, R. G., Weber, E., Barchas, J. D., and Chang, J.-K., 1983, Identification of gastrin releasing peptide-related substances in guinea pig and rat brain. Biochem. Biophys. Res. Commun., 112:528.

Seizinger, B. R., Liebisch, D. C., Gramsch, C., Herz, A., Weber, E., Evans, C. J., Esch, F. S., and Bohlen, P., 1985, Isolation and structure of a novel C-terminally amidated opioid peptide, amidorphin, from bovine adrenal medulla, Nature, 313:57.

Sonders, M., Barchas, J. D., and Weber, E., 1984, Regional distribution of metorphamide in rat and guinea pig brain, Biochem. Biophys. Res. Commun., 222:892.

Steiner, D. F., Kemmler, W., Tager, H. S., and Peterson, J. D., 1974, Proteolytic processing in the biosynthesis of insulin and other proteins, Fed. Proc., 33:2105.

Stern, A. S., Jones, B. N., Shively, J. E., Stein, S., and Udenfriend, S., 1981, Two adrenal opioid polypeptides: proposed intermediates in the processing of proenkephalin. Proc. Natl. Acad. Sci. USA, 78:1962.

Viveros, O. H., Diliberto, E. J., Hazum, E., and Chang, K-J., 1979, Opiate-like materials in the adrenal medulla: Evidence for storage and secretion with catecholamines, Mol. Pharm., 16:1101.

Weber, E., Evans, C. J., and Barchas, J. D., 1983b, Multiple endogenous ligands for opioid receptors, Trends in Neuroscience, 6:333.

Weber, E., Evans, C. J., and Barchas, J. D., 1982a, Opioid peptide dynorphin: predominance of the aminoterminal octapeptide fragment in rat brain regions, Nature, 299:77.

Weber, E., Evans, C. J., Chang, J-K., and Barchas, J. D., 1982b, Antibodies specific for α-N-acetyl β-endorphins: Radioimmunossays and detection of acetylated β-endorphins in pituitary extracts, J. Neurochem., 38, 436.

Weber, E., Esch, F. S., Bohlen, P., Paterson, S., Corbett, A. D., McKnight, A. T., Kosterlitz, H. W., Barchas, J. D., and Evans, J. C., 1983a, Metorphamide: Isolation, structure and biologic activity of a novel amidated opioid octapeptide from bovine brain, Proc. Natl. Acad. Sci. USA, 80:7362.

CONTROL MECHANISMS IN THE ENZYME HYDROLYSIS OF ADRENAL-RELEASED ENKEPHALINS

L. Giorgio Roda,[*] Gianna Roscetti,[°] Roberta Possenti,[°]
Francesca Venturelli,[°] and Fabrizio Vita[°]

Laboratorio di Farmacologia, University of Ancona, Ancona,
Italy.[*] Cattedra di Fisiologia Umana, "Tor Vergata"
University, Rome, Italy[°]

A: INTRODUCTION

Opioid peptides are secreted by the adrenal medulla where they are
stored within the chromaffin granule (1-3). Consequently, these peptides
are released into the blood stream together with the whole soluble content
of the granule during the physiological activity of the gland.

Once released, endogenous opioids are carried by the blood stream
towards their presumptive target organs. Such a fate is common to any substance released in blood by the endocrine glands. Notwithstanding, the
case if adrenal-released opioid peptides seems to be somewhat more complex.
Indeed, it is very difficult to demonstrate any pharmacological activity of
the smaller opioids when they are artificially administered under in vivo
conditions (406, see also 7). This appears--at least in part--to be
caused by the rapid inactivation of these peptides by plasma enzymes (8-10,
see also 11). In this respect, centrally and peripherally released opioid
peptides are in opposite situations: while a rapid inactivation is normal
for neurotransmitter-like substances released in the central nervous system,
the same phenomenon is hardly expected for hormone-like substances whose
activity is supposed to be a relatively long-lasting one.

Thus, there is an apparent discrepancy between blood as carrier of the
endogenous opioids and its capacity to degrade the carried substances. Yet,
in the last few years a good deal of evidence has been accumulated which
clearly indicates the existence of endogenous substances active in preventing a rapid hydrolysis óf the opioid peptides released into the blood
stream. These results may help to better organize the data available on the
stability of the peripheral enkephalins. This can certainly be useful.
Indeed, the concept that the immune response can at least partially be
influenced by the perpherally-released opioid peptides has been substantiated
by two sets of data: the first on the existence of interactions between
opioids and immunocompetent cells, and the second on the existence of
receptors for opioid peptides on the T-lymphocyte membrane. These data are
specifically reviewed elsewhere in this volume. Here, we will simply mention that the problem of the control of the active life of the serum-
released opioids is strictly related to the problem of the activity of
these peptides on the immunocompetent cells present in the blood stream.
The purpose of the following pages is to review the evidence on the hydrolysis of peripheral enkephalins, to add some new data and to extrapolate
from them concepts of more general interest.

B: ENKEPHALIN HYDROLYSIS

Unlike the hydrolysis by nervous system related enzymes, for which an extensive literature exists, relatively few works have been performed on the hydrolysis of enkephalins by plasma enzymes. However, this topic has been studied both in vivo and in vitro (8-10, 12) and the enzyme cleavage mechanism has been determined by separation and quantification of the hydrolysis by-products by chromatographic procedures (13).

The results known so far can be summarized as follows: i) enkephalins are hydrolyzed by several enzymes present both in plasma and in brain homogenates; ii) in both cases—at least in man, but not in all mammals—the first hydrolysis by-product is tyrosine (since the remaining tetrapeptide is biologically inactive, the tyrosine cleavage is also the most relevant step in the hydrolysis sequence; iii) the plasma half-life reported for enkephalins range from a few seconds (9) to 2-3 minutes (8), up to as long as 8-10 minutes (14). The enkephalin-hydrolyzing enzymes present in plasma seem to belong to the same classes, but not to be identical, to the related to the nervous tissue (13).

B1: REQUIREMENTS FOR ENKEPHALIN HYDROLYSIS

It is generally assumed that the rapid enzymatic degradation of the smaller opioids is a direct consequence of their relatively small size—that is, in the case of a molecule as short as a pentapeptide, the specificity of hydrolytic enzymes should necessarily be low. Indeed, no hydrolysis-susceptible bond can be shielded by steric effects, not can the conformation of the molecule hinder the accessibility of the active sites of the enzymes. From these considerations it follows that any proteolytic enzyme able to cleave the peptide bonds present in the molecule should in principle also be able to hydrolyze the enkephalins.

The real situation, however, is probably rather more complex than that. It seems indeed true that the degree of specificity necessary for the proteolytic enzymes to hydrolyze enkephalins is relatively high. Actually, we detected a considerable resistance of enkephalins to non-specific enzyme hydrolysis (submitted). From our data, only pronase is able to completely inactivate leu-enkephalin within minutes (the half-life of leu-enkephalin is 90 seconds in the presence of 1% enzyme w/w at pH 7.0). Of all the many other enzymes assayed, leucine aminopeptidase only was found to hydrolyze leu-enkephalin with measureable kinetics. On the other hand, papain, bommelain, and pepsin, forexample, are practically unable to hydrolyze leu-enkephalin.

These data can be at least partially explained by taking into account the structure of the peptide. Calculations of the minimal energy conformation (15-17), circular dichroism (18-20) and NMR data (19, 21-24), tend to suggest that both enkephalins have a degree of structure which is certainly unusually high for small peptides.

Indeed, a structure in which the C- and N-terminals are held close together has been suggested by several authors (e.g. 22,23). The existing data on enkephalins' structure, taken as a whole, make it highly probable that these peptides are rather rigidly constrained in a folded conformation with a I, I', II, or II'-bend involving the GLY[2], GLY[3], or PHE[4] residues. The band can also be stabilized by non-covalent backbone-backbone interactions and by one (23), two (25) or even three (19) hydrogen bonds. These data have been obtained mainly with the pentapeptides, but they may be extrapolated at least to the hectapeptide, met-enkephalin-ARG-PHE. Indeed, conformational features of the met-enkephalin molecule have been shown to be maintained even in beta-endorphin (26).

It seems therefore that the two sets of data (resistance to enzymatic hydrolysis and the existence of a well defined structure) can be related. Also, it is probably true that the conformation assumed by enkephalins is such as to partially protect the peptide bonds existing within the molecule from enzyme attack.

B2: MECHANISMS OF ENKEPHALIN HYDROLYSIS IN BLOOD

Enkephalin hydrolysis has been primarily studied in the case of nervous tissue-related enzymes. However, a few studies have been published on plasma hydrolysis. Among them, Hambrook et al. studied the kinetics and hydrolysis pattern of enkephalin in rat plasma(8); Hogu-Angeletti and Roda determined the same parameters in rabbit plasma(10); Dupont et al. studied with an in vivo technique the hydrolysis kinetics in rat blood(9); and Possenti et al. investigated enkephalin hydrolysis in human plasma(14). As detailed further on, some of the results of these studies are somewhat conflictual, and quite difficult to fit together in a consistent pattern.

B2a: Hydrolysis in human plasma

Detailed knowledge of the hydrolysis of enkephalins by plasma enzymes is obviously important for understanding protection from hydrolysis itself. Therefore, in this section, we report the experimental procedure which was used in our laboratory to study hydrolysis kinetics and the fragmentation pattern of leu-enkephalin upon cleavage by plasma enzymes.

Leu-enkephalin was incubated with whole plasma and the incubation mixture was fractioned by high pressure steric exclusion chromatography in order to remove the high molecular weight material. The enkephalin-containing low molecular weight fraction separated by the steric exclusion column was then fractioned by reverse phase chromatography, and the hydrolysis by-products were subsequently identified by their retention characteristics and by amino acid analysis(13). Figure 1 reports the kinetics of leuenkephalin degradation and that of the fromation and disappearance of the released fragments. Of the 13 fragments that are theoretically obtainable from pentapeptide, 8 final hydrolysis by-products were actually found: i) all the four possible monomers; ii) 2 dimers out of 4: GLY-GLY and PHE-LEU; iii) 1 trimer out of three: GLY-PHE-LEU; iv) 1 tetramer out of 2: GLY-GLY-PHE-Leu.

All the N-terminal tyrosine peptides are absent. This is due to the high activity of aminopeptidases in human blood. Also lacking are GLY-PHE and GLY-GLY-PHE, probably because of the lack of hydrolysis at the PHE-LEU-bond reported in the next section.

B2b: Enzymes in human plasma

The distribution of the enkephalin-degrading enzymes present in human blood was investigated as follows: whole plasma was fractioned by high pressure steric exclusion or ion exchange chromatography and labelled enkephalins were incubated in the presence of the pools thus obtained. The hydrolysis by-products were separated and identified by thin layer chromatography and quantified by scintillation counting of the thin layer-separated fragments(unpublished). This procedure permits one to identify indirectly and quantitate the enzymes from which the different fragments are generated. Figure 2 shows the pattern of enkephalin-hydrolyzing enzymes in human blood after separation by high pressure steric exclusion chromatography.

In addition, plasma was sequentially fractioned by steric exclusion and ion exchange chromatography. Under these conditions, and allowing for the limitation inherent to the lack of positive identification of the molecules themselves, six enzyme species were apparently separated, relative to the following enzyme activities: three aminopeptidases, one dipeptidylcarboxypeptidases and two dipeptidylaminopeptidases.

It should be noted that the results shown are valid only as far as human plasma is concerned. Indeed, as reported further on, the kinetics of enkephalin hydrolysis and the relative quantities and distribution of the enkephalin-hydrolyzing enzyme activities seems to be markedly dissimilar in man and in other animals.

B3: HYDROLYSIS BY BRAIN HOMOGENATES

The cleavage pattern described in the previous two paragraphs is consistent with inactivation schema followed by enkephalins when hydrolyzed by the soluble fraction of the nervous tissue. In this case too, three enzyme classes are responsible for enkephalin inactivation: aminopeptidase, dipeptidylaminopeptidase and dipeptidylcarboxypeptidase (11). The main difference between plasma and brain enzymes lies in the cleavage of the GLY-GLY bond which, in plasma, is considerably faster than that in the presence of brain soluble homogenates (13).

Although the inactivation of opioid peptides by central nervous system enzymes has been studied in considerable detail, an accurate molecular characterization of the enzyme systems involved is still lacking. Consequently, it is not as yet as easy to decide how similar are the plasma and brain enzyme systems.

Inhibition data may help to clarify this problem. The inhibition of both dipeptidylcarboxypeptidase and dipeptidylaminopeptidase activities by Tiorphan and Captopril in plasma is approximately 10-20% of the inhibition reported for the brain enzymes. Instead, the inhibition of plasma aminopeptidase activities by Bestatin tallies quite well with the values measured for the brain enzymes in the case of the higher molecular weight form. On the contrary, no inhibition at all was observed with the same substances in the case of the lower molecular weight form (unpublished). As a whole, these data tend to disprove the hypothesis of a strict similarity between the enzymes present in the two tissues. These data rather suggest that, while the enzyme activities in both tissues belong to the same class, they nevertheless represent different molecular forms.

B4: PLASMA LEVELS AND ADRENAL RELEASE

Enkephalins circulate as intact pentapeptides in blood, where they can be quantified by radioimmunoassay. In man, under physiologically base conditions, the enkephalin-like material present in the venous district is in the order of 1×10^{-12} to 1×10^{-13} moles/ml, viz. a total blood content of 3×10^{-7} to 3×10^{-6} g (27,28). The concentration in the adrenal vein is approximately 2×10^{-13} moles/ml (27). Since the blood flow through each adrenal vein is approximately 25 ml/min, the net enkephalin addition is 1×10^{-11} moles/minute, that is 6×10^{-9} g released per minute in the blood. Assuming degradation kinetics corresponding to half lives of 8 minutes (see paragraph C3), the inflow required to maintain a steady enkephalin concentration must be 2×10^{-8} to 2×10^{-7} g/minute.

Assuming that the values thus calculated are correct, the enkephalin released by the adrenal medulla is no more than 30% of the enkephalin needed to maintain a steady peptide concentration. Obviously, either a source for plasma enkephalins other than adrenal medulla can be found, or the degradation kinetics that may be determined under experimental condition are different from the ones which actually take place under physiological conditions.

C: MECHANISMS PROTECTING PERIPHERAL ENKEPHALINS

As described in the previous section, it is somewhat difficult to accord the data existing on enkephalin blood hydrolysis with the plasma levels of these peptides and with the data concerning adrenal release. The discrepancies percieved induced us to investigate specifically the possible existence of mechanisms acting in vivo, able to protect enkephalins from enzyme proteolysis. This on the assumption that protection mechanisms acting under physiological conditions might not be active on the enkephalins administered under experimental conditions. The results obtained since we started working on this hypothesis have certainly been encouraging, and by now the existence of these mechanisms is certain. The following paragraphs therefore deal with this topic, and primarily report the work carried out in our laboratory over the past few years.

C1: MECHANISMS WITHIN THE CHROMAFFIN GRANULE

The adrenal medulla chromaffin granule stores—within its seemingly uniform matrix- catecholamines(29,30), ions and several proteins(31-33), together with enkephalins and other opioid peptides(34-37), plus several peptides of a non-opioid nature(37-40). Among the proteins, proteolytic enzymes are also present(41,42). These enzymes could be able to hydrolyze other polypeptides present within the granule, notably precursors(43,44) of the opioid peptides(40-42. 45-46, see also 47), as well as enkephalins themselves. The peculiar physio-chemical milieu existing in the granules might alter the enzyme specificities. Yet, there is also a possibility that the smaller polypeptides, in particular enkephalins, are protected from the activity of these enzymes. Actually, we showed that enkephalins bind chromaffin granule components and that bound material is partially protected from enzyme hydrolysis(13-14,48). These data were obtained as described below.

Labelled leu-enkephalin was incubated in the presence of a chromaffin granule soluble lysate and the incubation mixture was fractionated by steric exclusion chromatography. From a column optimized for high molecular weight fractionation(figure 3), two peaks of bound radioactivity, plus one eluted at the free enkephalin volume, were separated. The first one eluted corresponds to a granule-contained lipoprotein, chromolipin(49), the second one was tentatively identified as chromogranin A(50). When the same material was fractioned with a Biogel P2 column(nominal fractionation range up to 2000 Daltons), a considerable amount of the radioactive label was found to be associated with a peptide-containing fraction(figur 4). This material was identified with a peptide family previously discovered in the chromaffin granule(51).

The enkephalins bound to the chromaffin granule—containing material are also partially protected from enzyme hydrolysis, as shown by the following data. Enkephalins - preincubated with chromaffin granule crude lysate - were incubated with whole human plasma and analyzed by ion exchange chromatography. Under these conditons, enkephalin hydrolysis kinetics were considerably altered. Specifically, at medium incubation times, the amount of intact enkephalin was higher than in the non-preincubated controls. After 5 minutes, the difference was 29.1%; after 15 minutes, 31.3%, while after 30 minutes it drops to 15.6%(10).

So far, two enkephalin binding systems - relative proteins and peptides - have been detected within the chromaffin granule. Two major roles may be attributed to these systems. The first one - as briefly outlined at the beginning of this section - is to protect enkephalins while they are still in the chromaffin granule. Indeed, the presence of opioid peptide precursors in the granule(43,44) also require proteolytic enzymes to cleave the parent molecules for the generation of the active peptides. The presence of these enzymes has been demonstrated(41,42), and it seems likely that they may also be able to hydrolyze the active opioid peptides contained in the granule. Thus the presence of enkephalin--binding systems might be instrumental in protecting enkephalins before their release into the blood stream.

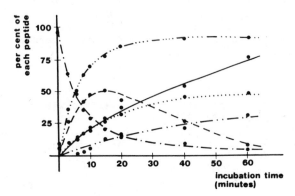

Figure 1. Kinetics of leu-enkephalin hydrolysis and of formation and disappearance of leu-enkephalin fragments by depeptidised plasma. Dash-dotted
line: leu-enkephalin; dash-four dots line: TYR; dashed line: GLY-GLY-PHE-LEU
and GLY-PHE-LEU; solid line: GLY and GLY-GLY; dotted line: PHE-LEU; dash-two
dots line: PHE and LEU. Solid circles indicate experimental points.

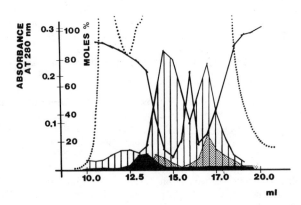

Figure 2. Enkephalin-degrading enzymes in human plasma as fractioned by high
pressure steric exclusion chromatography. Enzyme activites were determined
as described in the text. Dotted line indicates absorbance at 280 nm.
Solid line represents leu-enkephalin; the vertically ruled area represents
aminopeptidase; the dotted area represents dipeptidylaminopeptidase and the
dark shaded area represents dipeptidylcarboxypeptidase activity.

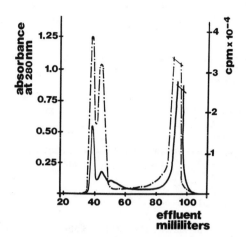

Figure 3: Steric exclusion chromatography(Biogel A 1.5m) of labelled leu-enkephalin incubated in the presence of a chromaffin granule crude lysate. Solid line represents absorbance at 280 nm. Dash-dotted line represents CPM per fraction.

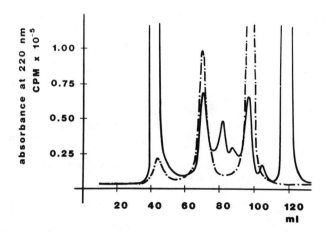

Figure 4: Steric exclusion chromatography of the same incubation mixture as in figure 3.

23

A second, perhaps more important, role of the chromaffin granule-contained protecting systems may be to contribute to the stability of opioid peptides once they are released into the blood stream. As described in the previous section, several enzymes present in blood are able to hydrolyze enkephalins. On the other hand, on the basis of the aforementioned data, the release of enkephalins is paralleled by the release of molecules able to protect them. If the binding is not destroyed in the different physio-chemical enviroment represented by plasma, this may well be a very effective way to protect the released enkephalins. The relevance of this topic will be discussed in more detail in the next section.

C2: PROTECTION MECHANISMS IN BLOOD

There is also the possibility that opioid peptides bind to plasma components which may act as carriers for these peptides, or that may protect them from enzyme hydrolysis. Indeed, a specific search for enkephalin-binding systems in human plasma revealed the existence of two systems with such an activity(48). The presence of enkephalin-binding substances was evidentiated as described below.

C2a: Binding systems in blood

Whole human plasma was incubated with labelled leu-enkephalin and the incubation mixture was fractioned by steric exclusion chromatography. Under these conditions several radioactive peaks were separated. Figure 5 shows the chromatogram obtained from a column separating high molecular weights. Figure 6 shows the same incubation mixture separated on a column optimized for fractioning low molecular weight material, as it is described further on. As shown by both figures, at least four different radioactive fractions can be separated with this technique. The first-eluted fraction represents serum albumin-bound material, the last-eluted one represents free enkephalin. The material eluted at intermediate volumes - approximately corresponding to molecular weights of 5-6000 and 2000 Daltons(pool 1 and 2 in figure 6) - represents enkephalin-binding material of a peptidic nature.

Enkephalin-binding activity quite naturally suggested the possibility that the bound material was protected from enzyme hydrolysis. Therefore, specific experiments were performed to ascertain this point.

Labelled leu-enkephalin was incubated with whole plasma. Albumin-bound enkephalin was separated from the free peptide by steric exclusion chromatography. The albumin-containing fraction(accounting from approximately 5% of the total radioactivity) was then incubated in 20% ethylene glycol to release bound enkephalin(60% of the albumin-bound enkephalin as released under these conditions after 30 minutes at 30°C). Intact enkephalin and hydrolysis by-products were separated and quantified by reverse phase chromatography. Under these conditions, over 90% of the labelled peptide was found to elute at the position of intact enkephalin, while the unbound enkephalin was almost completely(over 75%) degraded(48).

The same analyses were performed on the enkephalin bound to the peptidic fraction. Enkephalin-binding pools(1 and 2 in figure 6, approx-imately accounting for 5 and 15% of the labelled material) were incubated for 30 minutes at 37°C in 20%CH3CN. The incubation mixture was fractioned by reverse phase chromatography on a C-18 column. In this case, incubation and steric exclusion chromatography were found unnecessary since the enkephalin-bound peptides were separated from intact enkephalin by the reverse phase system. (This, in all likelihood, happened on account of the CH3CN-containing mobile phase used). Even in this case, though, the peptide-bound enkephalin was found to consist of intact pentapeptide for over 95%(14)

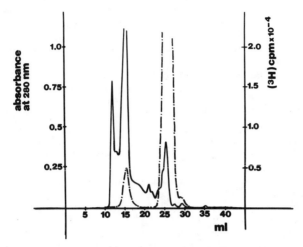

Figure 5. Steric exclusion chromatography (TSK G3000 SW) of labelled leu-enkephalin incubated in the presence of whole human plasma. Solid line represents absorbance at 280 nm; dash-dotted line represents CPM per fraction.

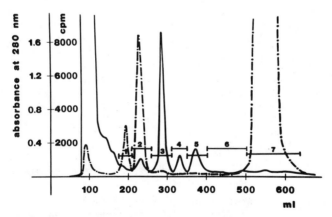

Figure 6. Steric exclusion chromatography of the same incubation mixture as in Figure 5, separated Fractogel HW40. Solid line represents absorbance at 280 nm; Dash-dotted line indicates CPM per fraction.

C2b: In vitro stability of enkephalins

The reliability of the aforementioned hypothesis is also confirmed by direct measurements of the half lives of enkephalins performed in the presence and in the absence of the plasma protection systems(serum albumin and peptides).

The hydrolysis kinetics of leu-enkephalin were determined with whole and de-peptidized human plasma, that is plasma fractioned by steric exclusion chromatography to serparate the peptides from the enzyme containing fractions (13). In the presence of plasma peptides the enkephalin half life is almost exactly three times as long as the one measured in the absence of the peptides (15 minutes instead of 5). In addition after 60 minutes of incubation, the intact enkephalin is approximately 25% in the first case and near to 0(3%) in the second case(13). So as to permit the identification of hydrolysis by-products by column chromatography, the reported values were obtained at enkephalin concentrations several orders of magnitude higher than those of the physiological resting level. Under these conditions, it may be hypothesized that the enkephalin-degrading enzymes are nearly saturated, or else that a high concentration of enkephalin hydrolysis by-products may be competing for the enzyme's active sites, and thus constituting an inhibitor. To circumvent these difficulties, we tried to determine leu-enkephalin plasma half life at a concentration as near to the physiological one as possible. Using a batch of labelled enkephalin of a particularly high specific activity, we were able to measure enkephalin hydrolysis kinetics at a concentration as low as 1×10^{-13} moles/ml, which is at the lower end of the physiologically steady-state concentrations of 1×10^{-13} to 1×10^{-12} moles/ml(27,28). Figure 7 actually shows the degradation kinetics of 1×10^{-10} M leu-enkephalin in the presence and in the absence of plasma peptides.

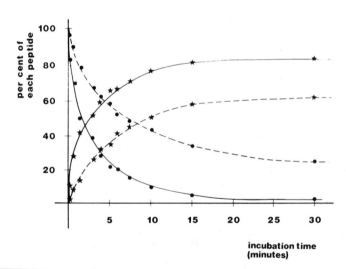

Figure 7. Degradation kinetics of leu-enkephalin in the presence of whole (dashed line) and de-peptidised(dashed line) human plasma. Solid circles represent tyrosine. Incubation and assay conditions as described in text.

Under these conditions, the half-life de-peptidized plasma is 2.5 minutes, while it is 8 minutes in whole plasma. This latter may be considered a reliable value for human plasma. This figure is in perfect accordance with the data previously determined in our laboratory. On the other hand, it strongly contradicts the values reported by other laboratories (8,9) as detailed in section D.

C2c Mechanisms of enzyme inhibition

The mechanisms of aforementioned enzyme inhibition are currently under study in our laboratory. However, some of the data available so far seem worth mentioning.

The peptides with enkephalin-binding and enzyme-degradation protections activities were fractioned as follows: to evidentiate enkephalin binding, whole plasma - preincubated with labelled leu-enkephalin - was fractioned by steric exclusion chromatography. To evidentiate protection from proteolysis, the plasma, not preincubated with enkephalin, was fractioned with the same steric exclusion column. The results of this experiment, combined, are shown in Figure 6. The obtained pools, indicated in Figure 6 by bars and numbers, were assayed for inhibition of the enkephalin-degrading enzymes as follows: the enzymes were fractioned from human plasma by steric exclusion chromatography as described in Section B2b. Labelled leu-enkephalin was incubated with the fractioned enkephalin-degrading enzymes obtained as indicated. The percent of degraded enkephalin was measured by thin layer and reverse phase chromatography. The results of these experiments are reported in Table I.

TABLE I

Inhibition of enkephalin-degrading enzyme activities by plasma components shown in figure 6, defined as percent of the inhibition due to an equimolar amount of leu-enkephalin.

POOL	AP	DAP	DCP
1	0	37	55
2	60	62	*
3	97	28	0
4	*	*	0
5	*	*	0
6	*	*	*
7	*	*	*

* Not significative, less than 10%.
AP = aminopeptidase
DAP = dipeptidyl-aminopeptidase
DCP = dipeptidyl-carboxypeptidase

The results shown indicate that the different peptide groups inhibit different amounts of the three enkephalin-degrading enzyme families. Moreover, the inhibition of the enzyme activities seems not to be due - as we originally supposed - to the binding of the enkephalin to the protecting peptides. Instead, from data available so far, the protection mechanism seems to be due to competition for the active sites of the degrading enzymes. While several of the peptide pools present in human plasma seem to inhibit some of the enkephalin-degrading enzyme systems present in the same tissue, only one of the fractioned pools seems to bind to enkephalin, and to partially inhibit only one(dipeptidylaminopeptidase) of the enzyme activities present in plasma. On the other hand, the data reported in paragraph C2a demonstrate that peptide-bound enkephalins are protected from enzyme hydrolysis. Therefore, two different protection mechanisms seem to be active: competitive inhibition of the enzymes, and a different mechanism acting through binding to the peptide or peptides, as indicated in Table 1.

D: ENKEPHALIN HYDROLYSIS IN DIFFERENT ANIMAL SPECIES

As already pointed out, the blood half-lives of enkephalins, such as they were measured by various authors, differ by a factor of approximately 200. That is, from 2-4 seconds reported by Dupont et al. in rat plasma(9) to the 8 minutes reported by us in human plasma(13). A span of this magnitude can hardly be accounted for by technical reasons alone. In addition, our interpretation of the physiological roles of opioid peptides in plasma can be quite strongly influenced by the degradation kinetics in blood one assumes to be true. Therefore - using the technical procedures listed in Section C3 we measured enkephalin hydrolysis kinetics in several laboratory animals and in man(52).

Figure 8 shows the hydrolysis kinetics of leu-enkephalin in human, rat and rabbit whole plasma. The corresponding half-lives are 8 minutes, 40 seconds and 90 seconds respectively. Specifically, the half-life measured for rat plasma is still one order of magnitude longer than the one measured by Dupont et al. But, these leatter values were obtained under completely different experimental conditions. Thus, it is possible that the discrepancies observed are mainly caused by technical reasons.

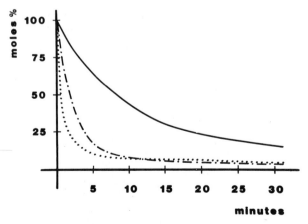

Figure 8. Hydrolysis kinetics of leu-enkephalin in the presence of human (solid line), rabbit(dash-dotted line) and rat(dashed line) plasma. Incubation and assay conditions as described in the text.

Summing up, it is evident that considerable care should be used in the
- frequently unavoidable - procedure of extrapolating data obtained with
laboratory animals to the human species. This even more so, since our
results indicate that the differences are not only quantitative but qualitative as well. That is, the relative amount of the different enkephalin-
hydrolyzing enzymes, as well as the total activity, is considerably different
in different mammals. This is evident by comparing Figure 9 and 10, which
show the pattern of enkephalin degrading enzymes in rabbit and rat plasma
respectively, to Figure 2, showing the distribution of the same enzymes in
human plasma.

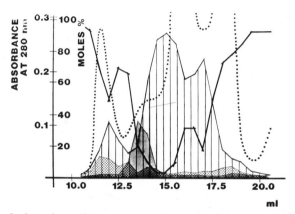

Figure 9. Enkephalin-degrading enzymes in rat plasma as fractioned by high
pressure steric exclusion chromatography. Enzyme activities were determined
as described in the text. Dotted line:absorbance at 280 nm. Solid line:Leu-
enkephalin, Vertically ruled area:aminopeptidase, Dotted area:dipeptidylamino-
peptidase. Dark shaded area:dipeptidylcarboxypeptidase activities.

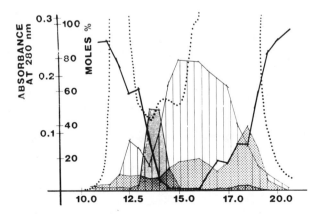

Figure10. Enkephalin-degrading enzymes in rabbit plasma. Symbols as in Fig.9.

29

E: CONCLUSION

The data reported in the previous sections may be summarized as follows: i) Once in the blood-strea, adrenal-released enkephalins are hydrolyzed by several enzyme groups cleaving TYR-GLY, GLY-GLY and GLY-LEU bonds. ii) The enzyme specificity necessary to hydrolyze enkephalins seems to be relatively high. This seems at least partially due to the unusually high degree of structural organization shown by these peptides. iii) Circulating enkephalins are protected from enzyme hydrolysis by binding to several goups of molecules all of a peptidic nature. Two such systems are present in the chromaffin granule, and two more in the plasma. iv) Taking into account the existence of the protecting systems, the half-lives of the enkephalins in man seem to be long enough to account for medium-lasting physiological effects. v) As far as enkephalin hydrolysis is concerned, the data obtained with a given animal species cannot be extended to other species.

On the whole, release, hydrolysis and protection of enkephalins seem to be a quite complex phenomena. The phylogenetic history of opioid peptides is a relatively long one, since these peptides are found in different, although related, phyla such as Mollusca, Annelida and Arthropoda, as well as in Chordata (53-55). A long molecular evolution can certainly account for the existence of complex interactions as well as for the existance of different physiological roles for the same molecule.

A certain degree of intrinsic naivete nothwithstanding, it seems worthwhile to attempt to interpret the existing data on enkephalins' hydrolysis in terms of the functional significance of the hydrolysis/protection mechanisms discovered so far. In this respect, the hypothesis that best fitls all the available evidence on opioid peptides' release, hydrolysis and protection seems to be the following: once enkephalins are released into the blood-stream. role of the degrading enzymes could be to terminate the physiological activit of these peptides, assuming that no such system exists in the target tissues. Moreover, the exostence in blood of two different systems with opposite functions - degradate as well as to protect enkephalins -- makes it appear that a homeostatic regulation of enkephalins' activity is measured through the opposite actions of these systems.

It is clear that the outlined hypothesis is nothing more than a tentative interpretation. Actually, it seems extremely difficult even to devise an experimental procedure to verify it. Yet, it is possible that the addition of more experimental evidence will show us - in the next few years - whether or not the outlined hypothesis can be correct.

ACKNOWLEDGEMENT

The work described in the present article has been carried out within the framework of an with partial support from the "Progetto Finalizzato Chimica e Secondaria" of the CNR (Italian National Council for Scientific Research).

REFERENCES

1. Terenius, L. and Wahlstrom, A. (1974) Inhibitor(s) of narcotic receptor binding in brain extracts and cerebrospinal fluid. Acta Pharmacol. Toxicol. (suppl. 1) 35, 55.
2. Hughes, J. (1975) Isolation of an endogenous compound from the brain with pharmacological properties similar to morphine. Brain Research 88, 295–308.
3. Pasternak, K.W., Goodman, R. and Snyder S.H. (1975) An endogenous morphine-like factor in mammalian brain. Life Sci. 16, 1765–1769.
4. Pert, C.B., Pert, A., Chang, J.K. and Fond, B.T.W. (1976) D-Ala^2-Met-Enkephalinide: a potent, long-lasting synthetic pentapeptide analgesic. Science 194, 330–32.
5. Buscher, H.H., Hill, R.C., Romer, D., Cardinaux, F., Closse, A., Hauser, D. and Pless, J. (1976) Evidence for analgesic activity of enkephalin in the mouse. Nature 261, 423–25.
6. Belluzzi, J.D., Grant, N., Garsky, V., Sarantakis, D., Wise, C.D., and Stein, L. (1976) Analgesia indiced in vivo by central administration of enkephalin in rat. Nature 260, 625–26.
7. Terenius, L., (1978) Endogenous peptides and analgesia. Ann. Rev. Pharmacol. Toxicol. 18, 189–204.
8. Hambrook, J.M., Morgan, B.A., Rance, M.J., and Smith, C.F.C., (1976) Mode of deactivation of the enkephalins by rat and human plasma and rat brain homogenates. Nature 262, 782–783.
9. Dupont, A., Cusan, L., Garon, M., Alvarado-Urbina, G. and Labrie, F. (1977) Extremely rapid degradation of ^{3}H methionine-enkephalin by various rat tissues in vivo and in vitro. Life Sci. 21, 907–914.
10. Hogue-Angeletti, R.A. and Roda, L.G. (1980) In vitro interaction of enkephalin with serum and chromaffin granule components. Experientia 36, 1420–1421.
11. Schwartz, J.C., Malfroy, B. and De La Baume, S. (1981) Biological inactivation of enkephalins and the role of enkephalin-dipeptidyl-carboxypeptidase ("Enkephalinase") as neuropeptidase. Life Sci. 29, 1715–1740.
12. Coletti-Previero, M.A., Matras, H., Descomps. B. and Previero, A. (1981) Purification and substrate characterization of a human enkephalin-degrading aminopeptidase. Biochem. Biophys. Acta 657, 122–127.
13. Roscetti, G., Possenti, R., Bassano, E. and Roda, L.G. (1984) Mechanisms of leu-enkephalin hydrolysis in human blood. Life Sci. in press.
14. Roda, L.G., De Marco, V. and Possenti, R. (1983) Stability of periphral enkephalins in "Degradation of Endogenous Opioid." S. Ehrenpreis and F. Sicuteri eds. pgs. 25–42 Raven Press, New York.
15. Loew, G.H. and Burt, S.K. (1978) Energy conformation study of met-enkephalin and its D-Ala^2 analogue and their resemblance to ridig opiates. Proc. Natl. Acad. Sci. USA 75, 7–11.
16. Momany, F.A.(1977) Conformational analysis of methionine-enkephalin and some analogs. Biochem. Biophys. Res. Comm. 75,1098–1103.
17. Isogai, Y., Nemethy, G. and Scherga, H.A.(1977) Enkephalin-conformational analysis by means of empirical energy calculations. Proc. Natl. Acad. Sci. USA 74,414–418.
18. Spirites, M.A.,Schwartz, R.W., Mattice, W.L. and Coy,D.H.(1978) Circular dichroism and adsorption study of the structure of methionine-enkephalin in solution. Biochem. Biophys. Res. Comm. 81,602–609.
19. Khaled,M.A., Long, M.M., Thompson, W.D., Bradley, R.J., Brown, G.B., and Urry, D.W. (1977) Conformational states of enkephalin in solution. Biochem. Biophys. Res. Comm. 76,224–231.
20. Fillippi, B. Gusti, P., Cima, L. Borin, G., Ricchielli, F. and Marchiori f. (1979) Synthetic enkephalins. Intl. J. Peptide Protein Res. 14,34–40.

21. Levine, B.A.,Rabenstein, D.L., Smith, D. and Williams, R.J.P.(1979) Proton magnetic resonance studies on methionine enkephalin and β-endorphin in aqueous solution. Biochem. Biophys. Acta 579, 279-291.

22. Garbay-Jaureguiberry, C., Marion, D., Fellion, E. and Roques, B.P.(1982) Refinement of conformational preferences of Leu-enkephalin and Tyr-Gly-Gly-Phe by ^{15}N NMR. Int. J. Peptide Protein Res. 20, 443-450.

23. Jones,C.R., Garsky, V. and Gibbons, W.A.(1977) Molecular conformations of met-enkephalin: comparition of the zwitterionic and cationic forms. Biochem. Biophys. Res. Comm. 76,619-625.

24. Garbay-Jaureguberry, C.,Roques, B.P. and Oberlin,R. (1977) ^{1}H and ^{13}C NMR studies of conformational behavior of leu-enkephalin. FEBS Letters 76,93-98.

25. Smith, G.D. and Griffin, J.F.(1978) Conformation of Leu[5] enkephalin from x-ray diffraction: features important for recognition at opiate receptor. Science 199,1214-1216

26. Cabassi, F. and Zetta, L. (1982) Human β-endorphin. Intl. J. Peptide Protein Res. 20,154-158.

27. Clement-Jones,V., Lovry, P.J.,Rees, L.H. and Besser,G.M.(1980) Conformation of Leu[5] enkephalin from x-ray diffraction: features important for recognition at opiate receptor. Nature 283,295-297.

28. Ryder, S.W. and Eng, J. (1982) Radioimmunoassay of leucine-enkephalin like substance in human and canine plasma. J. Clin. Endocrinol. and Metabolism 52,367-369.

29. Blaschko, H. and Welch, A.D.(1953) Localization of adrenaline in cytoplasmic particles of the bovine adrenal medulla. Naunyn Schmiedberg's Arch. Exp. Pathol. Pharmakol. 219, 17-22.

30. Hillarp, N.A., Lagenstedt, S. and Nilson, B. (1953) The isolation of a granular fraction from the suprarenal medulla, containing the sympathomimetic catechol amines. Acta. Phisiol. Scand. 29, 251-263.

31. Winkler, H. (1976) The conposition of adrenal chromaffin granules: an assessment of controversial results. Neuroscience 1, 65-80.

32. Njus, D. and Radda, G.K. (1978). Bioenergetic processes in chromaffin granules: a new prospective on some old problems. Biochem. Biophys. Acta. 463, 219-244.

33. Hogue-Angeletti, R.A., Roda, L.G., Nolan, J.A. and Zarenba, S. Catecholamine storage vesicles in "Protein of the Nervous System" R.A. Bradshaw and D.M. Schneider eds. Raven Press. New York 1980.

34. Schultzberg, M., Lundberg, J.M., Hokfelt, J., Terenius, L., Brandt, J., Elde, R.P. and Goldstein, M. (1978) Enkephalin-like immunoreactivity in gland cells and nerve terminals of the adrenal medulla. Neuroscience 3, 1169-1186.

35. Viveros, O.H., Diliberto, E.J.J., Hazum, E. and Chang, K.J. (1979) Opiate-like materials in the adrenal medulla: evidence for storage and secretion with catecholamines. Mol. Pharmacol. 16, 1101-1108.

36. Di Giulio, A.M., Yang, H.-Y.T., Fratta, W. and Costa, E. (1979). Decreased content of immunoreactive enkephalin-like peptide in peripheral tissues of spontaneously hypertensive rats. Nature 278 646-647.

37. Lewis, R.V., Stern, A.S., Rossier, J., Stein, S. and Udenfriend, S. (1979) Putative enkephalin precursor in bovine adrenal medulla. Biochem Biophys. Res. Comm. 89, 822-829.

38. Stern, A.S., Lewis, R.V., Kimura, S., Rossier, J., Stein, S. and Udenfriend, S. (1979) Isolation of the opioid heptapeptide met-enkephalin-Arg[6]-Phe[7] from bovine adrenal medullary granules and striatum. Proc. Natl. Acad. Sci. USA 76, 6680-6683.

39. Lewis, R.V., Stern, A.S., Kimura, S., Rossier, J., Brink, L., Gerber, L.D., Stein, S. and Udenfriend, S. Opioid peptides and precursor in the adrenal medulla in "Neural Peptides and Neural Communication." E. Costa and M. Trabucchi eds. Raven Press, New York 1980.

40. Yang, H.-Y.T., Di Giulio, A.M., Fratta, W., Hong, J.S., Majane, E.A. and Costa, E. (1980) Enkephalin in bovine adrenal gland: multiple molecular forms of Met[5]-enkephalin immunoreactive peptides. Neuropharmacology 19,209-215.

41. Troy, C.M. and Musacchio, J.M. (1982) Processing of enkephalin precursors by chromaffin granule enzymes. Life Sci. 31, 1717-1720.

42. Wallace, E.F., Evans, C.J., Jurik, S.M., Mafford, I.N. and Barchas, J.D. (1982) Carboxypeptidase B activity from adrenal medulla. Is it involved in the processing of proenkephalin? Life Sci. 31, 1793-1796.

43. Jones B.N., Shively J.E., Kilpatrick D.L., Stern A.S., Lewis R.V., Kojima K., Udenfriend S., Usa (1979) Adrenal opioid proteins of 8,600 and 12,600 daltons: intermediates in proenkephalin processing. Proc. Natl. Acad. Sci. 2096-2100.

44. Lewis, R.V., Stern, A.S., Kimura, S., Rossier, J., Stein, S. and Udenfriend, S., (1980). An about 50,000-dalton protein in adrenal medulla: a common precursor of Met- and Leu- enkephalin. Science 208, 1459-1461.

45. Fricker, L.D., Supattapone, S. and Snyder, S. (1982) Enkephalin convertase: a specific enkephalin synthesizing carboxypeptidase in adrenal chromaffin granules, brain, and pituitary gland. Life Sci. 31, 1841-1844.

46. Lindberg, I., Yang, H.-Y.T. and Costa, E. (1982) Characterization of a partially pufified trypsin-like enkephalin-generating enzyme in bovine adrenal medulla. Life Sci. 31, 1713-1716.

47. Lewis, R.V. and Stern, A.S. (1983) Biosynthesis of enkephalins and enkephalin-containing polypeptides. Ann. Rev. Pharmacol. Toxicol. 23, 353-372.

48. Possenti, R., De Marco, V., Cherubini, O. and Roda, L.G. (1983) Enkephalin-binding systems in human plasma. Neurochem. Res. 8, 423-432.

49. Hogue-Angeletti, R.A. and Sheetz, PxB. (1978) A soluble lipid protein complex from bovine adrenal medulla chromaffin granules. J. Biol. Chem. 253, 5613-5616.

50. Helle, K.B. (1966) Antibody formation against soluble protein from bovine adrenal medulla chromaffin granules. Biochem. Biophys. Acta 117, 107-110.

51. Roda, L.G. and Hogue-Angeletti, R.A. (1979) Peptides in the adrenal medulla chromaffin granule. FEBS Letters 107, 393-397.

52. Stefano, G.B. and Catapane, E.J. (1979) Enkephalins increase dopamine levels in the CNS of a marine mollusc. Life Sci. 24, 1617-1622.

53. Sundler, F., Hakanson, R., Alumets, J. and Walles, B. (1977) Neuronal localization of pancreatic polypeptide (PP) and vasoactive intestinal peptide (VIP) immunoreactivity in the earthworm (lubricus terrestris). Brain Research Bull. 2, 61-65.

54. Zipser, B. (1980) Identification of specific leech neurones immunoreactive to enkephalin. Nature 283, 857-858.

STUDIES OF THE ENDOGENOUS OPIOID SYSTEM

IN THE HUMAN STRESS RESPONSE

Martin R. Cohen[1], David Pickar[2], Michel Dubois[3], and Robert M. Cohen[4]

1. Ensor Foundation Research Laboratory, William S. Hall Psychiatric Institute, and the Department of Neuropsychiatry and Behavioral Sciences, University of South Carolina.
2. Section on Clinical Studies, Clinical Neuroscience Branch, NIMH, Bethesda, Md.
3. Department of Anesthesiology, Georgetown University School of Medicine, Washington, D.C.
4. Section on Brain Imaging, Laboratory of Psychology and Psychopathology, NIMH, Bethesda, Md.

During the last few years, our group has been actively engaged in clinical studies to understand the role of the endogenous opioid system (EOS) in human behavior. In this chapter, we review those of our studies that are most pertinent to our understanding of human behavior during stress and the implications of results from these studies on future strategies to understand and modify, for therapeutic purposes, the role of the EOS in the human stress response.

PLASMA BETA-ENDORPHIN AND HUMAN STRESS

When we began our studies in 1979, considerable evidence had already been gained from animal experimentation to support an important role for the EOS in the physiological response to stress [1]. Over the years, surgery had been one of the most intensively studied of human stressors. Thus, in our initial studies, we sought to determine whether activation of the EOS occurred with surgery.

The EOS is actually a complex of systems with unknown interrelations, different anatomical locations and different concentrations of endogenous opioids (endorphins) [2]. Nevertheless, due to practical considerations, we limited our study to the evaluation of patients' plasma levels of beta endorphin. This could only be considered a peripheral measurement of EOS activation, but changes in plasma levels of beta-endorphin could probably be attributed to alterations in pituitary secretion, a function known to play an important role in the physiological stress response [3]. In addition, by concomitantly measuring patients' plasma cortisol levels, we could assess the linkage, suggested in animal studies, of the hypothalmic-pituitary-adrenal axis (HPA) and the peripheral EOS during stress [4].

An initial pilot study in patients undergoing limb amputations suggested marked increases in plasma beta-endorphin levels but only in those patients who were administered anesthesia without opiates (exogenous opioids) [5]. We subsequently completed a study on a more uniform cohort [6] as follows:

Nine patients underwent laparotomy as part of a National Cancer Institute protocol for the assessment of testicular or ovarian malignancy. Patients were free of medical complications other than regional malignancy and were medication free for 72 hours before the surgical procedures. Premedication consisted of 100 mg. of pentobarbital administered intramuscularly. Induction of anesthesia was accomplished with thiopental and succinylcholine, and anesthesia was maintained with enflurane, nitrous oxide, and a muscle relaxant. All patients were intubated and had controlled ventilation. Surgery lasted between 2 and 4 hours. No exogenous opioids were administered before or during surgery.

Blood samples were collected from each patient before, 10 to 15 minutes after induction of anesthesia, 10 minutes after skin incision, at 30-minute intervals during surgery until skin closure and while the patient was conscious following surgery and before post-operative analgesia was initiated. A patient's mean surgery hormone level was calculated as the mean of values derived from samples obtained during surgery at the times just noted. Details of sample care are reported elsewhere.

Plasma cortisol and beta-endorphin levels were determined by radioimmunossay on unextracted samples with reagents supplied by New England Nuclear Corporation. There is in the beta-endorphin assay, 50 per cent crossreactivity to beta-lipotropin, $<$5 percent to ACTH, $<$ 0.01 per cent to alpha-endorphin and alpha-MSH, and $<$ 0.004 per cent to methionine and leucine enkephalin. Thus beta-endorphin (ir) as determined in the study was essentially the sum of circulating beta-endorphin (beta-lipotropin (61-91)) and beta-lipotropin; their ratio was not determined. Details of the assay method may be found in reference 5.

In summary, we found no change in plasma beta-endorphin (ir) following anesthesia and prior to surgical incision, but a marked increase in plasma beta-endorphin (ir) during surgery. Analogous effects of anaesthesia and surgery on plasma cortisol levels were found. In evaluating individual patient's hormone levels, we found across the 3 conditions of before, during and following surgery a strong positive correlation between plasma betaendorphin (ir) and cortisol levels ($r=0.61$, $p<0.01$). Individual hormone responses to surgery are illustrated in figure 1.

Thus we were somewhat comfortable that within the limitations of clinical design, we had been able to demonstrate an activation of the EOS during the human stress response. Similar to the findings in animal experimentation, this activation was concomitant with an activation of the HPA axis.

While we were engaged in our studies of surgical stress, we had the opportunity in collaboration with Drs. Nurnberger and Gershon of the NIMH to monitor the response of plasma beta-endorphin levels to an intravenous

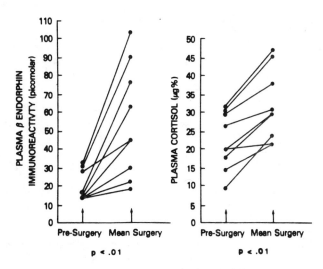

FIGURE 1: Individual patient plasma beta-endorphin (ir) and cortisol responses to surgery. Each line connects an individual's presurgery hormone level to mean-surgery hormone level. Presurgery beta-endorphin levels below the sensitivity of our radioimmunoassay (< 14.4 picomolar) were arbitrarily assigned the value of 14.4 picomolar to minimize any found increases with surgery. The group mean ±SEM were as follows: pre-surgery beta-endorphin 19.9±2.4 picomolar; mean surgery = 54.9±10.2 picomolar; presurgery cortisol = 22.1±2.6 ug per dl: mean surgery cortisol = 32.4±3.2 ug per dl. (From Cohen, M.R., Pickar, D., Dubois, M., et al.: Clinical and experimental studies of stress and the endogenous opioid system. In Verebey, K.: Opioids and Mental Illness. New York, New York Academy of Sciences. 1982)

amphetamine infusion [7]. We were intrigued by this opportunity since in animal models, amphetamine may simulate the effects of stress, and in humans, amphetamine is used in the treatment of behavioral disorders with apparent (narcolepsy) or hypothesized arousal abnormalities (hyperactivity and depression) [8,9].

As in our surgical studies, we found in response to amphetamine a concomitant activation of the EOS and the HPA axis. Although the response to amphetamine was considerably less than the response to surgery, it was demonstrable in a double-blind cross-over study, a design not practical with surgery. However, more recently in collaboration with Dr. C.H. Shatney of the Trauma Center of Baltimore, we have been able to demonstrate in patients coming to a trauma center markedly higher plasma beta-endorphin levels in patients with severe trauma and admission to the center compared to those patients referred elsewhere for treatment because of less severe trauma [10].

Concurrent and subsequent to our studies, many other groups have been able to demonstrate increases of plasma beta-endorphin (ir) in humans during physiological stress [11-13]. However, activation of the EOS only suggests that this system may be involved or may be an indicator of the physiological stress response.

The potential of the EOS to be involved in the behavioral adaptation to a stressor is suggested by the behavioral effects of narcotic alkaloids (exogenous opioids) which are presumed to function by activation of the EOS. In particular, the value of narcotic alkaloids to modify behavior to a continuing painful stimulus is well known [14]. The clinical application of this principle was the mainstay of post-operative analgesia at the NIH. Immediately following surgery, patients were taken to the Clinical Center Surgical Intensive Care Unit (SICU) where they stayed for a minimum period of 24 hours. During their stay, there was a standing routine clinical order for post-operative management of pain. Once patients were conscious (between first and third hour post awakening) they were administered intravenous morphine at 1.5 to 3.5 mg per hour as considered necessary by staff for relief of post operative pain.

We reasoned that if plasma beta-endorphin levels were an accurate indicator of the individual's arousal or stress response, i.e. the ability to physiologically adapt to a stressor, then individuals with high plasma beta-endorphin levels would require less morphine than those with low levels. This would be the clinical extension of the well documented laboratory phenomenon of stress induced analgesia.

A patient's morphine requirement was simply calculated as the total morphine administered to the individual during the first 24 postoperative hours in the SICU. This was obtained from the patient's clinical chart. The postsurgical morphine requirements of our patients ranged from 12 to 56 mg (mean ±SEM, 35.2±16.1). The validity of this simple measurement as a reflection of our patient's physiological need for relief of pain was supported by a positive (r=0.55), although not quite significant, correlation with patient weight (range = 47.5-85.5 kg) and a significant negative correlation (r = -0.69, p 0.05, 2 tail) with patient age (range = 21 to 60 years). This latter finding is expected from the slowing of morphine metabolism in the aged [15].

We were surprised however to find that not only did those patients with high surgery beta-endorphin (ir) have low morphine requirements (figure 2) but that they were also the patients with high pre-surgery beta-endorphin (ir) [16].

Our findings suggested that elevated plasma beta-endorphin (ir) could be considered a biologic marker of the human stress response much as plasma cortisol levels had previously been used to predict physiological and behavioral adaptation to a stressor. Further, our work suggested that even in the instance of an extreme physical stressor, a strong component of adaptation might lie in the individual's innate responsiveness to stress or his prior psychologic perception of this stress as patients' presurgical stress hormone levels were predictive of their levels during surgery as well as their postsurgery pain perception.

[17] Plasma beta-endorphin has not been directly implicated in analgesia but we might hypothesize that the larger morphine dose was required by some patients to substitute for a relatively poorly stress-activated physiological response. This is supported by the finding of Tamsen et al. of a negative relationship between lumbar CSF endogenous opioid levels

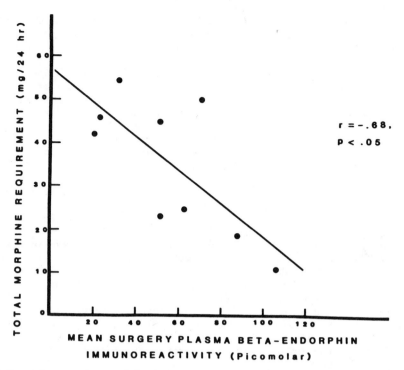

FIGURE 2: Nine patients (+) plotted two-dimensionally for the variables of
morphine requirement and mean (surgery) plasma beta-endorphin. Patient
morphine requirement can be predicted by the illustrated linear equation:
Morphine requirement = 54.9-0.36 x mean (surgery) plasma beta-endorphin.
Patient morphine requirement is the total morphine used during the first 24
postoperative hours. Mean (surgery) plasma beta-endorphin is the mean of
plasma beta-endorphin levels found in samples taken at 30-minute intervals
during surgery. (From Cohen, M.R., Pickar, D., Dubois, M., et al.: Stress
induced plasma beta-endorphin immunoreactivity may predict postoperative
morphine usage. Psychiatr. Res., 6:7-12, 1982).

measured prior to surgery and calculated 24 hour postsurgery CSF levels of
the self-administered opiate pethidine[18]. Further support for a role of
the EOS in surgical stress-induced analgesia is provided by the work of
Levine et al., demonstrating in the postsurgery period analgesia following
0.2 and 2 mg of naloxone but hyperalgesia following 7.5 and 10 mg doses[19].
A similar biphasic effect of naloxone on analgesia following exercise has
been reported[20].

NALOXONE AND HUMAN STRESS

Indeed a common clinical strategy to assess the role of the EOS in
human behavior is to evaluate the effect of the administration of naloxone.
Naloxone, which is considered a pure opiate receptor antagonist, is assumed
to affect an in vivo blockade of the EOS. Thus, if the EOS is involved in
an important role in the subject's present mood or behavior, then administration of naloxone should produce demonstrable alterations.

In contrast to the postive findings with stress induced analgesia, the

failure in some studies to find modification of the stress response following naloxone administration has led some investigators to exclude the
importance of the EOS in these human stress responses [21,22]. However the
EOS is a complex system such that parts of the system as a result of location and/or the involvement of different endogenous opioids and receptor
subtypes, or the need to be only intermittently active, may be relatively
resistant to functional blockade by naloxone. Thus investigators of the
stress response may well have generally used too low or restricted a dose
range of naloxone to fully assess EOS involvement. Conclusions regarding
the role of the EOS in pain perception following surgery or jogging would
have differed had not the experimenters increased the dose of naloxone
administered to their subjects [19,20].

In recent years, we have been able to demonstrate that bolus doses of
naloxone administered in the mg/kg range intravenously to normal volunteers
may produce behavioral and physiological responses that mimic responses
seen during the human stress response. These effects include an increase
in plasma levels of cortisol and growth hormone, an increase in systolic
blood pressure, and a behavioral syndrome of irritability, anxiety and
depression [23,24]. In addition, we have found that hospitalized patients
suffering from depression seem to be more sensitive to these naloxone
induced dysphoric symptoms [25]. One explanation of the pathogensis of
depression is based on physiological adaptation to stress in vulnerable
individuals [5]. We believe the previous reports of minimal or inconsistent
behavioral effects after naloxone administration to normals are directly
attributable to the lower doses of naloxone used in those studies.

The design of our initial study was complex due to the safety precautions that were necessitated by the administration of doses of naloxone not
previously administered to humans. The details may be found in reference
24.

> In brief, subjects were without physical illness or a
> personal history of psychiatric illness or drug abuse. In
> addition, all subjects were free from acute illness or drug
> intake for at least three days preceding any individual day
> of study and free from opiate intake for at least the three
> preceding weeks.

> Subjects participated in three separate days of study
> which were conducted at least a week apart. At 8:30 and
> 10:30 a.m. of each study day three-minute IV infusions of
> increasing doses of naloxone hydrochloride were adminis-
> tered: first day, 0.3 and 1 mg/kg; second, 1 and 2
> mg/kg; and third, 2 and 4 mg/kg. Subjects were blind to
> naloxone doses and sequence. Periodically during the course
> of the day, each volunteer completed self-rating scales and
> the non-blind attending psychiatrist the Brief Psychiatric
> Rating Scale (BPRS).

Results from the rating scales were quite consistent so that only the
scores on the self-rating mood adjective checklist are illustrated in
Figure 3. In summary, with the administration of increasing doses of
naloxone and presumeably increasing functional blockade of the EOS, normals
experienced dysphoric symptoms that were also manifest in their behavior
and apparent to the experimenters. The most prominent symptoms were
anxiety, irritability, depression, a general uncomfortable mental feeling
and difficulty with concentration and functioning. Although the effect was
found in almost every volunteer, its intensity, duration, and the dose
required for the effect was quite individually variable.

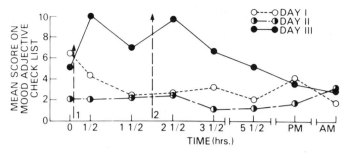

FIGURE 3: Normal volunteers participated in three separate days of study
at least one week apart. Bolus doses of naloxone were infused
intravenously at 0830 and 1030 hours (Arrows 1 and 2). Doses 1 and 2 were
as follows: first day 0.3 and 1 mg/kg, respectively; second day 1 and 2
mg/kg, respectively; and third day, 2 and 4 mg/kg respectively. Total
scores on the mood adjective checklist were found to have a main effect for
day (F=3.86, df=2,12, p = .05), no significant effect for time (F=1.25,
df=7,42, p=.3), but a very significant day x time interaction effect
(F=4.36, df=14,84, p<0.0001). The day x time effect was attributable to
significantly increased scores (increased symptoms) on day 3 compared with
day 1 after the first infusion and until discharge at 2 pm. Scores before
the first infusion were not significantly different between days. Negative
scores indicate a decrease in symptoms. The most prominent effects
indicated by volunteers were increasing anxiety, irritability and worry,
increasing difficulty with concentration and functioning, and an
uncomfortable mental feeling.

OPIOID AGONISTS AND HUMAN STRESS

The results from our investigations of opioid levels during surgery
and naloxone administration to normals led us to begin to assess the
potential therapeutic application of modifying the stress response by
activation of the EOS.

In 6 of the surgery patients, we were able to measure plasma beta-
endorphin (ir) following surgery, both prior to and following post-
operative morphine administration. The marked decrease in all of the
patients' hormone levels following morphine administration is illustrated
in Figure 4.

We have also been able to study the effect on EOS and HPA activation
during surgery of the addition of fentanyl (a synthetic opiate) to
anesthesia. Our methods and the results of this study are reported in
detail elsewhere [26].

> In brief, patient selection, anesthetic technique, blood
> collection, and assay methodology were as noted for the pre-
> viously presented study. However, in this study, 10 patients
> received, in addition to their premedication and anesthetic
> drugs, a single medium dose of fentanyl (10 to 20 ug per kg)
> given intravenously 5 minutes before the surgical incision.

The most important finding is illustrated in Figure 5. A single
administration of fentanyl completely blocks the plasma beta-endorphin and
cortisol responses early in surgery while partially blocking even the
responses late in surgery.

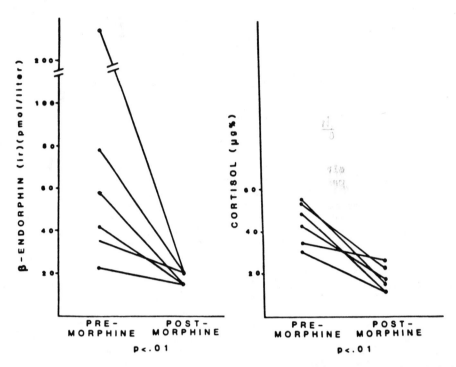

FIGURE 4: Changes in plasma levels of cortisol and beta-endorphin (ir) in six patients following the administration in the postoperative period of standard clinical doses of morphine. Samples were collected while patients were awake in the Surgical Intensive Care Unit. Patients had undergone laparotomy with enflurane as the primary anesthetic and without the aid of opiates. (From Pickar, D., Cohen, M., Naber, D., et al.: Clinical studies of the endogenous opioid system. Biol. Psychiatry., 17:1243-1276, 1981).

We have hypothesized that this suppression of hormone levels represents feedback inhibition from EOS activation. The effects of this activation on behavioral responses following surgery warrants study. What effect would such activation have on the development of phantom limb pain, a not infrequent complication of surgical amputation?

Because of the complexity of the EOS, the effects of its activation with an exogenous opioid do not necessarily demonstrate the potential therapeutic benefit of modifying the stress response by activation of the EOS with an endogenous ligand. Thus we have begun a preliminary study of the effect of intrathecal administration of beta-endorphin on the behavior of patients suffering from the chronic and severe pain of metastatic cancer[27]. The intrathecal route was chosen because of the apparent effect of the blood brain barrier to exclude from the central nervous system (CNS) peripherally administered beta-endorphin.

As expected, in the 2 patients who have undergone the study, beta-endorphin administration produced prolonged (>48 hrs.) complete relief from pain. However, one of the patients also experienced a marked generalized behavioral change characterized by confusion, hypomanic/manic behavior and psychosis that also persisted for more than 2 days. In patients undergoing the chronic stress of terminal metastatic cancer and persistent severe pain, it might prove difficult to assess the direct effects of an opioid agonist on behavior and mood from indirect effects resulting from

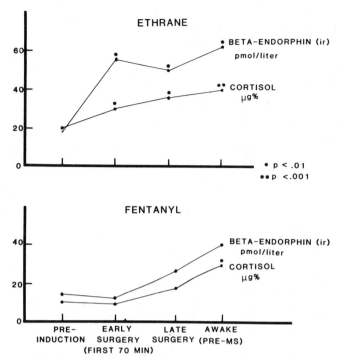

FIGURE 5: Nineteen patients, suffering only from regional malignancy, underwent laparotomy as part of a National Cancer Institute treatment rotocol. All patients received enflurane as the primary maintenance anesthetic. Ten patients received, in addition, 10 to 20 ug of fentanyl intravenously, per kg body weight, five minutes before surgical incision. Surgery lasted between two and four hours. Blood samples for hormone determinations were collected from each patient prior to anesthetic induction (preinduction), 10 minutes after skin incision, at 30-minute intervals during surgery, and when awake in the Surgical Intensive Care Unit, prior to administration of morphine sulfate (MS) for postoperative analgesia. The graphed points represent mean hormone values; p values report the statistical significance of differences from preinduction hormone levels.

pain-relief. However it would be difficult to attribute this patient's psychosis to such an indirect effect.

CONCLUSION

Our work and that of others strongly point to involvement of the EOS in stress induced analgesia. However following a stressful event the human responds with a cluster of behavioral and physiological symptoms. Many of these symptoms may be simulated by the administration of naloxone. If progress in medical science were to be considered the development of an increasingly accurate approximation of how the human body works, we suggest, as a first approximation, that stress disorders are attributable to an exhaustion of the EOS and that activation of the EOS should be helpful in relieving these symptoms. Future studies of this hypothesis must use a broad range of doses of naloxone to ensure functional blockade of the complex EOS. In addition, with the development of our ability to administer or measure various endogenous opioid ligands and to administer opioid antagonists specific to receptor subtypes, we should be able to further modify this first approximation.

REFERENCES

1. Amir, S., Brown, Z.W., and Amit, A., The role of endorphins in stress: Evidence and speculations, Neurosci. Biobehav. Rev. 4:77 (1980).
2. Frederickson, R., and Geary, L., Endogenous opioid peptides: Review of physiological, pharmacological and clinical aspects, Prog. Neurobiol., 19:19-69 (1982).
3. Rossier, J., French, E.D., Rivier, C., Ling, N., Guillemin, R., Bloom, F.E., Foot-shock induced stress increases B-endorphin levels in blood but not brain, Nature 270:618-620 (1977).
4. Guillemin, R., Vargo, T., Rossier, J., Minicck, S., Ling, N., Rivier, C., Vale, W., Bloom, F., Beta-endorphin and adrenocortiocotropin are secreted concomitantly by the pituitary gland, Science 197:1367-1369 (1977).
5. Cohen, M., Pickar, D., Dubois, M., Roth, Y., Naber, D., Bunney, W., Jr., Surgical stress and endorphins, Lancet I 213-214 (1981).
6. Dubois, M., Pickar, D., Cohen, M.R., Roth, Y., MacNamara, T., Bunney, W.E. Jr., Surgical stress in humans in accompanied by an increase in plasma B-endorphin immunoreactivity, Life Sciences 29:1249-1253 (1981).
7. Cohen, M.R., Nurnberger, J., Pickar, D., Gershon, E., Bunney, W., Jr., Dextroamphetamine infusions in normals results in correlated increases of plasma B-endorphin and cortisol immunoreactivity, Life Sciences 29:1243-1247 (1981).
8. Antelman, S., Caggiula, A., Stress-induced behavior: Chemotherapy without drugs in "Psychobiology of Consciousness," Davidson, J. and Davidson, R.M. eds. Plenum Press, New York 65-104 (1980).
9. Cohen, R.M., Campbell, I., Cohen, M.R., Torda, T., Pickar, D., Siever, L., Murphy, D., Pre-synaptic noradrenergic regulation during depression and antidepressant drug treatment, Psychiatr. Res. 3:93-105 (1980).
10. Shatney, C.H, Cohen, R.M., Cohen, M.R., Imagawa, D.R. Endogenous opioid activity in clinical hemorrhagic shock. Surgery, Gynecology and Obstetrics (in press).
11. Carr, D., Bullen, B., Skrinar, G., Arnold, M., Rosenblatt, M., Beitins, I., Martin, J.B., McArthur, J., Physical conditioning facilitates the exercise induced secretion of beta-endorphin and beta-lipotropin in women, N. Engl. J. Med., 305:560-563 (1981).
12. Colt, W., Wardlow, S., Frantz, A., The effect of running on plasma beta-endorphin, Life Sciences, 28:1637-1640 (1981).
13. Goland, R., Wardlaw, S., Stark, R., Frantz, A., Human plasma beta-endorphin during pregnancy, labor and delivery, J. Clin. Endocrinol. Metab., 52:74-78 (1981).
14. Jaffe, J.H., and Martin, W.R., Narcotic analgesics and antagonists. In The Pharmacological Basis of Therapeutics, Edition 6 Goodman, A.G., Goodman, A.S., and Gilman, L. (eds), Macmillian New York (1980).
15. Stanski, D., Greenblatt, D., and Lowenstein, E., Kinetics of intravenous and intramuscular morphine. Clin. Pharmacol. Ther., 24:52-59 (1978).
16. Cohen, M.R., Pickar, D., Dubois, M., Bunney, W.E., Jr., Stress induced plasma beta-endorphin immunoreactivity may predict post-operative morphine usage. Psychiatr. Res., 6:7-12 (1982).
17. Foley, K.M., Kourides, I.A., and Inturrisi, C.E., Kaiko, R., Zaroulis, C., Posner, J., Houde, R., Li, C.H., Beta-endorphin: Analgesic and hormonal effects in humans, Proc. Natl. Acad. Sci., 76:5377-5381 (1979).

18. Tamsen, A., Hartvig, P., Dahlstrom, B., Wahlstrom, A., Jerenics,L., Endorphins and on demand pain relief, Lancet, 1:769 (1980).

19 Levine, J., Gordon, N., and Field, H., Naloxone dose dependently produces analgesia and hyperalgesia in post-operative pain, Nature, 278:740-741 (1979).

20. Haier, R., Quaid, K., Mills, J., Naloxone alters pain perception after jogging, Psychiatr. Res., 5:231-232 (1981).

21. Spiler, I.J., and Molitch, M.E., Lack of modulation of pituitary hormone stress response by neural pathways involving opiate receptors, J. Clin. Endocrinol. Metab., 50:516-520 (1980).

22. Enquist, A., Hicquet, J. Saubrey, N., Blichert-Toft, M., Cortisol, glucose and hemodynamic responses to surgery after naloxone administration, Acta Anaesthesiol. Scand., 25:17-20 (1981).

23. Cohen, M.R., Cohen, R.M., Pickar, D., Murphy, D., Bunney, W.E., Jr., Physiological effects of high dose naloxone administration to normal adults, Life Sciences, 30:2025-2031 (1982).

24. Cohen, M.R., Cohen, R.M., Pickar, D., Weingartner, H., Murphy, D.L., High dose naloxone infusions in normals: dose-dependent behavioral, hormonal, and physiological responses, Arch. Gen. Psychiatry, 40:613-619 (1983).

25. Cohen, M.R., Cohen, R.M., Pickar, D., Sunderland, T., Mueller, E. III., Murphy, D.L., High Dose Naloxone in Depression, Biol. Psychiat., 19:6, 825-832 (1984).

26. Dubois, M., Pickar, D., Cohen, M.R., Gadde, P., Macnamara, T.E., Bunney, W.E., Jr., Effects of fentanyl on the response of plasma beta-endorphin immunoreactivity to surgery, Anesthesiology, 57:468-472 (1982).

27. Pickar, D., Dubois, M., and Cohen, M., Behavioral change in a cancer patient following intrathecal B-Endorphin Administration, American Journal of Psychiatry, 141:1, 103-104 (1984).

EXERCISE STRESS AND ENDOGENOUS OPIATES

Peter Farrell* and Anthony Gustafson**

Department of Human Kinetics* and Endocrine Metabolic Section**
University of Wisconsin-Milwaukee*Medical College of Wisconsin**

INTRODUCTION

The use of exercise to reveal physiological responses and adaptations
has a long history. Exercise can be quantified and repeated exertion
markedly alters body functions. Well established exercise procedures
such as the use of an individual's aerobic capacity have allowed exercise
stress to be used as an experimental model to investigate the endogenous
opiate system. A vast literature had accumulated prior to 1975
concerning the physiological effects of morphine. When the endogenous
opiates were discovered[1], researchers already had insights into
probable functions of the endogenous opiates. Therefore, it is not
surprising that many possible roles for endorphins/enkephalins have been
studied using the exercise model.

OPIATES AND MOTOR ACTIVITY

Opiates influence motor activity. Early investigations demonstrated
a relationship between spontaneous locomotor activity and exogenous
opiates. Goldstein and Sheehan[2] demonstrated the usefulness of
opioid-induced "running fit" as a measure of morphine-like drug actions
in mice. They showed that levorphanol tartrate (20 mg/kg, i.p.) resulted
in increased running activity which was constant for several hours post
injection. At higher doses (30 mg/kg) activity decreased. The L-(+)-
stereoisomer, dextrophan, had no effect on running activity and the
levorphanol effects were antagonized by nalorphine. Tolerance to a
repeated constant dose of 2 mg/kg injections of levorphanol over eight
hours was evident and this adaptation was shown to have cross-tolerance
with morphine.

Babbini and Davis[3] then demonstrated that low doses of morphine
sulfate, 1.25 to 5 mg/kg i.p., caused increased locomotor activity in
male rats while higher doses, 10 to 40 mg/kg, resulted in an initial
depression of activity followed by enhanced activity. However, Goldstein
and Sheehan[2] observed no activity change at doses up to 7 mg/kg. This
may represent an early indication of species differences.

Babbini and Davis[3] also reported a time-dependent effect of
morphine on locomotor activity. Activity was highest approximately 3
hours post injection, 20 mg/kg, i.p., and was followed by return to

47

normal 6 hours post injection. This response became exaggerated after 20 days of daily morphine injection.

Browne and Segal[4] provided two important observations. In rats and mice both exogenous alkaloids (morphine, methadone, etonitazene) and endogenous peptides (Beta-endorphin, as well as D-Ala^2-Met^5-enkephalinamide and D-Met^2-Pro^5-enkephalinamide) produced a biphasic, dose-dependent locomotor activity response. During the first hour following s.c. injection of opiate alkaloids, a decreased locomotor activity was observed while during hours 2-4 a dose dependent (1→10 mg/kg morphine, 0.25→2.5 mg/kg methadone, and 0.5→5.0 µg/mg etonitazene) increase was found. In like manner, intraventricular infusion of Beta-endorphin (1.0→5 µg/10 µl) reduced activity for the first hour followed by an increase over the next 2-4 hrs. Pre-treatment with naloxone (5.0 mg/kg s.c.) antagonized the effect of intraventricular Beta-endorphin. Recently Drust and Crawford[5] found that a low dose of D-Ala^2-Met- enkephalinamide (0.5 µg intracerebroventricular) enhanced locomotor activity in rats. There was no initial depression of activity suggesting that small doses may not result in a biphasic activity pattern as demonstrated by Browne and Segal.[4] This discrepancy may be caused by cannula placement; however, a decrease in spontaneous locomotor activity is not a uniform finding. Oka and Hosoya[6] found that 20 mg/kg morphine sulfate s.c. resulted in an increase in spontaneous locomotor activity in rats lasting several hours.

With the discovery of enkephalins the use of endogenous opiates quickly replaced exogenous opiates in studies examining the relationship between endorphins and activity. Katz et al[7] reported that D-Ala^2-Leu and Met enkephalinamide injections into brain ventricles of mice resulted in a dose-dependent increase in activity which was naloxone (4 or 8 mg/kg) reversible. The stereotyped running behavior produced in the mice was similar to that elicited by morphine injection. Naloxone (8 mg/kg) alone produced a decline of activity in mice who were hyperactive due to initial cage exposure. Amir et al[8] subsequently showed that naltrexone (1 or 2 mg/kg s.c.) reduced activity in rats. While route of administration, use of pharmacological doses, and the species differences tempers our conclusions, these and other studies[9,10,11] demonstrate that blockade of the endogenous opiate system causes decreased locomotor activity.

There is a genetic influence on the interaction between endogenous opiates and activity.[9,10,12,13] Castellano[9] demonstrated that FK 3-824, an enkephalin analogue, (0.25 → 40 mg/kg, i.p.) caused a dose-dependent reduction in locomotor activity in DBA/2J mice while the same enkephalin analogue (1.0 →. 40 mg/kg i.p.) produced a dose-dependent hyperactivity in C57BL/6J mice. In both strains naloxone reversibility was demonstrated. Castellano and Oliverio[12] observed that increasing doses of morphine i.p. caused an increased number of cage crossings. Doses ranged from 5 to 20 mg/kg and pawlick latency to hot plate-induced analgesia was also found to increase with increasing doses of morphine. This study also demonstrated strain differences in mice to both activity levels and analgesic responses. For example, DBA/2J mice showed no increase in crossing even at 20 mg/kg while C57BL/6J mice had an approximate 5-fold increase at this dose. However, C57BL/6J mice showed the least hot plate latency (pawlicking as the endpoint) when compared to either BDA/2J or BALB/CJ mice. Pharmacological manipulations do not necessarily imply physiological roles. However, it would appear that opiates are involved in the normal activity patterns of mice and rats.

Endogenous opiates modify immobility following forced exercise. Amir[8] observed that naloxone reduced the immobility time of BALB/CJ and C57BL/6J mice who swam at 22°C for 10 min. Naloxone injections (0.625→40 mg/kg i.p.) resulted in greater reductions in C57BL/6J compared to BALB/CJ mice. Morphine injections (0.15→10 mg/kg, i.p.) caused an increase in immobility during swimming only at the lowest dose (0.15 mg/kg) in both BALB/CJ and C57BL/6J mice. Even high doses of naloxone (40 mg/kg) did not completely block swimming-induced immobility suggesting involvement of non-opiate mechanisms in the survival-induced immobility response. Naloxone decreased cage crossing activity[14,11] but increased survival swimming activity[8] implying that the type or degree of stress influences the degree of endogenous opiate involvement in the physiological response.

Christie et al[15,16,17] examined the relationship between exercise and pain tolerance. Effects of chronic and acute exercise (3 min warm water swim) were compared to chronic and acute exposure to morphine in mice. Exposure to swimming resulted in an increase in tail-flick latency. After a schedule of one 3 minute swim over 48 hours, mice showed less antinociception when compared to naive mice. Cross tolerance with morphine was found since naive mice showed greater tail flick latency at any dose of morphine (1.1 → 8.9 mg/kg) compared to chronically-exercised mice. Christie's group[17] also demonstrated that naloxone-precipitated withdrawal behavior following cessation of chronic warm water swimming after 48 hours is similar to morphine withdrawal behaviors. This observation suggests that swimming elicits a release of endogenous opiates; and, as a result, chronic swimming may result in adaptations of endogenous opiate receptors leading to tolerance similar to that found after chronic exposure to morphine.

Shyu et al[18] provided compelling data to demonstrate that running in rats is associated with an early morning analgesia which persists for at least several hours after running. Rats were given free access to a running session (9 pm - 9 am). Squeak thresholds due to electrical stimulation increased at the end of the running period. Naloxone (1-2 mg/kg i.p.) blocked this exercise-induced analgesia. Non-running control rats did not show elevated pain thresholds. In a small group of rats (n=4) whose running wheels were locked the previous night, squeak thresholds were similar to control periods (mid afternoon). Additionally, the increased squeak threshold in spontaneously hypertensive running rats was positively related (r = 0.80, p < 0.001) to the distance run on the exercise wheel the preceding night. These data imply that endorphins are involved in exercise-induced analgesia. This analgesia may last for several hours or only for minutes[16] following exercise.

Few studies are available relating changes in endorphins in animals subjected to exercise. Pert and Bowie[19] demonstrated that binding of D-Ala^2-D-Leu-enkephalinamide is reduced in rat brain homogenates after 15 minutes of running or swimming. Further data revealed that the reduced binding was due to enhanced occupancy of opiate receptors by endogenous opiates. However, Metzer and Stein[20] found no change in pituitary, cerebral cortex, and posterior and anterior hypothalamic levels of Beta-endorphin in rats subjected to high intensity running. Significant increases in plasma Beta-endorphin were observed after the acute run. These studies suggest that running may differentially affect central Beta-endorphin and enkephalin systems although investigations using radioreceptor assays[19] cannot be compared directly with studies using radioimmunoassays.[20]

ADRENAL OPIATES

Enkephalins are present in the adrenal medulla.[14,21-28] Quirion et al[24] demonstrated ethyl ketocyclazocine binding sites in the adrenal gland. These sites were concentrated in the adrenal cortex with lower densities found in the medulla. Bindings sites for mu and delta ligands were not demonstrable. Human pheochromocytomas contain both kappa and benzomorphan opiate binding sites[23,29], but intra-tumor variation is large.[23] Yoshimasa et al[29] found enkephalin-like immunoreactivities in sixteen human pheochromocytomas. Epinephrine-producing pheochromocytomas contained high levels of Methionine enkephalin, Leucine enkephalin, and Methionine enkephalin - Arg^6 - Gly^7 - Leu^8 determined by ligand specific radioimmunoassays.

Kumakura et al[30] have provided _in vitro_ evidence for an interaction between adrenal medulla opiates and the release of catecholamines. They observed that nicotine-stimulated catecholamine release was reduced 50% by morphine ($10^{-5}M$) or Beta-endorphin ($10^{-6}M$) and this inhibition was blocked by $10^{-5}M$ naltrexone.

The presence of endogenous opiates in the adrenal gland suggests a possible role in adrenal function. Recently we reported[31] that naltrexone blockade of opiate receptors exaggerated the plasma epinephrine response to isotonic exercise at 70% of each subject's maximal oxygen consumption. Grossman et al[32] demonstrated that naloxone-sensitive endogenous opiates modulate the release of epinephrine during bicycle exercise at 40 and 80% VO_2 max. Plasma epinephrine and norepinephrine were significantly higher with naloxone compared to saline infusion. In like manner, exercise-induced elevations of plasma cortisol, renin activity, aldosterone, luteinizing hormone and prolactin were enhanced by naloxone (12.2 mg total dose). These data along with our study[31] indicate that the endogenous opiate system modulates the hormonal response to exercise. Interestingly, and in agreement with our results, naloxone had no significant effect on exercise heart rate, blood pressure, oxygen consumption or carbon dioxide production. Grossman et al[32] did find a significantly higher exercise ventilation with naloxone. While ventilation was increased in our study[31] by naltrexone (50 mg), the increase was not significant. These investigations reveal a probable relationship between adrenomedullary function and endogenous opiates.

HUMAN STUDIES

The release of hormones into the circulation is directly related to the intensity of aerobic exercise[33]. An important exception is plasma insulin which decreases during exercise. This exercise enhancement of hormone levels is intimately related to metabolic adaptations such as the availability of fuel substrates. The relationship of these metabolic adaptations to the exercise-induced alterations in blood or tissue levels of endorphins/enkephalins awaits elucidation.

Pre and post run plasma levels of Beta-endorphin/Beta-lipotropin-like activity have been reported by many groups and are shown in Table 1. These studies are similar in the following respects: 1) male subjects are in the majority, 2) RIA with antisera crossreacting with Beta-lipotropin from 10 to 50% on a weight basis were utilized, 3) plasma was extracted prior to RIA with the exception of Kelso et al[34], and 4) running protocols were used. However, intensity and duration of the running varied enormously. To provide a further frame of reference for the baseline values in Table 1, resting levels of Beta-endorphin are included which were determined using sequential immune affinity column chromatography prior to RIA which provides for the separation and quantification of Beta-endorphin distinct from Gamma-lipotropin and Beta-lipotropin[42]. Conclusions can be derived from the data in Table 1. All studies reported increases in plasma Beta-endorphin-like material after running. These increases do not appear to be related to intensity of exercise. Lastly, the elevations range from slight to about five-fold.

Immunoreactivity and biological activity are not synonymous for the RIA's employed.[43] Accordingly, we used a radioreceptor assay[44] to examine the effects of exercise on plasma ligands with opiate receptor activity.[45] Venous blood was obtained from 14 volunteers before and after a 10 mile road race. Conditions before and after the run were controlled in terms of diet, warm-up and time elapsed between the end of the race and the post race blood draw. Leucine Enkephalin-like radioreceptor activity (Leu-ERA) was 22.2 $\pm$13.7 pmol/ml (Mean $\pm$ SD) prior to the race and increased non-significantly to 26.1 $\pm$21.5 pmol/ml after the race, $p > 0.05$. However, post run Leu-ERA levels significantly correlated with race pace ($r = +0.52$, $p < 0.05$). No significant relationship was found between changes in mood state assessed by the Profile of Mood State (POMS) and Leu-ERA. These data suggest that no uniform change in Leu-ERA occurs after competitive running. Support for this finding has recently been provided by Grossman et al[32] who found no change in radioimmunoassayable Met-enkephalin after bicycle exercise at 40 and 80% VO_2 max.

Gender may influence the circulating endorphin response to aerobic exercise. In our studies[37,45] no sex difference was observed. However, Gambert et al[41] found a greater plasma Beta-Endorphin response in five men (51.7 $\pm$ 13 pg/ml) compared to four women (9.0 $\pm$ 4.6 pg/ml, $p < 0.05$) after a 20 minute treadmill run. In any event, interesting observations have been reported in studies solely using women.

Carr et al[40] studied seven women before, at mid point, and after an 8 week training program. Plasma Beta-endorphin increased at the end of 60 minutes of exercise at 85 percent of each woman's maximal heart rate. As training progressed, a larger increase in Beta-Endorphin was noted with a 38% increase at 8 weeks versus a 16% increase prior to training. It appears that the peripheral endorphin system may adapt to training in a manner opposite to the stress hormones[38]. Namely circulating opioids increase with training adaptations while the stress hormones diminish in plasma after training at the same absolute or relative workload.[33,46]

If these initial studies are corroborated by future longitudinal training studies, it would provide a strong impetus to training adaptation studies which could benefit from what is known concerning the development of tolerance and dependence on morphine.[48,49] It should be noted, however, that Carr et al[40] do not provide data which demonstrate that a cardiovascular training effect occurred during the training program.

Another investigation involving only female subjects suggests an interesting possibility that endogenous opiates are also involved in the cardiovascular and pulmonary responses to maximal exercise. McMurray et al[50] found no effect from an IV bolus of naloxone (0.4 mg) on submaximal cardiovascular and pulmonary variables. However, maximal ventilation (lower with naloxone), respiratory frequency (lower), end

Table 1

Summary of Human Studies Which Measured Beta-Endorphin/Beta-Lipotropin
During Isotonic Exercise. Values Are Means ± SEM.

Reference	Exercise Duration	Exercise Intensity	Exercise Mode	Cross-reactivity of anti-sera with B-LPH (%)	Beta-Endorphin/Beta-Lipotropin (pg/ml) Pre-exercise	Post-exercise	N
Fraioli (38)	8-15 min	exhaustive	run	Sephadex G-75 chomatography prior to RIA ≈ 0%	320±70	1620± 88	8
Colt (39)	6.4-12.8Km	"Comfortable"	run	10.8	11.8±1.8	17.6±3.1	20
Colt (39)	No data	"near maximal"	run	10.8	8.2±1.0	28.0±6.3	15
Gambert (41)	20 min	80% HR max (predicted)	run	20	increased by 51.7±13.0	increased by 9.0±0.4	5M 4F
Farrell (37)	30 min	60% VO_2 max / 80% VO_2 max / self-selected (X=75%)	run run	15	11.2±3.0 / 15.4±5.0 / 13.8±4.4	58.3±18.0 / 37.2±12.3 / 39.2±16.6	6 6 6
Elliot (36)	no data	exhaustive	run	1:1 molar crossreactivity	24.4±8.1	47.8±10.3	5
Elliot (36)	(45 min intermittent weight training)				20.8±10.3	52.0±27.2	5
Kelso (34) conditions	120	50% VO_2 max	bicycle	50			
Neutral environment euhydrated					25.1±4.1	32.8±4.8	6
Hot environment euhydrated					27.8±6.8	32.5±2.7	6
Hot environment dehydrated					21.7±3.1	40.3±2.8	6
Janal (35)	6.3 miles (43.9 min)	85.3% VO_2 max (estimated)	run	no data	63.±3 (estimated by author from graph in original article)	97.±5	12
Yamaguchi (42)	Resting Reference			0		7.6+0.38	19

52

tidal PCO_2 (higher), and heart rate (lower) were influenced by naloxone compared to placebo exercise or a control graded stress test. Endogenous opiates may become active regulators of vital physiologic functions with extreme stress levels.

The above _in vivo_ data conflict with a previous _in vitro_ report by Eiden and Ruth.[51] This investigation demonstrated that, using isolated spontaneously-beating rat atria, the maximal chronotropic effect of norepinephrine is greatly reduced by methionine or leucine enkephalin and several enkephalin analogues. This inhibition was abolished by naloxone. Interestingly, submaximal stimulation by norepinephrine was unaffected by either enkephalins or naloxone. These data show that _in vitro_ enkephalins reduce maximal heart rate which is opposite to the effect demonstrated _in vivo_ by McMurray et al.[50] Species differences and the pharmacological nature of the _in vitro_ study may explain these conflicting data.

Most of the investigations examined in Table 2 utilized a thermoneutral environment. Janal et al[35] and Colt et al[39] had their subjects run outdoors; however, neither excessively hot nor cool temperatures were noted. Kelso et al[34] tested their subjects under three different environmental conditions: 1) neutral temperature and humidity, euhydrated (24°C, 50% relative humidity), 2) hot temperature, euhydrated (35°C, 50% relative humidity), and 3) hot temperature, dehydrated (35°C, 50% relative humidity, no fluids, -2.6% body weight) Plasma Beta-endorphin/Beta-lipotropin increased to its highest level during the most environmentally stressful milieu, the hot temperature, dehydrated condition. Again, it would appear that the more stressful the situation, the greater the rise in plasma Beta-endorphin/Beta-lipotropin with exercise.

Haier et at[52] used naloxone infusion and running to determine if exercise-induced analgesia has an opiate basis. They demonstrated that exercise (one mile at a self-selected pace) significantly lengthens the time to the first report of pain due to a three pound weight on a fingertip. Ten mg naloxone completely blocked this exercise-induced analgesia while a 2 mg dose resulted in a significant hyperanalgesia, i.e., it took even longer for the subjects to notice pain after running one mile compared to placebo injection. Elucidation of the relationship between aerobic exercise and the endogenous opiate system will increase rapidly with the further use of opiate receptor blockade.

CONCLUSION

Pharmacological doses of exogenous and endogenous opiates affect locomotor activity in several species of mammals. Exercise stimulates the release of endorphin-like material into the human circulation, but physiological roles of these immunoreactive ligands are unknown. Brain levels of enkephalin-like material are increased after forced exercise in mice and rats, and opiate receptor blockade with naloxone alters post exercise-induced analgesia in both rats and man.

The importance of peripherally-released opiates during exercise may relate to their potential influence on hormonal and metabolic adaptations. Recent evidence suggests a modulating role for endogenous opiates in the adrenal medulla of man. While the metabolic and cardiovascular implications of this observation are unclear at present, elucidation of the physiological actions of the endogenous opioids during exercise should prove to be a fruitful and important area for future investigations.

Acknowledgement   This work was supported by NIH grants R03 MH/OA 36880-01 to PAF and General Clinical Research Center RR-00058; and TOPS Club, Inc., Obesity and Metabolic Research Program, Milwaukee, Wisconsin. Special thanks is extended to Catherine Ladd for her expert assistance in typing this review and to Lynn Cordell Breitlow for her valued assistance in our laboratory.

References

1. Hughes, J., T.W. Smith, H. Kosterlitz, L.A. Forthergill, B.A. Morgan and H.R. Harris. Identification of two related pentapeptides from the brain with potent opiate agonist activity. Nature 258:577-579, 1975.
2. Goldstein, A. and P. Sheenan. Tolerance to opioid narcotics. I. Tolerance to the "Running Fit" caused by levorphanol in the mouse. J. Pharmacol. and Exp. Therapeutics. 169:2, 175-184, 1969.
3. Babbini, M. and W.M. Davis. Time-dose relationships for locomotor activity effects of morphine after acute or repeated treatment. Br. J. Pharmac. 46:213-214, 1972.
4. Browne, R.G. and D.S. Segal. Behavioral activating effects of opiates and opioid peptides. Biol. Psychiat. 15:77-86, 1980.
5. Drust, E.G. and I.L. Crawford. Comparison of the Effects of TRH and Dl-Ala^2-Metenkephalinamide on hippocampal electrical activity and behavior in the unanesthetized rat. Peptides. 4:239-243, 1983.
6. Oka, T. and E. Hosoya. Effects of humoral modulators and naloxone on morphine-induced changes in spontaneous locomotor activity of the rat. Psychoparmacol. 47, 243-248, 1976.
7. Katz, R.J., B.J. Carroll and G. Baldrighi. Behavioral activation by enkephalins in mice. Pharmacol. Biochem. Behavior. 8, 493-496, 1978.
8. Amir, S., Z.H. Galina, R. Blair, Z.W. Brown and Z. Amit. Opiate receptors may mediate the suppressive but not the excitatory action of ACTH on motor activity in rats. Eur. J. Pharmacol. 66:307-313, 1980.
9. Castellano, C. Strain dependent effects of the enkephalin analogue FK 33-824 on locomotor activity in mice. Pharmacol. Biochem. Behav. 15:729-734, 1981.
10. Castellano, C. and S. Puglisi-Allegra. Effects of naloxone and naltrexone on locomotor activity in C57B1/6 and DBA/2 mice. Pharmacol. Biochem. Behav. 16:561-563, 1982.
11. Walker, J.M., G.G. Berntson, T.S. Paulucci and T.C. Champney. Blockade of endogenous opiates reduces activity in the rat. Pharmacol. Biochem. Behav. 14:113-116, 1981.
12. Castellano, C. and A. Oliverio. A genetic analysis of morphine-induced running and analgesia in the mouse. Psychopharmacologica. 41:197-200, 1975.
13. Oliverio, A. and C. Castellano. Genotype-dependent sensitivity and tolerance to morphine and herion dissociation between opiate-induced running and analgesia in the mouse. Psychopharmacologica 39:13-22, 1974.
14. Castanas, E., P. Giraud, Y. Audigier, R. Drissi, F. Boudouresque, B. Conte-Devolx and C. Oliver. Opiate binding sites spectrum on bovine adrenal medullas and six human pheochromocytomas. Life Sciences 33: Supp. 1, 295-298, 1983.
15. Christie, M.J. and G. Chesher. Physical dependence on physiologically released endogenous opiates. Life Sciences, 30:1173-1177, 1982.

16. Christie, J.J., G.B. Chesher and K.D. Bird. The correlation between swim-stress induced antinociception and [³H] Leu-enkephalin binding to brain homogenates in mice. Pharmac. Biochem. Behav. 15:853-857, 1981.

17. Christie, M.J., P. Trisdikoon and G.B. Chesher. Tolerance and cross-tolerance with morphine resulting from physiological release of endogenous opiates. Life Sciences. 31:839-845, 1982.

18. Shyu, B.C., S.A. Anderson and P.Toren. Endorphin-mediated increase in pain threshold induced by long-lasting exercise in rats. Life Sciences 30:833-840, 1982.

19. Pert, C.B. and D.L. Bowie. Behavioral manipulation of rats causes alterations in opiate receptor occupancy. In: E. Usdin, W.E. Bunney and N.S. Kline (Eds.) Endorphins in mental health research, 1979, New York: Oxford University Press, 93-104.

20. Metzer, J.M. and E.A. Stein. ß-endorphin and sprint training. Life Sciences 34:1541-1547, 1984.

21. Evans, C.J., E. Erdelyi, E. Weber, J.D. Barchas. Identification of pro-opiomelanocortin-derived peptides in the human adrenal medulla. Science 221:957-960, 1983.

22. Linnoila, R.I., R.P. Diaugustine, A. Hervonen and R.J. Miller. Distribution of [Met⁵]- and [Leu⁵]-enkephalin-, vasoactive intestinal polypeptide- and substance P-like immunoreactivities in human adrenal glands. Neuroscience 5:2247-2259, 1980.

23. Lundberg, J.M., B. Hamberger, M. Schultzberg, T. Höfelt, P.O. Grandbert, S. Efendic, L. Terenius, M. Goldstein and R. Luft. Enkephalin- and somatostatin-like immunoreactivities in human drenal medulla and pheochromocytoma. Proc. Natl. Acad. Sci. 76:4079-4083, 1979.

24. Quirion, R., M.S. Finkel, F.A.O. Mendelson and N. Zamir. Localization of opiate binding sites in kidney and adrenal gland of the rat. Life Sciences. 33: Supp. 1, 299-302, 1983.

25. Schultzberg, M., T. Höfelt, J.M. Lundberg, L. Terenius, L.G. Elfvin and R. Elde. Enkephalin-like immunoreactivity in nerve terminals in sympathetic ganglia and adrenal medulla and in adrenal medullary gland cells. Acta. Physiol. Scand. 103:475-477, 1978.

26. Viveros, O.H., E.J. Diliberto, E. Hazum and K.J. Chang. Enkephalins as possible adrenomedullary hormones: storage, secretion, and regulation of synthesis. In: Neural peptides and neuronal communication, ed. by E. Costa and M. Trabucchi. Raven Press, N.Y., vol. 22, 191-204, 1980.

27. Viveros, O.H., E.J. Diliberto, E. Hazum and K.J. Chang. Opiate-like materials in the adrenal medulla: evidence for storage and secretion with catecholamines. Mol. Pharmacol. 16:1101-1108, 1979.

28. Viveros, O.H., S.P. Wilson, E.J. Diliberto, E. Hazum. K.J. Chang. Enkephalins in adrenomedullary chromaffin cells and sympathetic nerves. Adv. Physiol. Sci. Vol. 14. Endocrinology, neuroendocrinology, neuropeptides-11, ed. by E. Stark, G.B. Markara, B. Halasz, G. Rappoy, 349-353.

29. Yoshimasa, T., K. Nakao, Y. Ikeda, M. Sakamoto, M. Suda and H. Imura. Methionine-enkephalin, Leucine-enkephalin, methionine-enkephalin-Arg⁶-Phe⁷ and methionine-enkephalin-Arg⁶-Gly⁷-Leu⁸ in human pheochromocytoma. Life Sciences. 33:85-88, 1983.

30. Kumakura, K., A. Guidotti, H.Y.T. Yang, L. Saiani and E. Costa. A role for the opiate peptides that presumably coexist with acetylcholine in splanchnic nerves. in: Neuronal Peptides and Neuronal Communication, ed. W. Costa and M. Trabucchi, Raven Press, New York, 1980, P. 571-580.

31. Gustafson, A.B., P.A. Farrell, T. Garthwaite and R. Kalkhoff. Endogenous opiates modulate the plasma epinephrine response to submaximal exercise in man. _Exerpta Medica_, International Congress Series 652:682, abstract 843, 1984.

32. Grossman, A., P. Bouloux, P. Price, P.L. Drury, K.S.L. Lam, T. Turner, J. Thomas, G.M. Besser and J.R. Sutton. Role of opioid peptides in the hormonal responses to acute exercise in man. _Clinical Science_ 67:483-491, 1984.

33. Galbo, H. Hormonal and metabolic adaptation to exercise. Georg. Thieme Verlag, Stuttgart, 1983.

34. Kelso, T.B., W.G. Herbert, F.C. Gwazdauskas, F.L. Goss and J.L. Hess. Exercise-thermoregulatory stress and increased plasma ß-endorphin/ß-lipotropin in humans. _J. Appl. Physiol.: Respirat. Environ. Exercise Physiol._ 57:444-449, 1984.

35. Janal, M.N., E.W.D. Colt, W.C. Clark and M.Glusman. Pain sensitivity, mood and plasma endocrine levels in man following long-distance running: Effects of naloxone, _Pain_ 19:13-25, 1984.

36. Elliot, D.L., L. Goldberg, W.J. Watts and E. Orwoll. Resistance exercise and plasma beta-endorphin/beta lipotropin immunoreactivity. _Life Sciences_ 34:515-518, 1984.

37. Farrell, P.A., W.K. Gates, W.P. Morgan, and M.G. Maksud. Increases in plasma ß-endorphin/ß-lipotropin immunoreactivity after treadmill running in humans. _J. Appl. Physiol.: Respirat. Environ. Exercise Physiol._ 52(5): 1245-1249, 1982.

38. Fraioli, F., C. Moretti, D. Paolucci, E. Alicicco, F. Crescenzi, and G. Fortunio. Physical exercise stimulates marked concomitant release of ß-endorphin and adrenocortiocotropic hormone (ACTH) in peripheral blood in man. _Experientia_ 36:987-989, 1980.

39. Colt, W.D., S.L. Wardlow, and A.G. Frantz. The effect of running on plasma ß-endorphin. _Life Science_ 28:1637-1640, 1981.

40. Carr, D.B., B.A. Bullen, G.S. Skrinor, M.A. Arnold, M. Rodenblatt, I.Z. Beitins, J.B. Martin and J.W. McArthur. Physical conditioning facilitates the exercise-induced secretion of Beta-endorphin and Beta-lipotropin in women. _N. Eng. J. Med._ 305:560-562, 1981.

41. Gambert, S.R., T.L. Garthwaite, C.H. Pontzer, E.E. Cook, F. Tristani, E.H. Duthie, D.R. Martinson, T.C. Hagen and D.J. McCarty. Running elevates plasma ß-endorphin immunoreactivity and ACTH in untrained human subjects. _Proc. Soc. Exp. Biol. Med._ 168:1-4, 1981.

42. Yamaguchi, H., A.S. Liotla and D.T. Krieger. Simultaneous determination of human plasma immunoreactive ß-Lipotropin, γ-Lipotropin, and ß-Endorphin using immune-affinity chromatography. _J. Clin. Endocrinol. Metab._ 51:1002-1008, 1980.

43. Li, C.H., A.J. Rao, B.A. Doneen and D. Yamashiro. ß-Endorphin: Lack of correlation between opiate activity and immunoreactivity in radioimmnoassay. _Biochem. Biophys. Res. Commun._ 75:576-590, 1977.

44. Naber, D., D.P. Pickar, R.A. Dionne, D.L. Bowie, B.A. Ewols, T.W. Moody, M.G. Sable and C.B. Pert. Assay of endogenous opiate receptor ligands in human CSF and plasma. _Sub. Alcohol Act./Misuse_. 1:113-118, 1980.

45. Farrell, P.A., W.G. Gates, W.P. Morgan and C.B. Pert. Leucine Enkephalin-like radioreceptor activity and tension – anxiety before and after competitive running. In: _Biochemistry of Exercise_, ed. H.G. Knuttgen, J.A. Vogel and J. Poortmans. Human Kinetics Publishers, Champaign, Illinois, 637-644, 1983.

46. Winder W.W., R.C. Hickson, J.M. Hagberg, A.A. Ehsoni and J.A. McLane. Training-induced changes in hormonal and metabolic responses to submaximal exercise. J. Appl. Physiol. Respirat. Environ. Exercise Physiol. 46:766-771, 1979.
47. Bullen, B.A., G.S. Skrinor, I.Z. Beitins, D.B. Carr, S.M. Reppert, C.O. Dodson, M. deM. Fencl, E.V. Gervino and J.W. McArthur. Endurance training effects on plasma hormonal responsiveness and sex hormone excretion. J. Appl. Physiol.: Respirat. Environ. Exercise Physiol. 56:1453-1463, 1984.
48. Kaymakcalan, S. and L.A. Woods. nalorphine-induced abstinence syndrome in morphine tolerant rats. J. Pharmac. Exp. Ther. 117:112-116, 1956.
49. Martin, W.R., A. Wikler, C.G. Eades and F.T. Pescor. Tolerance to and physical dependence on morphine in rats. Psychoparmacologia 4:247-260, 1963.
50. McMurray, R.G., D.S. Sheps and D.M. Guinan. Effects of naloxone on maximal stress testing in females. J. Appl. Physiol. Respirat. Envion. Exercise Physiol. 56:436-440, 1984.
51. Eiden, L.E. and J.A. Ruth. Enkephalins modulate the responsiveness of rat atria in vitro to norepinephrine. Peptides. 3:475-478, 1982.
52. Haier, R.J., K. Quaid, and J.C. Mills. Naloxone alters pain perception after jogging. Psychiatry Research 5:231-232, 1981.

EFFECTS OF COPING AND NONCOPING WITH

STRESSFUL EVENTS ON THE IMMUNE SYSTEM

Wolfgang H. Vogel

Departments of Pharmacology and
Psychiatry and Human Behavior
Jefferson Medical College
Thomas Jefferson University
Philadelphia, PA 19107

INTRODUCTION

All men and animals are continuously exposed to stressful events (stressors) which can affect and change the homeostasis of an organism. A change in homeostasis is usually called stress. Although man must have encountered stressful events and experienced stress from prehistoric times, a scientific concept of stress did not emerge until relatively late in history. Milestones in early stress research include the recognition of the "milieu interior" by C. Bernard as well as the response of the sympathetic-adrenal medullary system (epinephrine) by W.B. Cannon (1) and that of the pituitary-adrenal cortical system (steroids) by H. Selye (2) to stressful events.

Since this time, a large number of investigations have tried to investigate the chemical basis of stress in animals and to a more limited extent in man. In addition to the catecholamines and steroids, a wide variety of other chemicals has been investigated and significant changes have been observed with a number of enzymes, biochemicals and/or electrolytes during and after stress in plasma, brain and other organs of the body.

Stress is usually experienced in response to certain events in our daily environment which are perceived as unpleasant or threatening and which create feelings of tension, anxiety or fear. Experimentally, stress is produced by exposing the organism to a demanding or unpleasant situation. Animals are restrained, exposed to cold temperature, or subjected to an unpleasant footshock. The animal has no control over this situation. In humans, difficult, mental arithmetic is performed, the hand is submerged in ice-cold water or an unpleasant social situation is created. Again, the individual has no control over the experiment but is obliged to follow the instructions of the experimentors. In all these cases, the individual cannot control or cope with the particular situation. However, recent research has shown that not the stressful event per se but the ability or inability to cope with a stressor seems to be the most important determinant in the stress response of an organism. While coping with a stressful event produces few stress-induced changes, the inability to cope with the same event produces marked biochemical and physiological changes, including significant effects on the immune system and the immune response.

DEFINITION AND MEASUREMENT OF COPING

Coping can be defined as gaining and maintaining control over a situation which could otherwise be potentially dangerous, unpleasant or fearful. The ability to control a situation means in many, although not all, circumstances that the typical stress response of uncertainty, apprehension, anxiety or fear and its peripheral consequences such as sweating, tachycardia, rise in blood pressure might be attenuated or might not emerge at all.

The effects of coping and noncoping with a stressful situation can be measured in animals by using a pair of "yoked" animals exposed to a stressful situation. The "yoked" pair to be stressed is placed in a situation in which the pair receives foot or tail shock. However, one animal can press a lever and terminate the shock for both. The other animal has no way to terminate the shock. After onset of a sequence of shocks and rest periods, the first animal learns quickly to use the lever, respond and terminate the shock for both animals. This animal gains control over the unpleasant situation or can cope with it. The other animal can not terminate the shock, has no control and is unable to cope with the situation. Under these conditions, both animals receive the identical number of shocks with identical intensities and durations. Thus, the aversive situation (unpleasantness of footshock) is the same for both animals but the difference rests in the ability or inability to cope with the footshock. These measurements can also be compared with those obtained on a control animal which rests in its home cage. In humans, it is somewhat more difficult to measure coping. In a real life situation, individuals can be asked about their coping strategies and can be judged how successful they are in mastering environmental stressors. Experimentally, two individuals can be given a puzzle and be asked to assemble this "simple" puzzle as many times as they can in a given period of time. However, one individual receives a puzzle which indeed can be assembled easily and repeatedly whereas the other receives a puzzle which is an "unsolvable" puzzle and cannot be assembled. In both cases, a stressful situation exists except that the first individual can cope with this situation whereas the second individual cannot cope.

In experiments like this, a number of biochemical and physiological changes have been observed and a variety of specific pathological consequences have been found which were mostly related to the ability or inability of the individual to control the stressful event and not to the noxious or aversive nature of the stressor per se.

BIOCHEMISTRY OF COPING

Although stress-related chemical changes in noncoping animals have been extensively studied, very few biochemical studies have been performed on animals coping with a stressful event or a stressor. A few crucial studies will be cited because some of the chemicals which were studied may also be directly or indirectly involved in the immune response.

Rats were exposed to a footshock which could be terminated or controlled by one but not the other animal. Again, both animals received the same number of shocks with identical intensities and durations with the only exception that one animal could cope (terminate) whereas the other had no control (noncoping) over the shock. A third animal remained undisturbed in the home cage. Plasma norepinephrine, epinephrine and corticosterone levels rose in both animals as compared to the home cage animal. However, they rose significantly higher in noncoping rats during footshock and remained elevated longer after cessation of the footshock (3). Nor-epinephrine levels fell significantly in the hypothalamus of noncoping animals, while small or no changes were seen in this area in the coping rat during shock (3,4,5,6). In contrast, norepinephrine levels fell in the hippocampus of coping animals while no changes in this catecholamine were seen in noncoping animals (3). Dopamine levels were markedly affected in noncoping rats in the mesocortical and mesolimbic, but not the nigrostriatal, areas whereas no such changes were observed in animals capable of coping with the stressful event; dopamine levels of coping animals were the same as those in resting rats (7,8,9). Serotonin levels in the septum fell below normal levels in noncoping rats but increased above normal levels in coping rats (10). From experiments measuring pain threshold after exposure to controllable and uncontrollable shock, it was found that coping or noncoping can affect the opiate endorphin system differently. Uncontrollable electric shock exposure activates the opiate/endorphin system in the brain markedly and causes significant analgesia whereas controllable shock has only a slight effect on this system and causes only mild analgesia (11,12).

Coping must not necessarily imply gaining or controlling a stressful event directly or successfully. Directing one's attention away from the stressful situation can apparently serve as an alternate coping mechanism. Rats exposed to an uncontrollable footshock show the typical stress induced norepinephrine depletion in the hypothalamus. However, if 2 animals were exposed together to the same footshock and allowed to fight with each other what 2 rats will typically do under these circumstances than no norepinephrine depletion was observed (13) Similarly, wrong coping strategies can be adapted to prevent stress induced changes. Uncontrollable stress causes anxiety and hypothalamic NE depletion in rats. Alcohol can partially prevent this fall and, presumably, reduce stress-induced anxiety (14). Alcohol could now be used as a "wrong" coping strategy to correct temporarily a biochemical imbalance which, however, eventually might lead to alcoholism and related pathologies.

Thus, chemical changes produced in the brain and periphery do not seem to be the primary results of the aversive nature of the environmental event or situation but seem to depend to a much greater extent on the ability (coping) or inability (noncoping) of the organism to control the aversive nature of the potential stressor. Biochemical changes seem to be most marked in the uncontrollable situation whereas proper, or sometimes improper, coping seems to prevent such changes or, if they occur, seem to be of a different nature. Since evidence is available that some of the above mentioned chemicals are also involved in the regulation of the immune system, the occurrance or absence of such changes as determined by coping must then also exert a crucial role on the immune system.

Stressful events and the resulting stress have been implicated
in the pathogenesis of many diseases such as ulcers, hypertension,
myocardial infarctions, depression and, more recently, cancer.
Stressful events in man can include separation of spouses or
separation of children from parents, death of a beloved person as
well as loss of a job or unsurmountable work pressure. However, it
is well known that not all individuals who experience such stressful
events will become sick. Again, this suggests strongly that not
only the stressful event per se but other factors as well must play
a role in causing diseases. One factor which becomes more and more
important in the etiology of stress and stress-induced illnesses is
the particular coping behavior of the individual. And it might just
be this mechanism which will turn out to be rather crucial in the
response of the body and the potential health consequences to environmental insults. Rats which can escape or control electric shock
develop less ulceration than do "yoked" animals which can not
escape the identical shock situation (15). As mentioned later on,
tumor development is enhanced and tumor rejection is decreased in
rats receiving inescapable shock; coping animals show less tumor
development and better rejection similar to those found with
control animals (16,17). Again, coping must not necessarily mean
gaining direct control of the situation. Rats which could not
terminate or cope directly with a shock but could fight or chew
during a stressful experience developed less ulcers than rats which
can not use such alternative coping mechanisms (15). Thus, direct
or indirect coping can reduce or abolish the adverse health
consequences of a noxious environmental stimulus.

However, the ability to cope reduces detrimental health
consequences but must not necessarily mean the absence of pathology;
it can mean the occurrence of a different pathology. In "yoked"
squirrel monkeys, coping animals show a higher incidence of myo-
fibrillary changes and myocardial lesions whereas noncoping monkeys
show more general physical degeneration, bradycardia and ventricular
arrest (18). Monkeys which can avoid an electric shock ("executive
monkey") for themselves and "yoked" animals develope considerably
more gastric pathology than the animals which have no control (19);
in the latter case the shock was not terminated but could be
avoided which placed the additional stress of attention and pre-
paredness on the coping animal. Lowered cardiovascular activity
can be observed in individuals who can easily control an aversive
situation with a favorable outcome as compared with individuals who
can not (21). However, this beneficial effect seems to depend upon
the effort necessary to cope. Increased efforts to cope may
enhance and not reduce stress. Individuals who can not easily
control an aversive situation and need considerable effort for its
control show increased plasma epinephrine in comparison with their
noncoping counterparts (21).

Thus, the effects of coping on maintaining health or causing
diseases are quite complex. In general, they are beneficial but
depend on the particular physiological system studied as well as the
intensity of the coping effort.

COPING AND THE IMMUNE SYSTEM

The effects of stress, meaning inescapable or uncontrollable
stress, on the immune system have only received a limited amount of
attention in spite of the fact that all humans experience more or
less stress during their lifes. This might stem partly from the

opinion that stress and the brain do not affect the immune system.
However, more recent studies have clearly supported anecdotal
observations throughout history that stress can influence the body's
defense mechanisms and markedly affect the resistance to infections
and cancer. In this aspect, stress can increase, decrease or not
affect the immune response depending on a number of variables which
include the nature of the stressor used and the immunological
response studied (22,23,24,25). Unfortunately, only few studies in
animals and men have been performed on the effects of coping on the
immune system.

Tumor rejection was measured in rats which received 0.2 cm^2 of
a tumor (Walker 256 sarcoma) into the left flank (16). This tumor
piece induced tumors in 50% of unstressed control rats whereas the
other 50% of the animals rejected the implant. Sixty-three percent
of the rats which received escapable shock or could cope with the
stressor rejected the tumor and did not differ significantly from
the unstressed control animals (53%). However, only 27% of the
animals which received inescapable shock or could not cope rejected
the tumor implants. Thus, only inescapable, but not escapable,
shock decreased significantly the ability of an animal to reject a
tumor implant.

Mice received by subcutaneous injection 6.25 x 10^4 viable
syngenic P 815 mastocytoma cells which would result in tumor formation in all mice within 7-9 days (17). The animals were then
divided into 3 groups. One group received escapable shock, 1 group
received inescapable shock and 1 group received no shock. The day
of tumor appearance was earliest in the inescapable shock group and
delayed, but similar, in the other two groups. Survival time was
about 27 days in the group which could not escape the shock but was
about 30 days for the control and coping groups. These findings
indicate that the inability to cope was responsible for the detrimental effects seen whereas the ability to cope with the same
stressful event abolished the detrimental consequences of electric
shock.

A direct measure of coping on the immune system was published
recently (26). Rats were given a series of identical escapable and
inescapable shocks. Lymphocyte proliferation in response to the
mitogens phytohemagglutinin and concanavalin A was suppressed only
in the inescapable but not the escapable shock or coping group.
This correlates well with above mentioned studies.

In man, few measurements of coping on the immune system have
been attempted. Using ego strength as a measure of coping ability,
subjects received a high or low dose of a vaccine. Antibody titer
change was directly related to ego strength and coping ability (27).
In another study, undergraduate students were subjected to a
psychological evaluation including their coping behavior as well as
to influenza immunization. The students were then divided into good
and poor coping individuals and natural killer cells and antibody
titers were measured. Poor coping individuals showed fewer natural
Killer cells as compared to their better coping counterparts (28).
These studies were recently summarized as demonstrating that a
stressful event itself is not immunosuppressive but suppression of
the immune system occurs when the individual is unable to cope
effectively (21). In a somewhat reverse study, ego strength or the
coping ability of newly diagnosed cancer patient was investigated
(30). Patients with better coping abilities manifested less mood
disturbances, fewer symptoms, less vulnerability and a better course
of the disease.

It is tempting to speculate on the central mechanisms which become operative during coping and noncoping and how they affect the immune system. Although little evidence is available, it becomes more generally accepted that there is a strong interaction between the brain and the immune system; the brain can influence the immune system and the immune system can influence the brain. For instance, it has been shown that stimulation or depression of brain activity, in particular that of the hypothalamus, can modify humoral as well as cell-mediated immune responses (31). Often, a reduction in hypothalamic NE decreases the immune response. And, interestingly, the effects of coping and noncoping are most marked on norepinephrine levels in the hypothalamus. Only noncoping, but not coping, decreases NE levels in the hypothalamus. The decrease in NE could reduce immune activity and explain why noncoping rats develop more tumors and reject less tumor implants. This finding would also explain why depressed patients who have supposedly less coping strategies and lower norepinephrine levels (32), show a higher incidence of cancer (33). On the other hand, the immune system can also influence the brain. A decreased norepinephrine turn-over in the hypothalamus of rats can be observed during the peak of the immune response and a decrease in NE can also be produced by the injection of soluble mediators released by immunological cells (34).

Similar evidence is available for the enkephalins and endorphins. Endorphins have been shown to inhibit the immune response. For instance, splenic natural killer cells activity is markedly suppressed by endorphins (35). Inescapable shock increases endorphin levels which are probably less elevated in escapable shock. Thus, coping animals should have lower endorphin levels and a better functioning immune system than noncoping animals which should have higher levels. Again, these changes correlate well with the tumor experiments. Coping animals have lower endorphin levels and develop lighter tumors and reject more tumor implants whereas noncoping animals with high endorphin levels do worse in both cases. Enkephalins have been shown to stimulate the immune system (36). They also increase during stress and could mediate some of the beneficial effects.

TOWARDS A NEW DEFINITON OF STRESS INVOLVING COPING

The physical and psychological environment challenges organisms constantly with a series of events. In itself, these events are not stressful and are perceived as events only by the brain via sensory afferent nerves. The brain evaluates these events in "screening centers".

If the event has no specific meaning or requires only a minor biochemical or physiological adjustment, then the information will be sent directly to the appropriate brain centers necessary for this adjustment. As an example, pupils will constrict and blood vessels in the skin will dilate when an individual leaves a dark and cold room and enters a sunny, warm street. Other centers of the brain might not be aware of these processes or pay little attention to them. These changes should not be called stress but "adjustments".

If the event is judged important by the "screening centers" with possible consequences to the individual - either good or bad -, information is now channeled into "evaluation" centers. These centers evaluate the nature and intensity of the event. If the event is judged important, these centers will first evaluate if the organism can cope with this event and, second, how much effort is required for successful coping. For instance, an individual arrives at work in the morning and sees his desk loaded with work. Since he is totally indifferent to his work and since he has total job security, this sight is of no importance and does not provoke any stress response. A second person, arriving at his desk loaded with the hypothetically same amount of work, hates work and has experienced trouble to finish jobs in the past; the same sight will now be evaluated as a threat and a task with which he had trouble to cope with in the past and specific biochemical and physiological stress responses will be elicted. A third person who is a "workaholic" will also see the hypothetically identical load; he knows how quickly the job can be done, how easily he can cope with it and how much pleasure he gets out of this work. The event becomes a pleasurable stimuli and no chemical or physiological changes might occur or, if they do, will be different from the second individual. In each case, the event is the same but the response is different depending on its interpretation by the individual judged by its coping potentials.

Thus, the final response to an event will either be no or certain specific chemical and physiological changes which will depend greatly on the ability of the individual to cope with the outside stimuli. In turn, the ability to cope will depend on the individual's genetic background and environmental experiences. Any biochemical and physiological changes which occur during and after evaluation of the event should be called stress. Only events which cause stress should be called stressful events; the stressor is created in the "brain of the beholder".

The exact role of stress in health consequences is unknown. However, stress must not necessarily mean disease. Consequences can be good or bad. Jogging causes cardiac stress responses which are certainly beneficial to the individual. On the other hand, stress can cause ulcers, hypertension and heart attacks. Thus, the actual health consequences of stress must be determined individually before stress can be labelled as "eustress", that is good, or "distress", that is bad, for the individual.

Thus, stress are chemical and physiological changes created in the brain as a result of an evaluation of an environmental stimulus, the ability or inability to cope with this event and the effort required to cope. It is these considerations which make events stressful for certain individuals and which may cause no, negative, or positive health consequences.

CONCLUSION

Stress is usually defined as the chemical or physiological response of an organism to a stressful event. Stressful events and stress are then commonly implicated in the pathogenesis of a large number of diseases. However, stressful events do not produce stress and pathological consequences in all individuals. This controversy is probably due to the fact that stress and stressful events are too loosely defined.

A stricter definition of stressful events and stress must involve the coping mechanisms of the individual. Coping is defined as gaining control over a potentially threatening or unpleasant environmental event. It is a judgemental decision of an individual which derives from genetic factors as well as personal experiences. It is this decision which renders an environmental event either harmless with no or a minor stress response or threatening, uncontrollable and stressful with a major stress response of the organism. Although not all, but most health consequences and diseases seem to arise in the latter situation where the individual can or does not cope with the event.

Stress also affects the immune system. However, stress can inhibit, stimulate or not affect the immune system and its response. Infections and cancer are often less well controlled during stress. However, exposure to stressful events can also produce no or even beneficial effects on the defense system of the body. Again, the answer will probably not be found in the examination of the stressful event per se but in the ability or inability of the individual to cope with environmental challenges. And data are indeed available which suggest that not the aversive nature of the environmental stimulus, but the ability or inability to control the stressor, exerts the major influence on the immune system. It is the inability to cope with a stressor which seems to cause a major reduction in the immune response while the ability to control the same stressor protects the defense mechanisms from its impact.

REFERENCES

1. W.B. Cannon, The emergency function of the adrenal medulla in pain and major emotion, Am. J. Physiol. 33:356 (1914).
2. H. Selye, General adaptation syndrome and diseases of adaptation, J. Clin. Endocr. Metabl. 6:117 (1946).
3. R.M. Swenson and W.H. Vogel, Plasma catecholamine and corticosterone as well as brain catecholamine changes during coping in rats exposed to stressful footshock, Pharmac. Biochem. Behav. 18:689 (1983).
4. J.M. Weiss, H.J. Glazer and L.A. Pohorecky, Coping behavior and neurochemical changes: an alternate explanation for the original "learned helplessness" experiments, in: "Animal Models in Human Psychobiology," G. Serban and A. Kling, ed., Plenum Press, NY (1976).
5. J.M. Weiss, E.A. Stone and N. Harrel, Coping behavior and brain norepinephrine levels in rats, J. Comp. Physiol. Psychol. 72:153 (1970).
6. H. Anisman, A. Pizzino and L.S. Sklar, Coping with stress, norepinephrine depletion and escape performance, Brain Research 191:583 (1980).
7. A.J. Eichler and S.M. Antelman, Sensitization to amphetamine and stress may involve nucleus accumbens and medical frontal cortex, Brain Research 176:412 (1979).
8. A.M. Thierry, J.P. Tassin, G. Blanc and J. Glowinski, Selective activation of the mesocortical DA system by stress, Nature 263:242 (1976).
9. A.J. Maclennan and S.F. Maier, Coping and the stress-induced potentiation of stimulant stereotypy in the rat, Science 219:1091 (1983).
10. F. Petty and A.D. Sherman, A neurochemical differentiation between exposure to stress and the development of learned helplessness, Drug Development Research 2:43 (1982).
11. R.L. Hyson, L.J. Ashcraft, R.C. Drugan, J.W. Grace and S.F. Maier, Extent and Control of shock affects naltrexone sensitivity of stress-induced analgesia and reactivity to morphins, Pharm. Biochem. Behav. 17:1019 (1982).

12. S.F. Maier, R.C. Drugan and J.W. Grace, Controllability, coping behavior and stress-induced analgesia in the rat, Pain 12:47 (1982).
13. J.M. Stolk, R.L. Conner, S. Levine and J.D. Barchas, Brain norepinephrine metabolism and shock-induced fighting behavior in rats: Differential effects of shock and fighting on the neurochemical response to a common foot-shock stimulus, J. Pharmacol. Expt. Ther. 190:193 (1974).
14. K. DeTurck and W.H. Vogel, Effects of acute ethanol on plasma and brain catecholamine levels in stressed and unstressed rats: evidence for an ethanol-stress interaction, J. Pharm. Expt. Ther. 223:348 (1982).
15. J.M. Weiss, Effects of coping behavior in different warning signal conditions on stress pathology in rats, J. Comp. Physiol. Psychol. 77:1 (1971).
16. M.A. Visintainer, J.R. Volpicelli and M.E.P. Seligman, Tumor rejection in rats after inescapable or escapable shock, Science 216:437 (1982).
17. L.S. Sklar and H. Anisman, Stress and coping factors influence tumor growth, Science 205:513 (1979).
18. K.C. Corley, H.P. Mauck and F.O'M. Shiel, Cardiac responses associated with "yoked-chair" shock avoidance in squirrel monkey, Psychophysiol. 12:439 (1975).
19. J.V. Brady, Ulcers in executive monkeys, Scient. Americ. 199: 95 (1958).
20. D.E. DeGood, Cognitive control factors in vascular stress response, Psychophysiol. 12:399 (1975).
21. R.J. Contrada, D.C. Glass, L.R. Krakoff, D.S. Katz, K. Kehoe, C. Collins and E. Elting, Effects of control over aversive stimulation and type A behavior on cardiovascular and plasma catecholamine responses, Psychophysiol. 19:408 (1982).
22. R.J. Jamasbi and P. Nettesheim, Non-immunological enhancement of tumour transplantability in x-irradiated host animals, British Journal of Cancer 36:723 (1977).
23. R.C. LaBarba, Experiential and environmental factors in cancer, Psychosom. Med. 32:259 (1970).
24. S.N. Pradhan and P. Ray, Effects of stress on growth of transplanted and 7,12-dimethylbenz(a)anthracine-induced tumors and their modification by psychotropic drugs, Journal of the National Cancer Institute 53:1241 (1974).
25. P.R. Goldman and W.H. Vogel, Striatal dopamine-stimulated adenylate cyclase activity reflects susceptibility of rats to DMBA-induced mammary tumors, Carcinogens. (in press).
26. M.L. Laudenslager, S.M. Ryan, R.C. Drugan, R.L. Hyson and S.F. Maier, Coping and immunosuppression: inescapable but not escapable shock suppresses lymphocyte proliferation, Sci. 221:568 (1983).
27. R.J. Roessler, T.R. Cate and J.W. Lester, Ego strength, life change and antibody titers, Presented at the meeting of the American Psychosomatic Society in 1979.
28. S.E. Locke, M.W. Hurst and J.S. Heisel, The influence of stress on the immune response, Paper presented at the meeting of the American Psychosomatic Society in 1978.
29. S.E. Locke, Stress, adaptation and immunity studies in human. Gen. Hosp, Psychiatry 4:49 (1982).
30. J.W. Worden and H.J. Sobel, Ego strength and psychosocial adaptation to cancer, Psychosom. Med. 40:585 (1978).
31. M. Stein, R.C. Schiavi and M. Camerino, Influence of brain and behavior on the immune system, Sci. 191:435 (1970).
32. J. Mendels, S. Stern and A. Frazer, Biochemistry of depression,

Dis. Nerv. Syst. 37:3 (1976).

33. F.G. Surawitz, D.R. Brighwell, W.D. Weitzel and E. Othmer, Cancer, emotions and mental illness, Am. J. Psychiat. 133: 1306 (1976).

34. H. Besedovski, A. DelRey, E. Sorkin, M. DuPrada, R. Burri and C. Honegger, The immune response evokes changes in brain noradrenergic neurons, Sci. 221:564 (1983).

35. Y. Shavit, J.W. Lewis, G.W. Terman, R.P. Gale and J.C. Liebkind, Opioid peptides mediate the suppressive effect of stress on natural Killer cell cytotoxicity, Sci. 223: 188 (1984).

36. N.P. Plotnikoff and G.C. Miller, Enkephalins as immunomodulators, Int. J. Immunopharm. 5:437 (1983).

DEPRESSION, HORMONES AND IMMUNITY

Ziad Kronfol[1] and Janet Schlechte[2]

Departments of Psychiatry[1] and Internal Medicine[2]
University of Iowa College of Medicine
Iowa City, Iowa 52242

Introduction

The last decade or two have witnessed a sharp and steady increase in research and interest in the affective disorders. Clinically,
major depressive illness has been delineated from other psychiatric
disorders with depressed mood and clinical subtypes of depression
have been proposed to reflect the heterogeneity among subgroups of
depression. In addition to descriptive and clinical criteria, subtypes
of depression have also been differentiated by biological markers such
as sleep electroencephalography (EEG) records (1), urinary 3-methoxy-4-
-hydroxy phenylglycol (MHPG) excretion (2), cerebrospinal fluid
5-hydroxyindol acetic acid (HIAA) concentrations (3) and the dexamethasone suppression test (DST) (4). Particularly relevant to the
theme of this book are studies in neuroendocrine and immune regulation in depression. In this chapter we will first summarize major
advances in the study of hypothalamic-pituitary-adrenal (HPA) axis
activity in the depressive disorders, then review some of the preliminary work in the immunology of depression.

DEPRESSION AND THE HYPOTHALAMIC-PITUITARY-ADRENAL AXIS

A variety of hypothalamic and pituitary hormones have been
implicated in the etiology of affective illness but abnormalities of the
HPA axis are the most widely studied. Forty to fifty percent of
patients with depressive illness have abnormal parameters of cortisol
secretion. Failure to suppress serum cortisol after administration of
dexamethasone is the most widely investigated abnormality of HPA
function and has been extensively reviewed elsewhere (4-6). This
review will concentrate on other parameters of cortisol hypersecretion
and discuss studies of ACTH secretion and regulation in depression.
In addition, we will summarize some of the recent work on the relationship of endogenous opiates to depressive illness.

Cortisol

Abnormal cortisol metabolism in depression was first noted more than a quarter of a century ago when Board and colleagues reported elevated glucocorticoid values in depressed patients (7). Studies since then have largely confirmed the elevation in levels of cortisol or its metabolites in plasma (8), urine (9) and CSF (10) of patients with various forms of depression. Gibbons et al (11) used radioisotope dilution techniques to study the dynamics of cortisol secretion. They showed that both the production rate and metabolic clearance rate of cortisol were elevated during the acute phase of depression, and that following recovery the production rate fell while the metabolic clearance rate remained high. Such techniques are usually difficult to assess, but the elevated cortisol secretion rate corresponds with the elevated plasma cortisol level seen in depressed patients.

The nature of the 24 hour secretory pattern of cortisol in depressed patients was first elucidated when Sachar et al. analyzed plasma cortisol every twenty minutes for twenty-four hours in patients with psychotic depression (12). These investigators found that depressed patients secreted twice as much cortisol per day as normal subjects, and that during illness they had eleven to twelve major cortisol secretory episodes compared to seven to nine episodes seen in normal subjects. After treatment, the number of secretory episodes in the depressed patients returned to normal. They also found that the total time spent in active secretion of cortisol during the day was significantly elevated for the depressives to a mean of about 8 hours and 20 minutes compared to a mean of 6 hours and 20 minutes seen in normal subjects. The average biological half-life of cortisol in plasma both before and after treatment was close to the normal figure of 1 hour and 10 minutes.

Because these cortisol determinations all reflect total cortisol (protein-bound and free) and do not reflect the amount of biologically active cortisol present in the circulation, other parameters of cortisol secretion have been developed which offer an indirect estimate of circulatory free cortisol. One such parameter is urinary free cortisol (UFC) excretion. UFC reflects the effective level of circulating plasma cortisol over time and excreted free cortisol increases in direct proportion to plasma free cortisol (13). Despite the close relationship between urinary and plasma free cortisol, there have been remarkably few studies of this parameter of adrenal function in depressive illness. Using a competitive protein binding assay, Carroll measured UFC levels in 60 depressed patient and 35 non-depressed psychiatric controls (9). He found that depressed patients had mean urinary free cortisol excretion of 90 ug/24 hours vs. 47.6 ug/24 hours in the non-depressed group. Forty-three percent of those patients with elevated UFC had values greater than 100 ug/24 hours. Ferguson et al. (14) utilized a chromatographic technique and found high levels of urinary cortisol that returned to normal after electroconvulsive therapy in six patients with depression. Using a radioimmunoassay technique, we recently compared urinary free cortisol levels in depressed patients with those in normal subjects and in patients with Cushing's disease (15). Only individuals classified as nonsuppressors by the dexamethasone suppression test had urinary free cortisol that exceeded 50 ug/gm of creatinine, and in contrast to Carroll's results, less than 5% of the patients with depressive illness had UFC levels that were in the range seen in patients with Cushing's disease.

The best test of tissue exposure to cortisol is the measurement of plasma free cortisol, but this test of adrenal function has not been widely used in patients with depressive illness because assay methods are not applicable for routine clinical use. Using an equilibrium dialysis technique, Carroll (10) measured free cortisol in nine depressed subjects and five non-depressed psychiatric controls. The mean value for the depressed patients was 0.77 ug/dl compared to 0.31 ug/dl in the non-depressed group. In recent work, we measured plasma free cortisol in patients with depression, Cushing's disease and normal controls (15). Depressed patients who were classified as nonsuppressors after the dexamethasone suppression test had only slightly higher plasma free cortisol than the suppressor group. Although the nonsuppressors had significantly higher free cortisol levels than normal subjects, the levels were still 60% lower than those in patients with Cushing's disease. Furthermore, we found no significant difference in the binding capacity of corticosteroid binding globulin (CBG) in normal subjects and the depressed group. The role of the elevated cortisol values in the etiology of depression remains to be determined.

<u>Adrenocorticotrophic hormone (ACTH)</u>

The concept of hypothalamic-pituitary-adrenal regulation suggests that increases in plasma cortisol cause a decrease of the hypothalamic hormone corticotropin releasing factor (CRF) and a subsequent decrease in pituitary adrenocorticotrophic hormone (ACTH) secretion, thereby bringing circulating cortisol levels back to normal.

It has been assumed that the increased cortisol secretion in patients with depression is due to pituitary ACTH hypersecretion, but until recently plasma ACTH levels have not been studied systematically. High values were obtained by Berson and Yalow (16) in patients with "psycho-depressive disorders" but this was not corroborated by other early investigators (17). More recently, several investigators have begun a more detailed examination of plasma ACTH levels in patients with depression. Fang and co-workers (18) found no significant difference in plasma ACTH levels between depressed patients and control subjects at 8 a.m. before dexamethasone nor at 8 a.m. or 4 p.m. after 1 mg of dexamethasone the night before. Yerevanian and Wolff (19) had corresponding results in a different group of depressed patients and normal controls. Despite significant differences in plasma cortisol, depressed patients and normal controls showed no significant differences in plasma ACTH. Reus (20) and Kalin (21) compared ACTH levels in patients who were classified as suppressors and nonsuppressors after the dexamethasone suppression test. These investigators found significantly higher post-dexamethasone plasma ACTH levels in nonsuppressors. In a more detailed study, Pfohl et al. (22) measured ACTH levels every 20 minutes over a 24 hour period in 25 depressed patients and 21 normal controls. They found that the mean pre-dexamethasone plasma ACTH was higher in the depressives than in the normal subjects at each of the 72 sampling times during the 24 hour period. Pfohl's data support the idea that the increase in plasma cortisol in patients with depression is related to an increase in plasma ACTH. Pfohl et al. also showed that patients who are nonsuppressors after dexamethasone averaged greater elevations in plasma ACTH than suppressors and control subjects (23). While suppressors had cortisol values that were virtually identical to normal controls, they had significant elevations of ACTH compared to normal subjects. A time related analysis of the data revealed that the dexamethasone nonsuppressors also exhibited a blunting in the expected circadian rhythm of ACTH (23). The discrepancies among the studies of ACTH secretion in depressive illness have not been totally explained. While the data by Fang, Yerevanian and their colleagues raise the possibility of adrenal supersensitivity to ACTH, the more frequent sampling technique used by Pfohl and co-workers suggest ACTH hypersecretion in depression.

The whole issue of ACTH secretion can now be studied from a different angle, with the recent discovery of the structure and subsequent synthesis of corticotropin releasing factor (CRF), a hypothalamic neuropeptide thought to be the principal stimulus to ACTH secretion (24). Although work with CRF is still in its very preliminary phase, a recent review by Gold and co-workers (25) suggest that compared to normal controls, patients with depressive illness have a significantly lower ACTH response to CRF. The cortisol response to CRF however was similar in both groups. This decrease in the ratio of ACTH to cortisol response during CRF infusion in depressed patients was interpreted by Gold and colleagues as compatible with the hypothesis that the defect in HPA regulation in depression probably occurs at the hypothalamic level and may involve hypersecretion of endogenous CRF (25). More data are obviously needed to further clarify the relationship between CRF, ACTH and cortisol in depression.

Endorphin

If, as recent literature suggests, ACTH and β-endorphin are secreted concommitantly by the pituitary (26), an elevation in ACTH secretion in depressed patients should be accompanied by a similar increase in β-endorphin release. Previous chapters in this volume have concentrated on the localization and physiological significance of the endogenous opiate peptides and this review will be limited to a discussion of measurements of endorphin levels in patients with depressive disorders and the effects of opiate agonists and antagonists in depression.

Several investigators have attempted to measure circulating β-endorphin levels in patients with psychiatric illness and compare them with values in normal controls. Alexopoulos et al. (27) compared plasma β-endorphin levels in 10 patients with unipolar major depressive disorder and 16 psychiatrically normal controls. They found no difference in the basal levels in the two groups. They did however note a transient elevation in both ACTH and β-endorphin following electroconvulsive therapy in the depressed group. Brambilla and colleagues (28) measured plasma levels of β-endorphin, β-lipotropin and ACTH in patients with schizophrenia, primary and secondary depressions and normal controls. They found that both β-endorphin and β-lipotropin were significantly higher in depressed patients compared to normal controls. Risch (29) also reported higher basal levels of plasma β-endorphin in patients with schizoaffective or major depressive disorder compared to other psychiatric patients and normal controls. He also noted that physostigmine-stimulated release of β-endorphin was significantly greater in the depressed groups. Cohen and associates (30) measured basal plasma cortisol and plasma endorphin levels in patients with "major depression", "nonmajor depression" and normal controls. They noted lower plasma endorphin levels in the nonmajor group and found that a low ratio of plasma β-endorphin to cortisol characterized depressed patients in both groups. Pickar and colleagues (31) reported the case of a patient with manic-depressive illness whose switch from the manic phase to depression was accompanied by a significant decrease in plasma opioid activity.

A different approach to investigate the role of opiate peptides in mental illness is through the study of the behavioral effects of opiate agonists and antagonists in normal subjects and psychiatric patients. Pickar and colleagues (32) administered naloxone, an opiate antagonist, to normal volunteers and noted that at high doses, the behavioral effects consisted of irritability, anxiety, sadness and confusion.

Terenius and others (33) have administered naloxone to patients with primary depression. Results have been varied but the general concensus is that opiate antagonists are ineffective in treating depression. On the other hand, early reports have suggested that administration of β-endorphin may cause improvement in depressive symptoms (34). These reports however still await confirmation in larger samples. Thus, evidence for the involvement of endorphins in affective illness remains confusing and further well-controlled studies are needed to clarify many of the still outstanding issues.

In summary, the bulk of the evidence suggests increased cortisol secretion in many patients with depressive illness. Whether this is due to ACTH supersensitivity at the level of the adrenals or to increased production of pituitary ACTH and/or hypothalamic CRF is now the subject of intense investigation and controversy. The role of various neuropeptides is also being widely studied. While most researchers agree that many patients with depressive illness have high levels of biologically active circulating glucocorticoids, the biological significance of this hypercortisolemia is still unclear. Whether the high cortisol levels are etiologically related to depressive symptoms or whether they are just the by-product of central neurotransmitter disturbances remains to be clearly established. More work is also needed on the effects of hypercortisolemia on various physiological functions in depressed patients. The relationship between hypercortisolemia and different immune parameters in depression will now be discussed.

IMMUNE RESPONSE IN DEPRESSIVE ILLNESS

It is now well known, as evidenced by many chapters in this book, that the central nervous system and the immune system are closely associated. Animal studies have revealed intricate and highly complex interactions between stress, neuroendocrine secretion and immune function. The clinical implications of these phenomena have not been widely appreciated. In particular, the applications of immunological principles to the study of psychiatric illness have been very limited. In this section, we will first review the effects of human stress on a variety of immunological parameters, then discuss the immunological studies conducted so far in depressive illness.

Human stress and immunity

The notion that stress can affect the state of health of a person is not new. In 200 A.D., the Greek scientist Galen noted that melancholic women were more likely to develop cancer of the breast than sanguine women. More recently, several epidemiological studies have noted an association between negative life events, depression and cancer (35). Although work on specific pathophysiological pathways has been somewhat limited in the past, intensive research is presently underway to delineate specific biologic mediators between stress and physical illness. New areas of investigation such as psychoendocrinology and psychoimmunology have emerged to address those specific issues.

The effects of stress on the integrity of the human immune response have recently been the subject of excellent review articles (36,37). Palmblad and associates studied the effects of a prolonged experimental stress paradigm on different immune parameters. They found both a reduction in polymorphonuclear leukocyte phagocytic activity and an elevation in interferon production during the 77-hour vigil as compared to baseline values (38). In a different study,

Palmblad and his group also found a reduction in lymphocyte response to mitogen stimulation following 48 hours of sleep deprivation (39). They concluded that both lymphocyte and granulocyte activity can be altered by experimental stress involving sleep deprivation.

A number of investigators have studied the relationship between academic stress and immunological functioning. Dorian et al. (40) measured in-vitro lymphocyte response to mitogen stimulation in psychiatric residents before and after their Oral Fellowship Examination. They noted a reduction in lymphocyte mitogenic activity the morning before the exam, particularly among candidates who were "highly stressed". Jemmott et al. (41) measured the rate of secretion of salivary immunoglobulin A in dental students at different a priori high-stress and low-stress periods of the students' academic calendar. They found diminished secretion rate of Ig A during the high-stress period, suggesting reduced humoral immunity in relation to stress. Kiecolt-Glaser and associates (42) examined the relationship between academic stress and natural killer cell activity (NKCA). They found a significant decline in NKCA the morning of final exam compared to baseline values taken a month earlier. Locke and colleagues (43) also found lower NKCA among undergraduate students who scored high on both life change scales and psychiatric symptoms scales (poor copers), as opposed to students who scored high on the life change scales but not on the psychiatric symptoms scale (good copers). Baker et al. (44) compared the ratio of helper/suppressor T lymphocytes in medical students under varying degrees of academic stress. First year students had higher anxiety scores, higher plasma cortisol values and higher T_4 (helper T lymphocytes) percentages than second year medical students. The authors concluded that an increase in the percentage of T helper cells is part of the physiological reaction to stress.

Bereavement is another form of stress that has been of interest to psychoimmunologists. Two studies have examined the effects of bereavement on parameters of immune function. In 1977, Bartrop and associates (45) compared in-vitro lymphocyte blastogenesis in a group of bereaved subjects and normal controls. They found reduced lymphocyte mitogenic activity in the bereaved group. The number of T and B lymphocytes, serum immunoglobulin levels and the presence of autoantibodies did not differ in the two groups. These findings were later replicated by Schleifer and associates (46) who studied lymphocyte number and function in the spouses of women with advanced breast cancer. Compared to values obtained before the death of their spouses, lymphocyte responses to mitogen stimulation in the bereaved subjects were significantly reduced one or two months following bereavement. The total number of lymphocytes, T cells and B cells remained unchanged.

Depression and immune function

Indirect evidence for disturbed immunity in depressed patients comes from several sources. First, epidemiologic studies, although still inconclusive, suggest an association between depressive illness and a variety of immune related disorders such as infection, asthma, allergy and cancer. This topic has been reviewed in detail by Kronfol (47). If reports of such an association are confirmed, possible pathophysiological mechanisms may include an impairment of immune responses in depressed patients, thus rendering them more vulnerable to infection, autoimmune disease and cancer (47,48).

Another reason for the growing interest in the immunology of the depressive disorders is the documented disturbance in HPA regulation in many patients with acute depression. As discussed earlier (4-6), a

final common pathway of the HPA dysregulation is the excessive secretion of cortisol, an immunosuppressive hormone. The question then is
whether this excess in circulating cortisol would affect the integrity of
the immune response in depressed patients.

Furthermore, clinicians have often noted the similarities between
the reaction to intense stress such as bereavement and clinical depression. Common clinical manifestations include despondency, lack of
energy, lack of appetite, insomnia, crying spells, difficulty concen-
trating, etc. Since acute stress, and particularly bereavement, have
been associated with impairment in immunological functioning (45,46), it
is therefore reasonable to expect similar changes in depressed patients.

There is also growing direct evidence of impaired immunity in
patients with depressive illness. In 1972, vonBrauchitsch (49) reported that about 50% of patients hospitalized with mental depression
had positive serum antinuclear factor. These findings have later been
replicated by Debert et al. (50), but not by Plantey (51). However,
since most of these patients were on psychoactive medications, and
since some of these medications, particularly lithium, could produce
falsely elevated antinuclear antibodies (52), it is not clear to what
extent this positive antinuclear factor is related to depression per se
or is an artifact of treatment.

In 1971, Rimon and associates (53) noted an increase in herpes
simplex virus (HSV) antibodies in patients with psychotic depression.
These findings were replicated by Coppel et al. (54) who also noted an
increase in in-vitro lymphocyte response to HSV in psychotically
depressed patients. These authors suggested an association between
HSV and psychotic depression, and proposed that acute depression
may be related to a reactivation of a latent HSV infection with consequent dysfunction in CNS monoamine metabolism leading to depression.

In 1982, Sengar and associates (55) studied the frequency of T
and B lymphocytes and lymphocyte mitogenic responses in three groups
of subjects: 1) manic-depressive patients in remission, 2) psychia-
trically-well siblings and 3) normal controls. They found no significant differences in the distribution of T cells, B cells or lymphocyte
mitogenic activity among the three groups. However, since none of
the subjects studied was clinically depressed, the question of the
integrity of the immune response during the acute phase of depression
remained unanswered.

In 1983, Kronfol and associates (56) compared lymphocyte response
to mitogen stimulation in 26 drug-free acutely depressed patients and
20 normal controls. They found a generalized and marked reduction in
lymphocyte mitogenic activity among the depressive group. These
differences could not be explained on the basis of age, sex, diet,
diurnal variation or concommittant medical illness. The authors concluded that depression may be associated with an impairment in cell-mediated immunity that could explain the increased risk for immune-rela-
ted disorders among the depressive population. Kronfol's findings
were later replicated by Schleifer and co-workers (57), who also noted
a reduced number of both T and B cells in the depressed group,
although the percentage of these cells did not differ between depressed
patients and normal controls. The ratio of helper/suppressor T lymphocytes was examined by Kronfol and House (58). Depressed patients
had lower ratios than normal controls, but the difference was not
statistically significant. We are presently studying natural-killer cell
activity in depressed patients. Preliminary results from our lab do not
suggest major differences in NKCA between depressed and other

psychiatric patients (59). Data by Van Dyke and associates (60) however seem to indicate lower NKCA among depressed patients compared to normal controls. It is evident that more data is needed before definite conclusions can be drawn.

Another issue of major interest in this context is the relation of hypercortisolemia to lymphocyte number and function in major depression. In a large retrospective study of 178 untreated depressed patients and 179 untreated schizophrenic controls, Kronfol and associates (61) noted a significant increase in both the percentage and absolute neutrophil count, and significant decreases in both the percentage and absolute lymphocyte and eosinophil counts among the depressed group. These differences, the authors noted, were consistent with the expected hematologic effects of higher levels of circulating glucocorticoids in depressed patients. In a later, prospective study, Kronfol and colleagues (62) were able to confirm much of their earlier findings. In particular, depressed patients had lower concentrations of circulating lymphocytes than a schizophrenic control group. More interestingly, depressed patients with abnormal dexamethasone suppression test (DST) had lower lymphocyte concentrations than depressed patients with normal DST. Furthermore, a significant negative correlation was found between post-dexamethasone plasma cortisol levels and lymphocyte numbers among the depressed group.

The relationship between hypercortisolemia and lymphocyte function in depressed patients is less clear. Kronfol and associates (63) compared lymphocyte response to mitogen stimulation in 3 groups of subjects: 1) depressed patients with hypercortisolemia as indicated by elevated 24-hour UFC, 2) depressed patients without hypercortisolemia and 3) normal controls. Both depressed groups, regardless of UFC excretion, had lower lymphocytic responses than the normal control group. There were however no significant differences in lymphocyte mitogenic activity between the two depressive groups. Furthermore, there was no significant correlation between UFC excretion and lymphocyte mitogenic activity among the depressed group. The authors conclude that depression is associated with an impairment in lymphocyte function that cannot be explained solely on the basis of increased cortisol secretion.

Van Dyke and associates (60) studied two parameters of cellular immunity in depressed patients and patients with Cushing's disease. They found evidence of decreased mitogenesis and reduced NKCA in the depressed patients but not those with Cushing's disease. Within the depressed group, higher cortisol values were more likely to be associated with decreased mitogenesis than reduced NKCA. However, neither lymphocyte mitogenic activity nor NKCA were related to results of the DST. The authors thus concur with Kronfol and associates that immunosuppression in depressed patients is not solely dependent on abnormalities in cortisol secretion.

CONCLUSION

In summary, many patients with depressive illness have documented abnormalities in neuroendocrine and/or immune regulation. The endocrine abnormalities most widely investigated are abnormalities in HPA function. Briefly, these consist of disturbances in the circadian pattern of cortisol secretion, excessive cortisol production and impaired feedback regulation with dexamethasone. The role of ACTH, β -endorphin and CRF has not been adequately investigated. The immune abnormalities are much less know or understood. Lymphopenia, decreased lymphocyte mitogenic activity and a possible reduction of NKCA have

76

been noted. The relation between increased cortisol secretion and immunosuppression needs further investigation. Future research should also address the role of other hormones and/or neurotransmitters in the regulation of the immune response in patients with depressive illness. Special attention should be given to norepinephrine, serotonin, acetylcholine and β-endorphin which have been shown to play a role in the regulation of both mood and immunity. Traditionally, research in the psychobiology of the affective disorders has focused on the genetics, neurochemistry and neurophysiology of depression. More recently, the neuroendocrine approach has been adopted by several investigators. In the meantime, very rapid progress has been achieved in basic immunology and the pharmacology of the opiate peptides. The application of these new discoveries to the study of depression is now just starting.

References

1. D. Kupfer, G. Foster, P. Coble, R. McPartland and R. Ulrich, The application of sleep EEG for the differential diagnosis of affective disorders. Am J Psychiatry, 135:69 (1978).
2. J. Fawcett, J.W. Maas and H. Dekirmemjian, Depression and MHPG excretion: Responses to dextroamphetamine and tricyclic antidepressants. Arch Gen Psychiatry, 26:246 (1972).
3. M. Asberg, P. Thoren, L. Traskman, L. Bertillson and V. Ringberger, Serotonin depression - a biochemical subgroup within the affective disorders? Science, 191:478 (1976).
4. B.J. Carroll, M. Feinberg, J. Greden, J. Tarika, A. Albala, R. Haskett, N. James, Z. Kronfol, N. Lohr, M. Steiner, J.P. deVigne and E. Young, A specific laboratory test for the diagnosis of melancholia: standardization, validation and clinical utility. Arch Gen Psychiatry, 38:15 (1981).
5. B.J. Carroll and J. Mendels, Neuroendocrine regulation in affective disorders. in: "Hormones, Behavior and Psychopathology", E.J. Sachar, ed., Raven Press, New York (1976).
6. B.J. Carroll, The dexamethasone suppression test for melancholia. Br J Psychiatry, 140:292 (1982).
7. F. Board, R. Wadeson and H. Persky, Depressive affect and endocrine functions. Arch Neurol Psychiatry, 78:612 (1957).
8. E.J. Sachar, L. Hellman, D.K. Fukushima and T.F. Gallagher, Cortisol production in depressive illness. Arch Gen Psychiatry, 23:289 (1970).
9. B.J. Carroll, G.C. Curtis, B.M. Davies, J. Mendels and A.A. Sugerman, Urinary free cortisol excretion in depression. Psychol Med, 6:43 (1976).
10. B.J. Carroll, G.C. Curtis and J. Mendels, Cerebrospinal fluid and plasma free cortisol concentrations in depression. Psychol Med, 6:235 (1976).
11. J.L. Gibbons, Cortisol secretion rate in depressive illness. Arch Gen Psychiatry, 10:572 (1964).
12. E.J. Sachar, L. Hellman, H. Roffwarg, F. Halpern, D. Fukushima and T. Gallagher, Disrupted 24-hour patterns of cortisol secretion in psychotic depression. Arch Gen Psychiatry, 28:19 (1973).
13. F.H. Tyler and C.D. West, Laboratory evaluation of disorders of the adrenal cortex. Am J Med, 53:664 (1972).
14. H.C. Ferguson, A.C.G. Bartram, H.C. Fowlie, D.M. Cathro, K. Birchall and F.L. Mitchell, A preliminary investigation of steroid excretion in depressed patients before and after electroconvulsive therapy. Acta Endocrinol, 47:58 (1964).

15. J. Schlechte, B. Sherman and B. Pfohl, A comparison of adrenal corticol function in patients with depression and patients with Cushing's disease. (submitted).

16. S. Berson and R. Yalow, Radioimmunoassay of ACTH in plasma. J Clin Invest, 47:2725 (1968).

17. J.P. Allen, D. Denney, J. Kendall and P.H. Blachly, Corticotropin release during ECT in man. Am J Psychiatry, 131:1225 (1974).

18. V.S. Fang, B.J. Tricou, A. Robertson and H.Y. Meltzer, Plasma ACTH and cortisol levels in depressed patients: Relation to dexamethasone suppression test. Life Sci, 29:931 (1981).

19. B.I. Yerevanian, P.D. Woolf and H.P. Idel, Plasma ACTH levels in depression before and after recovery: Relationship to the dexamethasone suppression test. Psychiatry Res, 9:45 (1983).

20. V.I. Reus, M.S. Joseph and M.F. Dallman, M.F. ACTH levels after the dexamethasone suppression test in depression. N Engl J Med, 306:238 (1982).

21. N.H. Kalin, S.J. Weiler and S.E. Shelton, Plasma ACTH and cortisol concentrations before and after dexamethasone. Psychiatry Res, 7:87 (1982).

22. B. Pfohl, B. Sherman and J. Schlechte, Differences in plasma ACTH and cortisol between depressed patients and normal controls. Biol Psychiatry, in press.

23. B. Pfohl, B, Sherman and J. Schlechte, Pituitary-adrenal axis rhythm disturbances in major depression. Arch Gen Psychiatry, in press.

24. W. Vale, J. Spiess, C. Rivier and J. Rivier, Characterization of a 41-residue ovine hypothalamic peptide that stimulates secretion of corticotropin and beta-endorphin. Science, 213:1394 (1982).

25. P.W. Gold, G. Chrousos, C. Kellner, R. Post, A. Roy, P. Augerinos, H. Schulte, E. Oldfield and L. Lorianx, Psychiatric implications of basic and clinical studies with corticotrophin releasing factor. Am J Psychiatry, 141:619 (1984).

26. R. Guillemin, T. Vargo and J. Rossier, Beta-endorphin and ACTH are secreted concomitantly by the pituitary gland. Science, 197:1367 (1977).

27. G.S. Alexopoulos, C.E. Inturrisi, R. Lipman, R. Frances, J. Haycox, J.H. Dougherty, Plasma immunoreactive beta-endorphin levels in depression. Arch Gen Psychiatry, 40:181 (1983).

28. F. Brambilla, A.R. Genazzani, F. Facchinetti, D. Parrin, F. Petraglia, E. Sacchetti, S. Scarone, A. Guastalla and N. d'Antona, Beta-endorphin and beta-lipotropin plasma levels in chronic schizophrenia, primary affective disorders and secondary affective disorders. Psychoneuroendocrinology, 6:321 (1981).

29. S.C. Risch, Beta-endorphin hypersecretion in depression: possible cholinergic mechanisms. Biol Psychiatry, 17:1071 (1982).

30. M.R. Cohen, D. Pickar, I. Exstein, M. Gold and D. Sweeney, Plasma cortisol and beta-endorphin immunoreactivity in nonmajor and major depression. Am J Psychiatry, 141:628 (1984).

31. D. Pickar, N.R. Cutler, D. Naber, R. Post, C. Pert and W. Bunney, Plasma opioid activity in manic-depressive illness. Lancet, 1:937 (1980).

32. D. Pickar, M.R. Cohen, D. Naber and R.M. Cohen, Clinical studies of the endogenous opioid system. Biol Psychiatry, 17:1243 (1982).

33. L. Terenius, A. Wahlstrom and H. Agren, Naloxone (Narcan) treatment in depression: clinical observations and effects of CSF endorphins and monoamine metabolites. Psychopharmacology, 54:31 (1977).

34. J. Angst, V. Autenrieth, F. Brem, M. Koukkou, H. Meyer, H.H. Stassen and U. Storck, Preliminary results of treatment with beta-endorphin in depression. in: "Endorphins in Mental Health Research", E. Usdin, W. Bunney and N. Kline, eds., Oxford University Press, New York (1979).

35. R.B. Shekelle, W.J. Raynor, A.M. Ostfeld, D.C. Garron, L.A. Bieliauskas, C.L. Shuguey, C. Maliza and P. Ogelsby, Psychological depression and 17-year risk of death from cancer. Psychosom Med, 43:117 (1981).

36. M. Rogers, D. Dubey and P. Reich, The influence of the psyche and the brain on immunity and disease susceptibility: A critical review. Psychosom Med, 41:147 (1979).

37. M. Stein, S. Schleifer and S. Keller, Immune disorders. in: "Comprehensive Textbook of Psychiatry", Third Edition, H. Kaplan, A. Freedman and B. Sadock, eds., Williams and Wilkins, Baltimore, (1980).

38. J. Palmblad, K. Cantell, H. Strander, J. Froberg, C. Karlsson, L. Levi, M. Granstrom and P. Ungar, Stressor exposure and immunological response in man: interferon-producing capacity and phagocytosis. J Psychom Res, 20:193 (1976).

39. J. Palmblad, B. Petrini, J. Wasserman and T. Akerstedt, Lymphocyte and granulocyte reactions during sleep deprivation. Psychosom Med, 41:273 (1979).

40. B. Dorian, D. Garfinkel, G. Brown, A. Shore, D. Gladman and E. Keystone, Aberrations in lymphocyte subpopulations and function during psychological stress. Clin Exp Immunol, 50:132 (1982).

41. J. Jemmott, J. Borysenko, M. Borysenko, D. McClelland, R. Chapman and D. Meyer, Academic stress, power motivation and decrease in secretion rate of salivary secretory immunoglobulin A. Lancet, I:1400 (1983).

42. J. Kiecolt-Glaser, W. Garner, C. Speicher, G. Penn, J. Holliday and R. Glaser, Psychosocial modifiers of immunocompetence in medical students. Psychosom Med, 46:7 (1984).

43. S. Locke, M. Hurst and J. Heisel, J. The influence of stress on the immune response. Annual Meeting, American Psychosomatic Society, Washington, D.C. (1978).

44. G.H. Baker, N. Byrom, M. Irani, D. Brewerton, J.R. Hobbs, R.J. Woods and M. Nagvekar, Stress, cortisol and lymphocyte subpopulations. Lancet, I:574 (1984).

45. R. Bartrop, L. Lazarus, D. Luckhurst and L. Kiloh, Depressed lymphocyte function after bereavement. Lancet, I:834 (1977).

46. S. Schleifer, S. Keller, M. Camerino, J. Thornton and M. Stein, Suppression of lymphocyte stimulation following bereavement. J Am Med Assoc, 250:374 (1983).

47. Z. Kronfol, Depression and immune disease. Psychiatr Med, (in press).

48. Z. Kronfol, Cancer and depression. Br J Psychiatry, 142:309 (1983).

49. H. vonBrauchitsch, Antinuclear factor in psychiatric disorders. Am J Psychiatry, 128:1552 (1972).

50. R. Deberdt, J. VanHooren, M. Biesbrouch and W. Amery, Antinuclear factor-positive mental depression: A single disease entity? Biol Psychiatry, II:69 (1976).

51. F. Plantey, Antinuclear factor in affective disorders. Biol Psychiatry, 13:149 (1978).

52. E. Johnstone and K. Whaley, Antinuclear antibodies in psychiatric illness: their relationship to diagnosis and drug treatment. Br Med J, 2:724 (1975).

53. R. Rimon, P. Halonin, E. Anttinen and E. Evola, Complement fixing antibody to herpes simplex virus in patients with psychotic depression. Dis Nerv Sys, 32:822 (1971).
54. R. Coppel, F. Gregoire, L. Thiry and S. Sprecher, Antibody and cell-mediated immunity to herpes simplex virus in psychotic depression. J Clin Psychiatry, 39:266 (1978).
55. D. Sengar, B. Waters and J. Dunne, J. Lymphocyte subpopulations and mitogenic responses of lymphocytes in manic depressive disorder. Biol Psychiatry, 17:1017 (1982).
56. Z. Kronfol, J. Silva, J. Greden, S. Dembinski, R. Gardner and B.J. Carroll, Impaired lymphocyte function in depressive illness. Life Sci, 33:241 (1983).
57. S. Schleifer, S. Keller, A. Meyerson, M. Raskin, K. Davis and M. Stein, Lymphocyte function in major depressive disorder. Arch Gen Psychiatry, 41:484 (1984).
58. Z. Kronfol and J.D. House, Depression, cortisol and immune function. Lancet, I:1026 (1984).
59. H. Nasrallah, Z. Ballas, Z. Kronfol and S. Chapman, Natural-killer cell activity in major depression. in: "Viruses, Immunity and Mental Diseases", E. Kurstak, ed., Plenum Press, New York, (in press).
60. C. Van Dyke, K. McDaniel, V. Reus, W. Seaman and C. Kaufman, Immune response in depressed and Cushing's patients. American Psychiatric Association Annual Meeting, New Research Abstract #42, Los Angeles, CA (1984).
61. Z. Kronfol, R. Turner, H. Nasrallah and G. Winokur, Leukocyte regulation in depression and schizophrenia. Psychiatry Res, 13:13 (1984).
62. Z. Kronfol, H. Nasrallah, S. Chapman and J.D. House, Depression, cortisol metabolism and lymphocytopenia. J Affect Disord, (in press).
63. Z. Kronfol, J.D. House, J. Greden and B.J. Carroll, Depression, urinary free cortisol excretion and lymphocyte function. Br J Psychiatry, (in press).

ENDOGENOUS OPIOID SYSTEMS, STRESS, AND CANCER

Ian S. Zagon and Patricia J. McLaughlin

Department of Anatomy and Cancer Research Center
The Milton S. Hershey Medical Center
The Pennsylvania State University
Hershey, Pennsylvania 17033

INTRODUCTION

Opium's importance in both medicinal and social contexts dates back thousands of years (Blum, 1970; Terry and Pellens, 1928). Interest in opiates and opiate-like compounds (heretofore collectively referred to as "opioids") had been maintained throughout the years. A major breakthrough in our understanding of opioids came with the discovery of opioid receptors in 1973 by groups led by Simon (Simon et al., 1973), Snyder (Pert and Snyder, 1973), and Terenius (1973), along with the equally elegant finding of endogenous opioids by Hughes, Kosterlitz and colleagues (Hughes, 1975; Hughes et al., 1975) in 1975. Discovery of opioid receptors and the endogenous opioids (collectively referred to as "endogenous opioid systems") stands as a landmark of scientific achievement. Needless to say, this has stimulated intense research activity which has already culminated in important information as to the mechanisms and functions of opioids. One such exciting insight has been the discovery in 1983 that endogenous opioid systems are related to growth of both normal and abnormal cells and tissues (Zagon and McLaughlin, 1983a, b, c, d). This has led to a fascinating story concerning the fundamental nature of growth (Zagon and McLaughlin, 1984a, b, c; 1985a, b). The major purpose of this chapter is to review the evidence relating endogenous opioid systems to cancer. Since some aspects of stress may be associated with the endogenous opioid systems, and ACTH and some endogenous opioids share the same precursor (pro-opiomelanocortin), we have also included relevant information on the topic of stress and cancer in an attempt to provide perspective to the entire field of endogenous opioid systems and tumor biology.

ENDOGENOUS OPIOID SYSTEMS AND CANCER

To fully comprehend the role of endogenous opioid systems in cancer some background information is necessary. Although exogenous opioids such as morphine, methadone, and heroin have well-known analgesic and behavioral effects (Jaffe and Martin, 1980), these compounds have also been reported to alter cell function, particularly in developing neural systems (Zagon and McLaughlin, 1984d; Zagon et al., 1982, 1984). Exogenous opioids are known to be teratogenic in animals (Geber and Schramm, 1975; Harpel and Gautieri, 1968) and a review of the clinical and laboratory literature reveals that these agonists are antimitotic (Andersen, 1966; Simon, 1963), cytotoxic (Ma, 1931; Sinatra et al., 1978) and damaging to chromosomes (Falek and Hollingsworth, 1980; Fischman et al., 1977). Moreover, in vivo and in vitro studies have demonstrated that opioids can retard growth and development in many diverse organisms and cell types, with a suppression of cell division and alterations in poly-amine, nucleic acid, and protein synthetic systems thought to be involved (Hui et al., 1976; Slotkin et al., 1980; Zagon and McLaughlin, 1977, 1978).

In view of the growth retarding properties of exogenous opioids in normal tissues undergoing proliferation and development, we were prompted to determine whether these compounds were also effective in inhibiting carcinogenic processes. Since normal neural tissues are especially susceptible to exogenous opioids, we examined the effects of opioids on C1300 mouse neuroblastoma. As a point of information, the C1300 murine neuroblastoma has been widely used as an in vivo model for the study of human neoplasia, particularly in regard to the screening of therapeutic regimens (Arima et al., 1973; Finkelstein et al., 1973). The S20Y neuro-blastoma used in these experiments is a well-characterized cholinergic clone (Amano et al., 1972; Zagon and Schengrund, 1978) that contains opioid receptors (Klee and Nirenberg, 1974). We (Zagon and McLaughlin, 1981a) found that chronic administration of heroin (diacetylmorphine) to mice inoculated with 10^6 S20Y cells (a dosage that usually produces 100% tumor take in control mice) inhibited tumor growth and prolonged the life-span of tumor-inoculated mice. For example, in animals which began receiving heroin at dosages of 3,6,10, or 15 mg/kg starting 2 weeks prior to tumor cell inoculation, a prolongation in mean survival time of 32-39% and median survival time of 8-50%, was recorded. Tumor size of animals receiving heroin also was often smaller than controls but, on the day of death, tumor size of heroin- and saline-treated mice were comparable. In some instances (i.e., dosages of 6 and 15 mg/kg), at least 20% of the animals never developed a tumor. To examine whether the effect of heroin on tumor growth was specific for the opioid receptor, some mice inoculated with neuroblastoma received simultaneous injections of heroin and naloxone (an opioid antagonist). Tumor incidence, survival time, and tumor growth were similar in control and heroin/naloxone animals. The results of this study showed that dosages of heroin (3-15 mg/kg), which were above the analgesic dose of 1 mg/kg (Brands et al., 1975) but well-below the LD_{50} level of 158-190 mg/kg (Brands et al., 1975; Way et al., 1960) in mice, had an extraordinary effect on tumorigenesis that was related to opioid receptor interaction. This antitumor action appeared to be related to heroin's direct influence on tumor cells (presumably by way of the opioid receptors known to be present in these cells) rather than on which reflected a cascade of events from heroin's effects on the entire animal. For example, injections of heroin beginning 2 weeks prior to tumor inocu-lation, an interval in which tolerance to heroin's actions are known to develop, still altered the course of carcinogenesis. Indeed, an injection schedule beginning 2 weeks prior to tumor inoculation was even more effec-tive than a regimen that was initiated one week after tumor transplanta-tion, although tumor burden may have played a role in this difference.

Additional information which has important bearing on these in vivo experiments with heroin and neuroblastoma, comes from in vitro investiga-tions in which the effects of heroin on neuroblastoma cells in culture were examined (McLaughlin and Zagon, 1984; Zagon and McLaughlin, 1984c). The addition of heroin in concentrations ranging from 10^{-2}M to 10^{-8}M to S20Y cultures beginning 24 hr after seeding (new drug and media was pro-vided daily), produced a dose-dependent inhibition of growth. This growth retarding effect was reversible, since removal of heroin allowed cells to resume normal growth. Experiments with thymidine incorporation, as well as analyses of mitotic figures, revealed that heroin affected cell division. Morphological differentiation also was noted to be decreased in drug-treated cultures, but this activity was not necessarily dependent on heroin dosage. Quite importantly the action of heroin in perturbing cell growth was blocked by concomitant administration of an opioid antagonist, naloxone. Additionally, the sterospecific effects of opioid agonists were investigated by treating logarithmically growing cultures with equimolar concentrations of levorphanol or dextrorphan. Levorphanol is known to be the active isomer. Levorphanol-exposed S20Y neuroblastoma cell cultures were growth-inhibited in a fashion similar to that observed when heroin was applied, whereas dextrorphan had little effect on cell growth. Thus, these data extend in vitro investigations and show that the dose-dependent, sterospecific, and naloxone-reversible effects of opioids on neurotumor cells are the direct effects of opioid agonist action at the opioid receptor level.

Although these observations on the action of exogenous opioids on cancer were revealing, the ethical considerations of utilizing opioid drugs with addictive liability for cancer treatment were apparent. An intriguing observation in our study (Zagon and McLaughlin, 1981a) utilizing heroin was that chronic, once-daily, injections of naloxone (10 mg/kg), a non-addictive opioid antagonist, produced a significant increase (11%) in mean survival time. Additionally, 1 of the 8 mice inoculated with neuroblastoma never developed a tumor, despite a 100% tumor incidence in control animals. We decided to examine further the effects of naloxone on neuroblastoma (Zagon and McLaughlin, 1981a). In utilizing an injection regimen similar to that with heroin, mice inoculated with 10^6 S20Y neuroblastoma received daily subcutaneous injections of either 5, 10, 15, or 20 mg/kg naloxone hydrochloride; injections were initiated either 2 weeks prior to tumor cell inoculation (pre-treatment group) or one week after tumor transplantation (post-treated groups). All mice in the control (saline) and post-treated groups developed tumors within 3 weeks after tumor cell inoculation. In the naloxone pre-treated groups, 4 or 12 mice exposed to 20 mg/kg, 2 of 12 mice exposed to 15 mg/kg, and 1 of 12 mice exposed to 10 mg/kg, did not develop tumors within a 91-day period following tumor inoculation. Moreover, 3 animals in the 20 mg/kg naloxone pre-treated group developed tumors between 43 and 63 days after tumor cell inoculation. Tumor dimensions were often reduced in naloxone-treated mice, although at the time of death tumor sizes of control and naloxone-exposed animals were similar. In general, tumor-bearing mice receiving naloxone lived longer than saline-tumor controls, with animals receiving higher drug dosages surviving for the longest time. In contrast to a mean survival time of 27 days for controls, naloxone pre-treated mice had increases in survival times of 25-61%, whereas naloxone post-treated groups exhibited increases of 20-40%. The median day of death for all mice exposed to naloxone was prolonged by 21-75%, occurring 6-21 days after the 28-day median for saline-tumor controls.

The dosages of naloxone utilized in this study, 5-20 mg/kg, were not exceedingly high, being well-below the LD_{50} level of 252 mg/kg for mice, as well as below the maximum drug dose (i.e., 20 mg/kg) that can elicit evert effects such as ataxia and depression (Giering et al., 1974). The low general toxicity of the dosages employed was also reflected by the fact that tumor-bearing mice did not lose body weight. This observation also sets naloxone apart from many other antitumor agents that cause cachexia.

At this point, we suggested a number of interpretations as to naloxone's antitumor effect. Naloxone had long been regarded as a "pure" antagonist to the many biological actions of opioid substances and as devoid of significant intrinsic activity (Blumberg and Dayton, 1974;

Jasinski et al., 1967; Sawynok et al., 1979). However, an increasing number of reports indicated that naloxone may have a wide variety of pharmacological, physiological, and behavioral effects that are unrelated to opioid receptor blockade (Brown et al., 1980; Geber et al., 1976; Sawynok et al., 1979). Naloxone has been shown to reduce resting serum prolactin and growth hormone levels (Bruni et al., 1977) and to decrease serum titer of interferon (Geber et al., 1976), and these or other alterations in hormonal or immunologic functions may have been responsible for naloxone's antineoplastic activity. In reviewing the studies on heroin and naloxone, it appears that both compounds have a chemotherapeutic influence in mice with neuroblastoma. Yet concomitant administration of heroin and naloxone did not produce a greater (or cumulative) response, but rather simultaneous injections of these agents had little effect on neoplasia. Whether naloxone was capable of acting as an agonist when used alone, and as an antagonist when used in combination with opioid agonists, was unclear. Equally unclear were the mechanisms underlying naloxone's and heroin's ability to retard tumor growth and prolong survival. In this early paper, it was suggested that naloxone and heroin could activate a common mechanism (e.g., similar receptors) to elicit their effects, or these drugs may act through independent channels (e.g., different receptors for each drug). Somehow, in both of these hypotheses concomitant administration of these drugs removed one another's effectiveness. Finally, we suggested that administration of naloxone could provide an over compensating release of endogenous opioids; these endogenous opioids could act like heroin to inhibit cancer.

At this point we reasoned that if naloxone, a short-acting (half-life of 2 hours) opioid antagonist had such marked antitumor properties, we wondered what effect naltrexone, an opioid antagonist that is 8 times as active and 3 times as long-acting as naloxone (Blumberg and Dayton, 1973), would have on tumorigenesis. Once again choosing the neuroblastoma model, we initiated a schedule of chronic daily injections of naltrexone or sterile water. For these experiments, we began drug injections 2 days after inoculation of 10^6 S20Y neuroblastoma cells. Our results (Zagon and McLaughlin, 1983a) indicated that animals receiving the lowest drug dosage (0.1 mg/kg) had a 33% tumor incidence, a 98% delay in the time before the appearance of a palpable tumor, and a 36% increase in survival time of tumor-bearing mice. However, neuroblastoma-inoculated animals receiving the highest drug dosage (10 mg/kg naltrexone) had a 100% tumor incidence, a 27% reduction in the time before tumor appearance, and a 19% decrease in survival time. Inoculation of neuroblastoma cells in control subjects resulted in a 100% tumor incidence within 29 days. It appeared that naltrexone's major action was to modify the interval between tumor inoculation and tumor appearance. Remarkably, these effects occurred with dosages that were 0.01 to 2.0% of the LD_{50} (570 mg/kg; Blumberg and Dayton, 1973) and which did not elicit overt toxicological symptoms such as ataxia, convulsions, or loss of body weight. To examine whether the dosage effects were related to the extent of opioid receptor blockade, mice given 0.1 or 10 mg/kg naltrexone were challenge with an opioid antagonist (morphine). Animals demonstrate analgesia when placed on a hotplate following injection with morphine; when naltrexone is present it prevents the interaction of morphine with opioid receptors and the animals respond in a fashion similar to controls. Our results showed that a dosage of 0.1 mg/kg only blocked the opioid receptors for 4-6 hr per day, while a dosage of 10 mg/kg naltrexone invoked an opioid receptor blockade for at least 24 hr.

To further examine the relationship between tumor response, the pharmacological properties of naltrexone (e.g., ability to block the opioid receptor), and drug dosage a series of experiments were performed (Zagon and McLaughlin, 1984a). Mice were inoculated with S20Y neuroblastoma and injected with eigher (a) 0.1 mg/kg naltrexone given once daily, a dosage previously found to block the receptor for a short ime each day and to have antitumor effects, (b) 0.1 mg/kg naltrexone four times daily, a schedule that utilized a low dosage of drug but blocked the opioid receptor for an entire 24 hr period, or (c) 0.4 mg/kg naltrexone given once daily, a regimen which controlled for the effects of cumulative drug dosages in the four times daily 0.1 mg/kg naltrexone treatment schedule. The results showed that mice receiving 0.1 mg/kg naltrexone four times daily had a 100% tumor incidence, no deviation in time before tumor appearance, and a 17% decrease from control values in total survival time. In contrast, once daily injections of either 0.1 mg/kg naltrexone or 0.4 mg/kg naltrexone resulted in a tumor incidence of 20% and 60% respectively, delays in time prior to tumor appearance of 90% and 65%, respectively, and an increased total survival time of 10% and 24%, respectively, for tumor-bearing mice relative to control levels. Inoculation of neuroblastoma in control mice resulted in 100% tumor appearance within 16 days and a mean survival time of 36 days.

These data beautifully demonstrate the relationship between tumorigenesis and the pharmacological action of opioid antagonists, and show that opioid receptor perturbation is a key element in modulating neuroblastoma. Thus, exacerbation of tumor response is seen when the opioid receptor is blocked for an entire 24 hr period as demonstrated by the 0.1 mg/kg four times daily group in this study or in the study (Zagon and McLaughlin, 1983a) mentioned earlier with 10 mg/kg naltrexone once daily. However, antitumor activity was found at dosages which only blocked the opioid receptor for a short time each day as shown in the 0.1 and 0.4 mg/kg once daily groups and in previously mentioned studies (Zagon and McLaughlin, 1981b) with 0.1 mg/kg once daily or naloxone at dosages of 10-20 mg/kg once daily.

Another way to provide rigorous proof that opioid receptors mediate a particular tumor response, is to explore the stereospecificity of opioid antagonists. Opioid interactions at the receptor level have been shown to be stereospecific (Pert and Snyder, 1973), with isomeric forms showing markedly different affinities for opioid receptors. The (-) isomer of naloxone is known to be 3 or 4 orders of magnitude more active than the (+) isomer in its ability to bind to opioid receptors in rat brain membrane preparations, as well as in antagonizing physiological responses to opioids (Faden and Holaday, 1980; Gayton et al., 1978; Iijima et al., 1978). In fact, in these reports and others (Sawynok et al., 1979), demonstration of stereospecificity of opioid antagonist action has been recommended as a criteria for exclusion of pharmacological effects not due to interaction with opioid receptors. Utilizing the (+) and (-) isomers of naloxone, and providing daily subcutaneous injections of 15 mg/kg beginning 2 days after tumor cell inoculation, we (Zagon and McLaughlin, unpublished observations) found that mice given (-) naloxone had a 71% tumor incidence, a 33% delay in the interval before tumor appearance, and a 28% increase in survival time. Inoculation of neuroblastma cells in control subjects resulted in 100% tumor incidence within 13 days. Mice given the (+) isomer of naloxone were comparable to control subjects in all aspects of neural neoplasia. These data showing that the (-) isomer of naloxone, but not the (+) isomer, alters tumor incidence and survival time is consistent with the enantiomeric specificity of opioids.

An important question that needs to be addressed concerns the type(s) of opioid receptor that is(are) involved in neuro-oncogenesis. At least five different types have been proposed (Martin et al., 1976; Lord et al., 1977; Zukin and Zukin, 1981, 1984). Although the precise physiological function of distinct receptor types is unclear, recently developed selective antagonists (see Takemori and Portoghese, 1985) provide a unique opportunity to elucidate the importance of each receptor type. One such antagonist, β–funaltrexamine (β–FNA), is the fumaramate methyl ester derivative of naltrexone and binds selectively and irreversibly to μ receptors (Portoghese et al., 1980; Takemori et al., 1981; Ward et al., 1982a, b). This compound has been widely used in assessing the relative importance of μ receptors in various opioid actions (Ward and Takemori, 1983; D'Amato and Holaday, 1984). We (Zagon, McLaughlin, Takemori, and Portoghese, unpublished observations) ahve explored the effect of β–FNA in concentrations that antagonize morphine–induced analgesia, in mice inoculated with neuroblastoma. Presumably, tumor response should be altered if μ receptors sensitive to β–FNA were involved in neural neoplasia. We found that chronic injections of 2 mg/kg β–FNA every 48 hr beginning 2 days after tumor inoculation resulted in tumor incidence and survival times that were comparable to controls (i.e., a 100% tumor incidence within 16 days; mean and median survival times of 36 and 35 days, respectively, following tumor inoculation. These results suggest that, in and by themselves, μ receptors selectively antagonized by β–FNA do not play an important role in neuro–oncogenic events. Utilization of agonists that serve as prototypic ligands for particular receptors, as well as exploration of other selective antagonists, are currently being explored.

Another aspect of study in regard to endogenous opioid systems and neural cancer is whether neuro–oncogenesis that includes metastasis is regulated by endogenous opioid systems. In all of the studies described so far, a primary tumor model was used. However, by administering S20Y neuroblastoma cells by the intradermal, rather than subcutaneous, route a metastatic model of disease can be examined. Daily injections of 0.1 mg/kg naltrexone resulted in a 69% tumor take, 70% delay in time prior to tumor appearance, and a 60% increase in median survival time (Zagon and McLaughlin, 1983d). Inoculation of neuroblastoma in control mice resulted in 100% tumor take within 15 days. Mice receiving 10 mg/kg naltrexone were similar to the control group. The absence of detectable acceleration in tumorigenesis as observed earlier with primary tumors may have been due to the fact that a median survival of 50 days was recorded with the primary tumor model but a median survival of 30 days was noted in the metastatic tumor model. Thus, the stimulation of tumor growth by 10 mg/kg naltrexone seen earlier may not have had time to be expressed with the metastatic model. The importance of this study is that in a metastatic system closely resembling the clinical setting, naltrexone markedly influenced neuro–oncogenesis.

In summary, a number of lines of evidence have demonstrated that endogenous opioid systems regulate neural tumors. Exogenous opioid agonists inhibit neoplasia and this action can be completely blocked by concomitant administration of opioid antagonists such as naloxone. Results from in vitro studies reveal that opioid agonists exert a growth inhibitory effect on cells in culture that is dose-dependent, stereospecific, and blocked by naloxone. Moreover, at least 2 opioid antagonists, naloxone and naltrexone, have been shown to affect neural neoplasia. Experiments also demonstrate that the duration of opioid receptor blockade is crucial in determining the course of neuro-oncogenesis. In addition, opioid antagonists appear to alter carcinogenesis in a manner which suggest that opioid receptors and their ligands, rather than the specific antagonists, are the primary influence on cancer. Finally, investigations have demonstrated that opioid antagonists exert a stereo-specific action on neural cancer.

Based on evidence accumulated to this point, it is becoming clear that endogenous opioid systems function in the regulation of neural cancer. The endogenous opioids, as well as their exogenous counterparts, are capable of exerting an inhibitory influence on neoplasia. Data suggest that opioids retard cell proliferation by direct action on opioid receptors associated with neural tumor cells. Continuous occupation of the opioid receptors by opioid antagonists thereby preventing endogenous opioid-opioid receptor interaction, results in an acceleration in tumor development. This would imply that endogenous opioids mediate early events in the establishment of tumors as well as tumor growth. Precisely how opioid antagonists are involved with the growth of cells and tissues needs to be elucidated. It is known that chronic treatment with opioid antagonists results in a striking increase in plasma β-endorphin levels (Recant et al., 1980), an increase in the number of opioid binding receptor sites (Lahti and Collins, 1978; Zukin et al., 1980), and a super-sensitivity to opioid agonists (Tang and Collins, 1978). We have conjec-tured that daily intermittent opioid receptor blockade (e.g., 4-6 hr/day) exerts an anticancer effect by causing the production of more binding sites on tumor cells and a supersensitivity to basal (or elevated) levels of endorphins. The inhibitory action of the endogenous opioids takes place in the 14 to 18 hr interval when the opioid antagonist is no longer present.

Just how the opioid receptor is related to growth processes is an intriguing problem. Opioid receptors have been found to be associated with the amount and intracellular distribution of calmodulin (Simantov et al., 1982), known to be present in developing cells and tissues (Sano and Kitajima, 1983), and to regulate adenylate cyclase in nervous tissue (Bronstrom et al., 1977). In a related study, a calmodulin antagonist has been reported to inhibit tumor growth in mice inoculated with a sarcoma, and the authors suggest modulation of Ca^{++}-calmodulin-dependent processes (Ito and Hidaka, 1983). A link between opioid receptors and adenylate cyclase also has been reported (Sharma et al. 1975a, b). Endogenous (Lampert et al., 1976) and exogenous (Sharma et al., 1975b) opioids cause an inhibition of adenylate cyclase and a decrease in cAMP levels in con-fluent cultures of mouse neuroblastoma-rat glioma hybrid cells, but have little effect on parental cell lines (Sharma et al., 1975b). Although a connection between opioid receptors and adenylate cyclase would provide the basis of an attractive hypothesis as to how endogenous opioid systems control growth, it should be noted that treatment of neuroblastoma-glioma cultures with 10 μM morphine sulfate over a 9-day period did not alter total protein from control levels (Sharma et al., 1975b). This lack of effect by morphine on the growth of neuroblastoma-glioma cells stands in contrast to numerous reports (Zagon and McLaughlin, 1984c; McLaughlin and Zagon, 1984; Simon, 1971; North-Root et al., 1976) of opioid agonist-induced inhibition of growth that is naloxone-reversible and stereo-specific in other cell culture systems (including murine neuroblastoma). Thus, despite the abundance of opioid receptors in neuroblastoma-glioma hybrid cells, the special nature of these hybrid cells (two different cell types, neurons and glia from 2 different species, mice and rat) must be considered.

These results showing that endogenous opioid systems serve to regu-late growth of neuroblastoma raise a host of important questions. One of the most important is whether the endogenous opioid systems are involved in the development of other types of tumors. Presently, our laboratory is actively involved in addressing this issue. However, some information in this regard is available from other quarters. Frey and Kebabian (1984) have found opioid receptors in a prolactin-secreting tumor derived from a parent line isolated from the pituitary gland of a female Buffalo rat. In other experiments, Inoue and Hatanaks (1982), working with a rat pheo-chromocytoma cell line, found very low enkephalin binding in the absence of nerve growth factor but a dramatic increase when cells were cultured in the presence of nerve growth factor. Association of enkephalin with human pheochromocytoma has also been reported by a number of investigators

(Clement-Jones et al., 1980; Sullivan et al., 1978; Osamura et al., 1984).

Two other important studies need to be mentioned in regard to endogenous opioids and cancer. Aylsworth and colleagues (1979) have explored the effects of naloxone and naltrexone on mammary adenocarcinomas induced in rats by injection of 7, 12-dimethylbenz(a)-anthracene (DMBA). Apparently, the motivation for these experiments was that development and growth of mammary tumors in rats is dependent on prolactin and ovarian steroids, as well as growth hormone secretion, and that opioid antagonists are known to cause a decrease in these substances. Presumably, these opioid antagonist-induced changes would in turn influence mammary carcino-genesis. These authors found that both naloxone (0.2 mg/kg, 3 times daily) and naltrexone (1-2 mg/kg, twice daily) suppressed the growth of DMBA-induced mammary cancer, but did not induce regression of tumors. These inhibitory effects were reversible since resumption of growth followed withdrawal of drug treatment. Serum prolactin levels measured in rats receiving 2 mg/kg of naltrexone twice daily, were 50% lower than that of control animals. These investigators concluded by suggesting "that the endogenous opioid peptides may stimulate mammary tumor growth, via their ability to promote prolactin and growth hormone secretion" (Aylsworth et al., 1979, p. 19). In another report, Plotnikoff and Miller (1983) administered subcutaneous daily injections of methionine (met-) or leucine (leu-) enkephalin to mice inoculated with L1210 murine leukemia. Signifi-cant increases in the number of survivors were observed. Unfortunately, Plotnikoff and Miller did not try to block enkephalin's antitumor effect with an opioid antagonist in order to elucidate whether these alterations occurred at the receptor level.

ENDOGENOUS OPIOID SYSTEMS, CANCER, AND IMMUNITY

Although in vivo and in vitro studies with the neuroblastoma model argue strongly for a direct influence of opioids on cancer, and one mediated by opioid receptors, little is known about the presence of opioid receptors and responsivity to opioid agonists or antagonists in other tumor types. Additionally, the provocative findings relating endogenous opioid systems to the immune system suggests that immunological mechanisms may play a part in modulating some cancers. Given discussions of endoge-nous opioids, opioid receptors, and immunity that recur throughout this volume, along with some excellent reviews (Wybran, 1985; Chang, 1984; Fischer, in press; Faith et al., in press; Weber and Pert, 1984), I will not review all aspects of this subject. Rather, I would like to briefly recall some of the highlights in this field.

First, what is known about the effects of exogenous opioids on immunity? Viral hepatitis, endocarditis, bacteremia, cellulitis, injection-site abscesses, pulmonary infections, and other infections are common among individuals using opioids such as heroin (Hussey and Katz, 1950; Cherubin and Brown, 1968), and are frequently attributed to unsteri-lized needles or injection of contaminated materials. Despite a host of confounding variables that obfuscate interpretation of the results from studies in this area, some workers point towards a link between opioid addiction and susceptibility to infections (Cherubin and Brown, 1968). Brown and colleagues (1974) reported that heroin addicts display impaired in vitro responsiveness in culture studies to at least one of three mito-gens and suggested abnormalities occur in both the humoral and cellular immune systems of chronic heroin addicts. Methadone has also been found to have an immunosuppressive effect on the function of immunocompetent cells of human blood. Singh et al. (1980) discovered that methadone, in reaction mixtures of T- and B-cells, reduced T-rosette formation. More-over, investigations of the function of human lymphocytes, measured in

vitro by following the mitogen-induced proliferative response of lymphocytes, found that methadone suppressed the lymphocyte stimulation by mitogens. McDonough and co-workers (1980) recorded that opioid addiction
produces a significant depression in the absolute number of total T
lymphocytes in peripheral blood, an increase in the absolute number of
null lymphocytes, but no significant changes in B lymphocytes or total
white blood cell count. Naloxone reversed both T cell depression and null
cell increase.

A number of animal experiments concerned with exogenous opioids and
immunity should be noted. Lefkowitz and Chiang (1975) described the
immunosuppressive effect of morphine in mice using a plaque-forming cell
assay to evaluate antibody-forming efficiency. Nalorphine, an opioid
antagonist, did not diminish this morphine-induced suppression. Lefkowitz
and Nemeth (1976) reported that morphine and methadone have a depressive
effect in mice in a rosette forming cell test, while Ho and Leung (1979)
recorded a reduction in lymphocyte response to concanavalin A-mediated
blastogenesis in mice dependent on morphine that was only partially prevented by naloxone. Güngör and colleagues (1980) studied primary immune
response in mice chronically receiving morphine and estimated spleen/body
weight ratios and serum hemolysis production against sheep red blood
cells. They found morphine exerted a dose-dependent inhibitory effect on
the immune system which was antagonized by naloxone. In 1983, Tubaro and
colleagues (1983) demonstrated that exposure to morphine exacerbates
infections in mice. Morphine drastically reduces reticuloendothelial
system activity, phagocyte count, phagocytic index, killing properties,
and superoxide anion production in polymorphonuclear leukocytes and macrophages. Finally, Shavit et al. (1984) have shown that morphine causes a
dose-related suppression of natural killer cell activity in rats; opioid
specificity by the use of naloxone/naltrexone antagonism was not performed.

Even though the picture emanating from studies with exogenous opioids
generally conclude that these agents depress immunity, investigations
into endogenous opioid systems and immunity are less clear. In 1979,
Wybran and co-workers showed that normal human blood T lymphocytes have
opioid receptors. These investigators found that morphine and dextromoramide inhibited the percentage of active T-rosettes, and that this effect
was completely reversed by naloxone. Specificity was further demonstrated
by the absence of the effect of levomoramide, the inactive enantiomer upon
the rosette system. Interestingly, methionine-enkephalin increased the
percentage of T-rosettes and this action was antagonized by naloxone.
Evidence for opioid receptors on granulocytes and monocytes (Lopker et
al., 1980), mast cells (Yamasaki et al., 1983), the terminal complex of
human complement (Schweigerer et al., 1982), as well as lymphocytes
(McDonough et al., 1980; Wybran et al., 1979), has been established.
Hazum, Chang, and Cuatrecasas (1979) have also shown by a direct radioligand binding technique that transformed cultured human lymphocytes bind
β-endorphin in a manner which is not blocked by opioid agonists or antagonists suggesting the existence of a specific, non-opioid type of binding
site (receptor) for β-endorphin in these cells.

A number of laboratories have focused on endogenous opioids as
immunomodulators. Plotnikoff et al. (1982, 1985) and Plotnikoff and
Miller (1983) have found that endogenous opioids stimulate lymphocyte
blastogenesis in laboratory animals, and Miller et al. (1983, 1984) have
found a similar effect in lymphoma patients as well as normal patients.
The enkephalins were also observed to exhibit marked activity in
increasing natural killer cell activity in normal human volunteers (Faith
et al., 1984). Unfortunately, little is known about the ability to
antagonize these effects with opioid antagonists. Gilman et al. (1982)

have reported that β-endorphin enhances rat splenic lymphocyte proliferation in response to concananalin A and phytohemaglutin, although a
study my McCain et al. (1982) indicates that β-endorphin suppresses
lymphocyte proliferation. Other investigators have shown that β-endorphin
suppresses in vitro formation of antibodies (Johnson et al., 1982) and
stimulates natural killer cell activity (Mathews et al., 1983; Plotnikoff
et al., 1985). Van Epps and Saland (1984) have recently demonstrated
that β-endorphin and met-enkephalin interact with human mononuclear cells
and stimulate chemotaxis as measured by the in vitro leading front assay
for migration; this effect was blocked by naloxone. These investigators
also found that injection of β-endorphin into the rat cerebral ventricle
resulted in the immigration of macrophage-like cells into the third
ventricle.

    Another possible connection between opioid peptides and the immune
system involves the relationship between opioids and interferon.
Administration of opioid agonists such as morphine and methadone to mice
results in a dose-related decrease in the level of circulating interferon
following injection by polyinosinic:polycytidylic acid (poly I:C), a
double-stranded synthetic RNA capable of inducing interferon (Hung et al.,
1973; Geber et al., 1975, 1976). Naloxone did not eliminate this effect
(Hung et al., 1973). In a subsequent study (Geber et al., 1976), naloxone
was found to function as an antagonist to morphine-induced depression of
interferon, but acted as an agonist under some situations. Opioid
agonists were also tested on cells in vitro using poly I:C as an inducer,
and they did not appear to have a major effect on either the induction or
the action of interferon in vitro. In regard to endogenous opioids and
interferon, Blalock and Smith (1980) have reported that natural interferon
has structural and biological similarities to ACTH 1-13 and β-endorphin.
Subsequently, human peripheral lymphocytes were shown to be capable of
producing ACTH and endorphin-like substances(Smith and Blalock, 1981).
In another report (Blalock and Smith, 1981), human leukocyte interferon
was shown to bind to opioid receptors in vitro and, when injected intra-
cerebrally into mice, human leukocyte interferon caused potent endorphin-
like effects. All of these actions were preventable and reversible by
naloxone. Recombinant leukocyte A interferon has also been found to prevent naloxone precipitated abstinence in morphine-dependent rats (Dafny,
1983a), once again suggesting cross-reaction of interferon with opioid
systems. Some question as to the relationship of interferon with opioids
has been raised by Epstein and co-workers (1982) and Jörnvall and colleagues (1982). Epstein could not detect any functional or structural
homology between natural and recombinant inferferon-α with β-endorphin (or
ACTH), while Jörnvall excluded structural homologies in amino acid
sequence.

ENDOGENOUS OPIOID SYSTEMS, STRESS, AND CANCER

    The role of stress and psychological states in the etiology and
pathogenesis of neoplasia is an extraordinarily interesting, but complex,
subject. I refer the reader to a number of excellent reviews and discussions about this topic (LeShan, 1959; Perrin and Pierce, 1959; Sklar and
Anisman, 1980, 1981; Riley, 1981). Certainly there appears to be growing
evidence that stress can influence tumor development, as well as immune
competence. The results of this research are variable and often contradictory, with some studies reporting an acceleration of oncogenicity
(Seifter et al., 1973; Sklar and Anisman, 1979; Visintainer et al., 1982)
and others a suppression (Rashkis, 1952; Neuberry et al., 1972; Gershbein
et al., 1974; Pradhan and Roy, 1974). A number of factors have been suggested to account for these discrepancies, including the type of tumor
model utilized, type of stress applied, timing and duration of stress and

whether acute or chronic stress was administered. Exposure to stress can also release opioid peptides, and the purpose of this section is to review our knowledge concerning stress-related opioid activity and tumorigenesis.

Simon and co-workers (1980) have found that electrical stimulation of the midbrain mediates metastatic tumor growth. These investigators discovered that a single session of electrical stimulation of the mesencephalic periaqueductal gray (PAG) region (known to trigger endogenous opioid release) for 7 minutes following intravenous injection of Walker-256 carcinoma cells led to a dramatic increase in the number of "artificial" pulmonary metastases (metastatic-like aggregations which colonize the lung). Intraperitoneal injection of naloxone totally blocked the analgesic effects of the stimulation-produced analgesia (SPA), but did not appreciably block the metastatic effect. In a subsequent study, Simon and colleagues (1984) investigated the influence of the pain suppression system and its associated peptides on tumorigenesis by activating the pain suppressor system directly from the nucleus of the raphe magnus, a non-opioid subsystem. After inducing analgesia by giving a single injection of β-endorphin directly into the nucleus of the raphe magnus, Simon noted an increase in the number of "artificial" pulmonary metastases. This result could be abolished by pretreatment with naloxone. If the nucleus of the raphe magnus was activated by electrical stimulation sufficient to induce analgesia, the metastatic effect was still present but markedly attentuated.

Simon's work showing that SPA of the PAG enhances tumor metastasis, but which was not blocked by naloxone, suggested that the analgesia component was not importantly tied to the increase in neoplasia. However, as noted by Simon, naloxone may not block all opioid receptors. Moreover, opioid receptors on lymphocytes could be mediating some form of tumor enhancement by way of the immune system. To explore this question further, Brechner et al. (1983) designed an experiment in which Fischer 344 rats were implanted with either prolactin-sensitive (13762MT) or prolactin-insensitive (OR-163) tumors and received PAG stimulation. The rationale underlying this experiment was that if immunosuppression is induced by PAG-SPA, both types of tumors would have enhanced growth compared to nonstimulated animals. However, if other mechanisms such as prolactin release (known to be stimulated by opioids) were responsible for rapid tumor growth, then only the growth of prolactin-sensitive tumors would be enhanced compared to controls. Brechner found that the group with the prolactin-sensitive tumors had a statistically higher incidence of enhanced tumor growth than the non-PAG stimulated control group. No differences in tumor growth were observed in rats implanted with the prolactin-insensitive tumor, whether or not they had PAG stimulation. These results suggested that enhanced tumor growth with PAG stimulation may be related to hormonal release rather than immunosuppression.

Another segment of work involving stress-related endogenous opioid activity and cancer comes from studies utilizing the footshock technique. Inescapable foot shock causes a profound analgesia that is antagonized by naloxone (and dexamethasone) when shock is delivered intermittently, but not when it is applied continuously (Lewis et al., 1980). Thus, an equally potent analgesia could be induced by both techniques, but one appears to be mediated by opioid peptides ("opioid stress") and the other does not involve opioids ("nonopioid stress"). In a series of studies (Lewis et al., 1983a, 1983b, Shavit et al., 1983), the relationship between footshock induced stress on tumor growth has been examined. Fischer 344 rats injected with a mammary ascites tumor (13672B) and subjected to inescapable footshock of the "opioid" type manifest an enhanced tumor growth as indicated by decreased survival time and decreased percent survival as monitored over a 30-day post-tumor inoculation period. This

effect was prevented by an opioid antagonist, naltrexone. In a preliminary report (Shavit et al., 1983) the non-opioid stress did not
significantly affect tumor growth. In the absence of stress, naltrexone
(implanted as pellets) did not alter tumorigenicity. In another report,
Lewis et al. (1983b) showed that animals receiving morphine administration
for 4 days before or after tumor inoculation, or for 14 days after tumor
injection, had a decreased survival. The magnitude of morphine's effect
was similar to that caused by footshock of the "opioid" type. Interestingly, animals given morphine for 14 days before tumor inoculation did not
differ from nonstressed controls, suggesting that tolerance developed to
the effect of morphine. In the same study, exposure to footshock of the
"opioid" type for 4 or 14 days before or after tumor injection, or for 4
or 14 days after tumor inoculation, was found to produce equivalent and
significant decreases in the percent of animals surviving and median survival time. Animals receiving morphine treatment for 14 days before tumor
injection and footshock stress ("opioid" type) on the last 4 days of this
treatment still exhibited a significant reduction in survival time, indicating that cross-tolerance had not occurred. Thus, footshock stress (of
the "opioid" type) can alter tumorigenesis in a manner sharing characteristics of opioid involvement (e.g., responsivity to antagonism by
naltrexone) and non-involvement (e.g., no evidence of tolerance or cross-
tolerance). In a recent study, Shavit et al. (1984) has found that
splenic natural killer cell activity was suppressed by the "opioid", but
not the "nonopioid", form of stress and that this suppression was blocked
by naltrexone. A similar suppression of natural killer cell activity was
induced by high doses of morphine. Shavit suggests that immunological
mechanisms may be a common denominator in the alterations of tumorigenicity recorded in footshock stress ("opioid" type) and morphine experiments.

CONCLUSIONS

It is quite clear from this review that endogenous opioid systems
play an important role in tumor biology. As with most exciting new directions, we are only at the initial stages of gathering information and for
every question answered many more are raised. Are opioid receptors
associated with all tumor cells? What is the relationship of endogenous
opioids in the plasma and neoplastic tissues of animals with cancer? Is
endogenous opioid immunomoduation coincident or vitally important to neoplastic processes? Is "opioid stress" causally or coincidentally related
to cancer? Do endogenous opioid systems play a role in human cancer?

At this early junction in this new field, it is often difficult to
see an overall pattern to the pieces of information gathered to date. In
many ways it would seem that we have seemingly conflicting results that
often arrange themselves into two opposing camps: opioids either enhance
or retard carcinogenic processes. Alternatively, I would raise the
question of whether we are really looking at 2 sides of the same phenomenon?
I refer specifically to data gathered in studies with opioid antagonists
and neural tumors. Prevention of endogenous opioid binding to opioid receptors exacerbates neural cancer. Promotion of endogenous opioid-opioid
receptor interaction inhibits neuro-oncogenicity. Admittedly, most of the
evidence gathered so far is drawn from a neural tumor model, yet results
with other tumor systems (e.g., L1210 leukemia, mammary carcinoma), as
well as in vitro experimentation with neural tumor cells, appear to be
entirely consistent with this hypothesis. Support for the novel idea that
endogenous opioid systems regulate cancer also comes from other quarters.
Thompson et al. (1983) has found that gentically obese mice, which have
several times the level of β-endorphin compared to their lean littermates,
show increased resistance to metastasis of B16 melanoma. In a study by

Lee and Lin (1975), the effects of acupuncture (thought to trigger release of endogenous opioids) on the growth of Erlich ascites tumor was studied in mice. Tumor-inoculated mice receiving acupuncture exhibited slower tumor growth and had extended survival time in comparison to control animals. Moreover, it is now quite clear that endogenous opioid systems control the development of most cells and tissues in the body (Zagon and McLaughlin, 1983b, c, 1984b, 1985a, b), extending the concept from only abnormal tissue regulation.

How does one integrate studies utilizing footshock of the "opioid" type, or electrical stimulation of the brain, or direct injections of β-endorphins into the brain within this scheme? On the surface, the results of these studies appear to contradict the idea that endogenous opioids serve to suppress tumorigenicity. If in fact these situations are causally related to cancer, could it be that these procedures actually elevate endogenous opioids for a short time, but then the body goes through a period of readjustment during which time endogenous opioid levels are low. For example, direct injection of β-endorphin into the brain may lead to a compensatory decrease in endogenous opioids for some time. A decrease in endogenous opioid would permit tumor development to accelerate. Thus, influences on the opioid system, as well as reaction to these influences, must be kept in mind when assessing the role of endogenous opioid systems in cancer. Moreover, the repercussions on immunity by short- and long-term effects resulting from perturbations of endogenous opioid systems also need to be given full consideration.

In conclusion, exploration of endogenous opioid systems in regard to tumor biology is proving to be a fascinating and important new frontier of science. Future studies are certain to reveal fundamental insights into neoplasia, as well as normal cell and tissue development. The exciting information gathered from these studies should have an important bearing in designing strategies for prevention and therapeutic intervention of malignant diseases.

ACKNOWLEDGEMENTS

This research was supported by NIH grants NS 20500 and NS 20623 and a Pennsylvania Research Corporation grant.

REFERENCES

Amano, T. Richelson, E., and Nirenberg, M., 1972, Neurotransmitter synthesis by neuroblastoma clones, Proc. Nat'l Acad. Sci., USA, 69:258.

Andersen, N. B., 1966, The effect of CNS depressants in mitosis, Acta Anaesta Scand. Suppl., 22:7.

Arima, E., Byfield, J. E., Finkelstein, J. Z., and Fonkalsrud, 1973, An experimental model for the therapy of mouse neuroblastoma, J. Pediat. Surg., 8:757.

Aylsworth, C. F., Hodson, C. A., and Meites, J., 1979, Opiate antagonists can inhibit mammary tumor growth in rats, Proc. Soc. Exp. Biol. Med., 161:18.

Blalock, J. E. and Smith, E. M., 1980, Human leukocyte interferons: structural and biological relatedness to adrenocorticotropic hormone and endorphins, Proc. Nat'l Acad. Sci., USA, 77:5972.

Blalock, J. E. and Smith, E. M., 1981, Human leukocyte interferon (HuIFN-α): potent endorphin-like opioid activity, Biochem. Biophys. Res. Comm., 101:472.

Blum, R. H., 1970, A history of opium, in: "Society and Drugs. I.

Social and Cultural Observations," Jossey-Bass, Inc., San Francisco.

Blumberg, H. and Dayton, H. B., 1973, Naloxone and related compounds, in: "Agonist and Antagonist Actions of Narcotic Analgesic Drugs," H. N. Kosterlitz, H. O. J. Collins, and J. E. Villareal, eds., Raven Press, New York.

Blumberg, H. and Dayton, H. B., 1974, Naloxone, naltrexone and related noroxymorphones, in: "Narcotic Antagonists," M. C. Braude, L. S. Harris, E. L. May, J. P. Smith, and J. E. Villareal, Raven Press, New York.

Brands, M., Hirst, M., and Gowdey, C. W., 1975, Duration of analgesia in mice after heroin by two testing methods, Canad. J. Physiol. Pharmacol., 54:381.

Brechner, T., Motyka, D., and Sherman, J., 1983, Growth enhancement of prolactin-sensitive mammary tumor by periaqueductal gray stimulation, Life Sci., 32:525.

Brostrom, C. O., Brostrom, M. A., and Wolff, D. W., 1977, Calcium-dependent adenylate cyclase from rat cerebral cortex, J. Biol. Chem., 252:5677.

Brown, S. M., Stimmel, B., Taub, R. N., Kochwa, S., and Rosenfeld, R. E., 1974, Immunologic dysfunction in heroin addicts, Arch. Internal Med., 134:1001.

Brown, D. R., Blank, M. S., and Holtzman, S. G., 1980, Suppression by naloxone of water intake induced by deprivation and hypertonic saline in intact and hypophysectomized rats, Life Sci., 26:1535.

Bruni, J. F., Van Vugt, D., Marshall, S., and Meites, J., 1977, Effects of naloxone, morphine and methionine enkephalin on serum prolactin, luteinizing hormone, follicle stimulating hormone, thyroid stimulating hormone and growth hormone, Life Sci., 21:461.

Chang, K. J., 1984, Opioid peptides have actions on the immune system, Trends Neurosci., 7:234.

Cherubin, C. E. and Brown, J., 1968, Systemic infections in heroin addicts, Lancet, (i):298.

Clement-Jones, V., Corder, R., and Lowry, P. J., 1980, Isolation of human met-enkephalin and two groups of putative precursors from an adrenal medullary tumour, Biochem. Biophys. Res. Comm., 95:665.

Dafny, N., 1983a, Interferon modifies morphine withdrawal phenomena in rodents, Neuropharmacology, 22:647

Dafny, N., 1983b, Modification of morphine withdrawal by interferon, Life Sci., 32:303.

D'Amato, R. and Holaday, J. W., 1984, Multiple opioid receptors in endotoxic shock: evidence for δ involvement and μ - δ interactions in vitro, Proc. Nat'l Acad. Sci., USA, 81:2898.

Epstein, L. B., Rose, M. E., McManus, N. H., and Li, C. H., 1982, Absence of functional and structural homology of natural and recombinant human leukocyte interferon (IFN-α) with human α-ACTH and β-endorphin, Biochem. Biophys. Res. Comm., 104:341.

Faden, A. I. and Holaday, J. W., 1980, Naloxone treatment of endotoxin shock: stereospecificity of physiologic and pharmacologic effects in the rat, J. Pharmacol. Exp. Ther., 212:441.

Faith, R. E., Plotnikoff, N. P., and Murgo, A. J., Effects of opiates and enkephalins-endorphins on immune functions, NIDA Technical Meeting, Boston, in press.

Faith, R. E., Liang, H. J., Murgo, A. J., and Plotnikoff, N. P., 1984, Neuroimmunomodulation with enkephalins: enhancement of natural killer (NK) cell activity in vitro, Clin. Immunol. Immunopathol., 31:412.

Falek, A. and Hollingsworth, F., 1980, Heroin and chromosome damage, Arch. gen. Psychiat., 37:227.

Finkelstein, J. Z., Arima, E., Byfield, P. E., Byfield, J. E., and Fonkalsrud, E. W., 1973, Murine neuroblastoma: a model of human disease, Canc. Chemother, Rep., 57:405.

Fischer, E. G. and Falke, N. E., 1984, β-endorphin modulates immune

Functions - a review, Proc. of VIIth World Congress Intern. College of Psychosomatic Med.

Fischman, H. K., Roizin, L., Moralshoili, E., Joy, C., and Rainer, J. D., 1977, Effects of prolonged administration of "street heroin" on the chromosomes of Macaca mulatti (Rheses) monkeys, in: "Neurotoxicology", L. Roizin, H. Shirakii and N. Grecevic, Raven Press, New York.

Frey, E. A. and Krebabian, J. W., 1984, A μ-opiate receptor in 7315c tumor tissue mediates inhibition of immunoreceactive prolactin release and adenvlate cyclase activity, Endocrinology, 115:1797.

Gayton, R. J., Lambert, L. A., and Bradley, P. B., 1978, Failure of (+)naloxone to antagonize responses to opioid peptides, Neuropharmacology, 17:549.

Geber, W. F. and Schramm, L. C., 1975, Congenital malformations of the central nervous system produced by narcotic analgesics in the hamster, Am. J. Obstet. Gynec., 123:705.

Geber, W. F., Lefkowitz, S. S., and Hung, C. Y., 1975, Effect of morphine, hydromorphine, methadone, mescaline, trypan blue, vitamin A, sodium salicylate, and caffeine on the serum interferon level in response to viral infection, Arch. Int. Pharmacodyn, 214:322.

Geber, W. F., Lefkowitz, S. S., and Hung, C. Y., 1976, Action of naloxone on the interferon-lowering activity of morphine in the mouse, Pharmacology, 14:322.

Gershbein, L. I., Benuck, I., and Shurrager, P. S., 1974, Influence of stress on lesion growth and on survival of animals bearing parenteral and intracerebral leukemia L1210 and Walker tumors, Oncology, 30:429.

Giering, J. E., Davidson, T. A., Shetty, B. V., and Truant, A. P., 1974, in: "Narcotic Antagonists," M. C. Braude, L. S. Harris, E. L. May, J. P. Smith, and J. E. Villarreal, ed., Raven Press, New York.

Gilman, S. C., Schwartz, J. M., Miller, R. J., Bloom, F. E., and Feldman, J. D., 1982, β-endorphin enhances lymphocyte proliferative responses, Proc. Nat'l Acad. Sci., USA, 79:4226.

Güngör, M., Genc, E., Sugduyu, H., Eroglu, L., and Koyuncuoglu, H., 1980, Effect of chronic administration of morphine on primary immune response in mice, Experientia, 36:1309.

Harpel, H. S. and Gautieri, R. F., 1968, Morphine-induced fetal malformations, J. Pharm. Sci., 57:1590.

Hazum, E., Chang, K.-J. and Cuatrecasas, P., 1979, Specific nonopiate receptors for β-endorphin, Science, 205:1033.

Ho, W.K.K. and Leung, A., 1979, Effects of morphine addiction on concanavalin A-mediated blastogenesis, Pharmacol. Res. Comm., 11:413.

Hughes, J., 1975, Isolation of an endogenous compound from the brain with pharmacological properties similar to morphine, Brain Res., 88:295.

Hughes, J. A., Smith, T. W., Kosterlitz, H. W., Fothergill, L. A., Morgan, B. A., and Morris, H. R., 1975, Identification of two pentapeptides from the brain with potent opiate agonist activity, Nature, 258:577.

Hui, F. W., Krikun, E., Hirsh, E. M., Blaiklock, R. G., and Smith, A. A., 1976, Inhibition of nucleic acid synthesis in the regenerating limb of salamanders treated with dl-methadone or narcotic antagonists, Exp. Neurol., 53:267.

Hung, C. Y., Lefkowitz, S. S., and Geber, W. F., 1973, Interferon inhibition by narcotic analgesics, Proc. Soc. Exp. Biol. Med., 142:106.

Hussey, H. H. and Katz, S., 1950, Infections resulting from narcotic addiction: report of 102 cases, Am. J. Med., 9:186.

Iijima, I., Minamikawa, J., Jacobson, A.E., Brossi, A., and Rice, K.C., 1978, Studies in the (+)-morphinan series .5. Synthesis and biological properties of (+)-naloxone, J. Med. Chem., 21:398.

Inoue, N., and Hatankaka, H., 1982, Nerve growth factor induces specific enkephalin binding sites in a nerve cell line, J. Biol. Chem., 257:9238.

Ito, H. and Hidaka, H., 1983, Antitumor effect of a calmodulin antagonist on the growth of solid sarcoma-180, Cancer Lett., 19:215.

Jaffe, E. H. and Martin, W. R., 1980, Narcotic analgesics and antagonists, in: "The Pharmacologic Basis of Therapeutics," L. S. Goodman and A. Gilman, eds., MacMillan Publ. Co., New York, p. 494.

Jasinski, D. R., Martin, W. R., and Haertzen, C. A., 1967, The human pharmacology and abuse potential of N-allylnoroxymorphone (naloxone), J. Pharmacol. Exp. Ther., 159:420.

Johnson, H. M., Smith, E. M., Torres, B. A., and Blalock, J. E., 1982, Regulation of the in vitro antibody response by neuroendocrine hormones, Proc. Nat'l Acad. Sci., USA 79:4171.

Jörnvall, H., Persson, M., and Ekman, R., 1982, Structural comparisons of leukocyte interferon and pro-opiomelanocortin correlated with immuno-logical similarities, FEBS Letters, 137:153.

Klee, W. A. and Nirenberg, M., 1974, A neuroblastoma x glioma hybrid cell line with morphine receptors, Proc. Nat'l Acad. Sci., USA, 71:3474.

Lahti, R. A. and Collins, R. J., 1978, Chronic naloxone results in prolonged increases in opiate binding sites in brain, Eur. J. Pharmacol., 51:185.

Lampert, A., Nirenberg, M., and Klee, W. A., 1976, Tolerance and dependence evoked by an endogenous opiate peptide, Proc. Nat'l Acad. Sci., USA, 73:3165.

Lee, S.-C. and Lin, J.-H., 1975, An inhibitory effect of acupuncture on the growth of Ehrlich ascites tumor cells in mice, Chinese Med. J., 22:167.

Lefkowitz, S. S. and Chiang, C. Y., 1975, Effects of certain abused drugs on hemolysin forming cells, Life Sci., 17:1763.

Lefkowitz, S. S. and Nemeth, D., 1976, Immunosuppression of rosette-forming cells, Adv. Exp. Med. Biol., 733:269.

LeShan, L. L., 1959, Psychological states as factors in the development of malignant disease: a critical review, J. Nat. Cancer Inst., 22:1.

Lewis, J. W., Cannon, J. T., and Leibeskind, J. C., 1980, Opioid and nonopioid mechanisma of stress analgesia, Science, 208:623.

Lewis, J. W., Shavit, Y., Terman, G. W., Nelson, L. R., Gale, R. P., and Liebeskind, J. C., 1983a, Apparent involvement of opioid peptides in stress-induced enhancement of tumor growth, Peptides, 4:635.

Lewis, J. W., Shavit, Y., Terman, G. W., Gale, R. P., and Liebeskind, J. C., 1983b, Stress and morphine affect survival of rats challenged with a mammary ascites tumor (MAT 13762B), Nat. Immun. Cell Growth Regul., 3:43.

Lopker, H., Abood, L. G., Hoss, W., and Lionetti, F. J., 1980, Stereo-selective muscarinic acetylcholine and opiate receptors in human phagocytic leukocytes, Biochem. Pharm., 29:1361.

Lord, J. A. H., Waterfield, A. A., Huges, J., and Kosterlitz, H. W., 1977, Endogenous opioid peptides: multiple agonists and receptors, Nature, 267:495.

Ma, W. C., 1931, A cytological study of acute and chronic morphinism in albino rat, Clin. J. Physiol., 5:251.

Martin. W. R., Eades, C. G., Thompson, J. A., Huppler, R. E., and Gilbert, P. E., 1976, The effects of morphine and nalorphine-like drugs in the non-dependent and morphine-dependent chronic spinal dog, J. Pharmacol. Exp. Ther., 197:517.

Matthews, P. M., Froelich, C. J., Sibbitt, W. L., and Bankhurst, A. D., 1983, Enhancement of natural cytotoxicity by β-endorphin, J. Immunol., 130:1658.

McCain, H. W., Lamster, I. B., Bozzone, J. M., and Grbic, J. T., 1982, β-endorphin modulates human immune activity via-non-opiate receptor mechanisma, Life Sci., 31:1619.

McDonough, R. J., Madden, J. L., Falek, A., Shafer, D. A., Pline, M., Gordon, D., Bokos, P., Keuhule, J. C., and Mendelson, J., 1980, Alteration of T and null lymphocyte frequencies in the peripheral blood of human opiate addicts: in vivo evidence for opiate receptor sites on T lymphocytes, J. Immunol., 125:2539.

McLaughlin, P. J. and Zagon, I. S., 1984, Opioid regulation of tumor cell growth in vitro, Soc. Neurosci., 14th Annual Meeting, 10:111.

Miller, G. C., Murgo, A. J., and Plotnikoff, N. P., 1983, Enkephalins-enhancement of active T-cell rosettes from lymphoma patients, Clin. Immunol., Immunol., Immunopathol., 26:446.

Miller, G. C., Murgo, A. J., and Plotnikoff, N. P., 1984, Enkephalins-enhancement of active T-cell rosettes from normal volunteers, Clin. Immunol. Immunopath., 31:132.

Newberry, B. H., Frankie, G., Beatty, P. A., Maloney, B. D., and Gilchrist, J. C., 1972, Shock stress and DMBA-induced mammary tumors, Psychosom. Med., 34:295.

North-Root, H., Martin, D. W., and Toliver, A. P., 1976, Binding of an opiate, levorphanol, to intact neuroblastoma cells in continuous culture, Physiol. Chem. Physics, 8:221.

Osamura, R. Y., Watanabe, K., Yoshimasa, T., Nakao, K., and Imura, H., 1984, Immunohistochemical localization of met-enkephalin, met enkephalin-arg^6-gly^7-leu^8, met-enkephalin-arg^6-phe^7 and leu-enkephalin in human adrenal medulla and pheochromocytomas, Peptides 5:993.

Perrin, G. M. and Pierce, I. R., 1959, Psychosomatic aspects of cancer, Psychosom. Med., 21:397.

Pert, G. B. and Snyder, S. H., 1973, Opiate receptor: demonstration in nervous tissue, Science, 179:1011.

Plotnikoff, N. P. and Miller, G. C., 1983, Enkephalins as immuno-modulators, Int. J. Immunopharmacol., 5:437.

Plotnikoff, N. P., Miller, G. C., and Murgo, A. J., 1982, Enkephalins-endorphins: immunomodulators in mice, Int. J. Immunopharmacol., 4:366.

Plotnikoff, N. P., Murgo, A. J., Miller, G. C., Corder, C. N., and Faith, R. E., 1985, Enkephalins: immunomodulators, Fed. Proc., 44:118.

Portoghese, P. S., Larson, D. L., Sayre, L. M., Fries, D. S., and Takemori, A. E., 1980, A novel opiate receptor site directed alkylating agent with irreversible narcotic antagonistic and reversible agonistic activities, J. Med. Chem., 23:233.

Pradhan, S. N. and Ray, P., 1974, Effects of stress on growth of transplanted and 7, 12-dimethylbenz(α)anthracene-induced tumors and their modification by psychotropic drugs, JNCI, 53:1241.

Rashkis, H. A., 1952, Systemic stress as an inhibitor of experimental tumors in Swiss mice, Science, 116:169.

Recant, L., Voyles, N. R., Luciano, M., and Pert, C. B., 1980, Naltrexone reduces weight gain, alters "β-endorphin", and reduces insulin output from pancreatic islets of genetically obese mice, Peptides, 1:309.

Riley, V., 1981, Psychoneuroendocrine influences on immunocompetence and neoplasia, Science, 212:1100.

Sano, M. and Kitajima, S., 1983, Ontogeny of calmodulin and calmodulin-dependent adenylate cyclase in rat brain, Dev. Brain Res., 7:215.

Sawynok, J., Pinsky, C., and LaBella, F. S., 1979, Mini-review on the specificity of naloxone as an opiate antagonist, Life Sci., 25:1621.

Schweigerer, H., Bhakdi, S., and Teschemacher, H., 1982, Specific nonopiate binding sites for human β-endorphin on the terminal complex of human complement, Nature, 296:572.

Seifter, E., Rettura, G., Zisblatt, M., Levenson, S. M., Levine, N., Davidson, A., and Seifter, J., 1973, Enhancement of tumor development in physically stressed mice inoculated with an oncogenic virus, Experientia, 29:1379.

Sharma, S. K., Klee, W. A., and Nirenberg, M., 1975a, Dual regulation of adenylate cyclase accounts for narcotic dependence and tolerance, Proc. Nat'l Acad. Sci., USA, 72:3092.

Sharma, S. K., Klee, W. A., and Nirenberg, M., 1975b, Opiate-dependent modulation of adenylate cyclase, Proc. Nat'l Acad. Sci., USA, 74:3365.

Shavit, Y., Lewis, J. W., Terman, G. W., Gale, R. P., Liebeskind, J.C., 1983, Endogenous opioids may mediate the effects of stress on tumor growth and immune function, Proc. West. Pharmacol. Soc., 26:53.

Shavit, Y., Lewis, J. W., Terman, G. W., Gall, R. P., and Liebeskind, J. C., 1984, Opioid peptides mediate the suppressive effect of stress on natural killer cell cytotoxicity, Science, 223:188.

Simantov, R., Nadler, H., and Levy, R., 1982, A genetic approach to reveal the action of the opiate receptor in selected neuroblastoma-glioma cells. Interaction with α-adrenoreceptors, calmodulin and calcium ion ATPase, Eur. J. Biochem., 128:461.

Simon, E. J., 1964, Inhibition of bacterial growth by drugs of the morphine series, Science, 144:543.

Simon, E. J., 1971, Single cells, in: "Narcotic Drugs," D. H. Clouet, ed., Plenum Press, New York.

Simon, E. J., Miller, J. M., and Edelman, I., 1973, Stereospecific binding of the potent narcotic analgesic (^{3}H)etorphine to rat brain homogenate, Proc. Nat'l Acad. Sci., USA, 70:1947.

Simon, R. H., Lovett, E. J., Tomaszek, D., and Lundy, J., 1980, Electrical stimulation of the midbrain mediates metastatic tumor growth, Science, 209:1132.

Simon, R. H., Arbo, T. E., and Lundy, J., 1984, β-endorphin injected into the nucleus of the raphe magnus facilitates metastatic tumor growth, Brain Res. Bull., 12:487.

Sinatra, R. A., Milks, L. C., and Ford,D. H., 1978, Structural alterations in normal and axotomized facial nucleus neurons after treatment with morphine, Experientia, 35:1218.

Singh, V. K., Jakubovιc, A., and Thomas, D. A., 1980, Suppressive effects of methadone on human blood lymphocytes, Immunol. Lett., 2:177.

Sklar, L. S. and Anisman, H., 1979, Stress and coping factors influence tumor growth, Science, 205:513.

Sklar, L. S. and Anisman, H., 1980, Social stress influences tumor growth, Psychosom. Med., 42:347.

Sklar, L. S. and Anisman, H., 1981, Stress and cancer, Psychol. Bull., 89:369.

lotkin, T. A., Seidler, F. J., and Whitmore, W. L., 1980, Effects of maternal methadone administration on ornithine decarboxylase in brain and heart of the offspring: relationships of enzyme activity to dose and to growth impairment in the rat, Life Sci., 26:861.

Smith, E. M. and Blalock, J. E., 1981, Human lymphocyte production of corticotropin and endorphin-like substances: association with leukocyte interferon, Proc. Nat'l Acad. Sci., USA, 78:7530.

Sullivan, S. N., Bloom, S. R., and Polak, J. M., 1978, Enkephalin in peripheral neuroendocrine tumours, Lancet, 1:986.

Takemori, A. E. and Portoghese, P. S., 1985, Affinity labels for opioid receptors, Ann. Rev. Pharmacol., in press.

Takemori, A. E., Larson, D. L., and Portoghese, P. S., 1981, The irreversible narcotic antagonistic and reversible agonistic properties of the fumarate methyl ester derivative of naltrexone, Eur. J. Pharmacol., 70:445.

Tang, A. H. and Collins, R. J., 1978, Enhanced analgesic effects of morphine after chronic administration of naloxone in the rat, Eur. J. Pharmacol., 47:473.

Terenius, L., 1973, Stereospecific interaction between narcotic analgesics and a synaptic plasma membrane fraction of rat cerebral cortex, Acta Pharmacol. Toxicol., 32:317.

Terry, C. E. and Pellens, M., 1970, Pathology-tolerance-dependence-withdrawal, in: "The Opium Problem," C. E. Terry and M. Pellens, eds., Patterson Smith Publishing Corp., New York.

Thompson, C. I., Kreider, J. W., Black, P. L., Schmidt, T. J., and

Margules, D. L., 1983, Genetically obese mice: resistance to metastasis of B16 melanoma and enhanced T-lymphocyte mitogenic responses, Science, 220:1183.

Tubaro, E., Borelli, G., Croce, C., Cavallo, G., and Santiangeli, C., 1983, Effect of morphine on resistance to infection, J. Infectious Dis., 148:656.

Van Epps, E. E. and Saland, L., 1984, β-endorphin and met-enkephalin stimulate human peripheral blood monomuclear cell chemotaxis, J. Immunol., 132:3046.

Visintainer, M. A., Volpicelli, J. R., Seligman, N. E. P., 1982, Tumor rejection in rats after inescapable or escapable shock, Science, 216:437.

Ward, S. J. and Takemori, A. E., 1983, Relative involvement of mu, kappa, and delta receptor mechanisms in opiate-mediated antinociception in mice, J. Pharmacol. Exp. Ther., 224:525.

Ward, S. J., Portoghese, P. S., and Takemori, A. E., 1982a, Pharmacological profiles of β-funaltrexamine (β-FNA) and β-chlornal-trexamine (β-CNA) on the mouse vas deferens preparation, Eur. J. Pharmacol., 80:377.

Ward, S. J., Portoghese, P. S., and Takemori, A. E., 1982b, Pharmacological characteristics in vivo of the novel opiate β-funal-trexamine, J. Pharmacol. Exp. Ther., 220:494.

Way, E. L., Kemp, J. W., Young, J. M., and Grassetti, D. R., 1960, The pharmacologic effects of heroin in relationship to its rate of biotransformation, J. Pharmacol. Exp. Ther., 129:144.

Weber, R. J. and Pert, C. B., 1984, Opiatergic modulation of the immune system, in: Central and Peripheral Endorphins: Basic and Clinical Aspects, E. E. Muller and A. R. Genazzini, ed., Raven Press, NY, p. 35.

Wybran, J., 1985, Enkephalins, endorphins, substance P and the immune system, in:Neural Modulation of Immunity, R. Guillemin, M. Cohn, and T. Melnechuk, eds., Raven Press, NY, p. 157.

Wybran, J., Appelboom, T., Famaey, J.-P., and Govaerts, A., 1979, Suggestive evidence for receptors for morphine and methionine-enkephalin on normal human blood T lymphocytes, J. Immunol., 123:1068.

Yamasaki, Y., Shimamura, O., Kizu, A., Nakazawa, M., and Ijichi, H., 1983, Interactions of morphine with PGE isoproterenal, dopamine and aminophylline in rat mast cells: their effect on IgE-mediated ^{14}C-serotonin release, Agents and Actions, 13:21.

Zagon, I. S. and McLaughlin, P. J., 1977, The effects of different schedules of methadone treatment on rat brain development, Exp. Neurol., 56:538.

Zagon, I. S. and McLaughlin, P. J., 1978, Perinatal methadone exposure and brain development: a biochemical study, J. Neurochem., 31:49.

Zagon, I. S. and McLaughlin, P. J., 1981a, Heroin prolongs survival time and retards tumor growth in mice with neuroblastoma, Brain Res. Bull., 7:25.

Zagon, I. S. and McLaughlin, P. J., 1981b, Naloxone prolongs survival time or mice treated with neuroblastoma, Life Sci., 28:1095.

Zagon, I. S. and McLaughlin, P. J., 1983a, Naltrexone modulates tumor response in mice with neuroblastoma, Science, 221:671.

Zagon, I. S. and McLaughlin, P. J., 1983b, Increased brain size and cellular content in infant rats treated wtih an opiate antagonist, Science, 221:1179.

Zagon, I. S. and McLaughlin, P. J., 1983c, Naltrexone modulates growth in infant rats, Life Sci., 33:2449.

Zagon, I. S. and McLaughlin, P. J., 1983d, Opioid antagonists inhibit the growth of metastatic murine neuroblastoma, Cancer Lett., 21:89.

Zagon, I. S. and McLaughlin, P. J., 1984a, Duration of opiate receptor blockade determines tumorigenic response in mice with neuroblastoma:

a role for endogenous opioid systems in cancer, <u>Life Sci.</u>, 35:409.

Zagon, I. S. and McLaughlin, P. J., 1984b, Naltrexone modulates body and brain development in rats: a role for endogenous opioids in growth, <u>Life Sci.</u>, 35:2057.

Zagon, I. S. and McLaughlin, P. J., 1984c, Opiates alter tumor cell growth and differentiation <u>in vitro</u>, <u>NIDA Res. Monog.</u>, 49:344.

Zagon, I. S. and McLaughlin, P. J., 1984d, An overview of the neuro-behavioral sequelae of perinatal opioid exposure, <u>in</u>: Neuro-behavioral Teratology, J. Yanai, ed., Elsevier Science Publishers, Amsterdam.

Zagon, I. S. and McLaughlin, P. J., 1985a, Opiate antagonist induced regulation of organ development, <u>Physiol. Behav.</u>, in press.

Zagon, I. S. and McLaughlin, P. J., 1985b, Naltrexone's influence on neurobehavioral development, <u>Pharmacol. Biochem. Behav.</u>, in press.

Zagon, I. S., McLaughlin, P. J., Weaver, D. J., and Zagon E., 1982, Opiates, endorphins and the developing organism: a comprehensive bibliography, <u>Neurosci. Biobehav. Rev.</u>, 6:439.

Zagon, I. S., McLaughlin, P. J., and Zagon, E., 1984, Opiates, endorphins, and the developing organism: a comprehensive bibliography, 1982-1983, <u>Neurosci. Biobehav. Rev.</u>, 8:387.

Zagon, I. S. and Schengrund, C.-L., 1978, Neuronal and non-neuronal properties of neuroblastoma cells, <u>Exp. Cell Res.</u>, 114:159.

Zukin, R. S. and Zukin, S. R., 1981, Minireview: multiple opiate receptors: emerging concepts, <u>Life Sci.</u>, 29:2681.

Zukin, R. S. and Zukin, S. R., 1984, The case for multiple opiate receptors, <u>Trends Neurosci.</u>, 7:160.

Zukin, R. S., Sugarman, J. R., Fitz-Syage, M. L., Gardner, E. L., Zukin S. R., and Gintzler, A. R., 1982, Naltrexone-induced opiate receptor supersensitivity, <u>Brain Res.</u>, 245:285.

EFFECTS OF STRESS AND MORPHINE ON NATURAL KILLER CELL ACTIVITY
AND ON MAMMARY TUMOR DEVELOPMENT

James W. Lewis, Yehuda Shavit, Fredricka C. Martin,
Gregory W. Terman, Robert P. Gale, and John C. Liebeskind

Departments of Psychology and Medicine, University of
California, Los Angeles, CA 90024

At the time we began our investigations of the modulation of immune function and tumor development by neural and endocrine opioid systems, several findings suggested that this was a reasonable avenue to explore. For example, focal electrical stimulation of an opioid-rich brain region was found to increase tumor growth (Brechner et al., 1983; Simon et al., 1980), specific brain lesions alter immune functions (Cross et al., 1982; Stein et al., 1982), and immune responses have been correlated with changes in brain neural activity (Besedovsky et al., 1983). Also, evidence was accumulating from in vitro studies that opioids influence the functioning of the immune system (for reviews see Plotnikoff and Miller, 1983; Weber and Pert, 1984). It was our intent to use environmental stressors as stimuli for activating endogenous opioid systems and observe their effects on tumor development and immune competence. Examination of the literature pertaining to the effects of stress on these processes, however, presented us with a somewhat confusing picture. This literature contained a host of seemingly contradictory results: stress can either enhance, suppress, or not affect tumor development or immune function (e.g. Jensen, 1968; Newberry and Sengbush, 1979; Nieburgs et al., 1977; Riley, 1981; Sklar and Anisman, 1981).

This seemingly paradoxical situation was reminiscent of our experience with the phenomenon of stress-induced analgesia. Prior to 1980, several investigators had shown that exposure to stress could elicit an analgesic response in laboratory animals although there was no consensus on the involvement of opioid peptides in this analgesia (cf. Akil et al., 1976 and Hayes et al., 1978). In some cases stress analgesia appeared to be opioid-mediated, in others not. This lack of consensus was, in part, due to the heterogeneity of stressors used by different investigators rendering comparison of results difficult. We demonstrated that a single stressor, inescapable footshock, could cause either an opioid or a nonopioid form of stress analgesia depending upon the parameters of its application: Intermittent footshock stress causes analgesia that appears to be mediated by opioid peptides, whereas exposure to the same intensity of shock delivered in a continuous fashion causes an equipotent analgesia that is nonopioid in nature (Lewis et al., 1980, 1981). Moreover, the opioid analgesic response to intermittent footshock stress has been associated with activation of both central and peripheral opioid systems. Thus, multiple endogenous pain-inhibitory systems exist, and it appears that the temporal parameters of stress administration can critically define which system is activated.

Two general principles were illustrated by these stress analgesia experiments. First, stress is not a unitary phenomenon. The same stressor, inescapable footshock, can elicit qualitatively different responses, opioid- vs. nonopioid-mediated, depending upon the parameters of its application. Second, opioid peptides are not involved in all stress responses; but when they are, both central and peripheral opioid systems can be important. It was our goal, therefore, to begin systematic examination of the effects of stress on immune function and tumor development armed with the knowledge of the importance of stressor parameters and with some understanding of the physiological systems activated by these footshock procedures.

EFFECTS OF STRESS AND MORPHINE ON DEVELOPMENT OF A MAMMARY TUMOR

We investigated the effects of footshock stress on the development of a mammary ascites tumor (MAT 13762B) in Fischer 344 female rats. In accordance with our previous work, two footshock stress paradigms were used: intermittent footshock (2.0 mA, on 1 sec every 5 sec for 10 min), a procedure that releases opioids, and continuous footshock (2.0 mA, on continuously for 2 min), a procedure that elicits nonopioid-mediated analgesia. Note that the only apparent difference between these two stressors is the temporal pattern of their administration: In both cases, stimulus intensity and total "shock on" time are the same.

Groups of rats were subjected to either intermittent shock, continuous shock, or no shock, daily for four days. Three hours after the last stress session, all rats were injected intraperitoneally with MAT 13762B tumor cells. Animals were then returned to their home cages and survival was monitored for 30 days. Exposure to intermittent, but not continuous, footshock was found to cause a significant decrease in survival time and percent of rats surviving compared to nonstressed controls (Shavit et al., 1983b).

Considering our previous work on stress analgesia, the finding that development of MAT 13762B is enhanced by intermittent, but not continuous, footshock stress is suggestive of a role for opioid peptides. In order to establish the involvement of opioids in this, or any biological process, however, several criteria should be considered: the effect should be blocked by opiate antagonist drugs; the effect should be reproduced by administration of opiate drugs; and tolerance should develop upon repeated exposure. Subsequent experiments were conducted to address these issues.

Groups of rats were implanted subcutaneously either with pellets that slowly release naltrexone, a potent opiate antagonist drug, or with placebo pellets. Seven days later, half of the rats in each condition were exposed to 4 daily presentations of intermittent footshock and the remaining rats served as non-stressed controls. The tumor-enhancing effect of stress was prevented in rats implanted with naltrexone pellets (Lewis et al., 1983b). Placebo pellets did not alleviate the adverse effect of footshock stress, nor was there any effect of naltrexone on tumor lethality in non-stressed rats. Furthermore, we found that morphine could mimic the tumor-enhancing effect of intermittent footshock. That is, 4 daily injections of a high dose of morphine (50 mg/kg, s.c.) prior to tumor inoculation resulted in the same pattern of decreased survival time and percent survival as did exposure to intermittent footshock (Lewis et al., 1983a). Taken together, these results are compatible with the hypothesized role of opioids in the tumor-enhancing effect of stress.

Our attempts to satisfy the last criterion for opioid involvement, development of tolerance, were less conclusive. In the case of morphine, tolerance was apparent following 14 daily drug injections. Chronic exposure to intermittent footshock (14 sessions), however, did not diminish the impact of stress on mammary tumor development. In this regard, however, it should be noted that while many opioid-mediated behavioral effects of stress (e.g. analgesia, Lewis et al., 1981) do develop tolerance in 14 days, there is recent biochemical evidence indicating that after chronic stress exposure, stress-induced release of pituitary opioids is enhanced, not reduced, compared to control values (Akil et al., 1985).

Overall, these results suggest that opioid peptides are important mediators of stress-induced enhancement of tumor development. Several possible loci and/or mechanisms of action underlying this effect can be suggested. In our studies of stress analgesia we found that intermittent footshock stress caused the release of enkephalin-like peptides from the adrenal medulla (Lewis et al., 1982a, 1982b). It may be that in addition to their role in analgesia, these opioid peptides, circulating peripherally, interact with tumor cells to affect their proliferation. The occurrence of opioid receptors on MAT 13762B cells is, however, unknown. Alternatively, it may be that opioids enhance tumor development indirectly, via hormonal mechanisms. For example, opioids have been shown to modulate the stress-induced release of several hormones, including prolactin (e.g. Ragavan and Frantz, 1981) and corticosterone (Siegel et al., 1982), a hormone with potent immunosuppressant properties (e.g. Riley, 1981). Thus, it may be that enhanced tumor growth in stressed rats is due either to elevated levels of prolactin, a hormone known to facilitate the growth of MAT 13762B (Bogden et al., 1974), or to compromised immune function (Kreider et al., 1978).

EFFECTS OF STRESS AND MORPHINE ON IMMUNE FUNCTION

In parallel with our studies of the effect of footshock stress on tumor development, we have examined the effect of this same stress procedures on immune function. Since natural killer (NK) cells have recently been suggested to play an important role in immune surveillance against tumors (Herberman and Ortaldo, 1981), we elected to use NK cell cytotoxicity as an index of immunocompetence.

In our initial studies, rats were exposed to the same stressors and stress administration regimen as in the tumor experiments. Three hours after the last stress session, spleens were removed and lymphocytes prepared for use in a standard 4 hour chromium release assay (see Shavit et al., 1984a for details). Congruent with the results of the cancer studies, exposure to intermittent, but not continuous, footshock caused a significant suppression of NK cytotoxic activity. Administration of naltrexone prior to intermittent footshock attenuated this immunosuppression (Shavit et al., 1984a). Moreover, daily administration of morphine, at doses which enhanced tumor development, also reduced the cytotoxicity of NK cells. Finally, as before, tolerance developed to the immunosuppressive effects of morphine but not to that of footshock (Shavit et al., 1983a).

In our most recent work, we have continued to use morphine as a pharmacological probe for studying opioid regulation of NK activity. We have found that administration of a single high dose of morphine ($\geq$20 mg/kg, s.c.) induced NK suppression evident at three hours after drug injection, returning to normal values by 24 hours post-injection (Shavit et al., 1984b). This morphine-induced suppression of NK activity was blocked by naltrexone pretreatment. Several pieces of evidence suggest that the site of action of morphine in regulating NK activity is within the central nervous system: First, a very small amount of morphine, 20 µg, injected into the lateral cerebral ventricle causes as great an immunosuppression as is observed following systemic administration of 1000 times this dose (Shavit et al., 1985); Second, systemic administration of N-methylmorphine, an analog of morphine that does not readily penetrate the blood brain barrier, does not affect NK activity; Finally, the immunosuppressive effect of systemically administered morphine is prevented by intracerebroventricular application of naltrexone.

EFFECT OF OPIATES ON NATURAL KILLER CELL FUNCTION: COMPARISON OF IN VITRO AND IN VIVO STUDIES

Collectively the results of our experiments suggest that exposure to opioids in vivo causes enhanced tumor growth and suppression of NK function. This is in agreement with in vivo studies by others showing facilitatory effects of opioids on tumor development and adverse effects on several indices of immune competence (Cherubin and Brown, 1968; Cherubin and Millian, 1968; Brown et al., 1974; Ho and Leung, 1979; Tubaro et al., 1983; Zagon and McLaughlin, 1981). By contrast, using in vitro methods, others have shown that opioid peptides can either enhance or suppress the responsiveness of T lymphocytes (Chang, 1984; Gilman et al., 1982; McCain et al., 1982; Weber and Pert, 1984), and several opioid peptides appear to enhance the cytotoxic activity of NK cells (Faith et al., 1984; Froelich and Bankhurst, 1984; Kay et al., 1984; Mathews et al., 1983; Wybran, 1985).

In an attempt to resolve or clarify the disparities between in vivo and in vitro actions of opioids, we have carried out the following preliminary studies. Whereas we have reliably observed a suppression of NK cytoxicity 3 hours following injection of morphine in vivo, incubation of NK cells in morphine-containing media (concentrations ranging from 10^{-4} to 10^{-8} M) for 3 hours prior to the NK assay is without effect. These results and those of others (Kay et al., 1984; Mathews et al., 1983) suggest that morphine does not act directly upon NK cells (see however Wybran, 1985). In other work, we have compared the effects of the opiate alkaloid, levorphanol, with that of its opiate-inactive stereoisomer, dextrorphan. In vivo, only levorphanol (10 mg/kg) causes a suppression of NK activity. In vitro, however, it seems that both stereoisomers cause an equivalent, dose-dependent, reduction of NK cytotoxicity (Martin et al., 1985). It appears that the in vivo effects of opioids are mediated via opioid receptors since only morphine and levorphanol are effective. The in vitro effects of these drugs, however, is puzzling and apparently does not rely on opioid receptors since levorphanol and dextrophan, but not morphine, are active under these conditions.

SUMMARY AND CONCLUSIONS

In summary, it is apparent that some, but not all stressors are adequate stimuli for activation of neural and endocrine opioid systems and that opioid peptides released by stress have widespread physiological effects including analgesia, enhancement of tumor development, and immunosuppression. The parallels between the effects of intermittent footshock stress on tumor development and NK activity are striking: Thus far, every manipulation that caused an opioid-mediated effect on tumor development, also did so on measures of NK activity, thereby suggesting that these processes may be causally related.

One theme in psychoneuroimmunological research that has recently gained considerable support is the notion that the impact a particular stressor has on immunity or tumor growth is determined by the degree to which the organism can control the stressor. Originally, it was shown that exposure to inescapable, but not escapable, stressors resulted in a behavioral syndrome called "learned helplessness" (Maier and Seligman, 1976). More recently, work from several laboratories has indicated that exposure to inescapable stress suppressed the proliferative response of T-cells to mitogenic stimulation and facilitated tumor growth, whereas exposure to an equivalent amount of escapable stress is without effect (Laudenslager et al., 1983; Sklar and Anisman, 1979; Visintainer et al., 1982). In a collaborative study with Maier, Ryan, and Laudenslager, we have found that exposure to inescapable, but not escapable, tail-shocks suppresses NK activity (Shavit et al., 1983c). Moreover, it is possible that "perceived controllability" is one of the critical differences between the intermittent and continuous footshock stress procedures employed in our work. Although both stressors are technically inescapable, exposure to intermittent footshock, but not continuous footshock, causes learned helplessness (Maier et al., 1983). Thus, even though the two stressors we have studied have physically equivalent stimulus properties, it is only the stressor that is perceived as uncontrollable that adversely affects the organism.

Several summary messages may be gleaned from the data described in this chapter. For example, continued investigations of stress and immune function and cancer ought to carefully consider the stressors employed noting that a single stressor may cause markedly different effects depending on the particular parameters of its administration. Delineation of the role of opioid peptides in these stress-related phenomena must take into account the existence of multiple opioid systems and the possibility of both central and peripheral sites of action.

REFERENCES

Akil, H., Madden, J., Patrick, R.L., and Barchas, J.D., 1976, Stress-induced increase in endogenous opiate peptides; concurrent analgesia and its partial reversal by naloxone, in: "Opiates and Endogenous Opioid Peptides", H.W. Kosterlitz, ed., Elsevier, Amsterdam.

Akil, H., Shiomi, H., and Matthews, J., 1985, Induction of the intermediate pituitary by stress: Synthesis and release of a nonopioid form of ß-endorphin. Science, 227:424-426.

Besedovsky, H., Del Re, A., Sorkin, E., Da Prada, M., Burri, R., and Honegger, C., 1983, The immune response evokes changes in brain noradrenergic neurons. Science, 221:564-566.

Bogden, A.E., Taylor, D.J., Kuo, E.Y.H., Mason, M.M., and Speropoulos, A., 1974, The effect of perphenazine-induced serum prolactin reponse on estrogen primed mammary tumor-host systems, 13762 and R-35 mammary adenocarcinoma. Cancer Res., 34:3018-3025.

Brechner, T., Motyka, D., and Sherman, J.E., 1983, Growth enhancement of a prolactin-sensitive mammary tumor by periaqueductal gray stimulation. Life Sci., 32:525-530.

Brown, S.M., Stimmel, B., Taub, R.N., Kochwa, S., and Rosenfield, R.E., 1974, Immunologic dysfunction in heroin addicts. Arch. Intern. Med., 134:1001-1006.

Chang, K.-J., 1984, Opioid peptides have actions on the immune system. TINS, 7:234-235.

Cherubin, C.E. and Brown, J., 1968, Systemic infection in heroin addicts. Lancet, i:298-299.

Cherubin, C.E. and Millian, S.J., 1968, Serologic investingations in narcotic addicts I. Ann. Intern. Med., 69:739-742.

Cross, R.J., Brooks, W.H., Roszman, T.L., and Markesbery, W.R., 1982, Hypothalamic-immune interactions: effect of hypophysectomy on neuroimmunomodulation. J. Neurol. Sci., 53:557-566.

Faith, R.E., Liang, H.J., Murgo, A.J., and Plotnikoff, N.P., 1984, Neuroimmunomodulation with enkephalins: Enhancement of human natural killer (NK) cell activity in vitro. Clin. Immun. Immunopath., 31:412-418.

Froelich, C.J., and Bankhurst, A.D., 1984, The effect of ß-endorphin on natural killer cytotoxicity and antibody dependent cellular cytotoxicity. Life Sci., 35:261-265.

Gilman, S.C., Schwartz, J.M., Milner, R.J., Bloom, F.E., and Feldman, J.D., 1982, ß-endorphin enhances lymphocyte proliferative reponses. Proc. Natl. Acad. Sci. (USA), 79:4226-4230.

Hayes, R.L., Bennett, G.J., Newlon, P.G., and Mayer, D.J., 1978, Behavioral and physiological studies of non-narcotic analgesia in the rat elicited by certain environmental stimuli. Brain Res., 155:69-90.

Ho, W.K.K., and Leung, A., 1979, The effect of morphine addiction on concanavalin A mediated blastogenesis. Pharmacol. Res. Commun., 1:413-419.

Herberman, R.B., and Ortaldo, J.R., 1981, Natural killer cells: Their role in defenses against disease. Science, 214:24-30.

Jensen, M.M., 1968, Influence of stress on murine leukemia virus infection. Proc. Soc. exp. Biol. Med., 127:610-614.

Kay, N., Allen, J., and Morley, J.E., 1984, Endorphins stimulate normal human peripheral blood lymphocyte natural killer activity. Life Sci., 35:53-59.

Kreider, J.W., Bartllet, G.L., Purnell, D.M., and Webb, S., 1978, Immunotherapy of an established rat mammary adenocarcinoma (13762A) with intratumor injection of Corynebacterium parvum. Cancer Res., 38:689-692.

Laudenslager, M.L., Ryan, S.M., Drugan, R.C., Hyson, R.L., and Maier, S.F., 1983, Coping and immunosuppression: Inescapable but not escapable shock suppresses lymphocyte proliferation. Science, 221:568-570.

Lewis, J.W., Cannon, J.T., and Liebeskind, J.C., 1980, Opioid and nonopioid mechanisms of stress analgesia. Science, 208:623-625.

Lewis, J.W., Shavit, Y., Terman, G.W., Gale, R.P., and Liebeskind, J.C., 1983a, Stress and morphine affect survial of rats challenged with a mammary ascites tumor (MAT 13762B). Nat. Immun. Cell Growth Regul., 3:43-50.

Lewis, J.W., Shavit, Y., Terman, G.W., Nelson, L.R., Gale, R.P., and Liebeskind, J.C., 1983b, Apparent involvement of Opioid peptides in stress-induced enhancement of tumor growth. Peptides, 4:635-638.

Lewis, J.W., Sherman, J.E., and Liebeskind, J.C., 1981, Opioid and nonopioid stress analgesia: assessment of tolerance and cross-tolerance with morphine, J. Neurosci., 1:358-363.

Lewis, J.W., Tordoff, M.G., Liebeskind, J.C., and Viveros, O.H., 1982a, Evidence for adrenal medullary opioid involvement in stress analgesia. Soc. Neurosci. Abstr., 8:778.

Lewis, J.W., Tordoff, M.G., Sherman, J.E., and Liebeskind, J.C., 1982b, Adrenal enkephalin-like peptides may mediate opioid stress analgesia. Science, 217:557-559.

Maier, S.F. and Seligman, M.E.P., 1976, Learned helplessness: Theory and evidence. J. exp. Psychol. Gen., 105:3-46.

Maier, S.F., Sherman, J.E., Lewis, J.W., Terman, G.W., and Liebeskind, J.C., 1983, The opioid/nonopioid nature of stress-induced analgesia and learned helplessness. J. exp. Psychol. Anim. Behav., 9:80-90.

Martin, F.C., Shavit, Y., Terman, G.W., Pechnick, R.N., Oh, C., and Liebeskind, J.C., 1985, Stereospecificity of opiate immunosuppression in rats. Soc. Neurosci. Abstr., 11.

Mathews, P.M., Froelich, C.J., Sibbit Jr., W.L., and Bankhurst, A.D., 1983, Enhancement of natural cytoxicity by ß-endorphin. J. Immunol., 130:1658-1662.

McCain, H.W., Lamster, I.B., Bozzone, J.M., and Grbic, J.T., 1982, ß-endorphin modulates human immune activity via non-opiate receptor mechanisms. Life Sci., 31:1619-1624.

Newberry, B.H., and Sengbush, L., 1979, Inhibitory effects of stress on experimental mammary tumors. Cancer Detect. Prevent., 2:225-233.

Nieburgs, H.E., Weiss, J., Navarrete, M., Grillone, G., and Siedlecki, B., 1977, Inhibitory and enhancing effects of various stress on experimental mammary tumorigenesis. Cancer Detect. Prevent., 2:463-470.

Plotnikoff, N.P., and Miller, G.C., 1983, Enkephalins as immunomodulators. Int. J. Immunopharmac., 5:437-441.

Ragavan, V., and Frantz, A.G., 1981, Suppression of serum prolactin by naloxone but not anti-ß-endorphin antiserum in stressed and unstressed rats. Life Sci., 28:921-929.

Riley, V., 1981, Psychoneuroendocrine influences on immunocompetence and neoplasia. Science, 212:1100-1109.

Shavit, Y., Depaulis, A., Terman, G.W., Martin, F.C., Gale, R.P., and Liebeskind, J.C., 1985, Evidence for central mediation of morphine's immunosuppressive effects. Fed. Proc., 44:1489.

Shavit, Y., Lewis, J.W., Terman, G.W., Gale, R.P., and Liebeskind, J.C., 1983a, The effects of stress and morphine on immune function in rats. Soc. Neurosci. Abstr., 9:117.

Shavit, Y., Lewis, J.W., Terman, G.W., Gale, R.P., and Liebeskind, J.C., 1983b, Endogenous opioids may mediate the effects of stress on tumor growth and immune function. Proc. West. Pharmacol. Soc., 26:53-56.

Shavit, Y., Lewis, J.W., Terman, G.W., Gale, R.P., and Liebeskind, J.C., 1984, Opioid peptides mediate the suppressive effect of stress on natural killer cell cytotoxicity. Science, 223:188-190.

Shavit, Y., Ryan, S.M., Lewis, J.W., Laudenslager, M.L., Terman, G.W., Maier, S.F., Gale, R.P., and Liebeskind, J.C., 1983c, Inescapable but not escapable stress alters immune function. The Physiologist, 26:A-64.

Shavit, Y., Terman, G.W., Martin, F.C., Gale, R.P., and Liebeskind, J.C., 1984b, Naltrexone-sensitive suppression of the immune system's natural killer cells by morphine. Soc. Neurosci. Abstr., 10:726.

Siegel, R.A., Chowers, I., Conforti, N., Feldman, S., and Weidenfeld, J., 1982, Effects of naloxone on basal and stress-induced ACTH and corticosterone secretion in the male rat - site and mechanism of action. Brain Res., 249:103-109.

Simon, R.H., Lovett, E.J. III, Tomaszek, D., and Lundy, J., 1980, Electrical stimulation of the midbrain mediates metastatic tumor growth. Science, 209:1132-1133.

Sklar, L.S., and Anisman, H., 1979, Stress and coping factors influence tumor growth. Science, 205:513-515.

Sklar, L.S., and Anisman, H., 1981, Stress and cancer. Psychol. Bull, 89:369-406.

Stein, M., Keller, S.E., and Schleiffer, S.J., 1982, The role of brain and the neuroendocrine system in immune regulation - potential links to neoplastic diseases. In: Biological Mediators of Behavior and Disease: Neoplasia, S. Levy, ed., Elsevier, N.Y.

Tubaro, E., Borelli, G., Croce, C., Cavallo, G., and Santiangli, C., 1983, Effect of morphine on resistance to infection. J. Infect. Dis., 148:656-666.

Visintainer, M.A., Volpicelli, J.R., and Seligman, M.E.P., 1982, Tumor rejection in rats after inescapable or escapable shock. Science, 216:437-439.

Weber, R.J. and Pert, C.B., 1984, Opiatergic modulation of the immune system, in: "Central and Peripheral Endorphins: Basic and Clinical Aspects", E.E. Muller and A.R. Genazzani, eds., Raven Press, New York.

Wybran, J., 1985, Enkephalins and endorphins as modifiers of the immune system: Present and future. Fed. Proc., 44:92-94.

Zagon, I.S., and McLaughlin, P.J., 1981, Heroin prolongs survival time and retards tumor growth in mice with neuroblastoma. Brain Res. Bull., 7:25-32.

ENDOCRINE AND IMMUNOLOGICAL RESPONSES TO ACUTE STRESS

F. Berkenbosch, C.J. Heijnen[*], G. Croiset[*], C. Revers,[*]
R.E. Ballieux[**], R. Binnekade, and F.J.H. Tilders

Dept. Pharmacology, Medical Faculty, Free University,
1007 MC Amsterdam; [*]Dept. Immunology, University
Hospital for Children and Youth, Utrecht; [**]Dept.
Clinical Immunology, University Hospital, Utrecht

INTRODUCTION

Although the suggestion that the function of the immune system
is regulated by the endocrine system, was postulated some time ago
(see Selye, 1980; Besedovsky and Sorkin, 1977), the extent of this
interaction is now becoming more obvious by many recent technological
advances in the field of endocrinology and immunology. For instance,
regulation of the immune response by the hypothalamo-pituitary gonadal
axis has been proved to be of great importance (Grossman, 1984) and
also growth hormone (Grossman and Roselle, 1983; Michael et al., 1980)
prolactin (Bercze et al., 1981), glucocorticoids (Munck et al., 1984),
as well as peripheral circulating catecholamines (Johnson et al., 1981;
Del Rey et al., 1981) have been shown to have immunomodulatory capacities.
Recent studies have presented evidence that lymphocytes possess binding
sites for opiates such as morphine and its derivates (Wybran et al.,
1979; Gungor et al., 1980; Lopker et al., 1980). The presence of these
binding sites would indicate that opiates may be able to affect the
immune system directly. In this light, the discovery of the existence
of endogenous opiates such as the enkephalins and endorphins motivated
many workers to study the role of these peptides on immune function.
However, as in other areas of opioid peptide physiology, the effects
of opioid peptides in immune regulation are complex and often paradoxical.

Beta-endorphin and related peptides are produced in large quantities
in the anterior and intermediate lobe of the pituitary gland as cleavage
products from a precursor called pro-opiomelanocortin. It is of interest
that stress, which is known to affect immune function (Riley, 1981),
causes a rapid release of beta-endorphin and related peptides. In this
paper we briefly summarize our studies on the mechanisms involved in
stress-induced beta-endorphin secretion. In addition, effects of endorphins
on the primary immune response in vitro, and effects of acute stress on
the proliferative capacity of rat spleen lymphocytes will be presented.

CLEAVAGE PRODUCTS OF POMC IN CORTICOTROPHS AND MELANOTROPHS

The rat pituitary gland contains two cell types being the cortico-trophs of the anterior lobe and the melanotrophs of the intermediate lobe that both synthesize a precursor call pro-opiomelanocortin (POMC). After its formation POMC is processed by several enzymes resulting in glycosylation, phosphorylation, cleavage and formation of amidated and acetylated products (see for reviews, Eipper and Mains, 1980; Hope and Lowry, 1981; Roberts et al., 1982). The major POMC-derived peptides produced in the corticotrophs are different from those in the melanotrophs, suggesting cell-specific differences in the enzymatic machinery involved in processing of POMC. In both cell types the processing is started by cleavage of the glycosylated and/or phosphorylated precursor into three fragments being pro-gamma-MSH (16K fragment), ACTH and beta-LPH. The processing of POMC in the corticotrophs terminates at this stage, im-plicating that pro-gamma-MSH, ACTH and beta-LPH are major secretory products of this cell type, although beta-LPH can be partially processed to gamma-LPH and beta-endorphin.

In the melanotrophs, the processing proceeds to smaller fragments. For instance, ACTH is further cleaved to alpha-MSH and CLIP, whereas beta-LPH serves as an intermediate presursor for gamma-LPH, beta-endorphin-1-31 and smaller peptides being beta-endorphin-1-27, beta-endorphin-1-26, alpha- and gamma-endorphin. In this cell type the processing is completed by N-terminal acetylation of most of the end products (Mains, Eipper, 1981; Serzinger, Hollt, 1980). It is worth noting that the biological activity can be changed completely by N-acetylation. For instance, N-acetylation of beta-endorphin-1-31 causes a complete loss of its opiate activity (Smyth et al., 1979) and increases the melanotrophic activity of ACTH-1-13 approximately 10-fold (Hofman, Vajima, 1961).

SECRETION OF POMC-DERIVED PEPTIDES IN RESPONSE TO ACUTE STRESS

ACTH, alpha-MSH and beta-endorphin assays

Specific radioimmunoassays for the different POMC-derived peptides are required to obtain relevant information on circulating levels of POMC-derived peptides in the rat. Most of the ACTH immunoreactivity and alpha-MSH immunoreactivity as measured by our ACTH and alpha-MSH assays in samples of rat plasma, behaves chromatographically as ACTH-1-39 and alpha-MSH-1-13. In contrast, in our beta-endorphin assays as in most other beta-endorphin assays, acetylated and non-acetylated beta-endorphin-1-31, beta-endorphin-1-27 and beta-endorphin-1-26 and beta-LPH are measured with identical molar efficiencies (Tilders et al., 1984). In view of these considerations, we will refer only in the case of beta-endorphin to beta-endorphin immunoreactivity (beta-ENDi).

Experimental conditions

Experimental procedures such as handling, transport or injections cannot be avoided when rats are subjected to stress-stimuli such as ether, restraint, etc. Such experimental procedures can cause a complete endocrine stress response by itself, thereby complicating the interpreta-tion of the endocrine response to the actual stressor. In order to avoid such interference, the rats used in our experiments are always carefully adapted to experimental procedures by daily handling (transport, injection, etc.) at least 4 days prior to the experiment. Such adapted rats do not show a significant increase in ACTH, alpha-MSH and beta-ENDi in response to unavoidable experimental procedures (Berkenbosch et al., 1983; 1984).

Effects of acute stress

Expoaure of rats, adapted to experimental procedures as described above, to stressful conditions results in a rapid increase of plasma ACTH concentrations and a concomitant rise in plasma beta-ENDi (Berkenbosch et al., 1983; 1984). This observation is in line with those of others (Guillemin et al., 1977; Rossier et al., 1977) and is usually interpreted by assuming that the corticotrophs release ACTH and beta-endorphin and related peptides simultaneously in response to stress. However, it is not generally known that circulating alpha-MSH levels also rapidly increase after a variety of stress stimuli, indicating that stress also activates peptide secretion from the intermediate lobe (Berkenbosch et al., 1984). Therefore, its seems likely that beta-ENDi released during stress can also partially originate from the melanotrophs.

Analysis of the acute response of plasma alpha-MSH, lead us to conclude that stressors with a strong emotional impact (footshocks, passive avoidance, restraint) are good activators of the intermediate lobe, whereas more systemic stressors (ether, formalin or laparotomy under nembutal anesthesia) are rather poor in this respect (Berkenbosch et al., 1984). Studies with neurointermediate lobectomized rats and with dexamethason to selectively suppress corticotroph cell function show that most of circulating beta-ENDi after systemic stress (e.g. formalin) originates from the corticotroph cells, whereas most circulating beta-ENDi after emotional stress (e.g. restraint) originates from tha intermediate lobe (Berkenbosch et al., 1984).

FACTORS MEDIATING STRESS-INDUCED POMC SECRETION

Involvement of corticotropin releasing factor (CRF) and vasopressin (AVP)

Recently, a 41 amino acid has been isolated from bovine and rat hypothalami, that stimulates ACTH release from the anterior pituitary gland in vivo as well as in vitro (see for review Vale et al., 1983). Subsequently, CRF immunoreactivity has been localized in nerve cells from the paraventricular nucleus and in nerve fibres in the external zone of the median eminence in many species. Two lines of evidence indicate that this CRF peptide plays a key role in both the ACTH and beta-ENDi response to stress. First, anterolateral deafferentation of the hypothalamus, which lead to a loss of CRF-immunostaining in the median eminence (Tilders et al., 1982), completely prevents the ether-induced increase in circulating ACTH and beta-ENDi (Vermes et al., 1981). Second, immunoneutralization of CRF in rats with antisera raised to CRF prevent the increase of ACTH (Linton et al., in press; Tilders et al., 1985) and of beta-ENDi (Tilders, in prep.) to ether, formalin, and laparotomy. In contrast, in vivo administration of antisera to CRF partially inhibit peak beta-ENDi levels after emotional stressors, such as restraint stress and footshock, although the ACTH response to such stressors is completely prevented. In addition, no effect of immunoneutralization can be observed on peak levels of alpha-MSH in response to those stressors. Such observations lead us to conclude that CRF does not play a physiological role in the acute response of the intermediate lobe during emotional stress.

Several lines of evidence also indicate that vasopressin is involved in the control of corticotrophic activity (Gillies et al., 1982). Recently, we studied the physiological importance of AVP in stress-induced ACTH release by use of immunoneutralization with an antiserum to AVP (Linton et al., in press; Tilders et al., 1985). Since a marked attenuation is found of the increase in circulating ACTH in response to formalin and restraint, it could be concluded that AVP plays a role in stress-induced ACTH secretion independent of the type of stress stimulus employed.

Involvement of catecholamines

As pointed out above, a special relationship exists between emotional stimuli and reflex activation of the melanotrophs. Emotional stimuli are known to activate the sympatho-adrenomedullary system and lead to a rapid increase in circulating epinephrine (Kvetnansky et al., 1977) to a concentration which by itself can stimulate peptide secretion from the melanotroph (Berkenbosch et al., 1981; Tilders et al., 1982). The action of epinephrine on beta-ENDi and beta-MSH secretion involves beta-adrenoceptors which are known to be present in the intermediate lobe (Cote et al., 1982) and the activation of which leads to an increased peptide secretion (Tilders et al., 1981; Cote et al., 1982). Studies with propranolol to block beta-adrenoceptors lead us to conclude that catecholamines play an important role in stress-induced beta-ENDi and alpha-MSH secretion from the intermediate lobe (Berkenbosch et al., 1983; 1984). Although such studies do not discriminate between involvement of central or peripheral catecholamines, recent studies using rats subjected to extirpation of the adrenal medulla and/or destruction of the sympathetic nerves, suggest involvement of circulating catecholamines in the intermediate lobe response to acute stress(Kvetnansky et al., submitted).

IMMUNOMODULATORY EFFECT OF ENDORPHINS IN VITRO

In view of the suggested role of endorphins in immune regulation, we investigated the effect of endorphins on the primary antibody response of B-cells in vitro. Isolated human peripheral blood cells consisting of T-lymphocytes, B-lymphocytes and 10-15% monocytes (Boyum, 1968) were cultured with an optimal dose of the antigen ovalbumin (OA; 3 g/ml) (Heijnen et al., 1979) at 37°C in the presence or absence of beta- or alpha-endorphin. Alpha-endorphin represents an enzymatic breakdown product

TABLE 1. Effect of alpha- and beta-endorphin on the number of plaque-forming cells (PFC) in cultures of human peripheral blood.

	CONCENTRATION (M)	PFC/$10^6$1y*
Control	-	1563 ± 49
alpha-endorphin	0.005	1542 ± 37
	0.05	956 ± 28**
	0.5	656 ± 19**
	5.0	622 ± 25**
beta-endorphin	0.005	1822 ± 41**
	0.05	2978 ± 38**
	0.5	1608 ± 41
	5.0	1269 ± 29

For details of the methodology see Heijnen et al., 1979.
*Number of PFC are given per 10^6 lymphocytes recovered after 6 days of culture. Data represent mean ± SEM (n=3).

**Indicates significant difference in PFC formation between control and endorphin-treated cultures (P 0.01).

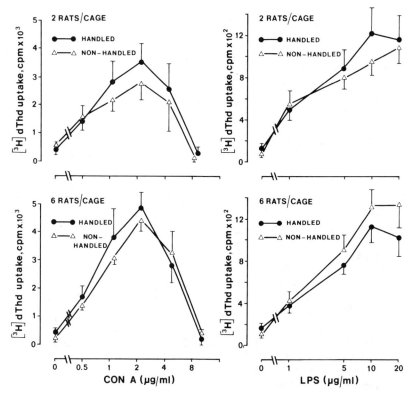

Fig. 1. CON A and LPS proliferation of splenic lymphocytes. Male
Wistar rats (140-160 g) were housed two or six per cage in an air-
conditioned room at 21-22° C for at least 5 days before the experiment. Food and water were freely available. The room was entered
twice daily for adaptation proceures for 4 days before the actual
experiment. These adaptation procedures consisted of opening the
cage, handling and transfering of animals to an adjacent room. On
the day of the experiment, rats were treated identically as
described under adaptation procedure except that they were decapitated
immediately after entering the adjacent room. Trunkblood was
collected in heparinized tubes (0° C) and after centrifugation plasma
was aliquoted and stored at -20°C until use or determination of corticosterone and ACTH. The spleen was removed by using sterile
scissors and immediately transferred to medium for further processing.
Results are expressed as [methyl-^{3}H]-thymidine uptake (cpm) (mean ±
SEM; n=4-6).

of beta-endorphin (1-16). When the antibody response of B-cells was
studied by enumerating the number of plaque-forming cells after 6 days
of culture (PFC) (Heijnen et al., 1979), it could be shown that alpha-
endorphin is capable of inhibiting the PFC-response in a concentration
of 0.05-0.5 M, whereas beta-endorphin possesses an enhancing effect
on the antibody response (see Table I). It is obvious from the results
obtained that the influence of alpha- and beta-endorphin on the PFC-
response occurs in the presence of relatively high concentrations. This
fact does not necessarily implicate that we are dealing with a non-

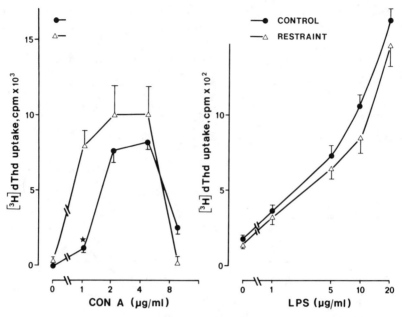

Fig. 2. CON A and LPS induced-proliferation of splenic lymphocytes. Male Wistar rats (140-160 g) were housed six per cage under identical experimental conditions as described in the legend of fig. 1. The adaptation procedure consisted of opening the cage, handling and transfer to an adjacent room. This procedure elsewhere in detail (Berkenbosch et al., 1983) with the exception of a prolonged period of restraining (5 min). Blood and the spleen were obtained in an adjacent room as described in legend 1. Results are expressed as [methyl-^{3}H]-thymidine uptake (cpm) (mean ± SEM; n=6).

physiological effect. The half life of endorphins in medium containing human serum has shown to be short (Burbach et al., 1979), which might explain the need for high concentrations of the peptides in order to exert their regulatory effect. Preliminary studies indicate that one important mechanism by which the endorphins regulate the PFC response is by blocking the production and/or secretion of soluble factors necessary for the differentiation of B-cells into antibody-secreting cells (PFC).

EFFECTS OF ACUTE STRESS ON THE IMMUNE RESPONSE

Experimental conditions

To our knowledge, no systematic studies are available which investigate the reaction of the immune system to short and relatively mild forms of emotional stress, although it can be anticipated that such situations reflect stress stimuli encountered in daily life. Anticipating that the reactivity of the immune system can be influenced by experimental procedures, we first studied the effects of daily handling of rats on the immune response. The reaction of the immune system was tested by measuring the proliferative response of spleen lymphocytes to stimulation in vitro with the T-cell mitogen Concanavalin A (CON A) as well as the B-cell mitogen Lipopolysaccharide (LPS) (Vos et al., 1980). As can be concluded from the experiment shown in fig. 1, a 4 day handling procedure does not significantly alter proliferative response to CON A and LPS. In addition, no marked differences are found between groups of rats that were housed 2 or 6 per cage. However, in some experiments handling introduced a slight but significant enhancement of the proliferative response to CON A. Although we cannot explain this observation as yet, it is feasible that manipulation of the non-handled rats sometimes induces a decrease in the proliferative response.

Effects of acute stress

Exposure of handled rats to the adverisve stimulus restraint during 5 minutes results in a marked enhancement of the proliferative response of isolated spleen cells to CON A (fig. 2), indicating that the response of T-cells to CON A is increased immediately in response to the stress stimulus. Since the effect of the stress stimulus was measured immediately after the restraint procedure, it can be deduced that the influence of the stress stimulus on the immune system is almost momentary. In contrast, the B-cell population does not change its reactivity in response to the restraint stress, as can be concluded from the proliferative response to LPS.

Not every type of acute emotional stress evokes an increase in the reactivity of the immune system. For instance, mild emotional stress caused by a retention session of 5 minutes duration, 24 hours after the delivery of an electric footshock in a passive avoidance paradigm induces a decrease in proliferative capacity of T-cells as well as of B-cells (C.J. Heijnen et al., 1985). The suppression is not only apparent in splenic lymphocyte cultures but also in peripheral blood cell cultures. It should be noted, that in control animals receiving only footshocks, a slight but significant increase in T-cell reactivity and no change in B-cell reactivity can be observed, indicating that the suppression of the T- and B-cell reactivity after the retention session is not caused by the footshock delivered 24 hours earlier. In addition, replacement of the retention session by a restraint stress of 5 minutes duration does not result in a decrease but in a dramatic potentiation of proliferating capacity of T-cells without affecting reactivity of the B-cell population. Therefore, the decrease of lymphocyte proliferation after the retention trial is not the result of summation of repeated stimuli but is related to the nature of the retention session itself. From these data the conclusion is warranted that short and mild emotional stress causes immediate changes in the reactivity of the immune system and that the reaction pattern is depending on the nature of the stress stimulus. We hypothesize that the emotional stress experienced in a conflict situation (e.g. passive avoidance) may lead to a prompt reduction of the immune system reactivity, whereas the adversive reaction induced by a sudden novel situation (e.g. restraint, footshock) may lead to a rapid increase in the reactivity of the immune system.

CONCLUDING REMARKS

From data presented in this paper it can be concluded that acute stress clearly affects the proliferative capacity of lymphocytes either originating from the spleen or from the circulation. However, it should be noted that such changes do not necessarily reflect alterations in humoral or cellular immunity. It would be of interest to know whether acute stress affects antibody synthesis or the delayed hypersensitivity to different antigens. Preliminary results in rats indeed indicate that the primary immune response to sheep red blood cells is affected by acute stress (personal observations).

The coincidence between changes in beta-ENDi release and changes in the immune reactivity in response to acute stress may suggest that these phenomena are interconnected. This suggestion finds support in the effects of endorphins on the primary immune response as demonstrated in vitro (Table I). However, it is worth noting that also other substances such as catecholamines, enkephalins and prolactin which are putative modulators of the immune system, are rapidly released in response to acute stress. Therefore, it can be anticipated that the reaction pattern of the immune response to acute stress may be the result of the interaction of many stress-labile substances on the level of the lymphocytes.

REFERENCES

Berezi, I., Nagy, E., Kovacks, K. and Horvath, E., 1981, Regulation of humoral immunity in rats by pituitary hormones, Acta Endocrinol., 98:506.

Berkenbosch, F., Tilders, F.J.H. and Vermes, I., 1983, Beta-adrenoceptor activation mediates stress-induced secretion of beta-endorphin and related peptides from intermediate but not anterior pituitary, Nature, 305:237.

Berkenbosch, F., Vermes, E., Binnkade, R. and Tilders, F.J.H., 1981, Beta-adrenergic stimulation induces an increase of plasma levels of immunoreactive alpha-MSH, beta-endorphin, ACTH and corticosterone, Life Sci., 29:2249.

Berkenbosch, F., Vermes, I. and Tilders, F.J.H., 1984, The beta adrenoceptor blocking drug propranolol prevents secretion of immunoreactive beta-endorphin and alpha-melanocyte stimuli, Endocrinology, 115:1051.

Besedovsky, H. and Sorkin, E., 1977, Network of immunoneuroendocrine interactions, Clin. Exp. Immunol., 27:1.

Boyum, A., 1968, The isolation of lymphocytes with density gradients, Scand. J. Clin. Lab. Invest., suppl. 97:77.

Burbach, H.P.G., Loeber, J.G., Verhoef, J., de Kloet, E.R. and de Wied, D., 1979, Biotransformation of endorphins by a synaptosomal plasma membrane preparation of rat brain and by human serum, Biochem. Biophys. Res. Comm., 86:1296.

Cote, T.E., Eskay, R.L., Frey, E.A., Grewe, C.W., Munemura, M., Stoof, J.C., Tsuruta, K. and Kebabian, J.W., 1982, Biochemical and physiological studies of the beta-adrenoceptors and the D-2 dopamine receptor in the intermediate lobe of the rat pituitary gland: A review, Neuroendocrinol., 35:217.

Del Rey, A., Besedovsky, H.O., Sorkin, E., Da Prada, M. and Arrenbrecht, S., 1981, Immunoregulation mediated by the sympathetic nervous system, II, Cel. Immun., 63:329.

Eipper, R.A., and Mains, R.E., 1980, Structure and biosynthesis of pro- adrenocorticotropin/endorphin and related peptides, Endocrine Rev., 1:1.

Gillies, G.E., Linton, E.A. and Lowry, P.J., 1982, Corticotropin releasing activity of the new CRF is potentiated several times by vasopressin, Nature, 299:355.

Grossman, C.J., 1984, Regulation of the immune system by sex steroids, Endocrine Rev., 5:435.

Grossman, C.J. and Roselle, G.A., 1983, The interrelationship of the HPG-thymic axis and immune system regulation, J. Steroid Biochem., 19 (1B):461.

Guillemin, R.T., Vargo. J., Rossier, J., Minick, S., Ling, M., Rivier, J., Vale and Bloom, F.E., 1977, Beta-endorphin and adrenocorticotropin are secreted concomitantly by the pituitary, Science, 197:1367.

Gungor, M., Genc, E., Sagduyu, H., Eroglu, L. and Koyunoglu, H., 1980, Effect of chronic administration of morphine in primary immune response in mice, Experientia, 36:1309.

Heijnen, C.J., Uytdehaag, F., Gmelig-Meyling, F.J.J., and Ballieux, R.E., 1979, Localization of human antigen-specific helper and suppressor function in distinct T-cell subpopulations, Cellular Immmnol., 43:282.

Heijnen, C.J., Croiset, G., Bevers, C., Veldhuis, H.D., de Wied, D. and Ballieux, R.E., 1985, Interactions between the central nervous system and the immune system. In: New concepts óf regulation of autonomic, neuroendocrine and immune systems, H.C. Hendrie, Ed. Martinus Nijhoff, The Hague.

Hofman, K. and Vajima, H., 1961, Studies on polypeptides XX: synthesis and corticotropin activity of a peptide amide corresponding to N-terminal tridecapeptide sequence of the corticotropins, J. Am. Chem. Soc. 83:2289.

Hope, J., Lowry, P.J., 1981, Pro-opiomelanocortin: The ACTH/LPH common precursor molecule, Front. Horm. Res., 8:44.

Johnson, D.L., Ashmore, R.E., and Gordon, M.A., 1981, Effects of beta-adrenergic agents on the murine lymphocyte response to mitogen stimulation, J. Immunopharmac., 3:205.

Kvetnansky, R., Sun, C.L., Lake, C.R., Thoa, N., Torda, R. and Kopin, I.J., 1977, Effect of handling and forced immobilization on rat plasma levels of epinephrine, norepinephrine and dopamine-beta-hydroxylase, Endocrinology, 103:1868.

Kvetnansky, R. Tilders, F.J.H., Van Zoest, I.D., Dobrakovova, M., Berkenbosch, F., Culman, J., Zeman, P. and Smelik, P.G., Sympatho-adrenal activity does not potentiate ACTH secretion but facilitates beta-endorphin and alpha MSH secretion during immobilization stress, submitted.

Linton, E.A., Tilders, F.J.H., Hodgkindon, S., Berkenbosch, F., Vermes, I. and Lowry, P.J., Stress-induced secretion of ACTH in rats is inhibited by administration of antisera to bovine corticotropin releasing factor and vasopressin, Endocrinology, in press.

Lopker, A., Abood, L.G., Moss, W. and Lionetti, F.J., 1980, Stereoselective muscarinic acetylcholine and opiate receptors in human phagocytic leukocytes, Biochem. Pharmacol., 29:1361.

Mains, R.E. and Eipper, R.A., 1981, Differences in posttranslational processing of beta-endorphin in rat anterior and intermediate pituitary, J. Biol. Chem., 256:5683.

Michael, S.D., Taguchi, O. and Nishizuka, Y., 1980, Effect of neonatal thymectomy on ovarian development and plasma LH, FSN, GH and PRL in the mouse, Biol. Reprod., 22:343.

Munck, A., Guyre, N.G. and Holbrook, N.G., 1984, Physiological functions of glucocorticoids in stress and their relation to pharmacological actions, Endocrine Rev., 5:25.

Riley, V., 1981, Psychoneuroendocrine influences on immunocompetence and neoplasia, Science, 212:1100.

Roberts, J.L., Chen, C.C., Eberwine, J.J., Eviner, M.J.A., Herbert, E. and Schachter, R.S., 1982, Glucocorticoid regulation of pro-opiomelanocortin gene expression in rodent pituitary, Rec. Prog. Horm. Res., 38:227.

Rossier, J., Grensch, E.D., Rivier, C., Ling, N., Guillemin, R. and Bloom, F.E., 1977, Footshock induces stress and increases beta-endorphin levels in blood but not in brain, Nature, 270:618.

Seizinger, B.R. and Hollt, V., 1980, In vitro biosynthesis and N-acetylation of beta-endorphin in pars intermedia of the rat pituitary gland, Biochem. Biophys. Res. Comm., 96:535.

Selye, H., 1980, ed. Selye's guide to stress research, Vol. I., Van Nostrand Reinhold Co., New York.

Smyth, D.G., Massey, D.E., Zakarian, S. and Finnie, M.D.A., 1979, Endorphins
are stored in biologically active and inactive forms: isolation of
alpha-N-acetyl peptides, Nature, 279:252.

Tilders, F.J.H., Berkenbosch, F., and Smelik, P.G., 1982, Adrenergic
mechanisms involved in the control of pituitary-adrenal activity in
the rat: a beta-adrenergic stimulatory mechanism, Endocrinology,
110:114.

Tilders, F.J.H., Berkenbosch, R. and Vermes, I., 1984, Stress-induced
secretion of immunoreactive beta-endorphin in rats: Role of a beta-
adrenoceptor mechanism, In: Central and perpheral Endorphins: Basic
and clinical effects, E.E. Muller and A.R. Ganazzani, ēds., 115.

Tilders, F.J.H., Berkenbosch, F., Vermes, I., Linton, E.A. and Smelik,
P.G., 1981, Beta-adrenergic stimulation of the release of ACTH- and
LPH-related peptides from the pars intermedia of the rat pituitary
gland, Acta Endocrinol., 97:343.

Tilders, F.J.H., Schipper, J., Lowry, P.J. and Vermes, I., 1982, Effect
of hypothalamic lesions on the presence of CRF-immunoreactive nerve
terminals in themedian eminence and on the pituitary-adrenal response
to stress, Reg. Pept., 5:77.

Vale, W., Rivier, C., Brown, M., Spiess, J., Koob, G., Swanson, L.,
Bilezikjan, L., Bloom, F. and Rivier, J., 1983, Chemical and biolo-
gical characterization of corticotropin releasing factor. Rec. Progr.
Horm. Res., 39:245.

Vermes,I., Berkenbosch, F., Tilders, F.J.H. and Smelik, P.G., 1981,
HYpothalamic deafferentation in the rat appears to discriminate
between the anterior loße and intermediate lobe response to stress,
Neurosci. Lett., 27:89.

Vos, J.G., Kreeftenberg, J.G., Kruijt, B.C., Kruizinga, W., and Stierenberg,
P.A., 1980, The athymic rat. II Immunological characteristics, Clin.
Immunol. Immunopathol., 15:229.

Wybran, J., Appelboom, T., Famaey, J.P. and Govaerts, A., 1979, Suggestive
evidence for receptors for morphine and methionine-enkephalin on
normal human blood T-lynphocytes, J. Immunol., 123:1068.

A COMPLETE REGULATORY LOOP BETWEEN THE IMMUNE AND NEUROENDOCRINE SYSTEMS

OPERATES THROUGH COMMON SIGNAL MOLECULES (HORMONES) AND RECEPTORS

Eric M. Smith and J. Edwin Blalock

University of Texas Medical Branch
Galveston, Texas 77550

INTRODUCTION

A link between an individual's psyche and ability to resist disease has been noted for a number of years but was largely based on anecdotal and phenomenological reports. While many mechanisms are possible, a large body of evidence has recently accumulated suggesting a circuit between the nervous, endocrine and immune systems, that operates in both directions. Both structural and functional evidence supports this relationship. Structural studies have shown the thymus, spleen, bone marrow, and possibly other lymphoid organs are innervated with both afferent and efferent nerve fibers (for review see reference 1). Specific perturbations of the central nervous system (CNS) such as brain lesioning (2) or sympathectomy (3) will enhance or suppress immune responses. Also, alterations in noradrenaline turnover and neuron firing rates have been observed in the hypothalamus at the height of an immune response (4,5). In addition to these "hard wired" connections, modulation of immune responses may occur indirectly through neuroendocrine hormones and neurotransmitters such as corticotropin (ACTH), endorphins (END), enkephalins (ENK), vasoactive intestinal peptide (VIP), as well as others (6-9; for review see 10). These hormones and neurotransmitters have been shown to modulate antibody production (7,11), T lymphocyte rosetting (6,12), natural killer (NK) cell activity (13-15), response to mitogens (16), and other examples reviewed in reference 10.

The interaction appears to be a complete circuit in that products of the immune system can also modulate nervous and neuroendocrine system responses. One way this appears to occur is through the production of neuroendocrine hormone-related peptides by stimulated lymphocytes. We recently found that virus-infected lymphocytes produce immunoreactive (ir) ACTH and END that appear identical to their pituitary counterparts on the basis of structure and function (17,18). Lolait et al. (19) found that non-stimulated mouse macrophages also synthesize ir ACTH and END. Furthermore, other products of the immune system such as the thymic hormone, thymosin (α-1) (20), or noncharacterized factors (21) are able to induce an endocrine response such as adrenal gland steroidogenesis. The production of neuroendocrine hormones by leukocytes and the effect of these hormones on primary antibody responses are major interests of our laboratory and thus will be the subject of this review. Two in vivo demonstrations of these responses will be described as an attempt to put this phenomena in a physiologic perspective.

Our prototype and best studied system of lymphocyte-derived hormones involves the production of the proopiomelanocortin (POMC) products ACTH and END in Newcastle disease virus (NDV)-infected lymphocytes (17,18). Initial screening for production of hormones by lymphocytes was accomplished by immunofluorescent staining with a variety of monospecific antisera to neuroendocrine hormones. Six to eight hours post infection with NDV, the lymphocytes began to stain positive for both ACTH and END (17). Interferon-α (IFN-α) was synthesized concomitantly with the ACTH and END (17). Presumably both T and B lymphocytes can synthesize these POMC-related products because, if 100% of the cells are infected and producing NDV antigens, 100% of the cells also synthesize ACTH and END. Lolait et al. (19) found ACTH and END were also produced constituitively by nonstimulated macrophages. If different inducers are used such as foreign cells, which primarily stimulate B lymphocytes (17,22), only 20-30% of the cells stained positive with anti-ACTH antiserum. The B-cell mitogen, lipopolysaccharide (LPS), also induces 20-30% of the lymphocytes to produce ACTH and END . Therefore, the majority of leukocytes appear able to synthesize ACTH and END when properly stimulated. These molecules are synthesized de novo, since the ir hormones can be inhibited by induction in the presence of actinomycin D and cycloheximide (23). Further evidence of de novo synthesis is that the peptides can be intrinsically labeled by inducing the lymphocytes in the presence of radiolabeled amino acids (18).

Structurally, the lymphocyte-derived ACTH and END are very similar if not identical to their pituitary counterparts. irACTH and pituitary ACTH share: antigenicity, molecular weight, resistance to inactivation by acid, and migration time on reverse phase HPLC (18). Sizing on SDS polyacrylamide gels shows the molecular weight of the ACTH-like molecule is 4.5 kd, which is identical with the full 39 amino acid ACTH molecule (17). The irEND, like β-END, has an apparent molecular weight of 3.6 Kd (24).

Functionally, lymphocyte-derived ACTH is also very similar to pituitary ACTH. The ir ACTH induces both steroidogenesis in mouse adrenal tumor cells and morphologic change (rounding) (17,24). Lymphocyte END also is biologically active, binding to opiate receptors both in vitro and in vivo (17,25). When analyzed by polyacrylamide gel electrophoresis (PAGE) the ir END had a molecular weight less than 5 kd. In vivo intracerebral inoculation of mice with the ir END induced a transient analgesia and catatonia (25). These effects could be immediately reversed or prevented by the opiate antagonist naloxone. Therefore, during an infection lymphocytes may be able to affect pain sensations, temperature regulation, neurotransmission, or other opiate-mediated functions by secretion of END.

Although, initially we thought the ACTH and IFN-α were products of the same gene (26), it is clear now that they are products of different genes which are induced concomitantly. The evidence for this is three-fold. First, the published cDNA sequences of the different IFN-α mRNA species do not contain any ACTH-related sequences. Secondly, the two polypeptides can be dissociated by acid treatment with full retention of IFN's antiviral activity and ACTH's steroidogenic activity (17). Finally, lymphocyte production of ACTH and END can be blocked by the synthetic glucocorticoid, dexamethasone, with no effect on IFN-α synthesis (23). Thus, the two genes can be differentially regulated. It appears that the same POMC gene expressed in pituitary cells is induced in leukocytes. POMC-related RNA can be detected in the BCL_1, B-cell line and in LPS stimulated murine splenocytes (27). This RNA is polyadenylated, but approximtely 200 base pairs longer than mRNA extracted from the AtT-20 pituitary tumor cell line.

Therefore, except for the final, conclusive characterization by sequence analysis, the lymphocyte ACTH and END polypeptides appear identical to their pituitary counterparts and to be products of the same gene.

Hormone production by the immune system is not limited to the POMC derived peptides but also includes immunoreactive (ir) thyrotropin (TSH) (28), vasoactive intestinal peptide (VIP)(29) and somatostatin (30). This laboratory is currently trying to determine the spectrum of peptide hormones which are made by the immune system and the stimuli which elicit their production. Preliminary immunohistochemical studies suggest that leukocytes, in addition to ACTH, END, and TSH also have the potential to produce chorionic gonadotropin (CG) when stimulated in a mixed lymphocyte culture (Table 1).

A Lymphoid Adrenal Axis

If the lymphocyte derived ACTH is biologically relevant, it should be able to replace pituitary ACTH and induce a "stress" response, such as adrenal corticosteroid release. This hypothesis was tested in a deletion type of experiment in which hypophysectomized mice were inoculated with NDV to induce ir ACTH. As a measure of stress the animal's serum was assayed for increases in corticosterone levels. There was a time-dependent increase in corticosterone and interferon which peaked approximately 8 h post inoculation (31). The splenocytes from the NDV infected hypophysectomized mice stained positive for both ACTH and END whereas control mouse splenocytes had no specific staining with either antiserum. Interestingly, if the mice were given dexamethasone per os 12h prior to the NDV there was no significant rise in circulating corticosterone and the splenocytes did not stain by IF with antiserum to ACTH. This experiment suggested that stimulated splenocytes can produce the ir ACTH in vivo and it is synthesized in biologically significant quantities. Furthermore, the inhibition by dexamethasone suggested that as in the pituitary, ACTH production by lymphocytes is under negative control by glucocorticoids (23,31). These findings strongly suggest the existence of a lymphoid-adrenal axis. An essentially identical time course of corticosterone production in response to NDV was observed in intact mice (data not shown). A similar system has also been observed in chickens (32) and humans. Specifically, we have preliminary data which shows that

Table 1. Leukocytes Produce Different Hormones Depending upon the Stimulus

Hormone	Stimulus	Reference
ACTH, END	Virus (NDV, HSV), Foreign cells, LPS Staph Protein A[a], CRF	17,18,19,24
TSH	T-lymphocyte mitogens (SEA[b])	28
CG	MLC[c]	–

[a]Staphylococcus protein A
[b]Staphylococcus enterotoxin A
[c]Mixed lymphocyte culture

typhoid vaccine induces lymphocyte ir ACTH in both normal and hypopituitary individuals (W.J. Meyer, E.M. Smith, G.E. Richards, A. Cavallo, A.C. Morrill, and J.E. Blalock, manuscript submitted for publication).

Preliminary studies of the effect of immunosuppression on virus induced increases in corticosterone in normal mice were done to determine whether the immune system or the pituitary gland caused the response. Beginning at birth, mice were depleted of B lymphocytes by treatment with rabbit antibody to the μ chain of mouse IgM. Whereas herpes simplex virus (HSV) infection of the eye caused a doubling in corticosterone levels in 5 out of 6 control mice, only 1 out of 6 of the B lymphocyte depleted mice showed an elevation of corticosterone relative to the uninfected controls. Thus, in addition to NDV, HSV can cause an increase in corticosterone levels in normal mice and this response seems to be mediated through lymphocytes rather than the pituitary gland (C. Jordan, E.M. Smith, G.J. Stanton, W.J. Meyer, and J.E. Blalock, unpublished observation).

Lymphocyte Derived END May be a Mediator in Endotoxic Shock

A pathogenic mechanism in which lymphocyte END may be a component has recently come to our attention. It seems that both lymphocytes and ENDs are involved in the pathophysiologic changes that occur during endotoxic shock. This is based on data showing that both naloxone (33), an opiate antagonist, and lymphocyte depletion (34) blocked the physiologic changes induced by LPS (endotoxin) administration. We wondered whether LPS induced lymphocyte END production as was seen with virus infection (17) and if that could be a mediator of endotoxic shock. Therefore, leukocytes were examined for the ability to produce ir END in response to LPS (35). Human peripheral blood lymphocytes and mouse spleen cells were cultured with LPS for 48h in the presence of radiolabeled amino acids. Culture supernatant fluids were passed over an anti-γ-END immunoaffinity column and the bound material sized by gel filtration chromatography. Radiolabeled ir END which eluted from the affinity column co-migrated with α and γ-END molecular weight standards at approximately 1800 daltons. The ir END also competed in a dose dependent fashion with dihydromorphine for opiate receptors in the in vitro receptor assay (25). These results indicated that LPS can stimulate lymphocytes to synthesize ir END. Thus, lymphocytes may be a peripheral source of END and responsible for some of the pathophysiologic changes induced during endotoxic shock. The result that a 1800d END was induced by LPS rather than the 3500d β-END size molecule seen in virus and CRF stimulated lymphocytes and a 2400d ACTH versus a 4500d molecule suggest that different stimuli may induce different processing mechanisms in the lymphocytes.

Immunoregulation by Neuroendocrine Hormones

Our laboratory and others have examined several neuroendocrine hormones for the ability to modulate immune responses. Our reasons for this were two-fold. One was to determine if pituitary hormones have a direct effect on the immune system. The other reason was the possibility that the ir hormones produced by leukocytes were immunoregulatory. Due to the lack of copious quantities of the ir hormones, their impure state, and the close similarity both functionally and structurally, pituitary derived hormones were used for these studies rather than the lymphocyte products. Both ACTH (1-39) and α-endorphin at a concentration of 0.5 μM suppressed over 80% of the in vitro antibody response to the T cell dependent antigen, sheep erythrocytes (SRBC) (7). ACTH also suppressed antibody production to a T-cell independent antigen, dinitrophenyl-Ficoll. Interestingly, only the full (39 amino acid) length ACTH suppresses the in vitro antibody response. Neither ACTH (1-24) or ACTH (1-13) are significantly active in this system (36). Furthermore, only the full ACTH (1-39) and not any shorter fragments will suppress the production of the lymphokine IFN-γ (36). In contrast to α-END, β and γ-END were minimal inhibitors (approximately 20% suppression) at 5-6 μM. However, (Met) and (Leu) enkephalins showed moderate suppression (approximately 60% suppression) at 0.2-2 μM. The interaction appeared to be specifically mediated through opiate receptors since naloxone and β-endorphin blocked the α endorphin mediated suppression of antibody production.

In contrast to ACTH and END, thyrotropin (TSH) enhances the in vitro antibody response to SRBC (11). Therefore, the alteration of each immune response is dependent upon the type and length of the hormone.

The immunomodulation appears to be mediated through specific receptors on the lymphocytes. Binding studies with ^{125}I-labeled ACTH suggest that mouse splenocytes possess approximately 3,000 high affinity (Kd 0.1 nM) and 50,000 lower affinity (5 nM) binding sites per average cell (7). This compares favorably with binding studies using isolated purified mouse adrenal cell ACTH receptors which had high and low affinity binding sites with Kds of 0.03 nM and 1 nM respectively (Bost and Blalock, submitted for publication). Binding studies with (^{3}H)-met-enkephalin showed mouse spleen cells possessed approximately 17,000 high affinity (kd=5.9x10^{-10} M) receptors per cell. The receptor binding assay was a membrane preparation of whole mouse spleen so the number of receptor sites per cell is an average of the whole spleen cell population. More than likely future studies of pure cell populations could demonstrate a greater number of receptors on limited cell types. Preliminary structural studies of the lymphocyte ACTH receptor show that it is composed of four subunits, totaling 225 Kd for the intact receptor and is very similar to adrenal cell ACTH receptors (Bost and Blalock, manuscript submitted for publication).

Thus it appears that immunoregulation by neuroendocrine hormones occurs through specific interaction with receptors, and varies with the particular hormone. Also, these results suggest that lymphocyte-derived hormones may play a role in regulating immune responses. The differential effects of various sized ACTH and END species puts a special emphasis on the apparent differential processing of the lymphocyte-derived hormones in response to different inducers. It suggests that differential processing of these molecules by the lymphocyte may be a way for inducers to alter in varied ways immune responsiveness.

Hypothalamic Modulation of the Immune System

During the in vivo studies of irACTH production in response to typhoid vaccine, we found that insulin tolerance testing would also induce irACTH synthesis. Since neither insulin or hypoglycemia treatment of lymphocytes was effective, corticotropin releasing factor (CRF) was evaluated as a possible mediator. In vitro, synthetic CRF was observed to cause the de novo synthesis and release of leukocyte derived ACTH and β-endorphin (24). While it occurred at about 10 fold higher concentrations, arginine vasopressin (AVP) alone was also observed to have intrinsic CRF activity. At concentrations (1-10nM) that are frequently used on cultured pituitary cells, CRF and AVP together acted in an additive fashion to induce these proopiomelanocortin (POMC) derived peptides and such induction was blocked by dexamethasone. Thus, leukocytes seem quite similar to anterior pituitary cells with respect to control of the POMC gene by positive hypothalamic signals (CRF and AVP) and feedback inhibition by a synthetic glucocorticoid hormone.

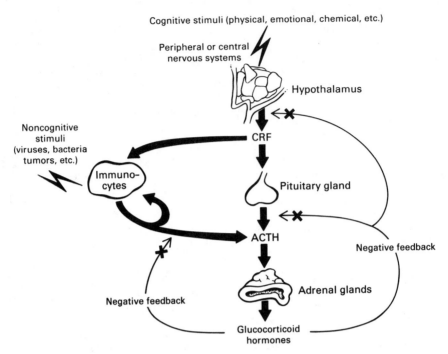

Fig. 1. A regulatory circuit between the immune and central nervous
systems mediated by ACTH reproduced with permission from
Blalock et al. (37).

A Complete Regulatory Circuit Betweens the Immune and Neuroendocrine Systems

The synthesis of neuroendocrine hormones and possession of high
affinity receptors for these same hormones by leukocytes provides the
molecules for a bidirectional regulatory circuit between the immune and
neuroendocrine systems. The ability of pituitary-derived ACTH, endorphins,
enkephalins, and adrenal corticosteroids to modulate immune responses
represents one direction of the circuit. Production of ir ACTH and ENDs by
lymphocytes, and their contribution to a stress response, represents a
pathway in the opposite direction and completes the loop. Figure 1 is a
simplified model depicting how a pathway between the immune and
neuroendocrine system could fit into the classic hypothalamic-
pituitary-adrenal axis. Because the hormones produced by each system can
feed back and regulate their own production, intrasystem regulatory loops
are included in the model. For example, a stimulus such as a virus
infection would induce lymphocyte ACTH and result in adrenal gland
steroidogenesis. Glucocorticoids alter host homeostasis as well as
suppress immune responses (for review see 10). Furthermore, the lymphocyte
ACTH may also suppress the immune response (7,36). Thus, a generalized
alteration in host homeostasis and immune response could be affected
through activation of the neuroendocrine system. Since different hormones
are produced by leukocytes, the particular alteration in homeostasis would

be a function of the induction stimulus. Another aspect of this model is that since hypothalamic products will activate leukocytes, there is a mechanism through which the central nervous system can directly modulate the immune system.

An indication that these interactions do occur and are physiologically relevant is that adrenalectomized rats subjected to stress demonstrate a suppressed immune response (38). This suggests that hypothalamic or pituitary hormones are directly immunomodulatory in vivo as well as in vitro (7,10). A naturally occurring case of leukocyte ACTH production in man has recently been reported by Dupont et al. (39). An individual with the clinical symptoms of ectopic ACTH syndrome was found to have normal inflammatory tissue which synthesized ACTH. Removal of the tissue dropped the individual's ACTH levels to normal and immunofluorescent staining showed the tissue to contain leukocytes positive for ACTH. Thus, in at least one instance leukocyte production of ACTH appears to be involved in a disease state.

In conclusion, it seems that the immune and neuroendocrine systems can interact in a regulatory manner by virtue of common ligands and receptors. Through these molecules, the immune system may be able to serve a sensory role, alerting the host of infections and tumors (40). Furthermore, an understanding of these interactions may help explain the pathophysiology of certain diseases and lead to new therapies.

REFERENCES

1. K. Bulloch, Neuroanatomy of lymphoid tissue: A review, in: "Neural Modulation of Immunity," R. Guillemin, M. Cohn, and T. Melnechuk, eds., Raven Press, New York (1983).
2. R.J. Cross, W.R. Markesbery, W.H. Brooks, and T.L. Roszman, Hypothalamic-immune interactions. I. The acute effect of anterior hypothalamic lesions on the immune response, Brain Res. 196:79 (1980).
3. H.O. Besedovsky, A. Del Rey, E. Sorkin, M. Da Prada, and H.H. Keller, Immunoregulation mediated by the sympathetic nervous system, Cell. Immunol. 48:346 (1979).
4. H.O. Besdovsky, A. Del Rey, E. Sorkin, and M. Da Prada, The immune response evokes changes in brain noradrenergic neurons, Science 221:564 (1983).
5. H.O. Besedovsky, E. Sorkin, D. Felix, and H. Haas, Hypothalamic changes during the immune response, Eur. J. Immunol. 7:323 (1977).
6. J. Wybran, T. Appelbroom, J.P. Famaey, and A. Govaerts, Suggestive evidence for receptors for morphine and methionine-enkephalin on normal blood T lymphocytes, J. Immunol. 123:1068 (1979).
7. H.M. Johnson, E.M. Smith, B.A. Torres, and J.E. Blalock, Neuroendocrine hormone regulation of in vitro antibody production, Proc. Natl. Acad. Sci. USA 79:4171 (1982).
8. R.E. Faith, N.P. Plotnikoff, and A.J. Murgo, Effects of opiates and enkephalins-endorphins on immune functions, Proc. Natl. Inst. Drug Abuse Technical Meeting on Mechanisms of Tolerance and Dependence (in press, 1983).
9. E.A. Beed, S. O'Dorisio, T.M. O'Dorisio, and T.S. Gaginella, Demonstration of a functional receptor for vasoactive intestinal polypeptide on Molt 4b T lymphoblasts, Regulatory Peptides, 6:1 (1983).

10. J.E. Blalock, E.M. Smith, and W.J. Meyer, III, The pituitary-adrenocortical axis and the immune system, in: "Clinics in Endocrinology and Metabolism," G.M. Besser and L. Rees, eds., W.B. Saunders Co. Ltd., East Sussex (in press, 1985).

11. J.E. Blalock, H.M. Johnson, E.M. Smith, and B.A. Torres, Enhancement of the in vitro antibody response by thyrotropin, Biochem. Biophys. Res. Commun. 125:30 (1985).

12. G.C. Miller, A. Murgo, and N.P. Plotnikoff, Enkephalins-enhancement of active T-cell rosettes from lymphoma patients, Clin. Immunol. Immunopath. 26:446 (1983).

13. H.W. McCain, I.B. Lamster, J.M. Bozzone, and J.T. Grbic, β-endorphin modulates human immune activity via non-opiate receptor mechanisms, Life Sciences 31:1619 (1982).

14. P.M. Mathews, C.J. Froelich, W.L. Sibbitt, Jr., and A.D. Bankhurst, Enhancement of natural cytotoxicity by β-endorphin, J. Immunol. 130:1658 (1983).

15. N. Kay, J. Allen, and J.E. Morley, Endorphins stimulate normal human peripheral blood lymphocyte natural killer activity, Life Sciences 35:53 (1984).

16. S.C. Gilman, J.M. Schwartz, R.J. Milner, F.E. Bloom, and J.D. Feldman, β-endorphin enhances lymphocyte proliferative responses, Proc. Natl. Acad. Sci. USA 79:4226 (1982).

17. E.M. Smith and J.E. Blalock, Human lymphocyte production of ACTH and endorphin-like substances: Association with leukocyte interferon, Proc. Natl. Acad. Sci. USA 78:7530 (1981).

18. J.E. Blalock and E.M. Smith, A complete regulatory loop between the immune and neuroendocrine systems, Fed. Proc. 44:108 (1985).

19. S.J. Lolait, A.T.W. Lim, B.H. Toh, and J.W. Funder, Immunoreactive β-endorphin in a subpopulation of mouse spleen macrophages, J. Clin. Invest. 73:277 (1984).

20. N.R. Hall, J.P. McGillis, B.L. Spangello, D.I. Healy, G.P. Chrousos, H.M. Schulte, and A.I. Goldstein, Thymic hormone effects on the brain and neuroendocrine circuits, in: "Neuromodulation of Immunity," P. Guillemin, M. Cohn, and T. Melnechuk, eds., Raven Press, New York (1985).

21. H.O. Besedovsky, A. E. Del Rey and E. Sorkin, What do the immune system and the brain know about each other,? Immunol. Today 4:342 (1983).

22. D.A. Weigent, M.P. Langford, E.M. Smith, J.E. Blalock, and G.J. Stanton, Human B lymphocytes produce leukocyte interferon after interaction with foreign cells, Infect. Immun. 32:508 (1981).

23. J.E. Blalock and E.M. Smith, Human lymphocyte production of neuro-endocrine hormone-related substances, in: "Human Lymphokines," A. Khan and N.O. Hill, eds., Academic Press, New York (1982).

24. E.M. Smith, A.C. Morrill, W.J. Meyer, and J.E. Blalock, Cortico-tropin releasing factor induction of leukocyte derived immuno-reactive ACTH and endorphins, Nature (in press, 1985).

25. J.E. Blalock and E.M. Smith, Human leukocyte interferon (HuIFN-α): Potent endorphin-like opioid activity, Biochem. Biophys. Res. Com. 101:472 (1981).

26. J.E. Blalock and E.M. Smith, Human leukocyte interferon: Structural and biological relatedness to adrenocorticotropic hormone and endorphins, Proc. Natl. Acad. Sci. USA 77:5972 (1980).

27. W.A. Kuziel, K.H Brooks, E.S. Vitetta, J.W. Uhr, and P.W. Tucker, Synthesis of pro-opiomelanocortin-related messenger RNA in normal and neoplastic B lymphocytes from the mouse, Science (in press, 1985).

28. E.M. Smith, M. Phan, D. Coppenhaver, T.E. Kruger, and J.E. Blalock, Human lymphocyte production of immunoreactive thyrotropin, Proc. Natl. Acad. Sci. USA 80:6010 (1983).

29. M.S. O'Dorisio, T.M. O'Dorisio, S. Cataland, and S.P. Balcerzak,

Vasoactive intestinal peptide as a biochemical marker for
polymorphonuclear leukocytes, J. Lab. Clin. Med. 96:666 (1980).

30. J. Lygren, A. Revhaug, P.G. Burhol, K.E. Giercksky, and T.G. Jenssen,
Vasoactive intestinal peptide and somatostatin in leukocytes,
Scand. J. Clin. Lab. Invest. 44:347 (1984).

31. E.M. Smith, W.J. Meyer, and J.E. Blalock, Virus-induced increases in
corticosterone in hypophysectomized mice: A possible lymphoid-
adrenal axis, Science 218:1311 (1982).

32. H.S. Siegel, N.R. Gould, and J.W. Latimer, Splenic leukocytes from
chickens injected with Salmonella pullorum antigen stimulate
production of corticosteroids by isolated adrenal cells, Proc.
Soc. Exper. Biol. Med. 178:523 (1985).

33. M.T. Curtis and A.M. Lefer, Protective action of naloxone in
hemorrhagic shock, Am. J. Physiol. 239:H416 (1980).

34. L.T. Bohs, J.C. Fish, T.H. Miller, and D.L. Traber, Pulmonary
vascular response to endotoxin in normal and lymphocyte depleted
sheep, Circ. Shock 6:13 (1979).

35. D.V. McMenamin, E.M. Smith, and J.E. Blalock, Bacterial lipopolysaccharide induction of leukocyte derived ACTH and endorphins,
Infect. Immun. (in press, 1985).

36. H.M. Johnson, B.A. Torres, E.M. Smith, L.D. Dion, and J.E. Blalock,
Regulation of lymphokine (γ-interferon) production by corticotropin, J. Immunol. 132:246 (1984).

37. J.E. Blalock, D.V. McMenamin, and E.M. Smith, Peptide hormone shared
by the neuroendocrine and immunological systems, J. Immunol.
(in press, 1985).

38. S.B. Keller, J.M. Weiss, S.J. Schleifer, N.E. Miller, and M. Stein,
Stress-induced suppression of immunity in adrenalectomized rats,
Science 221:1301 (1983).

39. A.G. Dupont, G. Somers, A.C. Van Steirteghem, F. Warson, and L.
Vanhaelst, Ectopic adrenocorticotropin production: Disappearance
after removal of inflammatory tissue, J. Clin. Endocrin. Met.
58:654 (1984).

40. Blalock, J.E., The immune system as a sensory organ, J. Immunol.
132:1067 (1984).

ACKNOWLEDGEMENTS

The authors wish to thank Dr. Walter J. Meyer, III, Dr. Howard M.
Johnson, and Ms. Audrey C. Morrill for their excellent contributions to
these studies. This research was supported in part by Office of Naval
Research grant N0014-84-K-0486, NIH research grant 1R01 AM 338-39-01A1.
We thank Diane Weigent and Rhonda Peake for their skillful typing of this
manuscript.

ENDORPHINS: A LINK BETWEEN PERSONALITY,

STRESS, EMOTIONS, IMMUNITY, AND DISEASE ?

George S. Solomon, Neil Kay, and John E. Morley

Geriatric Research, Education and Clinical Center
Sepulveda VA Medical Center (11E), 16111 Plummer Street
Sepulveda, CA 91343 and Minneapolis VA Medical Center
Minneapolis, MN 55417

A growing body of evidence - clinical and experimental, human and animal - that has been accumulating over the last 20 years since Solomon and Moos' then-speculative theoretical integration of emotions, immunity and disease (1) pointed to experiential influences on immune function mediated by the central nervous system and the neuro-endocrines, neurotransmitters, and neuropeptides controlled by it. The emerging field of psychoneuroimmunology (2), also referred to as neuroimmunomodulation (3), has rapidly expanded over the last few years due, in part, to the discovery that the endogenous opiods (endorphins), which are released from the anterior pituitary during stress, are potent immune system modulators.

Stress and emotions in the onset and course of immunologically resisted (infectious and neoplastic) and mediated (allergic and autoimmune) disease.   George Engel proposed the multifactoral biopsychosocial model of all disease (4). Wise clinicians since antiquity have recognized the role of emotions in disease. Galen is reputed to have said that melancholy women are more prone to cancer than sanguine women and Sir William Osler, the "father of modern medicine," remarked that it is as important to understand what is going on in a man's head as his chest in order to predict the outcome of pulmonary tuberculosis. A number of studies point to specific personality traits, stress and relative failure of psychological defenses and coping as predisposing factors relating to the onset and course of autoimmune diseases, particularly rheumatoid arthritis, but also to others such as systemic lupus erythrematosus and myasthenia gravis (5). [Deficiency of suppressor T-cell function is now felt to be related to autoimmunity (6).] Patients with autoimmune disease tend to be described as self-sacrificing, masochistic, conforming, self-conscious, shy, inhibited, perfectionistic, interested in sports, unexpressive of emotion (particularly anger), compliant, concerned about rejection, and prone to anxiety and depression (5). Poor prognosis relates to degree of anxiety, depression, alienation, and failure to cope (7,8). Similarly, personality studies of patients with cancer tend to report loss of an important relationship prior to development of the tumor with unresolved mourning and consequent depression, inability to express hostile feelings and emotions, unresolved tension about a parent figure and sexual disturbances (9,10). Emotional distress resulting from lack of mature acceptance of reality or from failure of denial defenses is associated with rapidity of death from mestastatic disease (11). [Immune resistance to cancer, an area of great complexity, is related to function both of sensitized cytotoxic T-cells and natural killer cells.] Allergies involve an interplay among genetic, psychological (particularly dependency conflict) and immune factors.

Stress, conditioning, early experience and behavioral effects on immunity in animals (12). Given observations on the relationship of emotional distress to onset and course of the diseases to which immune hypofunction or dysfunction can be related, it seemed rational to study the effects of stress and other experiential manipulations on immune function in animals. In 1969 Solomon first reported that overcrowding stress reduced primary and secondary antibody response to a novel antigen in rats (13). This immunosuppression depended on timing of stress in relation to administration of antigen and to the nature of stress, some stressors either having a lesser or absent effect. Duration of stress is relevant. Under prolonged stress, the immune response may be biphasic. In vitro lymphoproliferative response to T-cell and B-cell mitogens from animals subjected to sound stress is first decreased, followed after continuation of stress for 3 weeks by immunoenhancement (14). It is clear that stress can affect both humoral and cellular immunity (15). Controllability of the stressor appears critical since inescapable, but not the same amount of escapable shock ("controlled" by operantly conditioned lever pushing) leads to suppressed mitogen stimulation and NK cell activity (16,17). (Controllability may be an analogy of "coping" in humans.) Intensity of stress is important--graded stressors producing progressively greater immunosuppression (18). Stress in animals can also modify immunologically mediated disease. Group housing stress (high male/female ratio) significantly increaeses the intensity of adjuvant-induced arthritis and the incidence of spontaneous amyloidosis (19,20). Some separation studies in primates may more closely relate to effects of bereavement and depression on immunity in humans. The "agitation-depression reaction" exhibited by infant monkeys upon maternal or peer separation is associated with decreased lymphocyte stimulation by mitogens (21,22,23).

Russian investigators, in the tradition of Pavlov, claimed as early as 1926 that immunity could be influenced by classical conditioning, which, of course, would clearly implicate the CNS in immune regulation (24). [Editorially, we might comment that modulation of a physiological function, such as immunity, by the CNS is different from its control, as suggested by Eastern Europeans from the 1920s through the 1950s, and is also different from the autonomy of a physiological system, as implied by immunologists until very recent times.]

In elegant work reported in 1975, Ader and Cohen conditioned humoral immunosuppression using the immunosuppressive drug cyclophosphamide as the unconditioned stimulus and saccharin as the conditioned stimulus (saccharin alone reducing antibody response after prior pairing with cyclophosphamide) (25). The work has been confirmed in other laboratories including the utilization of other immunosuppressant agents. Cellular immunity and NK cell activity are also subject to conditioning, and conditioned immunosuppression can prolong the lives of mice with the autoimmune disease systemic lupus erythematosus (26,27,28,29).

There is little work demonstrating an ability experientially to enhance immunity. Rat pups picked up for 3 minutes a day from birth until weaning at 21 days show enhanced primary and secondary antibody response as adults (30). Such early experience seems to be "adaptive" behaviorally and physiologically, for example, leading to a briefer but more vigorous adrenal cortical hormone response to stress (31). [Moral: a good infancy promotes happiness and health!] Inbred female mice that spontaneously develop fighting behavior develop smaller virus-induced tumors, that are immunologically resisted, compared to their more placid "identical twin sisters" (32). [Moral: it is beneficial to express your anger even if you're a mouse!] Socially interactive hamsters develop smaller, less invasive melanomas with greater lymphocyte response than do passive animals (L. Temoshok, personal communication, 1985).

Human studies of stress and immunity. There is a considerable literature on the relationship of recent life changes requiring adaptation and coping and deleterious effects on health if such changes are of sufficient magnitude (33). More recently, life change stress has been correlated with reduction of NK cell activity (34). Social support appears to play a protective role in maintainance of health in the face of stress (35). Likewise, emotional "hardiness" characterized by a strong commitment to self, an attitude of vigorousness toward the environment, a sense of meaningfulness, and an internal locus of control (sense of responsibility for one's own destiny) appears "protective" against stress effects on health (36). (These studies have been done regarding health in general without study of intervening physiological mechanisms, including the immune system.) A large numer of studies point to stress events and/or decompensation of psychological defenses and adaptations as related to the onset of allergic, autoimmune, infectious, and neoplastic diseases (37,5,10).

Palmblad and associates carried out a number of experiments on the effects of food and sleep deprivation on immune mechanisms in humans with generally similar findings of immunosuppression, particularly lymphocyte response to PHA (38). New experiments aboard Spacelab 1 suggest that the decreased stimulability of lymphocytes by PHA from astronauts and cosmonauts after spaceflight is due to effects of weightlessness (39). Hypnosis, long observed to be able to alter the "efferent limb" of the immune response, such as skin response to tuberculin, has recently been claimed to alter mitogen responsiveness of lymphocytes from young, highly hypnotizable subjects (40,41). Bartrop was the first to demonstrate immunosuppression (decreased mitogen response) in bereaved spouses, work that has been confirmed in the laboratory of Schleiffer and Stein, who point out such immunosuppression tends to last up to a year (42,43). (That widowers have higher morbidity and mortality that similar aged married men during the year following their wives' deaths is a well-known observation.) In view of the well-accepted psychodynamic link between mourning and depression, first pointed out by Freud, it is not surprising that hospitalized patients with depressive disorders showed diminished lymphocyte responses to 3 mitogens and lower absolute numbers of T and B cells (44). Anxious college students with poor coping skills have reduced NK cell activity compared to asymptomatic students and those with high ego strength, who respond adaptively to life stress events (S. Heisel, personal communication, 1985).

Mechanisms of psychological and experimental effects on immunity

Neuroendocrines and neurotransmitters. The effect of hormones, which are subject to regulation by the hypothalamus, on immune response has been the subject of many reviews (29). Most clearly implicated, of course, have been adrenal corticosteroids. In vitro, low concentrations of corticosteroids stimulate lymphocyte proliferation and high concentrations inhibit (32). (Various influences on immune response, including stress, may be biphasic.) That stress and other experiential influences on immunity are not merely an adrenally-mediated pheonmenon has been made clear by recent work showing stress-induced suppression of immunity in adrenalectomized rats (33). [Earlier, Amkraut and Solomon had found that stress is more immunosuppressive in a graft vs. host model than is ACTH (15).] A variety of other experientially-influenced neuroendocrines affect immune response including growth, thyroid and sex hormones, insulin, the catecholamines, and histamine. Receptors for a number of CNS-controlled hormones and CNS-active compounds have been (and continue to be) found on lymphocytes or thymocytes by a number of investigators [reviewed by Solomon and Amkraut (45)]. Included are receptors for corticosteroids, insulin, testosterone, estrogens, B-adrenergic agents, histamine, growth hormone, acetylcholine, and B-endorphin as well as sites that seem to be receptors for bezodiazepine and haloperidol neuroleptic drugs (45,46,47). Presumably, the presence of receptor site implies a function for its substrate. Some sites have been identified as playing a role in differentiation of lymphocytes and in controlling their activity (48,49).

Catecholamines, which, of course, are both released into the general circulation and are neurotransmitters, have effects on immunity. Infusions of norepinephrine increase the activity of NK cells (50). Soviet work demonstrates that serotonin and 5-hydroxytryptophan (5-HTP) prolong the latent period of the primary immune response and lower the intensity of primary and secondary response (51). Hypophysectomy and lesions of the pituitary stalk abolish these inhibitory effects. Serotonergic structures of the hypothalamus appear to participate in the production of antibody. (Involvement of such mechanisms is likely in any psychological depression-induced immunosuppression.) Administration of the monoamine oxidase inhibitor antidepressant drug iproniazid, as well as serotonin or 5-HTP, delays involvement of T-cells participating in IgG response (helpers) (52). Similar serotonin-related drug effects are found on delayed hypersensitivity (53). There are claims that administration of serotonin can ameliorate autoimmune disease, both multiple sclerosis and its probable analogue, experimental allergic encephalomyelitis, affecting distribution and quantity of suppressor T-cells (54). Repeated mother-infant separations have persistent efects on serotonin levels (55). Growth hormone secretion is provoked by a variety of stimuli (56). Such responsiveness is diminished in patients with depressive illness, in whom (in contrast to animals) growth hormone can be simulated by thyrotropin-releasing hormone (57). Usually ACTH and growth hormone responses to stress are dissimilar (58). The responsivity of growth hormone to stress may be related to such personality characteristics as "neuroticism" (59) and "coronary-proneness" (60). Prolactin is responsive to stress in man, with a secretion pattern different from that of growth hormone (61). Direct measurement of TSH indicates small, if any, increase following psychological stress (62). However, clinical hyperthyroidism can be precipated by an acute emotional stress (63) (although some question exists whether these reports represent the dating phenomenon) and elevated thyroid hormone levels have been reported in patients with a variety of psychiatric diseases (63a). The thyrotropin response to TRH is blunted in up to one third of patients with bipolar depressive disorders (64). Most studies show a clear decrease in testosterone levels during stress, with poststress recovery to normal levels (65,66).

Important issues are how these multiple hormone responses may be interrelated and what their ultimate metabolic effect may be at the target level--in this case, the immunologically competent cell (67). The ultimate metabolic consequences of a given hormone are

influenced strongly by the existing overall "hormonal milieu" (68,69).
Endocrine responses to an acute stress seem to be organized in a cata-
bolic-anabolic sequence. The result is enhanced availability of energy
substrate (glucose) during the stress as a preparation for "fight or
flight," and then poststress restoration of protein and other tissue
stores (e.g., glycogen). Such a sequence may account for biphasic
immunologic responses to stress. Most hormones are secreted in a
pulsatile, episodic fashion. Many hormones have 24-hour secretory
rhythms; components of the immune system also show a 24-hour peri-
odicity. For example, stimulation of lymphocytes in vitro by mitogens
varies directly with the cortisol rhythm (70). Thus, timing of stress
in relation to naturally occurring rhythms may influence its immunologic
consequences.

   Nervous system and immunity: The hypothalamus, a small area of
the diencephalon, rich in neural connections to the limbic system of
the brain, that has receptors for humoral influences from blood and
cerebrospinal fluid and influences the pituitary through a variety of
polypeptide releasing factors (TRH, LHRH, CRF, and somatostatin), is
at the interface between the brain and a range of critical peripheral
regulatory functions. It is rich in neurohormones and neurotransmitters that may affect immune function and has been implicated in immune
function by direct research. Early work demonstrated alterations in
globulin levels as a result of the electrical stimulation of the
lateral hypothalamus of rats (71). Significant Soviet work revealed
that a destructive lesion in a specific portion of the dorsal hypothalamus of rabbits led to complete suppression of primary antibody
response, prolonged retention of antigen in the blood, and inability
to induce streptoccocal antigen myocarditis, as well as prolonged
graft retention (72); whereas, electrical stimulation of the same
region enhanced antibody resonse (73). Destruction of the posterior
hypothalamus aggravates experimental allergic polyneuritis, which is
related to the absence of antibodies to myelin that play a protective
role (74). Hypothalamic lesions also affect cell-mediated immunity.
Anterior lesions in the guinea pig suppress delayed cutaneous hypersensitivity to picrylchloride and tuberculin (75). Lesions decreased
and stimulation enhanced delayed cutaneous hypersensitivity (76).
Amkraut and Solomon found that electrolytic lesions of the ventromedial and posterior nuclei of the hypothalamus of hybrid rats impaired the graft versus host reaction in the recipient (unpublished
data, 1979). Guinea pigs with anterior hypothalamic lesions had
significantly smaller cutaneous tuberculin reactions than nonoperated
or sham-operated controls; and there was decreased stimulation in
vitro of lymphocytes from animals with hypothalamic lesions (77).
Epiphysectmony of the chick embryo leads to failure of development of
both thymus and bursa (78).

   Most interesting recent French work implicates the cerebral
cortex with lateral specificity in immunoregulation. Left cortical
lesions decrease T-cells and reduce T-mitogen and NK cell responses
(79).   B-cells and macrophages are not affected by cortical lesions.
Autoimmune and atopic diseases are more common in left-handed individuals (80).

   Portions of the immune system itself are significantly innervated
(81).   The thymus has fibers from the vagus and other sources (82).
The bone marrow also has a good neural supply (83). Brain lesions
affect marrow function (84). The autonomic nervous system also appears
significantly involved in modulation of the immune response. Noradrenaline decreases in the spleen, but not in non-lymphoid organs, during the
immune response (85). Further evidence that the hypothalamus is direct-

ly involved in regulation of immune response is provided by the work of Besedovsky and Sorkin in Switzerland and of Korneva in the U.S.S.R. (86,73). The firing rates of neurons (as determined by implanted electrodes) in the ventromedial nuclei of the hypothalamus increase following immunization (only in animals responding to antigen) (87).

Thymic hormones, important in T-cell maturation and function, are influenced by the CNS and may be true neuroendocrine modulators. Thymosin B 4 elicits release of lutenizing hormone-releasing factor, and, after intracerebroventricular injection, increases serum levels of luetinizing hormone (88). Thymectomy affects the hypophysis (89). Neuroendocrines influence the production of thymic hormones (90). "Lethargic" mutant mice suffer from a neurologic abnormality that develops before weaning, lasts 30-60 days, and then progressively disappears. The neurological disease is associated with thymic atrophy, which is reversed to normal as soon as the neural disturbances disappear (91). Both thymectomized and "nude" mice (that show thymic atrophy) display a profoundly disturbed neuroendocrine balance (92). Indeed, there is growing evidence of bidirectional interactions between the thymus and the neuroendocrine system. There is a report of the extraction from the anterior pituitary of a low molecular weight peptide with thymocyte-stimulating properties (93). Thymosin factor 5 increases levels of ACTH, cortisol, and β-endorphin (94). Hall suggests that thymic peptides down-regulate glucocorticoidal receptors enabling these to counteract potential suppressive effects of glucosteroids upon lymphocytes. Such an effect may occur in the brain as well, influencing the hypothalamic-pituitary-adrenal cortical feedback circuit including corticotropin-releasing factor (CRF), which, in turn, is influenced by serotonergic, adrenergic and cholinergic mechanisms (95).

Feedback mechanisms in immune regulation appear to act, at least in part, via CNS mediation. Serum cortisol levels are elevated in response to antigenic stimulation or graft rejection (presumably via hypothalamically-controlled ACTH) (86,96). This finding suggests a feedback loop between the immune system and the hypothalamic-endocrine system. Such an endocrine response was postulated as an explanation of the phenomenon of antigenic competition, in which response to one antibody inhibits that to another (97). Non-antigen-stimulated thymocytes are more sensitive to inhibitory effects of steroids than are sensitized T-cells, a probably modulating influence preventing inappropriate cells from being overstimulated by lymphokines released following antigenic stimulation (98). Recent work strongly suggesting such feedback is the finding of decreased noradrenaline turnover in the hypothalami of rats at the peak of immune response (99). This decreased noradrenergic activity was mimicked by injection of soluble mediators released by immunologic cells in vivo.

Stress, endorphins and immunity: Stress activates CRF, in turn leading to the release into the circulation of ACTH and β-lipotropin and β-endorphin from the anterior pituitary (100). In 1974 Brown et al. found that peripheral blood lymphocytes of heroin addicts had reduced proliferative responses to mitogens (101). A major interest in endorphins as physiological modulators of the immune system developed with the report by Hazum et al. (102) that the human lymphocyte cell line RPMI 6237 exhibited specific binding of (^{125}I) (D-Ala^2-1 β-endorphin and the finding of Blalock and Smith (103) that human peripheral blood lymphocytes produce a substance with immunoreactivity similar to γ-endorphin. Various studies established that opiod peptides modulate phytohemagglutin (PHA)-induced proliferation of peripheral blood lymphocytes. These findings were responsible for establishing a role for opioid peptides in the modulation of the immune system (104,105,106).

Recently, dynorphin and β-endorphin have been demonstrated to stimulate superoxide production by human polymorphonuclear leukocytes and macrophages in vitro (127). These findings show that a key metabolic response involved in the microbiodal function of phagocytic cells is triggered by opioids at concentrations in the physiological range.

β-endorphin was found to enhance NK activity (107). The dose response curve had an inverted U-shape. Of particular interest was the fact that this response could only be demonstrated in half the subjects tested. However, in those subjects in whom the response was present, it could be reelicited when lymphocytes from these subjects were tested on multiple other occasions. The β-endorphin effect could be reversed by the opioid antagonist, naloxone. β-lipotropin appeared to be equipotent to β-endorphin as an enhancer of NK activity, and γ-endorphin appeared to be more potent. The γ-endorphin effect was also reversed by naloxone. Morphine, α-endorphin and leucine-enkephalin did not significantly alter NK activity in the system developed by Kay and co-workers. Similar results were reported by Mathews et al., who found that both β-endorphin and methionine-enkephalin produced naloxone reversible enhancement of NK cell activity (108). They, too, found no effect of leucine enkephalin, α-endorphin and morphine. Faith et al. did, however, find effects of leucine-enkephalin as well as methionine-enkephalin on NK activity (109).

A number of Des-Tyr-endorphin fragments (2-16, 2-17, 6-17 and 2-9) have proved to be extremely potent stimulators of NK function with activities at concentrations as low as 10^{-15} M. The fragments (10-16) and (14-16) were inactive. These studies suggest that the ability of endorphins to stimulate NK activity rests predominantly in the (6-9) amino acid fragment. The activity, therefore, lies in the α-helix portion of the molecule (110) (Fig.1). However, the fact that methionine-enkephalin can enhance NK activity--combined with the discrepancy noted above between α- and γ-endorphin--suggests that more than one receptor site may be involved.

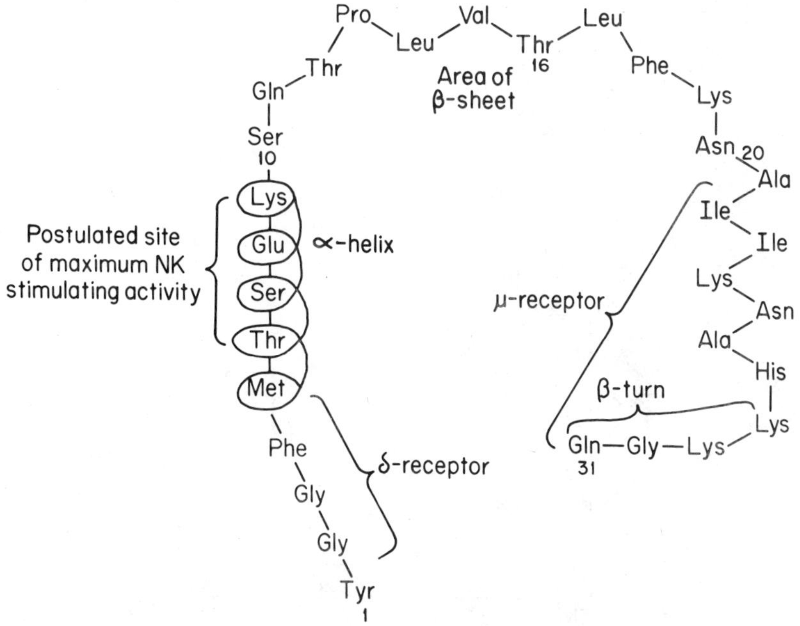

Fig. 1. Postulated sites of the β-endorphin molecule responsible for modulating NK-activity.

Activation of NK activity requires calmodulin (111). Calmodulin is a ubiquitous intracellular calcium binding protein which regulates a variety of intracellular processes and is important in the control of cell shape and cellular secretions. As a number of studies have suggested that opiates exert some of their effects through calmodulin modulation (112,113), Moon and co-workers examined the effect of calmodulin inhibition using the naphthelene sulfonamide W13, on β-endorphin-stimulated NK activity. The β-endorphin enhancement of NK activity was inhibited by W13 suggesting that the opioid stimulation of NK activity may be mediated by calmodulin.

Interferon is a potent stimulator of NK activity. Interferon levels can be altered by experiential manipulation (114). The level of NK enhancement produced by the endorphins is of the same magnitude as that produced by interferon. Interferon has been demonstrated to have a number of opioid-like effects (115). Thus, interferon may produce its enhancement of NK activity through opioid receptors. In support of the hypothesis, it was found that naloxone inhibited the interferon-mediated NK enhancement (107) (Fig. 2).

Interleukin-2 is another NK cell enhancer which has been shown to bind to opioid receptors (116). Preliminary studies suggest that naloxone can partially reverse the effect of interleukin-2 on NK cell activity. Since chronic administration of naltrexone did not affect NK cell activity or stimulability of lymphocytes by PHA, the question of the importance of endorphins in long-term regulation of the immune system remains open (117). Both interferon and interleukin-2 are released after an antigenic exposure or viral infection, making it important to determine if chronic opioid blockade blunts the increase in NK function after such challenges.

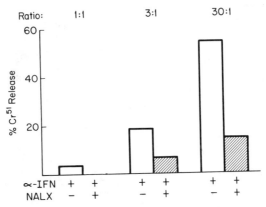

Fig. 2. Effect of naloxone on interferon-mediated NK enhancement.

Recently, the interest in the role of enkaphalins-endorphins in mediating stress effects on immunity has increased considerably. Both ACTH and β-endorphin are part of the precursor molecule pro-opio-melanocortin, and secretion of both is controlled by the hypothalamic corticotropin-releasing factor, CRF (118). In turn, the immune system secretes factors that influence CRF and opiocortin neurons. An anatomical substrate in the CNS exists for participation of peptide systems in autonomic, immune and other physiological homeostatic mechanisms, which tend to be disordered under conditions of stress, in disease and in aging. For example, both ACTH and β-endorphin are released simultaneously from the pituitary by disease or stress (119); the lymphocyte under "stress" (responding to antigen) also releases ACTH (120); the adrenal gland releases enkephalins, catecholamine and steroid hormones during stress (121).

Met-enkephalin-like, morphine-like, and β- and γ-endorphin receptors have been identified on lymphocytes (55). ACTH and β-endorphin can behave like lymphokines (122). As stated by Blalock, "Thus, it appears that the immune and neuroendocrine systems have the ability to signal each other through common or related peptide hormones and receptors." (122).

There is some direct evidence of opioid mediation of stress effects on immunity. Rats subjected to footshock stress develop analgesia; but, depending on its avoidability vs. nonavoidability, such analgesia is or is not reversed by naloxone--thus, is or is not opioid-dependent. Splenic NK cell activity and lymphocyte proliferation by mitogens PHA and ConA are suppressed by the opioid but not the nonopioid form of stress (123,17). Mice injected with enkephalins may have significant increases in thymic size and smaller spleens (125). In addition, BDF$_1$ mice inoculated with L1210 tumor cells and either Leu- or met-enkephalin have survival advantage over BDF$_1$ mice with tumor cells alone (126).

Conclusion: Psychoneuroimmunology, the developing field having to do with the effects of emotions and stress on immune function and thus on immunologically resisted and mediated diseases and with the role of the central nervous system (CNS) in modulation of immune function, is rapidly advancing especially because of the unraveling of mechanisms of bidirectional CNS-immune interaction, particularly understanding the role of endogenous opioids as immunomodulators (124).

REFERENCES:

1. Solomon, G.F., Moos, R.H. Emotions, immunity and disease: A speculative theoretical integration. Arch. Gen. Psychiat. 11:556-567, 1964.
2. Ader, R. (ed.). Psychoneuroimmunology, Academic Press, New York, 1981.
3. Guillemin, R., Chone, M., Melnechak, T. (eds.) Neural Modulation of Immunity. Raven Press, New York, 1985.
4. Engel, G.L. A unified concept of health and disease. Perspect. Biol. Med. 3:459-485, 1960.
5. Solomon, G.F. Emotional and personality factors in the onset and course of autoimmune disease, particularly rheumatoid arthritis. In: Ader, R.A. (ed.). Psychoneuroimmunology, Academic Press, New York, 1981, pp. 159-182.
6. Compston, A. Lymphocyte subpopulations in patients with multiple sclerosis. J. Neurol. Neurosurg. Psychiat. 46:105-114, 1983.

7. Moos, R.H. and Solomon, G.F. Personality correlates of the rapidity of progression of rheumatoid arthritis. Ann. Rheum. Dis. 23:145-151, 1969.

8. Solomon, G.F. and Moos, R.H. Psychologic aspects of response to treatment in rheumatoid arthritis. GP 32:113-119, 1965.

9. Le Shan, L.L. and Worthington, R.E. Personality as a factor in the pathogenesis of cancer: Review of the literature. Brit. J. Med. Psychol. 29:49-56, 1956.

10. Bahnson, C.B. Stress and cancer: State of the art. Psychosomatic 21:957-981, 1980.

11. Klopfer, B. Psychological variables in human cancer. J. Prof. Tech. 21:331-340, 1957.

12. Weiner, H. Bronchial Asthma. In: Psychobiology and Human Disease, Elsevier, pp. 223-317, New York, 1977.

13. Solomon, G.F. Stress and antibody response in rats. Int. Arch. Allergy 35:97-104, 1969.

14. Monjan, A.A. and Collector, M.I. Stress-induced modulation of the immune response. Science, 196:307, 1977.

15. Amkraut, A.A., Solomon, G.F., Kasper, P., Purdue, A. Effects of stress and of hormonal intervention on the graft versus host response. Adv. Exper. Med. Biol. 29:667-674, 1972.

16. Laudenslager, M.L., Rayan, S.M., Drugan, R.C., Hyson, R.L., Maier, S.F. Coping and immunosuppression: Inescapable but not escapable shock suppresses lymphocyte proliferation. Science 221:568-570, 1983.

17. Maier, S.F., Laudenslager, M.L., Ryan, S.M. Stressor controllability, immune function and endogenous opiates. Manuscript, 1983.

18. Keller, S., Weiss, J., Schleifer, S. et al. Suppression of immunity by stress: Effect of a graded series of stressors on lymphocyte stimulation in the rat. Science 221:1301-1304, 1981.

19. Amkraut, A., Solomon, G.F., Kraemer, H.C. Stress, early experience and adjuvant-induced arthritis in the rat. Psychosom. Med. 3:203-214, 1971.

20. Ebbesen, P. Spontaneous amyloidosis in differently grouped and treated DBA-2, BALB-C and CMA mice and thymus fibrosis in estrogen-treated BALB-C males. J. Exp. Med. 127:386-396, 1968.

21. Laudenslager, M.L., Reite, M., Harbeck, R.J. Suppressed immune response in infant monkeys associated with maternal separation. Behav. Neurol. Biol. 36:40-48, 1982.

22. Reite, M., Harbeck, R., Hoffman, A. Altered cellular immune response following peer separation. Life Sci 29:1133-1136, 1981.

23. Coe, C.L., Rosenberg, L.T., Levine, S. Immunological Consequences of Maternal Separation in Infant Primates. First international Workshop on Neuroimmunology, Bethesda, MD, November 28, 1984.

24. Metalnikov, S. and Chorin, V. The role of conditioned reflexes in immunity. Ann. Pasteu Inst. 11:1-8, 1926.

25. Ader, R. Behaviorally conditioned immunosuppression. Psychosom. Med. 37:333-340, 1975.

26. Kusnecov, A.W., Sivyer, M.G., King, A.J., Husband, A.W., Cripps, R.L. Behaviorally conditioned suppression of the immune response by antilymphocyte serum. J. Immunol. 189:2117-2120, 1983.

27. Borbjerg, D. and Ader, R. Acquisition and extinction of conditioned suppression of a graft versus host response in the rat. Psychosom. Med. 45:369 (Abstract), 1983.

28. Solvason, H.B., Ghanta, V., Hiramoto, R., Spector, N.H. Natural killer cell activity augmented by classical Pavlovian conditioning. First International Workshop on Neuroimmunology, Bethesda, MD, November 29, 1984.

29. Ader, R. Behaviorally conditioned immunosuppression and murine systemic iupus erythematosus. Science 215:1534-1536, 1982.

30. Solomon, G.F., Levine, S., Kraft, J.K. Early experience and immunity. Nature 220:821-822, 1968.

31. Levine, S. Plasma-free corticosteroid response to electric shock in rats timulated in infancy. Science 135:795-796, 1962.

32. Amkraut, A. and Solomon, G.F. Stress and murine sarcoma virus (Maloney) - Induced tumors. Cancer Res. 32:1428-1433, 1972.

33. Rahe, R.H. Life changes and illness studies: Past history and future direction. J. Hum. Stress 4:3-15, 1978.

34. Locke, S.E., Kraus, L., Leserman, J. Life change stress, psychiatric symptoms and natural killer cell activity. Psychosom. Med. 46:441-453, 1984.

35. Cobb, S. Social support as a moderator of life stress. Psychosom. Med. 38:300-314, 1976.

36. Kobasa, S.C. Stressful life events, personality and health: An inquiry into hardiness. J. Pers. Soc. Psychol. 37:1-11, 1979.

37. Solomon, G.F. and Amkraut, A.A. Emotions, immunity and disease. In: Temoshok, L., Van Dyke, C., Zegans, L.S. (eds.). Emotions in Health and Illness. Theoretical and Research Foundations. New York: Grun & Stratton, pp. 167-186, 1983.

38. Palmblad, J., Petrini, B., Wasserman, J., Akerstedt, T. Lymphocyte and granulocyte reactions during sleep deprivation. Psychosom. Med. 41:273-276, 1979.

39. Cogli, A. and Tschopp, A. Lymphocyte reactivity during space-flight. Immunol. Today 6:1-4, 1985.

40. Black, S., Humphrey, J.H., Niven, J.S. Inhibition of mantoux reaction by direct suggestion under hypnosis. Br. Med. J. 6:1649-1653, 1963.

41. Hall, H.H. Hypnosis and the immune system: A review with implications for cancer and the psychology of healing. Am. J. Clin. Hypnosis 25:92-103, 1983.

42. Barrop, R.W., Lazarus, L., Luckhurst, E. et al. Depressed lymphocyte function after bereavement. Lancet 1:834-836, 1977.

43. Schleifer, S.J., Keller, S.E., McKegney, F.P., Stein, M. Bereavement and lymphocyte function. Paper delivered at annual meeting of Am. Psychiat. Assn., 1980 and personal communication, 1983.

44. Schleifer, S.J., Keller, S.E., Meyerson, A.T. et al. Lymphocyte function in major depressive disorder. Arch. Gen. Psychiat. 41:484-486, 1984.

45. Solomon, G.F. and Amkraut, A.A. Psychoneuroendocrinologic effects on the immune response. In: Starr, M.P. (ed.) Annual Review of Microbiology 35:155-184, Annual Reviews, Palo Alto, 1981.

46. Weber, R.J., Smith, C.C., Norcross, M.A., Paul, S.M., Pert, C.B. Characterization and Distribution of "Peripheral Type" Benzodiazepine Receptors on Cells of the Immune System. First International Workshop on Neuroimmunology, Bethesda, MD, November 27, 1984.

47. Shaskan, E.G. Probable Lymphoid Cell Sites of Action for Immunomodulation by Haloperidol. First International Workshop on Neuroimmunology, Bethesda, MD, November 27, 1984.

48. Cantor, H. and Gershon, R.K. Immunological circuits. Cellular compositions. Fed. Proc. 39:2058-2064, 1979.

49. Helderman, J.H. and Strom, T.P. Specific binding site on T and B lymphocytes as a marker of cell activation. Nature 274:62-63, 1978.

50. Locke, S., Kraus, L., Kutz, S. et al. Altered Natural Killer Cell Activity During Norepinephrine Infusion in Humans. First International Workshop on Neuroimmunomodulation, Bethesda, MD, November 30, 1984.

51. Devoino, L.V., Eremine, O.F., Ilyutchenok R, Yu, R. The role of

the hypothalamo-pituitary system in the mechanism of action of reserpine and 5-hydroxytryptophan on antibody production. Neuropharmacology 9:67-72, 1970.

52. Devoino, L.V. and Idova, G.V. Influence of some drugs on the immune response. IV. Effect of serotonin, 5-hydroxytryptophan, iproniazid and p-chlorphenylalanin on the synthesis of IgM and IgG antibodies. Eur. J. Pharm. 22:325-331, 1973.

53. Devoino, L.V., Ilyutchenok, R., Yu, . Influence of some drugs on the immune response. II. Effects of serotonin, 5-hydroxytryptophan, reserpine and iproniazid on delayed hypersensitivity. Eur. J. Pharm. 4:449-456, 1968.

54. Abramchik, G.N. Clinical aspects of serotonin treatment for autoimmune diseases. Paper delivered at Soviet Academy of Sciences conference. "Regulation of Immune Homeostasis," Leningrad, 1982 (to be published in USSR, 1984).

55. Mybran, J. Enkephalins and endorphins as modifiers of the immune system: present and future. Fed. Proc. Vol. 44, No. 1, Part 1, pp. 92-94, January 1985.

56. Brown, G.M. and Reichlin, S. Psychologic and neural regulation of growth hormone secretion. Psychosom. Med. 34:45-61, 1972.

57. DeLaFuente, J.R. and Wells, L.A. Human growth hormone in psychiatric disorders. J. Clin. Psych. 42:270-274, 1981.

58. Yalow, R.S., Versano-Sharon, N., Echemendia, E., Berson, S.A. HGH and ACTH secretory responses to stress. Horm. Metab. Res. 1:3, 1969.

59. Miyabo, S., Hisada, T., Asata, T., Mizushima, No, Ueno, K. Growth hormone and cortisol responses to psychological stress. Comparison of normal and neurotic subjects. J. Clin. Endocrinol. Metab. 42:1158, 1976.

60. Friedman, M., Byers, S.O., Roseman, R.H., Newman, R. Coronary-prone individuals (Type A behavior patterns) growth hormone responses. JAMA 217:929, 1971.

61. Mirsky, A. The psychosomatic approach to the etiology of clinical disorders. Psychosom. Med. 19-424-430, 1957.

62. Mason, J.W., Hartley, L.H. Kotchen, T.A., Wherry, F.E., Pennington, L.L., Jones, J.G. Plasma thyroid-stimulating hormone response in anticipation of muscular exercise in humans. J. Clin. Endocrinol. Metab. 37:403, 1975.

63. Mandelbrote, B.M. and Wittkower, E. Emotional factors in Grave's disease. Psychosom. Med. 17:109-117, 1955.

63a. Morley, J.E. and Shafer, R.B. Thyroid function screening in new psychiatric admissions. Arch. Int. Med. 42:591-593, 1982.

64. Linkowski, P., Van Wetere, J.P., Kerhofs, M., Brauman, H., Mendlewicz, J. Thyrotrophin response to thyreostimulin in affectively ill women relationship to suicidal behavior. Brit. J. Psych. 143:401-405, 1983.

65. Kreuz, L.E., Rose, R.M., Jennings, J.R. Suppression of plasma testosterone levels and psychological stress. Arch. Gen. Psych. 26-469, 1972.

66. Hamanaka, Y., Kurachi, K., Aono, T., Mizutani, S., Matsumoto, K. Effects of general anesthesia and severity of surgical streee on serum LH and testosterone in males. Acta. Endocrinol. 65:258, 1975.

67. Mason, J.W. "Over-all" hormonal balance as a key to endocrine organization. Psychosom. Med. 30:791-808, 1968.

68. Mason, J.W. A historical view of the stress field. Hum. Stress 1(1):6, 1(2):22, 1975.

69. Mason, J.W. Levi, L. (ed.) In: Emotions - Their Parameters and Measurement. New York, Raven Press, pp. 143-181, 1975.

70. Tavadia, H.B., Fleming, K.A., Hume, P.D., Simpson, H.W. Circadian rhythmicity of human plasma cortisol and PHA-induced lympho-

cyte transformation. Clinb. Exp. Immunol. 22: 199, 1975.

71. Fessel, W.J. and Forsythe, R.F. Hypothalamic role in control of gamma globulin levels. Arth. Rheum. 6:770 (abstract), 1963.

72. Korneva, E.A. and Khae, L.M. Effects of destruction of hypothalamic areas on immunogenesis. Fiziol ZL SSSR 49:42-46, 1963.

73. Korneva, E.A. The effects of stimulating different mesencephalic structures on protective immune response pattern. Fiziol ZL SSSR 53:42-45, 1967.

74. Konovalov, G.F., Korneva, E.A., Khai, L.M. Effect of destruction of the posterior hypothalamic area on the experimental allergic polyneuritis. Brain Res. 29:283-286, 1971.

75. Macris, N.T., Schiavi, R.C., Camarino, M.S., Stein, M. Effect of hypothalamic lesions on immune processes in the guinea pig. Am. J. Physiol. 210:1205-1209, 1972.

76. Jankovic, B.D. and Isokovic, K. Neuroendocrine correlates of immune response: 1. Effects of brain lesions on antibody production, arthus reactivity, and delayed hypersensitivity in the rat. Int. and Allergy 45:360-372, 1973.

77. Keller, S.E., Shapiro, R., Schleifer, S.J., Stein, M. Hypothalamic influences on anaqhylaxis. Psychosom. Med. 44:302 (abstract), 1982.

78. Jankovic, B.D., Jankovic, D.LJ., Savovski, L. Effect of early epiphysectomy on the immune system of the chick embryo. First International Workshop on Neuroimmunology, Bethesda, MD, November 27, 1984.

79. Behan, P.O. and Geschwind, N. Hemisphere lateralization and immunity. In: Guillemin, R., Cohn, M., Melnechuk, T. Neural Modulation of Immunity. New York, Raven Press, pp. 73-80, 1985.

80. Biziere, K., Guillaumin, J.M., Degenne, D., Bardos, P., Renoux, M., Renoux, G. Lateralized Neocortical Modulation of the T-Cell Lineage. In: Guillemin, R., Cohn, M., Melnechuk, T. Neural Modulation of Immunity. New York, Raven Press, pp. 81-94, 1985.

81. Spector, N.H. Anatomic and physiological connections between the central nervous and immune systems (neuroimmunomodulation). In: Fabris, N., Garaci, E., Hadden, J., Mitchison, N.A. (eds.) Immunoregulation, New York, Plenum Press, 1983.

82. Bulloch, K. and Cullen, M.R. A Comparative Study of the Autonomic Nervous System Innervation of the Thymus in the Mouse and Chicken. At: First International Workshop on Neuroimmunomodulation. Lister Hill Center, NIH, Bethesda, MD, November 27-30, 1984.

83. Calvo, W. The innervation of the bone marrow in laboratory animals. Am. J. Anat. 123:315, 1968.

84. Bacui, I. La regulation nerveuse et humorale di l'erythropoiese. J. Physiol. (Paris) 54:441, 1962.

85. Besdovsky, H.O., Sorkin, E., DaPrada, M., Keller, H.H. Immunoregulation mediated by the sympathetic nervous system. Cell Immunol. 48:346, 1979.

86. Besedocsky, H.O. and Sorkin, E. Network of immune-neuroendocrine interactions. Clin. Exp. Immunol. 27:1-12, 1977.

87. Besedovsky, H.O., DelRey, A., Sorkin, E., DaPrada, M., Keller, H.H. Immunoregulation mediated by the sympathetic nervous system. Cell. Immunol. 48-346-355, 1979.

88. Rebar, R.W. Miyake, A., Low, T.L.K., Goldstein, A.L. Thymosin stimulates secretion of leuterinizing hormone-releasing factor. Science 213:669-671, 1981.

89. Jancovic, B.D. Immunomodulation of neural structures and functions. Paper delivered at Academy of Sciences of USSR conference (to be published in Russia, 1984), Leningrad, 1982.

141

90. Fabris, N. Endocrine control of thymic factor production in young adult and old mice. Paper prepared for Academy of Science of USSR conference, "Regulation of Immune Homeostasis," Leningrad, 1982.

91. Dung, H.C. Deficiency in the thymus - dependent immunity in "lethargic" mutant mice. Transplantation 23:39, 1977.

92. Fabri, N., Moccegianni, E., Muzzioli, M., Imberti, R. Thymus-neuroendocrine network. In: Fabris, N., Garaci, E., Hadden, J., Mitchison, N.A. (eds.). Immunoregulation, New York, Plenum Press, pp. 341-362, 1983.

93. Saxena, R.K. and Talway, G.P. An anterior pituitary factor stimulates thymide incorporation in isolated thymocytes. Nature 268:57, 1977.

94. Hall, H.R., McGullis, J.P., Spangelo, B.L. et al. Thymic hormone effects on the brain and neuroendocrine circuits. In: Guillemin, R., Cohn, M., Melnechuk, T. (eds.). Neural Modulation of Immunity. Raven Press, New York, pp. 179-193, 1985.

95. Jones, M.T., Hillhouse, E.W., Burden, J. Effects of various putative neurotransmitters on the secretion of corticotropia. J. Endocrinol. 69:1-10, 1975.

96. Besedovsky, H.O., Sorkin, E., Keller, H.H. Changes in the concentration of corticosterone in the blood during skin graft rejection in the rat. J. Endocrinol. 76:175-176, 1978.

97. Desedovsky, H.O., DelRey, A., Sorkin, E., DaPrada, M., Keller, H.H. Immunoregulation mediated by the sympathetic nervous system. Cell Immunol. 48:346-355, 1979.

98. Hall, N.R. and Goldstein, A.L. Role of thymosin and the neuroendocrine system in the regulation of immunity. In: Fabris, N., Garaci, E. Hadden, J., Mitchison, N.A. (eds.). Immunoregulation, New York, Plenum Press, pp. 141-163, 1983.

99. Besedovsky, H.O., DelRey, A., Sorkin, E., DaPrada, M., Burri, R., Honneger, C. The immune response evokes changes in brain noradrenergic neurons. Science 221-564-565, 1983.

100. Morley, J.E. The endocrinology of the opiates and the opioid peptides. Metabolism 30:195-209, 1981.

101. Brown, S.M., Stemmel, B., Taub, R.N., Kochwa, S., Rosenfeld, R.E. Immunologic dysfunction in heroin addicts. Arch. Int. Med. 134:1001-1006, 1974.

102. Hazum, E., Chang, K.J., Cautrecasas, P. Specific non-opiate receptors for B-endorphin. Science 205:1033-1035, 1979.

103. Blalock, J.E. and Smith, E.M. Human leukocyte interferon: Structural and biological relatedness to adrenocorticotropic hormone and endorphins. Proc. Natl. Acad. Sci. USA 77:5972-5974, 1980.

104. Gilman, S.C., Schwartz, J.M., Milner, R.J., Bloodm, F.E., Feldman, J.D. B-endorphin ehances lymphocyte proliferative responses. Proc. Natl. Acad. Sci. USA 79:4226-4230, 1982.

105. McCain, H.W., Lassiter, I.B., Bozzone, J.M., Grbic, J.T. B-endorphin modulates human immune activity via non-opiate receptor mechanisms. Life Sci. 31:1619-1624, 1982.

106. Plotnikoff, N. and Miller, G.C. Enkephalins as immunodilators. Int. J. Immunopharmacol. 5:437-441, 1983.

107. Kay, N.E., Allen, J., Morley, J.E. Endorphins stimulate normal human peripheral blood lymphocyte natural killer activity. Life Sci. 35:53-59, 1984.

108. Mathews, P.M., Froelich, C.J., Sibbit, W.L., Bankhurst, A.D. Enhancement of natural cytotoxicity by B-endorphin. J. Immunol. 130:1658-1662, 1983.

109. Faith, R.E., Liang, H.J., Murgo, A.J., Plotnikoff, N.P. Neuroimmunomodulation with enkephalins: Enhancement of natural killer (NK) cell activity in vitro. Clin. Immunol. Immunopathol.

31:412-481, 1984.

110. Li, C.H., Yamashiro, D., Tseng, L.F., Chang, W.C., Ferrara, P. B-endorphin omission analogs: Dissociation of immunoreactivity from other biological activities. Proc. Natl. Acad. Sci. USA 77:3211-3214, 1980.

111. Moon, T.D., Morley, J.E., Vesella, R.L., Lange, P.H. The role of calmodulin in human NK activity. Scand. J. Immunol. 18:255-258, 1983a.

112. Baram, D. and Simantov, R. Enkephalins and opiate antagonists control calmodulin distribution in neuroblastoma-glima cells. J. Neurochem. 40:55-63, 1983.

113. Clouet, D., Williams, N., Yonehara, N. Is a calmodulin-opiopeptide interaction related to the mechanism of opioid action. Life Sci. 33:727-730, 1983.

114. Solomon, G.F., Merigan, T.C., Levine, S. Variations in adrenal cortical hormones within physiologic ranges, stress and interferon production in mice. Proc. Soc. Exp. Biol. Med. 126:74069, 1967.

115. Dafny, N. Modification of morphine withdrawal by interferon. Life Sci. 32:303-305, 1983.

116. Ahmed, M.S., Llanos, J., Blatties, C.M. Interleukin-1 interacts with opioid binding sites. Proc. Soc. Neurosci. Abstr. 10:1109, 1984.

117. Morley, J.E., Baranetsky, N.G., Wingert, T.D., Carlson, H.E., Heshman, J.M., Melmed, S., Levin, S.R., Januson, K.R., Weitzman, R., Chang, R.J., Varner, A.A. Endocrine effects of naloxone-induced opiate receptor blockade. J. Clin. Endocrinol. Metab. 50:251-257, 1980.

118. Joseph, S.A., Pilcher, W.H., Knigge, K.M. Anatomy of the corticotropin-releasing factor and opiomelanocortin systems of the brain. Fed. Proc. Vol.44, No. 1, Part 1, pp. 100-107, January 1985.

119. Guillemin, R., Vargo, T., Rossier, J., Minick, S., Ling, N., Rivier, C., Vale, W., Bloom, F. B-endorphin and adrenocorticotropin are secreted concomitantly by the pituitary gland. Science 197:1360-1372, 1977.

120. Smith, E.M. and Blalock, J.E. Lymphocyte Production of Neurally Active Pituitary Hormone-like Molecules. First International Workshop on Neuroimmunomodulation, Bethesda, MD, November 27, 1984.

121. Hanbauer, I., Kelly, G.D., Saini, L., Yang, H.Y.T. (Met5)-enkephalin-like peptides of the adrenal medulla: Release by nerve stimulation and functional implications. Peptides 3:469-473, 1982.

122. Blalock, J.E. and Smith, E.M. A complete regulatory 1-op between the immune and neuroendocrine systems. Fed. Proc. Vol. 44, No. 1, Part 1, pp. 108-111, January 1985.

123. Shavit, Y., Lewis, J.W., Terman, G.W. et al. Opioid peptides mediate the suppressive effect of stress on natural killer cell cytotoxicity. Science 223:188-190, 1984.

124. Solomon, G.F. The Emerging Field of Psychoneuroimmunology: Hypotheses, Supporting Evidence and New Directions. Advance (in press).

125. Plotnikoff, N.P., Murgo, A.J., Miller, G.C., Cordev, C.N., Faith, R.E. Enkephalins-Immunomodulation. Fed. Proc. 44:118-122, 1985.

126. Plotnikoff, N.P., Kasten, A.J., Coy, D.M., Christensen, C.W., Schally, A.V., Spirtes, M.A. Neuropharmacological actions of enkephalin after systemic administration. Life Sci. 19:1283-1288, 1976.

127. Sharp, B., Keane, W.F., Suh, H.J., Gekker, G., Peterson, P.K.

Opioid peptides stimulate superoxide production by human polymorphonuclear leukocytes and macrophages. Clin. Res. (in
press), 1985.

INVOLVEMENT OF NON-OPIATE PEPTIDES IN PSYCHONEUROIMMUNOLOGICAL MODULATIONS

V. Kluša, R. Muceniece, Š. Svirskis, E. Kukaine, M. Ratkeviča,
G. Rosenthal, and G. Afanasyeva

Institute of Organic Synthesis, Latvian SSR Academy
of Sciences
Riga, USSR

INTRODUCTION

At present, several teams of investigators have provided evidence that endogenous opiate peptides play an important role in interactions between the nervous, endocrine and immune systems, their dysfunctions being intimately associated with stress (Arrigo-Reina and Ferri, 1980). Hence, the rapid growth of psychoneuroimmunology, a new field of neurobiology, largely relies on investigation of opiatergic modulations of these systems. Non-opiate peptides, however, are equally involved in regulating the integrity of biochemical and physiological processes responsible for homeostasis.

It should be emphasized in this connection that a number of non-opiate analgesic peptides, e.g. substance P, participate in stress adaptation syndromes triggering the release of other peptide hormones, such as vasopressin and oxytocin(Haldar et al.1980), stimulate histamine liberation from mast cells, etc. (Oehme et al., 1981). Vasopressin, which similarly to ACTH is implicated in learning and memory consolidation processes (De Wied, 1979), elicits analgesia (Bertnson and Berson, 1980) and like opiate peptides becomes released during pain-induced stress (Kendler et al., 1978) and serves as a potent regulator of immune homeostasis (Bukharin et al., 1982; Block et al., 1981; Whitefield et al., 1970).

The two posterior pituitary hormones, vasopressin and oxytocin can replace interleukin functions during gamma-interferon (IFNγ) production by lymphocytes (Johnson, 1983).

Analgesia, influence on immunocompetent cell transmitters, central effects, etc. are also characteristic of other non-opiate peptides - insulin, neurotensin, bradykinin, vasointestinal polypeptide, etc. (Kluša, 1984).

Enhanced release of numerous opiate and non-opiate peptides during stress implies increased biosynthesis of their precursors - protein molecules whose fine processing with proteinases determines the release of oligopeptides of varying specificity (Ashmarin, 1983). Since different protein groups may be related in evolution (Jörnvall et al., 1981) allowing their classification within the same family, several precursors can exist for a single protein. It is interesting to note that hyperglobulinemia (increased IgM and IgG concentration) has been reported in opiate addicts

(Faith and Plotnikoff, in press), while anti-IgE antibody production is affected during stress (Yoshinori et al., 1983). Our knowledge of protein molecules (immunoglobulins, interferons, albumins, enzymes, haemoglobins and so forth) as precursors of physiologically active endogenous protein fragments is very limited. In the past years, special attention has been attracted by IgG fragments: tuftsin (Thr-Lys-Pro-Arg-OH), IgG 289-292 (Najjar and Nishioka, 1970) and rigin (Gly-Gln-Pro-Arg-OH), IgG 341-344 (Chipens et al., 1980) showing immuno- and neuromodulatory properties (see also Kluša, 1984).

Finally, little is known about peptide hormone fragments, i.e. their natural metabolites formed as a result of proteolytic cleavage of intact hormone molecules. Our own findings (Kluša et al., 1982; see also Kluša, 1980) indicate that C-terminal fragments carrying a terminal $-CONH_2$ group (the gastrin, substance P, oxytocin, luliberin fragments) elicit neurotropic effects characteristic of regulatory peptides, possess various immunomodulating properties and can be classified as regulatory peptides with independent functions in the regulation of CNS activities.

We will confine ourselves to the effects exerted by the short non-opiate peptides - protein fragments (tuftsin, rigin), peptide fragments (gastrin, substance P), neuropeptides (TRH and MIF), on neuro- and immuno-modulation by comparing their action with the similar effects produced by the short opiate peptides, enkephalins.

The structure-functional organization of peptide hormones is characterized by certain features such as the specific active fragments represented by the common amino acid sequences of the long molecules, e.g. ACTH 4-10, ACTH 4-7 (as well as for α- and ß-MSH, ß-lipotropin) (De Wied, 1979) or by the common C-terminal sequences in tachykinins, caerulein-like and bombesin-like peptides, etc., which in most cases correspond to the principal metabolites of the full-length hormone molecules (see also Kluša, 1984).

Moreover, apart from the native ACTH 4-10 present in the organism (Ashmarin et al., 1981), high concentrations of some C-terminal hormone fragments considerably exceeding the amounts of the parent hormone in the brain have been demonstrated. For instance, a high cerebral level of the C-terminal tetrapeptide of gastrin was noted in the hog, the fragment being also predominant in the cholecystokinin-producing regions of the gastro-intestinal tract (Rehfeld and Golterman, 1979). The C-terminal tripeptide of gastrin was identified as the shortest fragment exhibiting biological activity (Lin, 1972). Furthermore, the possibility of peptide bond breakage in cholecystokinin (gastrin) between 30 and 31 amino acid sequences resembling metalloendopeptidases that cleave enkephalins (Deschodt-Lanckman and Strosberg, 1983):

$$Tyr^1-Gly^2-Gly^3 \longrightarrow Phe^4-Met^5-OH$$
$$-Met^{28}-Gly^{29}-Trp^{30}-Met^{31}-Asp^{32}-Phe^{33}-NH_2$$

enkephalinase A

The structure of the C-terminal tripeptide (MAF) and met-enkephalin is strikingly similar (Kluša, 1984) as evidenced by the common Met and Phe and equifunctional amino acid residues Gly and Asp (Chipens, 1971). On intracerebral administration to rats, MAF exhibits equal antinociceptive activity in the tail-flick test as the enkephalins (300-400 nmol), but is characterized by a longer duration of action (60-90 min, as compared to 5-7 min in the case of enkephalins. The maximum level of activity is attained 15-30 min following injection. Pentagastrin (BOC-ß-Ala-Trp-Met-Asp-Pre-OH), a protected analogue of the C-terminal fragment, was even more analgesic (150 min, 37.5 nmol) in this test; its peak of activity was attained 30 min following administration.

Unlike the enkephalins that elicit only central analgesia, MAF is also analgesic on peripheral (intraperitoneal) administration in a 5 mg/kg dose. The effect, lasting 15-20 min, is observed 10 min following the injection (Kluša et al., 1984).

Structural similarity has been revealed by us between the non-opiate peptide, substance P, and the immunopeptide tuftsin (Kluša et al., 1984), as the amino acid sequence Lys-Pro-Arg of tuftsin coincides with the retro-sequence of the N-terminal tripeptide in substance P. However tuftsin, though evoking a longer duration (15-30 min) of analgesia i. c. v. than the enkephalins, appears less effective in the tail-flick test in rats. Applied in a 300-400 nmol dose it prolongs the latent period of a nociceptive response only by 20%, as compared to controls. The other immunopeptide under study, rigin, resembles tuftsin in its activity. This effect of tuftsin is similar to that of substance P eliciting analgesia in a 5 nmol dose. At the same time, the C-terminal tetra- (Phe-Gly-Leu-Met-NH_2) and tripeptides (Gly-Leu-Met-NH_2) of substance P, sharing common structural elements with the enkephalins, are equally analgesic at 50 and 100 nmol as the full-length substance P molecule at 5 and 100 nmol (Kluša et al., 1981b).

It should be noted that on intracisternal injection to mice, tuftsin, rigin, MAF and the TRH are much more active in the tail-pinch test than the enkephalins (Takagi et al., 1979), but show the same duration (5 min) of action (Kluša et al., 1984) - see Table 1.

Analysis of analgesia mechanisms in the enkephalins and the above peptides reveals both significant differences and similarities in the character of their action. For instance, naloxone (1 mg/kg) given intraperitoneally 5 min prior to peptide injection reversed enkephalin-induced analgesia, but failed to alter the effects of other examined peptides. The radioreceptor assay used for analysis of competitive stereospecific binding of ^{3}H-naloxone and ^{3}H-DADL to synaptic membranes in the rat brain revealed the ability of rigin to bind to opiate receptors (Table 2). However, this effect is attained at very high rigin concentrations considerably exceeding those of Leu-enkephalin.

However, the parallel linearized dose-response curves suggest a comparable intrinsic activity for rigin. Rigin shows binding to δ-opiate recepotrs in concentrations greater by one order of magnitude than those in the case of μ-receptors. Tuftsin fails to bind to opiate receptors in a concentration as high as 5 mmol (Kukaine et al., 1984).

Evidence for rigin binding to opiate receptors in the brain is well-correlated with the findings obtained during a study of its binding to opiate receptors in the smooth muscle (electric stimulation of isolated strips of guinea-pig ileum, GPI, and mouse vas deferens, MVD). In concentrations (IC_{50} = 300 mM) exceeding by 3-4 orders of magnitude the concentration of enkephalins, rigin binds to the GPI μ-receptors and is capable of potentiating by a factor of two the effect of morphine. Neither rigin, nor tuftsin show binding to the MVD δ-receptors (Kukaine et al., 1984). Consequently, despite the low affinity of rigin for opiate receptors, the propensity of rigin for the μ-receptors is in contrast with the prevailing affinity of enkephalins for the δ-receptors. It is difficult to give a straightforward answer to the question as to rigin's identification with opiate peptides.

Table 1. Comparative Analgesic Activity of
Peptides on Their Intracisternal
Administration in Mice

Peptide	ED_{50} nmol/animal $(M \pm m)$
Met–enkephalin	146 (99.0–215.0)
Leu–enkephalin	223.0 (160.0–310.0)
Tuftsin	46.0 (31.5–66.7)
Rigin	68.0 (46.9–99.3)
MAF	50*
TRH	54.0 (31.8–91.8)

*ED_{50} could not be determined for lack of
dose-response effect

An interesting finding is the dualism of action observed by us for
rigin, tuftsin and MAF, e.g. the central analgesic and peripheral anti-
morphine (naloxone-like) effects (see also Kluša et al., 1984). It follows
from Fig. 1 that antagonism to morphine (15 mg/kg, ip) of these peptides
(10 and 100 mg/kg ip), as judged from the tail-pinch test in mice is analogous to that of the naloxone-like peptides TRH and MIF described in the
literature (Kastin et al., 1980; Bhargava, 1981), tuftsin and rigin being
superior to MIF and TRH in their duration of action. The dualism of tuftsin,
rigin and MAF action bears some resemblance to the effects of enkephalin.
For example, Met-enkephalin given intracerebroventricularly in subanalgesic
doses (40 µg) weakens morphine-induced analgesia (Vaught et al., 1982).
The non-opiate peptide hormone, bradykinin, when administered centrally
elicits analgesia (Ribeiro et al., 1968), whereas on peripheral administration it acts as a pain-producing peptide (Walaszek, 1970) acting like TRH,
somatostatin, melanotropin, ACTH and its fragments (Bulaev, 1982), cholecystokinin (Parviz, 1978) as opiate antagonist (see also Bulaev, 1982).

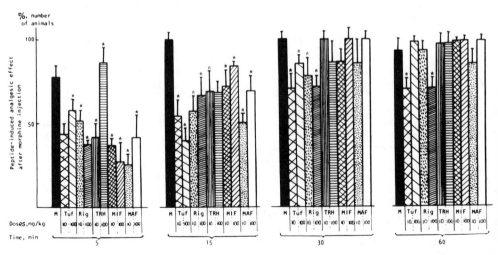

Fig. 1. Anti-morphine action of peptides in mice (ip). M – morphine
(control), Tuf – tuftsin, Rig – rigin. (*p ⩽ 0.05 with respect to morphine-induced effects.)

Table 2. Opiate Activity of Peptides Assayed by
Radioreceptor Method in the Rat Brain

Peptide	^{3}H-naloxone	^{3}H-DADL
Leu-enkephalin	0.0103 ± 0.0016	0.0117 ± 0.007
Rigin	32.65 ± 6.79	272.0 ± 70.0
Tuftsin	>5000	>5000

Thus, the examined fragments of IgG and gastrin are apparently involved in pain induction and hence can be placed in the family of endogenous factors regulating pain perception. It is conceivable that these peptides elicit conformational changes in opiate receptors, thereby affecting the mechanism of association during receptor-effector coupling and regulating the analgesic effects of opiates (Vaught et al., 1982).

When analyzing the mechanisms of analgesic effects exerted by peptides, the important implications of the monoaminergic system in regulating pain perception must be borne in mind (Sewell and Spencer, 1977). Relying on our own data as to the effect of peptides on the rat brain content of monoamines and their metabolites obtained by using inhibitors of monoamine biosynthesis and postsynaptic monoamine inhibitors (Kluša, 1984) and on the literature data concerning the monoaminergic mechanism of action of TRH (Agarwal et al., 1976), tuftsin (Waldman, 1982) and MIF (Dolzhenko and Komissarov, 1982) we made an attempt to elucidate the principal sites of their involvement in presynaptic monoaminergic transmission. Each peptide in these processes has a unique multidirectional profile as illustrated by Fig. 2. However, these

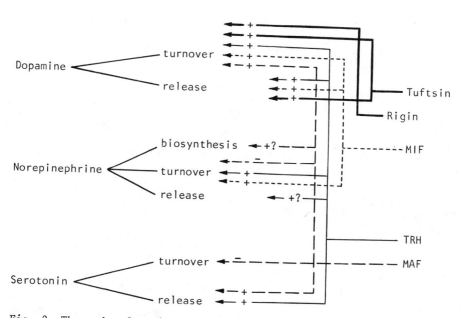

Fig. 2. The mode of action of peptides on presynaptic monoaminergic processes (+ stimulation, - inhibition).

Table 3. Variation in the Analgesic Activity of Compounds (Administered Intracisternally to Mice) in Response to Diethyldithiocarbamate (DDC)

Compound	ED_{50}, nmol/animal	
	Without DDC	In response to DDC
Met-enkephalin	146.0 (99.0–215.0)	18.7 (15.5–21.9)*
Leu-enkephalin	223.0 (160.0–310.0)	20.0 (15.8–24.2)*
Morphine	1.2 (0.6–2.2)	0.015 (0.009–0.024)*
Tuftsin	46.0 (31.5–66.7)	31.2 (27.9–34.5)*
TRH	54.0 (31.8–91.8)	12.5 (9.9–15.1)*

*$p \leqslant 0.05$ with respect to effects without DDC

interactions alone fail to provide a satisfactory explanation of the intricate neurochemical involvements of the peptides and call for more extensive studies. The membrane-affinity (binding to model bilayer phospholipid membranes) of peptides has been recently implicated in their modulating influence (Waldman, 1982): the largest increment in the fluorescence of the probe was induced by MAF, the smallest by tuftsin. Tuftsin was found to enhance GABA-ergic processes in the brain (Nikitina et al., 1983). The monoaminergic mechanism of enkephalins according to our data (Kluša, 1984) is mainly directed towards enhancement of the serotonin turnover. Despite the different neurochemical features of structurally distinct peptides, common pathways do exist by which their analgesic properties are effectuated. A striking example is provided by the fact that preliminary inhibition of dopamine-ß-hydroxylase with diethyldithiocarbamate (600 mg/kg 1.5 h prior to peptide administration) potentiates the central analgesic effects of both the enkephalins, morphine and TRH, tuftsin given intracisternally (Table 3) suggesting a significant role of the catecholaminergic system in the analgesic response to opiate and non-opiate peptides. Monoamines themselves are known to elicit analgesic activity on subarachnoidal administration.

Thus, the results discussed above indicate that the non-opiate peptides under examination affect both the pre- and postsynaptic monoaminergic transmission which allows to qualify them as neuromodulatory peptides. They are also capable of behavioural modulations.

More structurally related peptides (enkephalins, MAF, the C-terminal tetra- and tripeptides of substance P) on intracerebroventricular administration to rats in analgesic doses elicit more uniform locomotor responses: a moderate sedative effect with occasional shakes. Tuftsin enhanced appreciably the locomotor activity, induced grooming and wet-dog shakes resembling the same responses following substance P (25 nmol) and MIF (200 nmol) administration. Increased CNS-activity after rigin administration (marked enhancement of locomotor activity, head shakes, wet-dog shakes and grooming) reminds the effects of TRH (Kluša, 1984).

Our fragments, similarly to the classical neuropeptides, appear to exert both regulatory and modulatory properties (Kluša et al., 1982), which may account for their adaptational role in extremal and stress conditions. Upon peripheral (ip) administration these fragments in a 5 mg/kg dose decreased the immobilization time and increased the swimming time of animals (Table 4) to the same extent as the known neuropeptides when tested under behavioural dispair conditions after the method described by Porsolt et al., 1977. The highest activity was detected for tuftsin, MAF and substance P

Table 4. Comparative Effects of Peptides (5 mg/kg, ip),
on Immobilization Time in Mice (Porsolt's Test)

Compound	Immobilization time, %	Difference with respect to control, %Δ
Saline (control)	100.0 ± 5.2	
Tuftsin	50.5 ± 3.9*	−49.5
Rigin	64.5 ± 9.8*	−35.5
MAF	48.4 ± 15.6*	−51.6
MIF	57.3 ± 12.5*	−42.7
TRH	78.6 ± 4.6*	−21.4
Leu-enkephalin	87.26 ± 12.27	−12.74
Met-enkephalin	60.37 ± 4.76*	−39.63
Substance P	48.2 ± 6.1*	−51.8
Substance P C-terminal tripeptide	83.7 ± 6.1*	−16.3

*$p \leqslant 0.05$ with respect to control ($100\% = 199.2 \pm 8.4$ s)

(Kluša et al., 1984). Tuftsin in this test was found active also in lower (200-500 µg/kg) doses (Kozlovskaya et al., 1982).

The peptides also show activity in acute emotional stress (Kozlovskaya et al., 1982), thereby behavioural avoidance of a stressful situation under the influence of peptide fragments (Henderson's test, 1970) is dependent on initial emotional reactivity of rats. In other words, the peptides elicit different responses in various subclasses of animals with different emotional backgrounds. For instance, whereas tuftsin given intraperitoneally (200 µg) improves the behaviour of animals in all subclasses, the optimizing effect of MAF (5 mg/kg) is to a lesser extent observed in animals with polar emotional responses (unemotional intact and emotional animals receiving 6-hydroxydopamine). At the same time, the neuropeptide MIF interferes with avoidance behaviour due to enhanced emotional responses of the rats developing in parallel to the high initial level of emotional reactivity.

These data support our assumption that enhanced release of proteins including immunoglobulins and peptide hormones, capable of producing short peptides and fragments active in the regulation of adaptational reactions, occurs in stress reactions. In 1981, we advanced a hypothesis postulating a functional relationship between the neuro-, immuno- and glucoregulating peptides which were shown to involve various aspects of homeostatic regulation (Kluša et al., 1981a). An extensive investigation of immunomodulating action of peptides (Kukaine et al., 1982) has revealed that, similarly to tuftsin and rigin stimulating humoral immunity responses in mice (10-20 mg/kg, ip.), the titre of haemagglutinating antibodies is increased in response to leu-enkephalin (20 mg/kg), MAF (10 mg/kg) and, in particular, to MIF (20 mg/kg). Leu-enkephalin used in a high concentration (100 mg/kg) acts as immunosuppressant. Met-enkephalin in doses below 100 mg/kg fails to affect antibody production (Fig. 3). The in vivo results are somewhat different from in vitro findings (Johnson et al., 1982) where the two enkephalins suppress antibody production in spleen lymphocyte cultures in the presence of sheep erythrocytes.

TRH causes suppression in very high doses (from 100 mg/kg onwards). Generally the immunomodulating properties of peptides are only manifest in doses exceeding those affecting the CNS on peripheral administration (Kluša, 1984). It is interesting to note that TRH inhibits antibody production not only on peripheral administration but also if given centrally (intracisternally, 100–200 μg) when the peptide is not readily accessible to the immunocompetent blood and lymphoid tissue cells but has access to brain neurotransmitters. Neurotransmitters administered in the same manner to animals are also known to affect antibody production by acting either as stimulants (dopamine and serotonin, 10 mg/kg) or inhibitors (noradrenaline, 100 μg/kg) (Kukaine, 1981). Our suggestion that immunopharmacological characteristics of peptides are largely dependent on the activated state of the brain monoaminergic system is supported by the fact that a prior injection of haloperidol, a dopamine receptor inhibitor, (5 mg/kg given ip. 15 min prior to TRH administration) reversed the central immunosuppressive action of TRH (100–400 μg per mouse, intracisternally) (Kukaine et al., 1982).

A study of tuftsin and rigin in T- and B-cell immunity systems (Zālītis et al., 1982) has demonstrated that the two peptides stimulate delayed-type hypersensitivity and are capable of binding the specific antibodies produced against these substances. Rigin (10^{-4} mg/ml in vitro and 20 mg/kg in vivo) is more effective than tuftsin in stimulating rosette-formation in T- and B-lymphocytes from healthy subjects and cirrhotic liver patients; it promotes the adhesive properties of blood monocytes from chronic carriers of hepatitis virus antigen and from mammary tumour patients (Chipens et al., 1982).

As for the immunostimulating role of neuropeptides allowing to predict their effect on resistance to infection and tumours, the first evidence has been obtained of the antitumour activity of MIF in transplantable animal tumours derived from hormone-dependent tissues such as mammary adenocarcinoma Ca-755, cervical carcinoma CCM-5 and melanoma B-16 (Sof'ina et al., 1982).

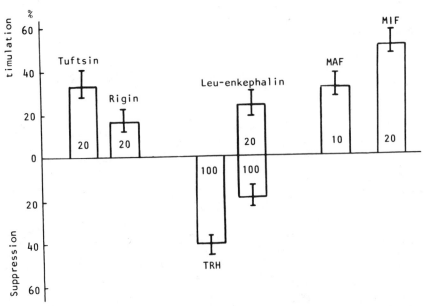

Fig. 3. Effect of peptides on antibody production in mice. Figures in the columns denote the dose of peptides given intraperitoneally. Abscissa corresponds to the control values of haemagglutinating antibody titre (saline = 100%). The peptides were administered 3 days prior to intraperitoneal injection of sheep erythrocytes ($5 \cdot 10^7$ cells per 1 ml of saline).

Experimental evidence accumulated on opiate and non-opiate peptides and the mechanisms of their action is indicative of their universality. A convincing proof is provided by the recent data demonstrating the immuno-modulating properties of opiate peptides: enhancement of T-rosettes by enkephalins (Miller et al., 1983), a certain γ-endorphin and interferon similarity, endorphin binding to T-lymphocyte receptors (Weber and Pert, 1984), and so forth. To date, opiate receptors have been located on various immunocompetent cells including the mast cells (DiAugustine et al., 1980), polymorphonuclear leukocytes, and macrophages (Lolait et al., 1984). On the other hand, numerous of receptor populations exist on the membranes of immunocompetent cells (Waksman, 1979) that comprise receptors both for opiate and non-opiate peptides (insulin, ACTH), for prostaglandins, adrenand cholinergic agents, etc. Therefore, it is not surprising that such immunological transmitters as histamine and serotonin are released by immunocompetent cells, e.g. the mast cells, in response to a large number of agents. Morphine was found to release histamine from the mast cells as far back as the late 1940's (Feldberg,1949), in the 1980's the release of serotonin has been demonstrated in response to morphine and endorphins (Yamasaki et al., 1982). Histamine can be also released from the mast cells in response to substance P (Oehme et al., 1981), neurotensin (Rossie and Miller, 1982) and bradykinin. According to our data, tuftsin (10^{-6}-10^{-5}M) released histamine, whereas rigin and enkephalin were fairly ineffective in the test devised by May et al., 1970. So far, the only hormone known to suppress histamine release is the vasointestinal polypeptide (Said, 1984).

At present, histamine is viewed not only as local messenger for immunocompetent cells, but also as neuroendocrine transmitter in the brain (Donoso and Alvarez, 1984), being involved not only in the immunobiological reactions, but also in the regulation of central pain mechanisms (Bulaev, 1982). The universal principles of membrane-associated processes (from changes in adenylate cyclase activity to protein phosphorylation, etc.) mediated by cyclic nucleotides also apply to histamine (Greengard, 1979). Moreover, histamine has been recently demonstrated to affect isolated adrenal chromaffin tissues. Histamine injected intracerebroventricularly enhances ACTH, vasopressin, prolactin and corticosteroid secretion, especially under immobilization stress conditions (see also Donoso and Alvarez, 1984). The above findings suggest that the effects of neuronal histamine are associated with stress.

CONCLUSION

It follows from the aforesaid that both opiate and non-opiate peptides affect all aspects of homeostatic regulation. However, the principles of their action are not identical, although sharing some similarity. Depending on its structural peculiarities each peptide exerts its unique effect on presynaptic neuromediation. The common effects are apparently mediated at the level of postsynaptic receptors, largely monoaminergic, where their interaction takes place with a definite concentration of monoamines being altered by the neuromodulating effects of each particular peptide. Aggregation of various receptor populations on immunocompetent cells plays an equally important role. The effects of peptides on multiple interrelated peptidergic and neurotransmitter interactions mediating universal intracellular processes regulate practically all cellular functions. Variations in the enzyme profiles of tissues, cells and cellular subpopulations account for the prevailing physiological responses.

The immunomodulating properties of non-opiate neuropeptides, on the one hand, and the neurotropic properties on the short IgG and peptide hormone fragments, on the other, as well as their common manifestations, as compared to the short opiate peptides (enkephalins) allow not only classification of natural metabolites as endogenous adaptational agents but also to predict the possible usefulness of their exogenous administration for psychoneuro-immunological homeostasis control, especially in stress-induced disturbances.

REFERENCES

Agarwal, R. A., Rastogi, R. B., and Singhal, R. L., 1976, Changes in brain catecholamines and spontaneous locomotor activity in response to thyrotropin releasing activity, Res. Comm. Chem. Pathol. Pharmacol., 15:743-752.

Ashmarin, I. P., 1983, Neuropeptide complexes, in: Rational Search for New Neurotropic Agents, Zinātne, Riga.

Ashmarin, I. P., Antonova, L. V., Burbaeva, G. Sh., and Kamensky, A. A., 1981, On the possibility of native $ACTH_{4-10}$ being present in the rat, in: Abstr. 4th USSR Symp. on Drug Design, Riga.

Arrigo-Reina, R., and Ferri, S., 1980, Evidence of an involvement of the opioid peptidergic system in the reaction to stressful conditions, Eur. J. Pharmacol., 64:885-888.

Berntson, G. G., and Berson, B. S., 1980, Antinociceptive effects of intra-ventricular or systemic administration of vasopressin in the rat, Life Sci., 26:255-259.

Bhargava, H. N., 1982, Dissociation of tolerance to the analgesic and hypo-thermic effects of morphine using thyrotropin releasing hormone, Life Sci., 29:1015-1020.

Block, L. H., Locher, R., and Tenschest, W., 1981, ^{125}J-8-L-Arginine vasopressin binding to human mononuclear phagocytes, J. Clin. Investig., 68:374-381.

Bulaev, V. M., 1982, Opiate receptors and their ligands, in: Advances in Science and Technology, Series: Pharmacology. Chemotherapeutic Drugs. "Opioid Peptides and Their Receptors", I. P. Ashmarin, Ed., Moscow.

Bukharin, O. V., Vasiliev, N. V., and Volodina, E. P., 1982, Oxytocin and vasopressin - regulators of immune homeostasis, in: Abstr. 3rd USSR Symp. on Regulation of Immune Homeostasis, Leningrad, 129-130.

Chipens, G., 1971, Similarity of signature carriers in some physiologically active peptides, in: Chemistry and Biology of Peptides, Zinātne, Riga.

Chipens, G., Blüger, A., Wechsler, H., Timoshenko, Zh., Baumanis, E., Iriste, A., Daija, D., Mergina, G., Poluektova, L., Veretennikova, N., 1982, Comparative study of immunobiochemical effect of tuftsin and rigin, in: Abstr. USSR Symp. on Bioorganic Chemistry and Drug Design, Riga.

Chipens, G. I., Veretennikova, N. I., Zālītis, G. M., Atare, Z. A., Afana-syeva, G. A., and Kukaine, E. M., 1980, New IgG fragments and their analogus possessing immunostimulating and immunoinhibitory activity, in: Abstr. 3rd Intern. Colloquium on Physico-Chemical Information Transfer of Reproduction and Ageing, Varna, Bulgaria, 22-23 Sept.:20.

De Wied, D., 1979, Pituitary and brain peptides and behaviour, in: Brain Peptides: a New Endocrinology, A. M. Gotto, ed., Elsevier/North Holland Biomed. Press, Amsterdam.

Deschodt-Lanckman, M., and Strosberg, A. D., 1983, In vitro degradation of the C-terminal octapeptide of cholecystokinin by enkephalinase, Febs Let., 152:109-183.

DiAugustine, R. P., Lazarus, L. H., Jahnke, G., Khan. M. N., Erisman, M. D., and Linnoilar, R. I., 1980, Corticotropin/ß-endorphin immunoreactiv-ity in rat mast cells. Peptide or protease? Life Sci., 27:2663-2668.

Dolzhenko, A. T., and Komissarov, I. V., 1982, A comparative study of the modulating effect of thyroliberin and melanostatin on neuromediator release by rat brain slices, in: Abstr. USSR Symp. on Bioorganic Chemistry and Drug Design Riga.

Donoso, A. O., and Alvarez, E. O., 1984, Brain histamine as neuroendocrine transmitter, TIPS, March: 98-100.

Faith, R. E., Plotnikoff N. P., Murgo, A. J. (In press), Effects of opiates
and enkephalins-endorphins on immune functions.
Feldberg, W., and Paton, W. D. M., 1949, Release of histamine by morphine
alkaloids, J. Physiol. (Lond.), 111:19P.
Greengard, P., 1979, Cyclic nucleotides, phosphorylated proteins, and the
nervous system, Federat. Proc., 39:2208-2217.
Haldar, J., Hofman, D. L., Nilaver, G., and Zimmerman, E. A., 1980, Oxytocin
and vasopressin release by substance P injected into the cerebral
ventricles of rats, in: Abstr. 9th Annu. Meet. Atlanta, Georgia,
Nov. 2-6, 1979, Bethesda, Soc. Neurosci., 5:447.
Henderson, N. D., 1970, Behavioural reactions of Wistar rats to conditioned
fear stimuli, novelty and noxious stimulation, J. Psychol., 75:19-34.
Johnson, H. M., 1983, Neuroendocrine polypeptide hormone regulation of
lymphokine production and lymphocyte function, Lymphokine Research,
2:49-56.
Johnson, H. M., Smith, E. M., Torres, B. A., and Blalock, J. E., 1982, Regulation of the in vitro antibody response by neuroendocrine hormones,
Proc. Natl. Acad. Sci., 79(13):4171-4174.
Jörnvall, H., Carlström, A., Pettersson, T., Jacobsson, B., Persson, M., and
Mutt, V., 1981, Structural homologies between prealbumin gastrointes-
tinal prohormones and other proteins, Nature, 291:261-263.
Kastin, A. J., Olson, R. D., Ehrensing, R. H., Berzas, M. C., Schally, A. V.,
and Coy, D. H., 1980, MIF-I differential actions as an opiate antagonists, Pharmacol. Biochem. Behav., 11:721-723.
Kendler, K. S., Weitzman, R. E., and Fisher, D. A., 1978, The effect of pain
on plasma arginine vasopressin concentration in man, Clin. Endocrinol.,
8:89-94.
Kluša, V., 1984, Peptides as Regulators of Brain Functions, Zinātne, Riga.
Kluša, V., Abissova, N., Kukaine, E., Afanasyeva, G., Misiņa, I., Myshlia-
kova, N., Muceniece, R., and Svirskis, Š., 1981a, Possible functional
relationship between neuro-, immuno- and glucomodulating peptides: A
hypothesis, in: Abstr. 4th USSR Symp. on Drug Design, Riga.
Kluša, V., Abissova, N., Muceniece, R., Svirskis, Š., Bienert, M., and
Lipkowski, A., 1981b, Comparative study of substance P and its fragments: analgesic properties, effects on behaviour and monoaminergic
processes, Byul. eksp. biol. i med., 12:692-694.
Kluša, V., Muceniece, R., and Svirskis, Š., 1982, Fragments of peptide hormones as possible central regulation factors, in: Neuropharmacology
of Peptides, A. V. Waldman, Ed., Moscow.
Kluša, V., Praulīte, G., Svirskis, Š., Muceniece, R., Kukaine, E., and
Abissova, N. A., 1984, Comparative study of the central effects of
the immunopeptides tuftsin and rigin, LPSR Zin. Akad. vēstis, 12:103-
109.
Kozlovskaya, M., Kluša, V., and Bondarenko, N., 1982, A comparison of psychotropic and neurochemical effects of short peptides, in: Neurochemical
aspects of psychotropic action, A. V. Waldman, Ed., Moscow.
Kukaine, E., 1981, Effects of neuropeptides and neurotransmitters on the
humoral immune system, in: Abstr. 4th USSR Symp. on Drug Design, Riga.
Kukaine, E., Muceniece, R., and Kluša, V., 1982, Comparison of neuro- and
immunomodulating properties of low-molecular neuropeptides, Byul.
eksp. biol. i med., 8:79-82.
Kukaine, E., Rosenthal, G., and Kluša, V., 1984, Tuftsin and rigin - opiate
or non-opiate peptides? in: Abstr. Conf. on Synthesis and Properties
of Physiol. Active Agents, Vilnius, 70-71.
Lin, T. M., 1972, Gastrointestinal actions of the C-terminal tripeptide of
gastrin, Gastroenterology, 63:922-923.
Lolait, S. J., Lim, A. T. W., Toh, B. H., and Funder, J. M., 1984, Immunoreactive ß-endorphin in a subpopulation of mouse spleen macrophages,
J. Clin. Invest., 73(1):277-280.
May, Ch. D., Lyman, M., Alberto, R., and Cheng, J., 1970, Procedures for
immunochemical study of histamine release from leukocytes with small

volume of blood, J. Allerg., 46:12-20.

Miller, G. C., Murgo, A. J., and Plotnikoff, N. P., 1983, Enkephalins - enhancement of active T-cell rosettes from lymphoma patients, Clin. Immunol. Immunopathol., 26(3):446-451.

Najjar, V. A., and Nishioka, K., 1970, Tuftsin, a natural phagocytosis stimulatory peptide, Nature, 228:672-673.

Nikitina, Z. S., Batuner, A. S., and Sytinsky, I. A., 1983, Activity of gamma-glutamine transferase in the brain following tuftsin administration, in: Abstr. 4th USSR Conf. on Biochemistry and Nervous System, Yerevan, 216-217.

Oehme, P., Bienert, M., Hecht, K. B., and Bergman, J., 1981, Substance P. Ausgewählte Probleme der Chemie, Biochemie, Pharmacologie, Physiologie und Pathophysiologie, Berlin.

Parviz, M. A., 1978, Psychopharmacology of morphinomimetic peptides in relation to schizophrenia, Gen. Pharmacol., 9:221-222.

Porsolt, R. D., Bertin, A., and Jalfre, M., 1977, Behavioral despair in mice: a primary screening test for antidepressants, Arch. Intern. Pharmacodyn., 229:327-336.

Rehfeld, J. F., and Golterman, N. R., 1979, Immunochemical evidence of cholecystokinin tetrapeptides in hog brain, J. Neurochemistry, 32: 1339-1341.

Ribeiro, S. A., Corrade, A. P., and Graff, F. G., 1968, Analgesia induced by intraventricular administration of bradykinin in the rabbit, Acta Physiol. Latinoam., 18:78-81.

Rossie, S. S., and Miller, R. J., 1982, Regulation of mast cell histamine release by neurotensin, Life Sci., 31:509-516.

Said, S. J., 1984, Vasoactive intestinal polypeptide (VIP): Current Status, Peptides, 5:143-150.

Sewell, R. D. E., and Spencer, P. S. J., 1977, The role of biogenic agents in the actions of centrally-acting analgesics, in: Progress in Medicinal Chemistry, G. P. Ellis, G. B. West, Eds., Elsewier/North Holland Biomedical Press, Amsterdam.

Sof'ina, Z. P., Lagova, N. D., and Kalashnikova, N. M., 1982, Hypothalamic peptide factors as potential antitumour agents, in: Abstr. USSR Symp. on Bioorgan. Chemistry and Drug Design, Riga, 53.

Tagaki, H., Shiomi, H., Ueda, H., and Amano, H., 1979, A novel analgesic dipeptide from bovine brain is a possible Met-enkephalin releaser, Nature, 282:410-413.

Vaught, J. C., Rothman, R. B., and Westfall, T. C., 1982, Mu and delta receptors: their role in analgesia and in differential effects of opioid peptides on analgesia, Life Sci., 30:1443-1455.

Waksman, B. H., 1979, Adjuvants and immune regulation by lymphoid cells, Springer Seminar of Immunopathology, 2:5-33.

Walaszek, E. J., 1970, Effect of bradykinin on the central nervous system, in: Handbook of Experimental Pharmacology, v. 25, Bradykinin, Kallidin and Kallikrein, E. G. Erdös, Ed., Springer Verlag, Berlin - Heidelberg - New York.

Waldman, A. W., 1982, Peptides as modulators of monoaminergic processes, in: Pharmacology of Neropeptides, A. V. Waldman, Ed., Moscow.

Weber, R., and Pert, C., 1984, Opiatergic modulation of the immune system, in: Central and Peripheral Endorphins: Basic and Clinical Aspects, E. E. Müller, A. R. Genazzani, Eds., Raven Press, New York.

Whitefield, J. F., Mac Manus, J. P., and Rixon, R. H., 1970, Potentiation by antidiuretic hormone (vasopressin) of the activity of parathyroid hormone to stimulate the proliferation of rat thymic lymphocytes, Hormone Metabol. Research, 2:235-237.

Yamasaki, Y., Shimamura, O., Kizu, A., Nakagawa, M., and Ijichi, H., 1982, IgE-mediated ^{14}C-serotonin release from rat mast cells modulated by morphine and endorphins, Life Sci., 31:471-478.

Yoshinori, I., Kazunori, M., Yukihiro, A., Tetsuya, N., Michihiro, F., and
   Showa, U., 1983, Attact stress and IgE antibody production in rats,
   Pharmacol. Biochem. and Behav., 19:883-886.
Zalitis, G., Afanasyeva, G., G., Golubeva, V., Veretennikova, N., and Chipens,
   1981, Immunochemical properties of rigin and tuftsin and their ef-
   fects on cellular and humoral immunity, in: Abstr. of USSR Symp.
   Bioorg. Chemistry and Drug Design, Riga, 49.

REGULATION OF HUMAN CELLULAR IMMUNE RESPONSES BY GLUCOCORTICOSTEROIDS

George C. Tsokos and James E. Balow

Arthritis and Rheumatism Branch
National Institute of Arthritis, Diabetes, and Digestive
   and Kidney Diseases
Building 10, Room 3N114
National Institutes of Health
Bethesda, Maryland 20205

INTRODUCTION

That glucocorticosteroids (GCS) are involved in the regulation of
the immune response was implied by Dr. Addison as early as the 1850's,
in his observations on disease states which today carry his name. It
was not until the 1930's when it was demonstrated that GCS exhibit
powerful thymolytic and lympholytic activities in vivo and later on
(1940's) in vitro. During the decade of 1940 Hench and his colleagues
reported spectacular therapeutic effects of cortisone in patients with
rheumatoid arthritis (1). During the next decade GCS were used
extensively in the treatment of various immune diseases including
systemic lupus erythematosus. During the 1960's several investigators
started intensive studies aimed at the dissection of the metabolic
effects of GCS on several cells (2-4). The decade of 1970's saw elegant
studies which addressed the question of the immunoregulation associated
with GCS both in vitro and in vivo (5-8). GCS have been found to
modulate every phase of human and animal immune responses. Several
described effects of GCS on different phases of the immune response
cannot be easily integrated to define the precise mechanism(s) of action
of these agents. Studies in animals have helped significantly the
understanding of the mode of action of GCS. The ultimate understanding
of the modulation of the human immune response has been impeded by the
different concentration ranges which obtain optimal effects in vivo and
in vitro. In addition the interspecies differences in tissue
sensitivity to GCS makes extrapolation of results from animal studies to
humans difficult (8,9). The present chapter will update the current
knowledge of the effects of GCS on the cellular immune response, i.e.
effects on peripheral mononuclear cells, cytotoxic and proliferative
responses, suppressor cell function, lymphokine production and B
lymphocyte responses.

MECHANISM OF ACTION

The mechanisms of action of GCS at a subcellular level have been
previously reviewed (2,3,7) and are elaborated elsewhere in this book.

A main contributor to the observed effects of GCS on cell-mediated immune responses pertains to the shift of the traffic of circulating human leucocytes. These traffic patterns have been dissected in elegant studies and have been reviewed elsewhere (8,10). In brief, the absolute number and the relative proportion of eosinophils, basophils, monocytes and lymphocytes are decreased 4 to 8 hours after the administration of pharmacologic doses of GCS and recover to the previous baseline levels within 24 to 72 hours. In contrast, neutrophils, both in absolute and relative numbers, increase 4-6 hours after administration of GCS and normalize 24 hours later. In particular, among the lymphocytes the thymus (T) derived cells are more sensitive than the bone marrow (B) derived. In regard to the subpopulations of the T lymphocytes, Tμ cells (carrying receptors for the Fc portion of the IgM molecule, helper subpopulation) are more sensitive than the Tγ cells (carrying receptors for the Fc portion of the IgG molecule, suppressor subpopulation) to GCS (11). Parallel studies of the effects of GCS on T lymphocyte subsets defined by monoclonal antibodies found that OKT4 cells (helper subpopulation) are more sensitive than OKT8 cells (suppressor subpopulation)(12).

EFFECT ON SURFACE MEMBRANE RECEPTORS

The reticuloendothelial system (RES) is currently thought to play a major role in the pathogenesis of immune and autoimmune diseases. Humoral elements interact with the receptors on the RES surface membranes for the Fc portion of the IgG molecule and receptors for breakdown products of the third component of the complement, particularly C3b (13). Corticosteroid treatment of guinea pigs prolonged the circulation of IgG and IgM sensitised autologous erythrocytes probably by decreasing the numbers of Fc and C3b receptors on the surface membranes of the cells of the RES (14). Similarly, GCS treatment of mice delayed the clearance of polymeric immune complexes of human serum albumin and corresponding antibody (15). In vitro studies using human peripheral monocytes showed that hydrocortisone (at concentrations 10^{-3} to 10^{-4} M) treatment for 30 minutes inhibited the binding of IgG sensitized erythrocytes as well as the binding of erythrocytes coated with C3 (16). In potentially related studies involving surface receptors, GCS have been found to inhibit the expression of Fc receptors on a human granulocytic cell line (27).

In vivo administration of GCS in normal individuals and in patients with autoimmune hemolytic anemia resulted in a significant decrease of the number of receptors for the Fc portion of IgG1 on the cell surface membrane of peripheral monocytes. The affinity binding constant (Ka) was not affected by GCS treatment (18). The above findings herald the salutory therapeutic effects of GCS in patients with autoimmune hemolytic anemia. However, the interactions of surface membrane receptor, immune complexes and GCS are far from simple. Thus, in other disease states, such as rheumatoid arthritis (19) and systemic lupus erythematosus (20), where the numbers of the Fc receptors are high, still the clearance of immune complexes is decreased (13) and the role of therapeutic GCS is far from clear.

EFFECTS ON MONOCYTE FUNCTION

GCS have been found to affect multiple functions of the human monocytes, including antigen presentation, lymphokine production, differentiation and phagocytosis. Monocyte chemotaxis is particularly sensitive to pharmacologic doses of glucocorticoids as measured by skin-window tests (21,22).

160

GCS inhibit the expression of surface Ia antigens by murine peritoneal macrophages both in vitro and in vivo, reduce the production of interleukin-1 (IL-1) and inhibit antigen presentation for T cell proliferation by macrophages (23). Similarly in man, it has been shown that GCS inhibit production of pyrogen (now known as IL-1) (24), interleukin-1 production and antigen (e.g. keyhole limpet hemocyanin) presentation (25), responses of macrophages to migration inhibitory factor (26,27) and macrophage mitogenic factor production (27). The latter in vitro effects of GCS on macrophages have been associated with their in vivo observed anti-inflammatory effects, namely decreased number of mononuclear cells in the inflammatory site and decreased "inflammatory" substances release. In contrast to the observations in mice, GCS increase instead of decreasing Ia antigen expression on the cell surface membrane of monocytes (28). Similar inhibitory effects exerted by GCS were described on the Langerhans cells in the skin (antigen presenting cells) (29). Thus, GCS are clearly involved in the initial phases of the immune response, i.e. antigen presentation.

Upon antigenic challenge monocytes are transformed to macrophages; this differentiation is associated with increased cell size, number of lysosomes, rough endoplasmic reticulum, increased acid phosphatase and 5' nucleotidase content; hydrocortisone inhibits all the above events if present at a concentration of 2.5 μM or higher (30). At the biochemical level, at least in mice, GCS inhibit the incorporation of leucine, glucose uptake and CO_2 production by peritoneal macrophages (31) which might account for the above described effects of GCS on human monocytes and macrophages.

EFFECTS ON THE PROLIFERATIVE RESPONSES OF T-LYMPHOCYTES

GCS inhibit the proliferative response of human T cells to several mitogens and antigens. Proliferative responses to phytohemagglutinin (PHA) are inhibited in vitro, manifested by a rightward shift of the dose-response curve (32). Removal of the phagocytic cells from the cell preparations greatly (100 fold) enhances the sensitivity to GCS (33). Cell cycle studies of human cells stimulated with PHA have indicated that GCS either prevent resting cells from entering the G1 phase (34) or arrest the progression of activated lymphocytes from G1 to S phase (35). In vivo administration of GCS inhibits the proliferative responses of peripheral mononuclear cells to PHA (32,36,37). Pokeweed mitogen (PWM) induced proliferative responses of human T cells (estimated usually by tritiated thymidine uptake on day 3 of the culture) is suppressed by GCS (38,39). GCS also inhibit the proliferative responses to antigens such as PPD (40).

Human allogeneic reactions are markedly decreased by GCS both in vitro (41-44) and after in vivo administration (45,46). The significance of the inhibition of the allogeneic mixed lymphocyte reaction may be relevant to their therapeutic usage in organ transplantation.

The mechanism of inhibition of cell proliferation by GCS can be understood considering the role of interleukin-2 (IL-2) production in T cell proliferation. Mitogenic or antigenic stimulation of T cells leads to the production of IL-2 (previously T cell growth factor) (41,47,48) which is necessary for the proliferation of T cells, sustenance of T cell lines and generation of cytotoxic T cells (49-51). Dexamethasone at concentrations of 1 μM, produces an almost complete inhibition of T cell growth factor production by human peripheral lymphocytes stimulated with PHA (4). GCS also inhibit the production of IL-2 in the human autologous mixed lymphocyte reaction (52). That GCS inhibit the production of T cell growth factor after stimulation with PHA, has also been extensively studied in mice (53,54) and underscores the potential importance of this mechanism in GCS-induced immunosuppression.

EFFECTS ON B LYMPHOCYTE RESPONSES

GCS have various effects on the immunoglobulin production by human B cells. In vivo administration of high doses of methylprednisolone for 3 to 5 days results to 22% decrease in serum IgG, 43% in IgA and 14% in IgM levels. Nadir levels are achieved 3 weeks after the end of the treatment (55). Increased catabolism during the treatment and decreased synthesis were postulated to be responsible for the observed results. GCS significantly depressed the primary IgG and IgM responses in asthmatic children immunised with keyhole limpet hemocyanin, but had no effect on the secondary antibody response (56). Similarly, IgE levels were depressed in asthmatic patients treated with GCS (57).

Mononuclear cells taken from individuals who were given a single dose (58) or 3-5 doses (12) of GCS exhibit diminished immunoglobulin secretion measured by plaque forming cell response after stimulation with pokeweed mitogen (PWM). This is probably due to the redistribution of the helper subpopulation of T lymphocytes caused by GCS treatment, and contrasts with the enhanced spontaneous B cell immunoglobulin production observed in these individuals (12).

In contrast to the suppressive effects of GCS administration in vivo on immunoglobulin production are the effects of GCS in in vitro systems. Addition of prednisolone at concentrations of 10^{-6} M in culture of human mononuclear cells with PWM (59-61) resulted in increased immunoglobulin production in the culture supernatants. This increase was attributed to direct action of GCS on B cells rather than through action on T cells (60). Similarly, in vitro corticosteroids enhance a PWM-driven direct anti-sheep red blood cell response (62), while plaque forming cell responses to trinitrophenyl-polyacrylamide are inhibited (63). The mechanism by which GCS cause enhancement of the PWM-induced immunoglobulin production is not clear. PWM stimulation requires accessory cells, and helper T cells. Recently it was found that nanomolar concentrations of hydrocortisone in vitro induce the generation of immunoglobulin producing cells from human mononuclear cells which peaks after 8-10 days (64). Of note is that these cultures were carried out in fetal calf serum. This immunoglobulin induction is T cell dependent and furthermore it was found that T cells stimulated with dexamethasone produce a lymphokine which has characteristics of T cell replacing factor (65). In short, it appears that GCS have major physiological roles at low concentrations and immunosuppressive effects at pharmacologic levels which is well demonstrated by their effects on B lymphocyte functions.

EFFECTS ON SUPPRESSOR CELL FUNCTION

GCS have been found to affect the suppressor cell limb of the immunoregulatory circuit. Waldmann et al initially described that the suppressor T cells which circulate in patients with common variable immunodeficiency are sensitive to hydrocortisone treatment both in vivo and in vitro. Pretreatment of the T cells from these patients with hydrocortisone abrogated their ability to suppress immunoglobulin

production by autologous and allogeneic B cells stimulated with pokeweed
mitogen (66,67). Administration of GCS to normal volunteers leads to a
temporary loss of suppressor cells generated in vitro after stimulation
of the peripheral MNC by PWM (58) but not with concanavalin A (Con A)
(68). The difference is apparently due to the fact that Con A is a more
potent stimulus of human suppressor cells than PWM. Pharmacologic
concentrations of GCS inhibit Con A induced suppressor cells if added
prior to initiation of cultures but they cannot modulate the expression
of suppressor activity of cells precultured with Con A (69).

The mechanism of expression of suppressive function by Con A
stimulated cells seems to be multiple. It has been suggested that Con A
stimulated cells can absorb interleukin 2, depriving the culture media
of necessary growth factors (70). It is possible that GCS inhibit the
expression or the function of interleukin-2 receptors on Con A blasts in
a way similar to that by which GCS inhibit the function of Fc and
complement receptors on cell surface membranes (16). Another way of
expression of suppressor cell function is by secretion of a 70 KD
suppressor factor (72) which either directly or indirectly (through
monocytes) inhibits immunoglobulin secretion by B cells. Blockage of
action of this suppressor factor has been postulated as one mechanism of
inhibition of suppressor cell function by GCS (72).

Besides the Con A-associated suppressor cell system, other more
specialized suppressor cells are inhibited or abrogated by GCS.
Hydrocortisone blocks the expression of suppressor cell activity which
is generated by culture in vitro of human mononuclear cells (7,73).
Similarly, GCS also abrogate the naturally occurring suppressor cell of
the PWM-stimulated anti-sheep red blood cell PFC response (68,69), and
the generation of suppressor cells in the human allogeneic mixed
lymphocyte reaction (74). Further delineation of the precise nature of
the suppressor cell mechanisms and functions is needed prior to
understanding their modulation by GCS.

EFFECTS ON AUTOLOGOUS MIXED LYMPHOCYTE REACTION (AMLR)

Human peripheral blood T lymphocytes respond with vigorous
proliferation when cultured in vitro with irradiated non-T peripheral
mononuclear cells. The presence of hydrocortisone during the culture at
concentrations equivalent to those found in normal plasma inhibits this
proliferative response (42-45,75). Treatment of adult volunteers with
intravenous methylprednisolone led to significant depression of the AMLR
(43,46). Interleukin-2 but not interleukin-1 is able to abrogate the
suppressive effect of hydrocortisone in these cultures, indicating that
suppression is exerted either by inhibition of the production of
interleukin-2 or by rendering the interleukin-2 producing T cells
unresponsive to interleukin-1 (52). AMLR is an important immune
reaction in vitro as it represents the ongoing autoreactivity in vivo.
Suppression of AMLR by physiologic concentrations of GCS indicates that
the generation of autoreactive cells in vivo is under such control.

EFFECTS ON CELL MEDIATED CYTOTOXICITY

Several forms of cell mediated cytotoxicity responses have been
found to be altered by GCS. Allo-specific cytotoxic T cells can be
generated in vivo or in vitro. Addition of GCS to cultures during the
cytolytic-effector phase has been shown to have little inhibitory effect
(76-79). The presence of GCS during the sensitization of cytotoxic
cells most consistently reduces the number of cytolytic T cells

generated during the culture (77,79), but in some systems also appears
to impair generation (76) as well as effector capacity (78) during
prolonged incubations. Peripheral blood mononuclear cells taken from
normal volunteers infused with hydrocortisone demonstrated enhanced
natural killer cell activity on a per cell basis during the nadir of
lymphopenia (80,81). The enhancement of natural killer cell activity
appears to be due to a selective depletion of non-cytotoxic cells from
the blood. Antibody-dependent cell-mediated cytotoxicity is similarly
enhanced by in vivo administration of GCS (81,82). As with cell
mediated lympholysis, GCS are generally unable to inhibit the cytolytic
phase of natural killer and antibody-dependent cellular cytotoxicity in
vitro (68). Lectin-mediated cytotoxicity is variably inhibited by GCS
(40,83).

CONCLUSION

      GCS participate in the human immunoregulation through a variety of
mechanisms. The need for elucidation of the mechanisms of action is
self-evident given that GCS are normal constituents of living organisms
and by the extent GCS are used today in the treatment of various disease
states. In Table I we summarise the effects of GCS on several facets of
the human cellular immune responses which have been described rather
unanimously as inhibitory. In Table II we list effects of GCS
on lymphoid cells which have an enhancing character. Despite the fact
that an enormous amount of information has been collected so far, the
definitive characterization of the mechanism of GCS-induced
immunoregulation depends on further knowledge of the regulation of the
human immune response in normal individuals and in patients.

Table I: Capitulation of the Inhibitory Effects of GCS on Human

Cellular Immune Responses

1. Effects on lymphocyte traffic

     a. Lymphopenia 4-6 hours after GCS treatment.
     b. T μ lymphopenia.

2. Effects on surface membrane receptors

     a. Fc receptor mediated immune clearance.
     b. C3b mediated immune clearance.

3. Effects on the proliferative responses of T cells

     a. Soluble antigens.
     b. Alloantigens and autoantigens.

4. Effects on lymphokine production

     a. IL-2 production in AMLR.
     b. IL-1 production.
     c. T-cell growth factor production after mitogenic stimulation.

5. Effects on monocytes

    a. Ia-antigen presentation.
    b. Interleukin-1 production.
    c. Migration inhibitory factor responsiveness.
    d. Differentiation to macrophages.

6. Autologous mixed lymphocyte reaction

7. Suppressor cells

    a. Spontaneously occurring suppressor cells in normal human peripheral blood.
    b. Spontaneous occurring suppressor cells in diseases (i.e., common variable immunodeficiency).
    c. Spontaneously developing after in vitro culture of human MNC.
    d. Generation of suppressor cells after stimulation in vitro with Con A, PWM, autoantigens.

8. Effects on cytotoxic responses

    a. PHA induced cellular cytotoxicity.
    b. Allogeneic cell mediated lympholysis.

9. Effects on B cell responses

    a. Serum immunoglobulins.
    b. Anti-trinitrophenyl plaque forming cell responses.
    c. PWM induced plaque forming cell responses following in vivo treatment with GCS.

Table II: Enhancing Effects of GCS on Lymphoid Cell Responses

A. Enhancement of PWM-induced plaque forming cell responses in vitro.

B. Immunoglobulin synthesis induction in vitro by GCS at nanomolar concentrations.

C. Induction of production of T cell replacing factor.

D. Enhancement of natural killer and antibody-dependent cell-mediated cytotoxic responses in vivo.

REFERENCES

1. P. S. Hench, E. D. Kendall, C. H. Slocumb, and H. F. Polley, Effect of a hormone of the adrenal cortex (17-hydroxy-11-dehydrocorticosterone: Compound E) and of pituitary adrenocorticotropic hormone on rheumatoid arthritis. Proc. Staff Meet. Mayo Clin. 24:181 (1949).

2. A. Munck, and K. Leuny, Glucocorticoid receptors and mechanisms of action receptors and mechanism of action of steroid hormones. Part II. Edited by J. R. Pasqualin; New York, Marcel Dekker Inc., p. 311.

3. A. Munck, and D. Young, Corticosteroid and lymphoid tissue, in "Handbook of physiology," Section 7, Vol. VI, Washington, D.C., American Physiological Society, p. 231.

4. G. R. Crabtree, K. A. Smith, and A. Munck, Glucocorticoids and immune responses, Arthritis Rheum. 22:1246 (1979).

5. A. S. Fauci, D. C. Dale and J. E. Balow, Glucocorticosteroid therapy: mechanisms of action and clinical considerations. Ann. Intern. Med. 84:304 (1976).

6. A. M. Dannenberg, The anti-inflammatory effects of glucocorticosteroids. A brief review of the literature. Inflammation 3:329 (1979).

7. J. E. Parrillo, A. S. Fauci, Mechanisms of glococorticoid action on immune processes. Ann. Rev. Pharmacol. Toxicol. 19:133 (1979).

8. T. R. Cupps, and A. S. Fauci, Corticosteroid-mediated immunoregulation in man. Immunological Rev. 65:133 (1982).

9. H. N. Claman, Corticosteroids and lymphoid cells. N. Engl. J. Med. 287:388 (1972).

10. A. S. Fauci, Immunosuppressive and anti-inflammatory effects of glucocorticoids. Monographs in endocrinology. Vol. 12. Glucoroticoid hormone action. Edited by J. D. Baxter and G. G. Rousseau, p. 449-465. Springer-Verlag Berlin Heidelberg.

11. B. F. Haynes, and A. S. Fauci, The differential effects of in vivo hydrocortisone on kinetics of subpopulations of human peripheral blood thymus-derived lymphocytes. J. Clin. Invest. 61:703 (1978).

12. T. F. Cupps, L. C. Edgar, C. A. Thomas, and A. S. Fauci, Multiple mechanisms of B cell immunoregulation in man after administration of in vivo corticosteroids. J. Immunol. 132:170 (1984).

13. M. M. Frank, T. J. Lawley, M. I. Hamburger, and E. J. Brown, Immunoglobulin G Fc receptor-mediated clearance in autoimmune diseases. Ann. Intern. Med. 9o8:206 (1983).

14. J. P. Atkinson, A. D. Schreiber, and M. M. Frank, Effects of corticosteroids and splenectomy on the immune clearance and destruction of erythrocytes. J. Clin. Invest. 52:1509 (1973).

15. A. O. Haakenstad, J. B. Case, and M. Mannik, Effect of cortisone on the disappearance kinetics and tissue localization of soluble immune complexes. J. Immunol. 114:1153 (1975).

16. A. D. Schreiber, J. Parson, P. McDermott, and R. A. Cooper, Effect of corticosteroids on the human monocyte IgG and complement receptors. J. Clin. Invest. 56:1189 (1975).

17. G. R. Crabtree, A. Munck, and K. A. Smith, Glucocorticoids inhibit expression of Fc receptors on the human granulocytic cell line HL-60. Nature 279:338 (1979).

18. L. F. Fries, C. M. Brickman, and M. M. Frank, Monocyte receptors for the Fc portion of IgG increase in number of autoimmune hemolytic anemia and other hemolytic states and are decreased by glucocorticoid therapy. J. Immunol. 131:1240 (1983).

19. S. Katayama, D. Chia, H. Nasau, and D. W. Knutson, Increased Fc receptor activity in monocytes from patients with rheumatoid arthritis: a study of monocyte binding and catabolisms of soluble aggregates of IgG in vitro. J. Immunol. 127:643 (1981).

20. L. F. Fries, W. W. Mullins, K. R. Cho, P. H. Plotz, and M. M. Frank, Monocyte receptors for the Fc portion of IgG are increased in systemic lupus erythematosus. J. Immunol. 132:695 (1984).

21. D. C. Dale, A. S. Fauci, D. Guerry, and S. M. Wolff, Comparison of agents producing a neutrophilic leucocytosis in man. Hydrocortisone, prednisone, endotoxin, and etiocholanolone. J. Clin. Invest. 56:808 (1974).

22. J. J. Rinehart, S. P. Balcerzak, A. L. Sagone, and A. F. Lobuglio, Effects of corticosteroids on human monocyte function. J. Clin. Invest. 54:1337 (1974).

23. D. S. Synder, and E. R. Unanue, Corticosteroids inhibit murine macrophage Ia expression and interleukin-1 production. J. Immunol. 129:1803 (1982).

24. G. M. Dillard, and P. Bodel, Studies on steroid fever. II. Pyrogenic and antipyrogenic activity in vitro of some endogenous steroids of man. J. Clin. Invest. 49:2418 (1970).

25. T. L. Gerrard, T. R. Cupps, C. H. Jergensen, and A. S. Fauci, Hydrocortisone-mediated inhibition of monocyte antigen presentation: Dissociation of inhibitory effect and expression of DR antigens. Cell. Immunol. 85:330 (1984).

26. J. E. Balow, and A. S. Rosenthal, Glucocorticoid suppression of macrophage migration inhibitory factor. J. Exp. Med. 137:1031 (1973).

27. M. R. Duncan, J. R. Saklik, and J. W. Hadden, Glucocorticoid modulation of lymphokine-induced macrophage proliferation. Cell. Immunol. 67:23 (1982).

28. T. L. Gerrard, T. R. Cupps, C. H. Jurgensen, and A. S. Fauci, Increased expression of HLA-DR antigens in hydrocortisone-treated monocytes. Cell. Immunol 84:311 (1984).

29. D. V. Belsito, T. J. Flotte, H. W. Lim, R. L. Baer, G. J. Thorbecke, and I. Gigli, Effect of glucocorticosteroids on epidermal Langerhans cells. J. Exp. Med 155 (1982).

30. J. J. Rinehart, D. Wuest, and G. A. Ackerman, Corticosteroid alteration of human monocyte to macrophage differentiation. J. Immunol. 129:1436 (1982).

31. J. M. Norton, and A. Munck, In vitro actions of glucocorticoids on murine macrophages: Effects on glucose transport and metabolism growth in culture and protein synthesis. J. Immunol. 125:259 (1980).

32. A. S. Fauci, Mechanisms of corticosteroid action on lymphocyte subpopulations. II. Differential effects of in vivo hydrocortisone, prednisone and dexamethasone on in vitro expression of lymphocyte function. Clin. Exp. Immunol. 24:54 (1976).

33. H. Blomgren, Steroid sensitivity of the response of human lymphocytes to phytohemagglutinin and pokeweed mitogen: Role of phagocytic cells. Scand J. Immunol. 3:655 (1974).

34. A. J. Robertson, J. H. Gibbs, R. C. Potts, R. A. Brown, M. C. K. Browning, and J. S. Back, Dose-related depression of PHA-induced stimulation of human lymphocytes by hydrocortisone. Int. J. Immunopharmacol. 3:21 (1981).

35. J. C. Sloman, and PO. A. Bell, Cell cycle-specific effects of glucocorticoids on phytohemagglutinin-stimulated lymphocytes. Clin. Exp. Immunol. 39:503 (1980).

36. J. L. Webel, R. E. Ritts, H. F. Taswell, J. V. Donadio Jr., and J. E. Woods, Cellular immunity after intravenous administration of methylprednisolone. J. Lab. Clin. Med. 83:383 (1974).

37. J. L. Webel, and R. E. Ritts Jr., The effects of corticosteroid concentrations on lymphocyte blastogenesis. Cell. Immunol. 32:287 (1977).

38. D. H. Heilman, Failure of hydrocortisone to inhibit blastogenesis by pokeweed mitogen in human leukocyte cultures. Clin. Exp. Immunol. 11:393 (1972).

39. D. H. Heilman, M. Gambrill, and J. P. Leichner, The effect of hydrocortisone on the incorporation of tritiated thymidine by human blood lymphocytes cultured with phytohemagglutinin and pokeweed mitogen. Clin. Exp. Immunol. 15:203 (1973).

40. A. E. Butterworth, Nonspecific cytotoxic effects of antigen-transformed lymphocytes. II. Inhibition by drugs. Cell. Immunol. 16:60 (1975).

41. J. C. Rosenberg, M. P. Kaplan, K. Lysz, Mechanisms of steroid suppression of immune function: Effect of methylprednisolone on lymphocyte activation and proliferation. Surgery. 88:193 (1980).

42. D. M. Ilfeld, R. S. Krakauer, and R. M. Blaese, Suppression of the human autologous mixed lymphocyte reaction by physiologic concentrations of hydrocortisone. J. Immunol. 119:428 (1977).

43. D. T. Y. Yu, S. J. Ramer, and P. J. Clements, Effect of methylprednisolone on autologous mixed lymphocyte cultures. Transplantation. 163:165 (1978).

44. R. P. MacDermott, and M. C. Stacey, Further characterization of the human autologous mixed leucocyte reaciton (MLR). J. Immunol. 126:729 (1981).

45. P. Katz, and A. S. Fauci, Autologous and allogeneic intercellular interaction. Modulation by adherent cells, irradiation and in vitro and in vivo corticosteroids. J. Immunol. 123:2270 (1979).

46. B. H. Hahn, R. P. MacDermott, Burkholder, S. Jacobs, J. L. Pletscher, and M. G. Beale, Immunosuppressive effects of low doses of glucocorticoids: Effects on autologous and allogeneic mixed lymphocyte reactions. J. Immunol. 124:2812 (1980).

47. D. A. Morgan, F. W. Ruscetti, and R. Gallo, Selective in vitro growth of T-lymphocytes from normal human bone marrows. Science 193:1007 (1976).

48. J. D. Watson, L. A. Aarden, and I. Lefkovitz, The purification and quantitation of helper T-cell replacing factors secreted by murine spleen cells activated by concanavalin A. J. Immunol. 122:204 (1979).

49. S. Gillis, D. A. Smith, Long-term culture of tumor-specific cytotoxic T-cells. Nature 268:154 (1977).

50. W. L. Farrar, H. M. Johnson, and J. J. Farrar, Regulation of the production of immune interferon and cytotoxic T lymphocytes by interleukin-2. J. Immunol. 126:1120 (1981).

51. S. Gillis, and J. Watson, Interleukin-2 induction of hapten-specific cytolytic T cells in nude mice. J. Immunol. 126:1245 (1981).

52. R. Pelacios, and I. Sugawara, Hydrocortisone abrogates proliferation of T cells in autologous mixed lymphocyte reaction by rendering the interleukin-2 producer T cells unresponsive to interleukin-1 and unable to synthesize T cell growth factor. Scand. J. Immunol. 15:25 (1982).

53. E. L. Larsson, Cyclosporin A and dexamethasone suppress T cell responses by selectively acting at distinct sites of the triggering process. J. Immunol. 124:2828 (1980).

54. S. Gillis, G. R. Crabtree, and K. A. Smith, Glucocorticoid induced inhibition of T cell growth factor production. I. The effect on mitogen-induced lymphocyte proliferation. J. Immunol. 123:1624 (1979).

55. W. T. Butler, and R. G. Rossen, Effects of corticosteroids on immunity in man. I. Decreased serum IgG concentration caused by 3 or 5 days of high doses of methylprednisolone. J. Clin. Invest. 52:2629 (1973).

56. M. Tuchinda, R. W. Newcomb, and B. L. De Vald, Effect of prednisone treatment on the human immune response to keyhole limpet hemocyanin. Int. Arch. Allergy 42:533 (1972).

57. W. C. Posey, H. S. Nelson, B. Banch, and D. S. Pearlman, The effects of acute corticosteroid therapy for asthma on serum immunoglobulin levels. J. Allergy Clin. Immunol. 62:340 (1978).

58. A. Saxon, R. H. Stevens, S. J. Ramer, P. J. Clement, and D. T. Y. Yu, Glococorticoids administered in vivo inhibit human suppressor T lymphocyte function and diminish B lymphocyte responsiveness in in vitro immunoglobulin synthesis. J. Clin. Invest. 61:922 (1978).

59. D. A. Cooper, M. Duckett, V. Petts, and R. Penny, Corticosteroid enhancement of immunoglobulin synthesis by pokeweed mitogen-stimulated human lymphocytes. Clin. Exp. Immunol. 37:145 (1979).

60. D. A. Cooper, M. Duckett, P. Hansen, V. Petts, and R. Penny, Glucocorticosteroid enhancement of immunoglobulin synthesis by pokeweed mitogen-stimulated human lymphocytes. Clin. Exp. Immunol. 37:145 (1979).

61. D. A. Cooper, P. Hansen, M. Duckett, J. B. Ziegeler, and R. Penny, Glucocorticosteroid enhancement of immunoglobulin synthesis by pokeweed mitogen-stimulated human lymphocytes. III. Common variable immunodeficiency. Clin. Exp. Immunol. 45:399 (1981).

62. A. S. Fauci, K. R. Pratt, and G. Whalen, Activation of human B lymphocytes. IV. Regulatory effects of corticosteroids on the triggering signal in the plaque-forming cell reponse of human peripheral blood B lymphocytes to polyclonal activation. J. Immunol. 119:598.

63. P. Galanaud, M. C. Crevon, D. Hillion, and J. F. Delfraissy, Hydrocortisone sensitivity of human in vitro antibody response: Different sensitivity of the specific and the nonspecific B cell responses induced by the same agent. Clin. Immunol. Immunopathol. 18:68 (1981).

64. J. Grayson, N. J. Dooley, I. R. Koski, and R. M. Blaese, Immunoglobulin production induced in vitro by glucocorticoid hormones. T cell-dependent stimulation of immunoglobulin production without B cell proliferation in cultures of human peripheral blood lymphocytes. J. Clin. Invest. 68·1539 (1981).

65. F. M. Orson, J. Grayson, S. Pike, V. DeSean, and R. M. Blaese, T cell-replacing factor for glucocorticosteroid-induced immunoglobulin production. A unique steroid-dependent cytokine. J. Exp. Med. 158:1473 (1983).

66. T. A. Waldmann, S. Broder, R. Krakauer, R. P. MacDermott, M. Durm, C. Goldman, and B. Meade, The role of suppressor cells in the pathogenesis of common variable hypogammaglobulinemia and the immunodeficiency associated with myeloma. Fed. Proc. 35:2067 (1976).

67. T. A. Waldmann, R. M. Blaese, S. Broder, and R. S. Krakauer, Disorders of suppressor immunoregulatory cells in the pathogenesis of immunodeficiency and autoimmunity. Ann. Intern. Med. 88:226 (1978).

68. B. F. Haynes, P. Katz, and A. S. Fauci, Mechanisms of corticosteroid action on lymphocyte subpopulations. V. Effects of in vivo hydrocortisone on the circulatory kinetics and function of naturally occurring and mitogen-induced suppressor cell in man. Cell. Immunol. 44:169 (1979).

69. B. F. Haynes, A. S. Fauci, Mechanisms of corticosteroid action on lymphocyte subpospulations. IV. Effects of in vitro hydrocortisone on naturally occurring and mitogen-induced suppressor cells in man. Cell. Immunol. 44:157 (1979).

70. R. Palacios, and G. Moller, T cell growth factor abrogates concanavalin A-induced suppressor cell function. J. Exp. Med. 153:1360 (1981).

71. T. A. Fleisher, W. C. Greene, R. M. Blaese, and T. A. Waldmann, Soluble suppressor supernatants elaborated by concanavalin A-activated human mononuclear cells. II. Characterization of a soluble suppressor B cell immunoglobulin production. J. Immunol. 126:1192 (1981).

72. D. Ilfeld, and R. S. Krakauer, Hydrocortisone reverses the suppression of immunoglobulin synthesis by concanavalin A-activated spleen cell supernatants. Clin. Exp. Immunol. 48:244 (1982).

73. P. E. Lipsky, W. W. Ginsburg, F. D. Finkelman, and M. Ziff, Control of human B lymphocyte responsiveness enhanced suppressor T cell activity after in vitro incubation. J. Immunol. 120:902 (1978).

74. B. M. Frey, F. J. Frey, K. C. Cochrum, and L. Z. Benet, Induction kinetics of human suppressor cells in the mixed lymphocyte reaction and influence of prednisolone on their genesis. Cell. Immunol. 56:225 (1980).

75. G. Opelz, M. Kinchi, M. Takasugi, and P. I. Terasaki, Autologous stimulation of human lymphocyte subpopulations. J. Exp. Med. 142:1327 (1975).

76. J. C. Rosenberg, and K. Lysz, Suppression of the immune response by steroids. Comparative potency of hydrocortisone, methylprednisolone, and dexamethasone. Transplantation 29:425 (1980).

77. J. E. Balow, G. W. Hunninghake, and A. S. Fauci, Corticosteroids in human lymphocyte-mediated cytotoxic reactions. Effects on the kinetics of sensitization on the cytolytic capacity of effector lymphocytes in vitro. Transplantation 23:322 (1977).

78. R. P. Scheimer, A. Jacques, S. H. Shin, L. M. Lichtenstein, and M. Plant, Inhibition of T cell-mediated cytotoxicity by anti-inflammatory steroids. J. Immunol. 132:266 (1984).

79. L. M. Muul, and M. K. Gately, Hydrocortisone suppresses the generation of nonspecific "anomalous" killers but not specific cytolytic T lymphocytes in human mixed lymphocyte-tumor cultures. J. Immunol. 132:1202 (1984).

80. M. Onsrud, and E. Thorsby, Influence of in vivo hydrocortisone on some human blood lymphocyte subpopulations. Scand. J. Immuno. 13:573 (1981).

81. P. Katz, A. M. Zaytoren, and J. H. Lee, The effects of in vivo hydrocortisone on lymphocyte-mediated cytotoxicity. Arthritis Rheum. 27:72 (1984).

82. J. W. Parrillo, and A. S. Fauci, Comparison of the effector cells in human spontaneous cellular cytotoxicity and antibody-dependent cellular cytotoxicity: Differential sensitivity of effector cells to in vivo and and in vitro corticosteroids. Scand. J. Immunol. 8:99 (1978).

83. J. R. Clarke, R. F. Gagnon, F. M. Gotch, M. R. Heyworth, I. M. C. MacLennan, S. C. Truelove, and C. A. Waller, The effect of prednisolone on leucocyte function in man. Clin. Exp. Immunol. 28:292 (1977).

ESTROGEN-MEDIATED IMMUNOMODULATION

Oscar J. Pung, Anne N. Tucker, and Michael I. Luster

National Institute of Environmental Health Sciences
Systemic Toxicology Branch, TRTP, P.O. Box 12233
Research Triangle Park, NC 27709

INTRODUCTION

Early anatomic observations demonstrating that ovariectomy enhanced thymic weights while thymectomy modulated uterine weight provided an impetus for numerous studies which established a relationship between sex hormones and the immune system (see rev. by Ahlquist, 1976; Kalland, 1982; Luster et al., 1985). These studies suggested that pharmacological and to some extent physiological levels of estrogens, as well as inadvertent exposure to estrogenic compounds in the environment, may modulate immune function. Consistent with the immunological alterations, clinical and laboratory studies demonstrated that altered estrogen levels can modulate host resistance to a variety of infectious agents. Illustrative of this are the findings that estrogens precipitate a dramatic increase in Listeria monocytogenes susceptibility (Dean et al., 1980; Pung et al., 1984), impair the intestinal expulsion of adult nematode Trichinella spiralis (Dean et al., 1980; Luebke et al., 1984) and increase the susceptibility of mice to both transplantable and methylcholanthrene-induced tumors (Dean et al., 1980; Morahan et al., 1984; Kalland and Forsberg, 1981). Estradiol has also been shown to induce more intense chlamydial (Rank et al., 1982) and staphylococcal (Toivanen, 1967) infections. Pharmacological doses of diethylstilbestrol (DES), a nonsteroidal synthetic estrogen, or 17β-estradiol increase the severity of experimental toxoplasmosis in mice (Pung and Luster, submitted). In other instances, estrogen treated mice are less susceptible to bacterial infection, examples being Pneumococcus Type I, Pasteurella spp. and Salmonella spp. (Nicol et al., 1964). Rodents exposed to DES are also less susceptible to the formation of transplantable lung melanoma tumors (Fugmann et al., 1983) as well as to certain plasmodial, babesial and trypanosomal infections (Cottrell et al., 1977; Kierszenbaum et al., 1974; Mankau, 1975).

A number of chemical xenobiotics, including DDT, isomers of poly-chlorinated biphenyls (PCB's) and chlordecone (Kepone), demonstrate both estrogenic activity, as determined by the rat uterine bioassay (rev. by Katzenellenbogen et al., 1980) and immunotoxicity (rev. by Luster et al., 1985). Naturally occurring environmental estrogens, including Δ^9-tetrahydrocannabinol, the mycotoxin zearalenone and its derivative zearalenol, a commercial anabolic agent, have also been reported to affect the immune system (rev. by Luster et al., 1985). While these xenobiotics are only weakly estrogenic, they have relatively long half-lives and may exert a chronic influence on normal ovulatory cycles (Eroschenko and Palmiter, 1980). DES, one of the most potent synthetic estrogens, has widespread agricultural and therapeutic use, having been employed as a growth promoting agent in the sheep and cattle industries as well as therapeutically in humans in estrogen replacement, as anti-abortive agents and in the treatment of breast and prostate cancer (rev. by McMartin et al., 1978; McLachlan et al., 1976). More importantly, the therapeutic use of DES has been associated with adenosquamous carcinoma of the uterus (Culter et al., 1972) and clear-cell adenocarcinoma of the vagina in young women exposed to DES in utero (Herbst et al., 1971).

INFLUENCE OF ESTROGENS ON IMMUNE FUNCTION

Pharmacological Levels

Estrogens induce multiple effects on the immune system of laboratory animals when administered in pharmacological quantities, many of which are listed in Table 1. Suppression of cell-mediated immunity by DES and estradiol has been well documented. In mice, both compounds depress cutaneous delayed hypersensitivity (Kalland and Forsberg, 1978; Rifkind and Frey, 1974; Luster et al., 1980), allograft rejection (Franks et al., 1975; Waltman et al., 1971) and the in vitro lymphoproliferative response to mitogens or allogeneic leukocytes (Luster et al., 1980; Kalland et al., 1979; Ways et al., 1980). Immunosuppression following perinatal exposure, i.e. during periods of immune ontogenesis, appears to persist, whereas adult exposure induces more transient responses (Kalland 1982; Luster et al., 1981). Estrogens are reported to decrease the number of splenic T-helper cells (Kalland, 1980) and inhibit the production of interleukin 2 (Henriksen and Frey, 1982) which suggests that they affect T cell maturation. Depressed cellular immunity has been reported in women taking oral contraceptives (Barnes et al., 1974). Studies by Ablin et al. (1979) have also demonstrated depressed cellular immunity in prostate cancer patients receiving estrogen therapy.

Humoral immunity is also modulated in mice administered estrogen, although the alteration does not appear to be at the level of the B cell. Suppression of humoral immunity may occur as a result of stimulation of the RES and subsequent antigen sequestering and/or increased hepatic uptake and clearance of antigen from the blood (Sljivic and Warr, 1974; Bick et al., 1984). Suppression of the antibody response observed in mice exposed perinatally to DES has been reported to occur as a result of altered regulatory cell function, specifically depletion of T-helper cell function (Kalland, 1980a). Several investigators have provided evidence that estrogens enhance antibody synthesis (Kenny et al., 1976), which may be due to a general depletion of T-suppressor cells (Paavonen et al., 1981). It is also evident from clinical observations that the thera-peutic use of estrogens can affect humoral immune responses in humans. For example, women taking oral contraceptives exhibit enhanced humoral immunity (Bole et al., 1969).

In contrast to suppression of T-cell functions, pharmacological levels of estrogen stimulate mononuclear phagocyte activity. This is illustrated by enhanced vascular clearance of antigen from the cir-culation of estrogen-treated animals (Nicol et al., 1964). The rapid clearance is due to hyperphagocytosis and increased division of Kupffers cells (Den Dulk et al., 1979; Kelly et al., 1962). The effects of

Table 1

Altered Host Resistance and Immunity in Laboratory Animals Exposed to Pharmacological Doses of Estrogens

	References
Increased Resistance To: Pneumococcus, Pasteurella, Salmonella Lung melanoma tumors plasmodial, babesial and trypanasomal infections	Nicol et al., 1964 Fugmann et al., 1983; Morahan et al., 1984 Cottrell et al., 1977; Kierszenbaum et al., 1974
Decreased Resistance To: Listeria monocytogenes Trichinella tumors (transplantable and chemically induced) chlamydial infections staphylococcal infections toxoplasmosis	Dean et al., 1980; Pung et al., 1984 Dean et al., 1980; Luebke et al., 1984 Dean et al., 1980; Kalland and Forsberg, 1981 Rank et al., 1982 Toivanen, 1967 Kittas and Henry, 1980; Pung and Luster, 1984
Altered Immune Functions: enhanced mononuclear phagocytic activity stimulation of antigen clearance depressed delayed hypersensitivity response depressed allograft rejection depressed mixed leukocyte response depressed T cell lymphoproliferative response decreased number of splenic T-helper cells inhibition of interleukin-2 production decreased numbers of bone marrow stem cells depressed erythropoiesis deficient NK activity	Boorman et al., 1980; Dean et al., 1984 Loose and DiLuzio, 1976; Nicol et al., 1964; Sljivic et al., 1975 Kalland and Forsberg, 1978; Luster et al., 1980 Franks et al., 1975; Waltman et al., 1971 Luster et al., 1980 Kalland et al., 1979; Luster et al., 1980; Kalland, 1980a Henriksen and Frey, 1982 Boorman et al., 1980; Fried et al., 1974 Boorman et al., 1980; Fried et al., 1974 Seaman et al., 1979; Kalland, 1980b; Kalland and Forsberg, 1981

estrogens on circulating mononuclear phagocytic cells are less clear. While chronic estrogen exposure decreases the number of circulating monocytes (Loose and DiLuzio, 1976), moderate increases in circulating (Kelly et al., 1962) and resident peritoneal macrophages (Boorman et al., 1980) occur following subchronic exposure, in addition to hyperphagocytosis, increased production of plasminogen activator, and increased inhibition of tumor cell growth, i.e., cytostasis (Boorman et al., 1980; Dean et al., 1984). On the other hand, characteristics of fully activated macrophages such as cytolytic protease secretion and tumor cell binding or lysis are lacking (Dean et al., 1984). Consequently, these cells more closely resemble an inflammatory macrophage population.

Spleen cells from mice treated with estradiol or DES are deficient in natural killer (NK) cell activity (Kalland et al., 1980b; Kalland and Forsberg, 1981; Seaman et al., 1979). DES also impairs natural killer cell activity in humans during treatment for prostatic cancer (Kalland and Haukaas, 1981).

Exposure to pharmacological doses of estrogen depresses hematopoiesis in rodents (Reisher, 1966). Estrogen induced myelotoxicity is characterized by bone marrow hypocellularity and depressed numbers of CFUs (Fried et al., 1974; Boorman et al., 1980). Decreased bone marrow erythropoiesis also occurs although a compensatory increase in splenic erythropoiesis is observed several days following cessation of estrogen administration (Fried et al., 1974). Splenic compensation does not occur for CFU-S or CFU-GM progenitor cells which remain depressed in both the bone marrow and spleen for several weeks (Fried et al., 1974; Boorman et al., 1980; Luster et al., 1984a). Myelotoxicity occurs in the absence of estradiol-induced osteoproliferation, indicating that cell kinetics are not simply due to decreases in marrow volume (Luster et al., 1984a).

Physiological Levels

Pregnancy, age, ovariectomy and the ovulatory cycle influence serum estrogen levels. These quantitative alterations in the serum often correlate with changes in the immune system which may be more regulatory in nature than pathological. However, pregnancy, age, ovariectomy and the ovulatory cycle are also accompanied by fluctuations in a variety of other hormones and serum proteins which are also potential immunoregulators, including human chorionic gonadotrophin (Carter, 1976), corticosteroids (Heslop et al., 1954) and pregnancy-associated α-macroglobin (Stimson, 1976). Thus, in vivo data correlating immunological changes with variations in physiological estrogen levels may not represent a direct relationship. Ovulation, pregnancy and ovariectomy influence the number of peripheral leukocytes; for instance, lymphocyte counts are lowest in women at the midpoint of the menstrual cycle when estradiol levels are maximal (Mathur et al., 1979). The number of peripheral lymphocytes and eosinophils progressively declines during pregnancy as estradiol levels rise and then return to normal following partuition (Sturgis and Bethell, 1943; Valdimarsson et al., 1983). Polymorphonuclear leukocyte (PMN) numbers increase throughout pregnancy whereas peripheral monocyte numbers rise during the first and early second trimester and then return to normal levels (Sturgis and Bethell, 1943; Valdimarsson et al., 1983). The number of endometrial macrophages is decreased by ovariectomy and restored by estrogen treatment (Fluhmann, 1932) and increased during proestrus and metestrus when serum estradiol reaches peak levels (Nicol and Abou-Zikry, 1953).

With regards to the physiological effects of estrogens on immune function, the blastogenic response of murine splenic lymphocytes to B cell and T cell mitogens, as well as the number of IgM plaque forming cells, increases during proestrus and estrus (Krzych et al., 1981). Relative enhancement of antibody production reported in females (Batchelor, 1968; Rifkind and Frey, 1972; Stern and Davidsohn, 1955) may be due to an absence of immunosuppressive androgenic hormones rather than of physiological estrogen. The X chromosome may also play a role in regulation of the humoral response, as suggested originally by Washburn et al. (1965). This idea is supported by familial studies comparing IgM levels among parents and offspring (Grundbacher, 1972). On the other hand, pregnancy depresses the contact allergic reaction to picryl chloride (Carter, 1976). Depression of contact allergic reactions also occurs in ovariectomized pregnant mice reconstituted with estradiol and progesterone (Carter, 1976). Allograft rejection (Heslop, 1954) and the lymphoproliferative response to T-cell mitogens (Purtilo et al., 1972; Valdimarsson, 1983) are depressed during pregnancy, as is IgM antibody production (Suzuki and Tomasi, 1979).

Changes in physiological estrogen levels may also affect the mono-nuclear phagocyte system. For example, macrophages from female mice are more phagocytic than those from male mice (Fruhman, 1973), and cyclic increases in estradiol during proestrus and metestrus correlate with augmented antigen clearance by macrophages, as well as increased macrophage activity and numbers (Nicol and Vernon-Roberts, 1965; Vernon-Roberts, 1969). Enhanced phagocytosis also correlates with increases in uterine weight during estrus (Vernon-Roberts, 1965), whereas ovariectomy decreases phagocyte activity (Nicol and Vernon-Roberts, 1965).

The effects of cyclic changes in serum estradiol concentrations on resistance to infection appear to be consistent with alterations in the immune system. For example, decreased resistance to viral (Mendelow and Lewis, 1969), bacterial (Kass, 1960; Luft and Remington, 1982) and fungal infections (Vaughan and Ramirez, 1951) have been reported to occur in pregnant women. Furthermore, pregnant mice are more susceptible to L. monocytogenes and Toxoplasma gondii (Luft and Remington, 1982) and Plasmodium berghei (van Zon et al., 1982). Bodel et al. (1972) reported that the bactericidal activity of PMNs is inhibited during pregnancy. In contrast, Mitchell et al. (1966) found PMNs from pregnant women to be hyperphagocytic and highly bactericidal. They also observed (1970) that hexose monophosphate shunt and myeloperoxidase (MPO) enzyme activity was augmented in PMNs from pregnant women. These data suggest that estradiol regulates PMN activity during pregnancy.

Regulation of the immune response by physiological estrogen levels is also suggested by contrasting males and females, although in many studies the sex differences are minimal and require large numbers of experimental animals to achieve statistical significance (rev. by Alquist, 1976). Females are generally considered to have augmented humoral immunity as opposed to males (Terres et al., 1968; Krzych et al., 1981; Kenny and Gray, 1971) although, as mentioned before, this may be due to chromosomal and not hormonal sex differences (Rhodes et al., 1969). In humans, cell-mediated immunity is depressed in females relative to males as evidenced by an increased incidence of autosomal disorders (Inman, 1978) and depressed cell-mediated cytotoxic events (Santoli et al., 1976). The blastogenic response of spleen cells from female mice to B-cell and T-cell mitogens is generally higher than that of male mice (Krzych et al., 1981).

Environmental Estrogens

As mentioned previously, several environmental xenobiotics demonstrate both estrogenic activity, as determined by the rat uterine bioassay, and immunotoxicity (rev. by Luster et al., 1985). Although intriguing, there is no evidence that their immunotoxicity is related to estrogenic activity. In fact, DDT and chlordecone (Kepone), both of which appear to induce persistent uterotrophic activity in the rat (rev. by Katzenellenbogen et al., 1980), induce decreased antibody production and thymic atrophy only at near lethal doses (rev. by Luster et al., 1985). The immunological effects of Δ^9-THC are typical of those seen by other estrogens in that lymphocyte reactivity is depressed and CMI is more affected than HMI, but atypical with respect to the lack of effect on the RES (Munson et al., 1976).

MECHANISMS OF ACTION

Subcellular Mechanisms

Unlike peptide hormones, where effects are often mediated through second messengers such as cyclic AMP, estrogens exert their effects on target cell chromatin to initiate the response. Translocation of estrogen into the nucleus and its association with chromatin is regulated by a specific intracellular receptor (Gorski et al., 1968). While many mammalian tissues contain estrogen receptors, including lymphocytes (Cohen et al., 1983; Luster et al., 1984a) and eosinophils (Tshernitchin, 1983), in general, only certain tissues, usually those that possess relatively high receptor concentrations, have been shown to be responsive. In this respect, accumulating evidence suggests that the thymus, and specifically thymic epithelium, is an estrogen responsive tissue, and some manifestations of estrogen-induced immunotoxicity are clearly related to thymic alterations. Although it was only recently demonstrated that the binding of estrogens to thymic tissue could alter the immune response (Grossman et al., 1982; Luster et al., 1984a,b; Stimson and Hunter, 1980), the existence of an interaction between the thymus and the gonads has been known for many years. For example, both pregnancy (Jolly and Lieure, 1930) and lactation (Bompiani, 1914) are known to decrease thymic weights. Chiodi (1940) observed that age-related thymic involution also occurs in castrated animals suggesting that the phenomenon is not totally due to gonadal involvement. Just as gonadal dysfunction was known to affect the thymus, it was long suspected that the thymus, in turn, could affect the gonads. For example, perinatal thymectomy delays vaginal opening by several days (Besedovsky and Sorkin, 1974). Also, the uterus of athymic nude mice is atrophied by comparison with normal litter mates, a condition which is reversed by thymic tissue transplants (Besedovsky and Sorkin, 1974). These observations, demonstrating a relationship between the gonads and the thymus, were confirmed by Chiodi (1940), who described a dose dependent thymic involution in castrated rats following exposure to either estradiol or testosterone. Estrogen induced thymic atrophy is primarily characterized by a reduction in the number of cortical lymphocytes (Boorman et al., 1980; Scheiff and Haumont, 1979). Castration, on the other hand, induces cellular hypertrophy (Chiodi, 1940). Allen et al. (1984) demonstrated that the injection of thymosin fraction 5 in mice increased circulating levels of serum estradiol and advanced the time to vaginal opening, while administration of estrogen decreased both thymic weight and circulating levels of thymosin $\alpha 1$. Thus, it is probable that both sex hormones and thymic hormones are feedback regulators of thymic and gonadal function.

In 1978, Reichman and Villee demonstrated that rat thymus homogenates contain macromolecular components capable of binding estradiol. Grossman et al. (1979a) later confirmed the presence of estrogen receptors in both bovine and rat thymus and, using crude thymic fractions, suggested that the estrogen binding component was present in cytosols from thymic epithelium. In another study, Grossman et al. (1979b) used autoradiography to demonstrate the binding of tritium-labeled estradiol to the thymic epithelium of exposed rats. Luster et al. (1984b) reported that, although estrogen binding occurred in density gradient enriched mouse thymocytes, estrogen receptors prepared from primary cultures of mouse thymic epithelial cells possessed 10-fold greater concentrations. This suggested that thymic epithelial cells, not thymocytes, are a primary target cell for estrogen.

Several lines of evidence directly support a link between estrogen-induced immunomodulation and the thymus. Stimson and Hunter (1980) observed that serum from estrogen exposed rats inhibited the lymphocyte blastogenic response to PHA and the BCG-induced suppression of leukocyte migration. These effects were not observed when serum from estrogen-exposed, thymectomized rats were added to the cell cultures, suggesting that estrogen exposure induced soluble immunoregulatory products from the thymus. In a related series of experiments, Grossman et al. (1982) observed that serum from castrated rats supported the blastogenic response of thymocytes to Con A and PHA while serum from castrated rats exposed to physiological doses of estradiol inhibited blastogenesis. Thymectomy also abolished the inhibitory effects of serum from estrogen-treated rats on lymphoproliferation (Grossman et al., 1982). Additional evidence supporting a role for the thymus in estrogen mediated immunoregulation was provided in experiments utilizing adult thymectomized mice (Luster et al., 1984a,b). It was found that thymectomy inhibited the ability of estradiol or DES to modulate a number of immune functions. Additionally, adult thymectomy inhibited the effects of estrogens on host resistance to L. monocytogenes infection and transplantable tumor cell growth (Pung, et al., 1984). Evidence that estrogen-induced immunomodulation is partially mediated through the binding of estrogens to thymic epithelium, resulting in alterations in the quality and/or quantity of thymic hormones, is also available. Supernatant fluids obtained by culturing thymic epithelial cells in the presence of estradiol, in contrast to cultures not containing estradiol, are deficient in their ability to support T cell maturation (Luster et al., 1984a) and lymphocyte blastogenesis (Stimson and Crilly, 1981). The products in these supernatants have not been characterized and any relationship with known thymic peptide remains to be determined.

Molecular Mechanisms

Certain responses to estrogens, such as those which occur in smooth muscle (Batra and Sjogren, 1983) and selected neoplastic mammary tissues (Gorlich et al., 1981), are mediated by nonspecific events which are independent of the estrogen receptor. In this respect, there is evidence that at least part of immunotoxicity by estrogens, particularly cytotoxic events observed at higher doses, is related to metabolism of the parent compound to reactive quinone intermediates (Pfeifer and Patterson, submitted; Mendelsohn et al., 1977). These metabolites are believed to partition into the lymphocyte membrane and alter cell surface interactions such as response to growth or regulatory factors or cell to cell interaction. In this respect, the catechol estrogen, 2-OH estrone, is present at fairly high levels in plasma, approximating that of estradiol and exceeding that of estriol (Fishman and Martucci, 1980). Recently, it has been shown that catechol estrogen metabolites are more potent compared to other metabolites or the parent compound at suppressing PHA-induced lymphocyte activation in vitro (Pfeifer and Patterson, submitted). A distinctive role for catechol estrogens has previously been described in regulating neuroendocrine feedback response to estrogens (Fishman and Martucci, 1980). Although catechol estrogens demonstrate significant binding to the estrogen receptor, they do not undergo significant nuclear translocation and, therefore, have negligible uterotrophic activity (Fishman and Martucci, 1980). These data suggest a role for these metabolites in modulating the early events of lymphocyte activation at the cell surface, probably independent of a specific estrogen receptor-mediated mechanism. This is further supported by the observation that splenic lymphocytes from mice exposed to DES demonstrate a reduced percentage of cells undergoing lectin-induced capping, suggesting interference with cytoskeletal structures at the cell surface (Kalland, 1982).

Cellular Mechanisms

A number of studies have provided data suggesting that altered regulatory cell functions contribute to estrogen-induced immunoregulation. As described earlier, a relationship has been established between increased phagocytic activity of the RES and antibody responses, suggesting that depressed antibody responses occur as a result of altered antigen redistribution or increased antigen sequestering by the RES (Sljivic and Warr, 1974: Sljivic et al., 1975; Bick et al., 1984). Furthermore, macrophages from estrogen-treated mice are deficient in their ability to support lymphocyte mitogenesis (Luster et al., 1980). Several studies have indicated that production or inhibition of lymphocyte-derived regulatory factors are also influenced by estrogens. Estrogens have been reported to increase T suppressor cell activity in spleen cells of pregnant mice (Suzuki and Tomasi, 1979) while perinatal exposure to DES in mice decreases the number of regulatory cells, specifically T-helper cells (Kalland, 1980a). More recently it has been shown that estrogens reduce the synthesis of interleukin 2 (IL2), a second signal for T-cell proliferation (Henriksen and Frey, 1982). It must be remembered, however, that alterations in growth or regulatory factors may be a manifestation of an earlier lesion in cell maturation or cellular metabolism.

Hormonal Influences

There is evidence demonstrating the presence of estrogen receptors in the brain and the pituitary, particularly in the anterior hypothalamus, the median eminence and the adenohypophysis (rev. by Kato, 1977). The mechanism of action of these receptors is similar to that of the uterine estrogen receptor (Kato, 1977) and, under normal conditions, they serve as sites for the initiation of feedback regulation of reproductive behavior (Pfaff, 1983) and the onset of maturation (Kato, 1977). Estrogen binding to receptors in the hypothalamus or adenohypophysis stimulates the release of gonadotropin releasing factors, pituitary gonadotropins (Kato, 1977; Pfaff, 1983), prolactin (Neill, 1980) and adrenocorticotrophic hormones (ACTH) (Kitay et al., 1965). While there is little evidence that the binding of estrogens to receptors in the brain or the pituitary is responsible for the immunoregulatory effects of estrogenic hormones, certain of the hormones released by these organs are potentially immunosuppressive. Prolactin exposure, for example, reduces resistance to nematode infection (Kelly and Dineen, 1973) and inhibits the ability of lymphocytes to respond to PHA (Karmali et al., 1974). Thus, it is conceivable that estrogens may act as a secondary signal for immunoregulation by stimulating the release of other hormones such as prolactin.

Estrogen binding to receptors in the pituitary and/or adrenals may also induce the release of immunosuppressive glucocorticosteroids. Prior to the discovery of translocatable cytoplasmic estrogen receptors in the pituitary (Kato, 1977) and the adrenals (Muller and Wotuj, 1978; Calandra et al., 1978), it was accepted that estrogens affected various components of the pituitary-adrenocortical axis. Early work demonstrated that ovariectomy caused adrenal atrophy which could be reversed by estrogen treatment (Carter, 1956). Ovariectomy diminishes the secretion of pituitary ACTH and adrenal corticosterone (Kitay, 1963). The levels of both hormones can be restored by estrogen treatment (Kitay, 1963). Estrogens may stimulate glucocorticoid release by acting directly on the adrenals, or indirectly by stimulating ACTH release, or both (Kitay, et al., 1965; Colby and Kitay, 1974). Increased levels of corticosterone occur in ovariectomized, hypophysectomized rats following treatment with both estrogen and ACTH but not estrogen alone, suggesting that estrogens can act directly on the adrenals to alter corticosterone levels only in the presence of pituitary ACTH (Colby and Kitay, 1974). Estrogen binding to adrenal receptors may affect corticosterone levels by inhibiting its metabolism to inactive metabolites (Kitay et al., 1970). However, while physiological amounts of estrogen may induce increased serum levels of glucocorticosteroids, pharmacological amounts of estrogen have the opposite effect (Kitay et al., 1970). Additionally, the effects of pharmacological levels of estrogen on immunity are not altered by adrenalectomy (Luster, 1984a).

SUMMARY AND CONCLUSIONS

Extensive evidence indicates that supraphysiological levels of estrogens alter immune function. Suppression of cell-mediated immunity and stimulation of the RES appear to be the primary effects. The effects of physiological levels of estrogens on the immune system are less clear and probably perform more of a regulatory rather than pathological role. Several mechanisms may be responsible for estrogen-induced immune alterations, particularly at supraphysiological levels (Table 2). In this respect, estrogens are similar to corticosteroids, which also influence immune function by multiple mechanisms (rev. by Cupps and Fauci, 1982). The bulk of evidence presently available indicates that the effects of estrogen on immunity are hormonal in nature and indirectly mediated through the release of immunoregulatory hormones by estrogen responsive lymphoid tissues, particularly the thymic epithelium. Although intracellular estrogen receptors have been described in leukocytes, there is no evidence to suggest that they modulate cell function. Estrogen binding to receptors in the hypothalamus, pituitary and adrenals also influences the release of a variety of potentially immunoregulatory hormones. The metabolism of estrogens to membrane reactive intermediates suggest that under appropriate circumstances estrogens may also have direct impact on cell function.

Table 2

Potential Mechanisms of Estrogen Induced Immunotoxicity

- Cell Membrane Perturbations
- Altered T Cell Maturation (Thymic Microenvironment)
- Alterations in Regulatory Cell Numbers
- Secondary Hormonal Influences
- Inhibition of Interleukin Synthesis

ACKNOWLEDGEMENTS

The authors are indebted to Mrs. S. Wilkins for her assistance in preparing the manuscript.

REFERENCES

Ablin, R.J., Bhatti, R.A., Guinan, P.D., and Khin, W., 1979, Modulatory effects of oestrogen on immunological responsiveness. Clin. Explt. Immunol., 38:83-91.

Ahlquist, J., 1976, Endocrine influences on lymphatic organs, immune responses, inflammation and autoimmunity. Acta Endologica. (Supp. 206), 83:1-136.

Allen, L.S., McClure, J.E., Goldstein, A.L., Barkley, M.S., and Michael, S.D., 1984, Estrogen and thymic hormone interactions in the female mouse. J. Reprod. Immunol., 6:25-37.

Barnes, E.W., Loudon, N.B., MacCuish, A.C., Jordan, J., and Irvine, W.J., 1974, Phytohaemagglutinin-induced lymphocyte transformation and circulating autoantibodies in women taking oral contraceptives. Lancet, May 11, 898-900.

Batchelor, J.R., 1968, Hormonal control of antibody formation, in "Regulation of the Antibody Response", B. Cinader, ed., pp. 276-295, Thomas, Springfield.

Batra, S., and Sjogren, C., 1983, Effect of estrogen treatment on calcium uptake by the rat uterine smooth muscle. Life Sci., 32:315-319.

Besedovsky, H.O., and Sorkin, E., 1974, Thymus involvement in female sexual maturation. Nature, 249:356-358.

Bick, P.H., Tucker, A.N., White, K.L., Jr., and Holsapple, M., 1984, Effects of subchronic exposure to diethylstilbestrol on humoral immune functions in female B6C3F1 mice. Immunopharmacology, 7:27-39.

Bodel, P., Dillard, G.M., Kaplan, S.S., and Malawista, S.E., 1972, Antiinflammatory effects of estradiol on human blood leukocytes. J. Lab. Clin. Med., 80:373-384.

Bole, G.G., Friedlaeuder, M.H., and Smith, C.K., 1969, Rheumatic symptoms and serological abnormalities induced by oral contraceptives. Lancet, 1:323-326.

Bompiani, G., 1914, Der einfluss der sangens auf die restitutions - fahigheit des thymus nach der schwangerschaft. Zbl. Allg. Pathol. u. pathol. Anat., 25:929-935.

Boorman, G.A., Luster, M.I., Dean, J.H., and Wilson, R.E., 1980, The effect of adult exposure to diethylstilbestrol in the mouse on macrophage function and numbers. J. Reticuloendothel. Soc., 28:547-559.

Calandra, R.S., Naess, O., Purvis, K., Attramadal, A., Djoseland, O., and Hansson, V., 1978, Oestrogen receptors in the rat adrenal gland. J. Steroid Biochem., 9:957-962.

Carter, J., 1976, The effect of progesterone, oestradiol and HCG on cell-mediated immunity in pregnant mice. J. Reprod. Fert., 46:211-216.

Carter, S.B., 1956, The influence of sex hormones on the weight of the adrenal gland in the rat. J. Endocrin., 13:150-160.

Chiodi, H., 1940, The relationship between the thymus and the sexual organs. Endocrinology, 26:107-116.

Cohen, J.H.M., Danel, L., Cordier, G., Saly, S., and Revillard, J.P., 1983, Sex steroid receptors in peripheral T cells: absence of androgen receptors and restriction of estrogen receptors to OKT8-positive cells. J. Immunol., 131:2767-2771.

Colby, H.D., and Kitay, J.I., 1974, Interaction of estradiol and ACTH in the regulation of adrenal corticosterone production in the rat. Steroids, 24:527-536.

Cottrell, B.J., Playfair, J.H.L., and de Sousa, B., 1977, Plasmodium yoelii and Plasmodium vinckei: the effects of nonspecific immunostimulation on murine maleria. Exp. Parasitol., 43:45-53.

Cupps, T.R., and Fauci, A.S., 1982, Corticosteroid-mediated immunoregulation in man. Immunol. Rev., 65:133-155.

Cutler, B.S., Forbes, A.P., Ingersoll, F.M., and Scully, R.E., 1972, Endometrial carcinoma after stilbestrol therapy in gonadal dysgenesis. N. Engl. J. Med., 287:628-631.

Dean, J.H., Boorman, G.A., Luster, M.I., Adkins, B., Lauer, L.D., and Adams, D.O., 1984, Effect of agents of environmental concern on macrophage function, in "Mononuclear Phagocyte Biology", A. Volkman, ed., pp. 473-485, Marcell Dekker, Inc.

Dean, J.H., Luster, M.I., Boorman, G.A., Luebke, R.W., and Lauer, L.D., 1980, The effect of adult exposure to diethylstilbestrol in the mouse: alterations in tumor susceptibility and host resistance parameters. J. Reticuloendothel. Soc., 28:571-583.

Den Dulk, M.M.C.D., Crofton, R.W., and Van Furth, R., 1979, Origin and kinetics of Kupffer cells during an acute inflammatory response. Immunology, 37:7-18.

Eroshenko, V.P., and Palmiter, R.D., 1980, Estrogenicity of kepone in birds and mammals, in "Estrogens in the Environment", J.A. McLachlan, ed., pp. 305-325, Elsevier North Holland, New York.

Fishman, J., and Martucci, C., 1980, Dissociation of biological activities in metabolites of estradiol, in "Estrogens in the Environment", J.A. McLachlan, ed., pp. 131-145, Elsevier/North-Holland, New York.

Fluhmann, C.F., 1932, The influence of sex hormones on the reticuloendothelial cells of the uterus and a possible application to the treatment of pelvic inflammatory conditions. Am. J. Obstet. Gynecol., 24:654-655.

Franks, C.R., Perkins, F.T., and Bishop, D., 1975, The effect of sex hormones on the growth of Hela tumor nodules in male and female mice. Brit. J. Cancer, 31:100-110.

Fried, W., Tichlee, T., Dennenberg, I., Bacone, J., and Wang, F., 1974, Effects of estrogens on hematopoietic stem cells and on hematopoiesis of mice. J. Lab. Clin. Med., 83:807-815.

Fruhman, G.J., 1973, Peritoneal macrophages in male and female mice. J. Reticuloendothel. Soc., 14:371-379.

Fugmann, F.A., Aranyi, C., Barbera, P.W., Bradof, J.N., Gibbons, R.D., and Fenterro, J.D., 1983, The effect of diethylstilbestrol as measured by host resistance and tumor susceptibility assays in mice. J. Toxicol. Environ. Health, 11:827-841.

Gorlich, M., Hecker, D., and Heise, E., 1981, Comparison of estradiol receptor investigations and histochemical investigations on enzymes in human mammary cancers. J. Natl. Cancer Inst., 67:521-527.

Grossman, C.J., Sholiton, L.J., and Nathan, P., 1979a, Rat thymic estrogen receptor. I. Preparation, location and physiochemical properties. J. Steroid Biochem., 11:1233-1240.

Grossman, C.J., Sholiton, L.J., Blaha, G.C., and Nathan, P., 1979b, Rat thymic estrogen receptor. II. Physiological properties. J. Steroid Biochem., 11:1241-1246.

Grossman, C.J., Sholiton, L.J., and Rosselle, G.A., 1982, Estradiol regulation of thymic lymphocyte function in the rat: mediation by serum thymc factors. J. Steroid Biochem., 16:683-690.

Grundbacher, F.J., 1972, Human X chromosome carries quantitative genes for immunoglobulin M. Science, 176:311-312.

Henriksen, O., and Frey, J.R., 1982, Control of expression of interleukin-2 activity. Cell. Immunol., 73:106-114.

Herbst, A.L., Ulfelder, H., and Poskanzer, D.C., 1971, Adenocarcinoma of the vagina. Association of maternal stilboestrol therapy with tumor appearance in young women. N. Engl. J. Med., 284:878-881.

Heslop, R.W., Krohn, P.L., and Sparrow, E.M., 1954, The effect of pregnancy on the survival of skin homografts in rabbits. J. Endocrin., 10:325-332.

Inman, R.D., 1978, Immunologic sex differences and the female predominance in systemic lupus erythematosus. Arthritis Rheum., 21:849-852.

Jolly, J., and Lieure, C., 1930, Influence de la gestation sur le thymus. C.R. Soc. Biol., 104:451-454.

Kalland, T., 1980a, Decreased and disproportionate T-cell population in adult mice after neonatal exposure to diethylstilbestrol. Cell. Immunol., 51:55-63.

Kalland, T., 1980b, Reduced natural killer cell activity in female mice after neonatal exposure to diethylstilbestrol. J. Immunol., 124:1297-1321.

Kalland, T., 1982, Long-term effects on the immune system of an early life exposure to diethylstilbestrol, in "Environmental Factors in Human Growth and Development", Banbury Report 11, pp. 217-242.

Kalland, T., and Forsberg, J.G., 1978, Delayed hypersensitivity response to oxazolone in neonatally estrogenized mice. Cancer Lett., 4:141-146.

Kalland, T., and Forsberg, J.G., 1981, Natural killer cell activity and tumor susceptibility in female mice treated neonatally with diethylstilbestrol. Cancer Res., 41:5134-5140.

Kalland, T., and Haukaas, S.A., 1981, Effect of treatment with diethylstilbestrol-polyestradiol phosphate or estramustine phosphate (Estracyt®) on natural killer cell activity in patients with prostatic cancer. Invest. Urol., 18:437-441.

Kalland, T., Strand, O., and Forsberg, J.G., 1979, Long-term effects of neonatal estrogen treatment on mitogen responsiveness of mouse spleen lymphocytes. J. Natl. Cancer Inst., 63:413-421.

Karmali, R.A., Lauder, I., and Horrobin, D.F., 1974, Prolactin and the immune response. Lancet, July (II):106-107.

Kass, E.H., 1960, Bacteriuria and pyelonephritis of pregnancy. Arch. Int. Med., 105:194-198.

Kato, J., 1977, Steroid hormone receptors in brain, hypothalamus, and hypophysis, in "Receptors and Mechanisms of Action of Steroid Hormones", J.R. Pasqualini, ed., pp. 603-671, Marcel Dekker, New York.

Katzenellenbogen, J.A., Katzenellenbogen, B.S., Tatee, T., Robertson, D.W., and Landvatter, S.W., 1980, in "Estrogens in the Environment", J.A. McLachlan, ed., pp. 33-51, Elsevier, North Holland.

Kelly, J.D., and Dineen, J.K., 1973, The suppression of rejection of Nippostrongylus brasilunsis in Lewis strain rats treated with ovine prolactin. Immunology, 24:551-558.

Kelly, L.S., Brown, B.A., and Dobson, E.L., 1962, Cell division and phagocytic activity in liver reticuloendothelial cells. Proc. Soc. Exp. Biol. Med., 110:555-559.

Kenny, J.F., and Gray, J.A., 1971, Sex differences in immunologic response: studies of antibody production by individual spleen cells after stimulus with Escherichia coli antigen. Pediat. Res., 5:246-255.

Kenny, J.F., Pangburn, P.C., and Trail, G., 1976, Effect of estradiol on immune competence: in vivo and in vitro studies. Infect. Immun., 13:448-456.

Kierszenbaum, F., Knecht, E., Budzko, D.B., and Pizzimenti, M.C., 1974, Phagocytosis: a defense mechanism against infection with Trypanosoma cruzi. J. Immunol., 112:1839-1844.

Kitay, J.I., 1963, Pituitary-adrenal function in the rat after gonadec-
    tomy and gonadal hormone replacement. Endocrinology, 73:253-260.
Kitay, J.I., Cayne, M.D., Newsom, W., and Nelson, R., 1965, Relation of
    the ovary to adrenal corticosterone production and adrenal enzyme
    activity in the rat. Endocrinology, 77:902-908.
Kitay, J.I., Cayne, M.D., and Swygert, N.H., 1970, Influence of gonadec-
    tomy and replacement with estradiol or testosterone on formation of
    5α-reduced metabolites of corticosterone by the adrenal gland of the
    rat. Endocrinology, 87:1257-1265.
Krzych, U., Strausser, H.R., Bressler, J.P., and Goldstein, A.L., 1981,
    Effects of sex hormones on some T and B cell functions, evidenced by
    differential immune expression between male and female mice and
    cyclic pattern of immune responsiveness during the estrous cycle in
    female mice. Am. J. Repro. Immunol., 1:73-77.
Loose, L.D., and DiLuzio, N.R., 1976, Dose related reticuloendothelial
    system stimulation by diethylstilbestrol. J. Reticuloendothel. Soc.,
    20:457-460.
Luebke, R.W., Luster, M.I., Dean, J.H., and Hayes, H.T., 1984, Altered
    host resistance to Trichinella spiralis infection following
    subchronic exposure to diethylstilbestrol. Int. J. Immunopharmacol.,
    in press.
Luft, B.J., and Remington, J.S., 1982, Effect of pregnancy on resistance
    to Listeria monocytogenes and Toxoplasma gondii infections in mice.
    Infect. Immun., 38:1164-1171.
Luster, M.I., Boorman, G.A., Dean, J.H., Lawson, L.D., Wilson, R., and
    Haseman, J.K., 1981, Immunological alterations in mice following
    adult exposure to diethylstilbestrol, in "Biological Relevance of
    Immunosuppression", J.H. Dean and M.L. Padarathsingh, eds., pp.
    153-175, Van Nostrand, New York.
Luster, M.I., Boorman, G.A., Dean, J.H., Luebke, R.W., and Lawson, L.D.,
    1980, The effect of adult exposure to diethylstilbestrol in the
    mouse: alterations in immunological functions. J. Reticuloendothel.
    Soc., 28:561-569.
Luster, M.I., Boorman, G.A., Korach, K.S., Dieter, M.P., and Hong, L. ,
    1984a, Mechanisms of estrogen-induced myelotoxicity: evidence of
    thymic regulation. Int. J. Immunopharmacol., 6:287-297.
Luster, M.I., Hayes, H.T., Korach, K., Tucker, A.N., Dean, J.H.,
    Greenlee, W.F., and Boorman, G.A., 1984b, Estrogen immunosuppression
    is regulated through estrogenic responses in the thymus. J.
    Immunol., 133:110-116.
Luster, M.I., Pfeifer, R.W., and Tucker, A.N., 1985, Influence of sex
    hormones on immunoregulation with specific reference to natural and
    synthetic estrogens, in "Endocrine Toxicology", J.A. McLachlan,
    K. Korach, and J. Thomas, eds., pp. 67-83, Raven Press, New York.
MacMartin, K.E., Kennedy, K.A., Greenspan, P., Alam, S.N., Greiner, P.,
    and Yum, J., 1978, Diethylstilbestrol: a review of its toxicity and
    use as a growth promotant in food producing animals. J. Environ.
    Pathol. Toxicol., 1:297-313.
Mankau, S.K., 1975, Host sex and sex hormones as a factor affecting
    Trypanosoma lewisi population in white rats. Jap. J. Parasitol.,
    24:379-384.
Mathur, S., Mathur, R.S., Goust, J.M., Williamson, H.O., and Fudenburg,
    H.H., 1979, Cyclic variations in white cell subpopulations in the
    human menstrual cycle: Correlations with progesterone and estradiol.
    Clin. Immunol. Immunopath., 13:246-253.
McLachlan, J.A., and Dixon, R.L., 1976, Transplacental toxicity of
    diethylstilbestrol: A special problem in safety evaluation, in
    "Advances in Modern Toxicology", M. Mehlman, and R.E. Shapiro, eds.,
    Vol. 1, pp. 423-448, Hemisphere Publ. Corp., New York.

Mendelow, D.A., and Lewis, G.C., 1969, Varicella pneumonia during
    pregnancy. Obstet. Gynecol., 33:98-99.
Mendelsohn, J., Multer, M.M., and Bernheim, J.L., 1977, Inhibition of
    human lymphocyte stimulation by steroid hormones: Cytokinetic
    mechanisms. Clin. Exp. Immunol., 27:127-134.
Mitchell, G.W., Jacobs, A.A., Haddad, V., Paul, B.B., Strauss, R.R., and
    Sbarra, A.J., 1970, The role of the phagocyte in host-parasite
    interactions. XXV. Metabolic and bactericidal activities of
    leukocytes from pregnant women. Am. J. Obstet. Gynecol.,
    108:805-813.
Mitchell, G.W., McRipley, R.J., Selvaraj, R.J., and Sbarra, A.J., 1966,
    The role of the phagocyte in host-parasite interactions. IV. The
    phagocytic activity of leuocytes in pregnancy and its relationship to
    urinary tract infections. Am. J. Obstet Gynecol., 96:687-697.
Morahan, P.S., Bradley, S.G., Menson, A.E., Duke, S., Fromtling, R.A.,
    and Marciano-Cabral, F., 1984, Immunotoxic effects of diethylstil-
    bestrol on host resistance: comparison with cyclophosphamide. J.
    Leukocyte Biol., 35:329-341.
Muller, R.E., and Wotiy, H.H., 1978, Estrogen-binding protein in mouse
    and rat adrenal glands. J. Biol. Chem., 253:740-745.
Munson, A.E., Levy, J.A., Harris, L.S., and Dewy, W.L., 1976, Effects of
    Δ^9-tetrahydrocannabinol on the immune system, in "Pharmacology of
    Marihuana", M.C. Braude, and S. Szara, eds., pp. 187-197, Raven
    Press, New York.
Neill, J.D., 1980, Neuroendocrine regulation of prolactin secretion, in
    "Frontiers in Neuroendocrinology", L. Martini, and W.F. Ganong, eds.,
    6:129-155, Raven Press, New York.
Nicol, T., and Abou-Zikry, A., 1953, Influence of eostradiol benzoate and
    orchidectomy on the reticuloendothelial system. Brit. Med. J.,
    i:133-134.
Nicol, T., Bilbey, D.L.J., Charles, L.M., Cordingley, J.L., and
    Vernon-Roberts, B., 1964, Oestrogen: the natural stimulant of body
    defense. J. Endocrinol., 30:277-291.
Nicol, T., and Vernon-Roberts, B., 1965, The influence of the estrus
    cycle, pregnancy and ovariectomy on RES activity. J. Reticulo-
    endothel. Soc., 2:15-29.
Paavonen, T., Andersson, L.C., and Aldercreutz, H., 1981, Sex hormone
    regulation of in vitro immune response. J. Exp. Med., 154:1935-1945.
Pfaff, D.W., 1983, Impact of estrogens on hypothalamic nerve cells:
    ultrastructural, chemical and electrical effects. Rec. Prog. Hormone
    Res., 39:127-179.
Pung, O.J., Luster, M.I., Hayes, H.T., and Rader, J., 1984, Influence of
    steroidal and nonsteroidal sex hormones on host resistance in the
    mouse: Increased susceptibility to Listeria monocytogenes following
    exposure to estrogenic hormones. Infect. Immun., 46:301-307.
Purtilo, D.T., Hallgren, H.M., and Yunis, E.J., 1972, Depressed maternal
    lymphocyte response to phytohaemagglutinin in human pregnancy.
    Lancet, i:769-771.
Rank, R.G., White, H.J., Hough, A.J., Pasley, J.N., and Barrow, A.L.,
    1982, Effect of estradiol on chlamydial genital infection of female
    guinea pigs. Infect. Immun., 38:699-705.
Reichman, M.E., and Villee, C.A., 1978, Estradiol binding by rat thymus
    cytosol. J. Steroid Biochem., 9:637-641.
Reisher, E.H., 1966, Tissue culture of bone marrow. II. Effect of
    steroid hormones on hematopoiesis in vitro. Blood, 27:460.
Rhodes, K., Scott, A., Markham, R.L., and Monk-Jones, M.E., 1969,
    Immunological sex differences. Ann. Rheum. Dis., 28:104-119.
Rifkind, D., and Frey, J., 1972, Sex difference in antibody response of
    CFW mice to Candida Albicans. Infect. Immun., 5:695-698.

Rifkind, D., and Frey, J.A., 1974, Influence of androgen and estrogen on delayed skin test reactivity to Candida albicans. Infect. Immun., 10:971-974.

Santoli, D., Trichieri, G., Amijewski, C.M., and Koprowski, H., 1976, HLA-related control of spontaneous and antibody-dependent cell-mediated cytotoxicity in humans. J. Immunol., 117:765-770.

Scheiff, J.M., and Haumont, S., 1979, The effect of oestradiol on thymic epithelial cells in the mouse. J. Clin. Lab. Immunol., 2:225-234.

Seaman, W.F., Merigan, T.C., and Talal, N., 1979, Natural killing in estrogen-treated mice responds poorly to poly I.C despite normal stimulation of circulating interferon. J. Immunol., 123:2903-2905.

Sljivic, V.S., and Warr, G.W., 1974, Activity of the reticuloendothelial system and the antibody response. III. The fate of Type III pneumococcal polysaccharide and the antibody response. Immunology, 27:1009-1022.

Sljivic, V.S., Clark, D.W., and Warr, G.W., 1975, Effects of estrogens and pregnancy on the distribution of sheep erythrocytes and the antibody response in mice. Clin. Exp. Immunol., 20:179-186.

Stern, K., and Davidsohn, I., 1955, Effect of estrogen and cortisone on immune hemeoantibodies in mice of inbred strains. J. Immunol., 74:479-486.

Stimson, W.H., 1976, Studies on the immunosuppressive properties of a pregnancy-associated alph-macroglobulin. Clin. Exp. Immunol., 25:199-206.

Stimson, W.H., and Crilly, P.J., 1981, Effects of steroids on the secretion of immunoregulatory factors by thymic epithelial cell cultures. Immunology, 44:401-407.

Stimson, W.H., and Hunter, I.C., 1980, Oestrogen-induced immunoregulation mediated through the thymus. J. Clin. Lab. Immunol., 4:27-33.

Sturgis, C.C., and Bethell, F.H., 1943, Quantitative and qualitative variations in normal leukocytes. Physiol. Rev., 23:279-303.

Suzuki, K., and Tomasi, T.B., 1979, Immune responses during pregnancy. Evidence of suppressor cells for splenic antibody response. J. Exp. Med., 150:898-908.

Tshernitchin, A.N., 1983, Eosinophil-mediated non-genomic parameters of estrogen stimulation - a separate group of responses mediated by an independent mechanism. J. Steroid Biochem., 19:95-100.

Terres, G., Morrison, S.L., and Habicht, G.S., 1968, A quantitative difference in the immune response between male and female mice. Proc. Soc. Exp. Biol. Med., 127:664-667.

Toivanen, P., 1967, Enhancement of staphylococcal infection in mice by estrogens. I. Effect of timing, quantity and quality of the hormone. Ann. Med. Exp. Fenn., 45:138-146.

Valdimarsson, H., Mulholland, C., Fridriksdottir, V., and Coleman, D., 1983, A longitudinal study of leucocyte blood counts and lymphocyte responses in pregnancy: a marked early increase of monocyte-lymphocyte ratio. Clin. Exp. Immunol., 53:437-443.

van Zon, A.A.J.C., Eling, W.M.C., Hermsen, C.C.R., and Koekkoek, A.A.G.M., 1982, Corticosterone regulation of effector function of malarial immunity during pregnancy. Infect. Immun., 36:484-491.

Vaughan, J.E., and Ramirez, H., 1951, Coccidiorodomycosis as a complication of pregnancy. Calif. Med., 74:121-125.

Vernon-Roberts, B., 1969, The effect of steroid hormones on macrophage activity. Int. Rev. Cytol., 25:133-151.

Waltman, S.R., Burde, R.M., and Berrias, J., 1971, Prevention of corneal homograft rejection by estrogens. Transplantation, 11:194-196.

Washburn, T., Medearis, D., and Childs, B., 1965, Sex differences in susceptibility to infections. Pediatrics, 35:57-64.

EFFECTS ON THE IMMUNE SYSTEM OF LESIONING AND STIMULATION OF THE NERVOUS SYSTEM: NEUROIMMUNOMODULATION

Branislav D. Janković
Immunology Research Center
Vojvode Stepe 458
11221 Belgrade, Yugoslavia

Novera Herbert Spector
Fundamental Neurosciences Program
National Institutes of Health, NINCDS
Federal Building, Room 916
Bethesda, Maryland 20892, USA

INTRODUCTION

The ancient Egyptians and Greeks, among others, knew that defense against disease involved "mind." Today as monists, many scientists (including the authors of this chapter) believe that "mind" is a function of the nervous system, most particularly the brain. More than a few specialists in science today have developed severe tunnel vision: they see only a small piece of the whole integrated biological entity (the organism). The organism itself does not know that it is supposed to be divided like the departments of a medical school, so it functions as a unit. Thus the ancients were correct on this aspect of life, whereas some educated researchers of today fail to appreciate the connections between the brain and the immune system (Spector, 1980).

Today we are in a much better position than were the ancient philosophers. We need speculate no longer. The evidence for neuroimmunomodulation (NIM) is overwhelming. This entire book details only a part of it. Modern research in this area probably began with Metalnikov and his colleagues at the Pasteur Institute in Paris in the 1920's, and today there is a virtual "information explosion" in solid data on NIM (Spector, 1985).

The data comes from molecular biology, genetics, neurochemistry, cellular immunology, neurophysiology, neuroanatomy, physiology and the behavioral sciences, among others. This chapter will outline that portion of the evidence that derives from experiments using the techniques of partial lesioning (mechanical, chemical, electrical, electromagnetic) of the nervous system and from experiments utilizing stimulation (electrical, mechanical, chemical) of discrete neural loci.

BRAIN LESIONS IN MATURE ANIMALS

Data from brain lesion and brain stimulation experiments (Tables 1 and 5) give us important clues to solving the fascinating puzzle of fitting the details to the "big picture." Based on a number of experimental findings, we could suggest at least seven more detailed possible pathways, all of these always involving the two major routes (see below).

Lesion and stimulation experiments, as well as single-unit recordings from neurons in specific brain nuclei (e.g. Klimenko, 1972; Korneva & Klimenko, 1976; Besedovsky, et al, 1977; Spector and Korneva, 1981) help us to orient ourselves within the myriad pathways of the central nervous system, but the exact "centers" in the hypothalamus and elsewhere and the exact fiber tracts that modulate, regulate or initiate (?) immune responses are still not precisely known. Indeed, depending on the species, the laboratory, the antigen, the time of day, and other variables, experimental results are frequently different (for a fuller and historical discussion of this problem, see Spector, 1979).

It is important also to appreciate both the phylogeny and the ontogeny of these systems (see below for a brief discussion of embryonic brain lesions). Early - in-life lesions do not always have the same effects as lesions in adults (e.g. Paunovic, et al., 1976). Brain lesions in embryos trace the ontogeny of neuroimmunomodulation to even earlier stages .

The timing of a lesion with respect to the immune challenge is likewise critical. We have discussed this in other reviews so let us just mention it here as a reminder to those who wish to design new experimental protocols.

Table one outlines the history of experiments in brain lesioning. Not all papers are listed. Nor do we attempt to list the voluminous literature on lesions of the pituitary (hypophysectomies, partial or total), adrenals or other glands. We will, however, say a few words (below) about epiphysectomies or lesions of the pineal, since this "organ" rests squarely in the brain and is part of the brain itself, both anatomically and physiologically.

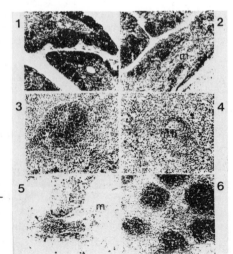

Fig. 1   Normal-looking thymus of a sham-lesioned rat. c, cortex; m, medulla. Haematoxylin and eosin, X 30.

Fig. 2   Profound changes in the thymus from a hypothalamus-lesioned rat. Haematoxylin and eosin, X 80.

3   Normal-looking spleen of a sham-lesioned rat. mb, Malpighian body. Haemotoxylin and eosin, X 100.

Fig. 4   Invòlved Malpighian body (mb) in the spleen of a hypothalamus-lesioned rat. Haematoxylin and eosin, X 100.

Fig. 5   Large area of plasmacellular elements (arrows) in the thymus of a rat with lesioned amygdaloid complex. Methyl green and pyronin, X 80.

Fig. 6   Numerous modules (n) in the lymph node of a rat with lesions in the amygdaloid complex. Methyl green and pyronin, X 80.

Table 1

BRAIN LESIONS (SAMPLING OF EXPERIMENTS)
Hypophysectomy not Included

DATE	AUTHORS	SITE OF LESION	ANIMAL	ANTIGEN	Immune Response ASSAY	Immune Response RESULTS
1920s	Speranskii	Rupture of meninges: subarachnoid space	Dog	Many pathogens	Disease symptoms	Alleviated
1930s	Speranskii	Rupture of meninges: subarachnoid space	Human	Many pathogens	Disease symptons	Alleviated
1942	Kopeloff et al.	Cortex	Monkey	Chemical lesions	Production of autoanti-bodies	
1958	Szentivanyi & Filipp	Tuberal region of hypothalamus	Guinea pig	Horse serum	Anaphylaxis	Protection
1958	Szentivanyi & Szekely	Tuberal region of hypothalamus	Guinea pig	Histamine	Histamine shock	Histamine resistance
1958	Freedman & Fenichel	Midbrain reticulum at superior colliculus	Guinea pig	Egg albumin	Anaphylaxis	Protection
1963	Korneva & Khai	Anterior hypothalamus	Rabbit	Horse serum	Complement binding	Reduction in circulatory antibodies
1964	Khai et al.	Posterior hypothalamus	Rabbit	Horse serum	Complement-fixation reaction	Suppression of antibody production
1964	Luparello et al.	Anterior hypothalamus	Rat	Ovalbumin	Anaphylaxis	Protection
1964	Luparello et al.	Posterior hypothalamus	Guinea pig	Ovalbumin	Anaphylaxis	No effect
1966	Schiavi et al.	Anterior hypothalamus	Guinea pig	Histamine	Histamine shock	Histamine resistance
1968	Bowen	Cortex	Rabbit	Cryogenic lesions	Production of autoantibodies	
1969	Polyak et al.	Posterior hypothalamus		Plague capsule	Antibody formation	Suppression
1969	Thakur & Manchanda	Hypothalamus	Cat		Phagocytosis	Diminution
1969	Thakur & Manchanda	Cingulate gyrus	Cat		Phagocytosis	No effect
1970	Macris et al.	Anterior hypothalamus	Guinea pig	Picryl chloride	Antibody production, delayed sensitivity	Suppression
1970	Macris et al.	Posterior hypothalamus	Guinea pig	Picryl chloride	Antibody production, delayed sensitivity	No effect
1971	Thrasher et al.	Hypothalamus, anterior, medial, or posterior	Rat	Egg albumin	Antibody production	No effect
1972	Macris et al.	Anterior hypothalamus	Guinea pig	Ovalbumin	Passive anaphylaxis	Protection
1972	Macris et al.	Posterior hypothalamus	Guinea pig	Ovalbumin	Passsive anaphylaxis	No effect
1972	Tyrey & Nalbandov	Anterior hypothalamus	Rat	Ovalbumin	Antibody production	Decrease
1973	Janković & Isaković	Hypothalamus and reticular formation	Rat	Bovine serum albumin	Antibody production, Arthus and delayed skin reactions	Decrease
1973	Isaković & Janković	Hypothalamus, reticular formation, thalamus, superior colliculus, caudate nucleus and amygdaloid complex	Rat	Bovine serum allbumin	Thymus	Involution, plasmacytic reaction

(Continued)

Table 1 (Continued)

BRAIN LESIONS (SAMPLING OF EXPERIMENTS)

Year	Author	Site	Animal	Antigen	Parameter	Effect
1973	Isaković & Janković	Hypothalamus	Rat	Bovine serum albumin	Spleen, lymph nodes	Lymphocyte depletion
1974	Spector et al.	Several nuclei of hypothalamus	Rat	Plasmodium berghei	Parasitemia Ab to Plasmodium	Increase
1975	Schiavi et al.	Anterior hypothalamus	Guinea pig	Ovalbumin	Antibody production	No effect
1975	Spector et al.	Anterior hypothalamus	Rat	Ovalbumin	Antibody production	Decrease
1976	Goldstein	Medial hypothalamus	Rabbit	Ovalbumin	Anaphylaxis	Increase
1976	Paunović et al.	Medial and posterior hypothalamus	Rat*	Bovine serum albumin	Antibody production, Arthus and delayed skin reactions	Decrease
1977	Plezitiy	Dorsal hypothalamus	Rabbit	Bovine serum	Arthus reaction	Decrease
1977	Spector et al.	Several nuclei of hypothalamlus	Mouse	Newcastle disease virus	Interferon, Antibody to NDV	No significant change
1978	Goldstein	Anterior and posterior hypothalamus & thalamus	Rat	Sheep red blood cells	Plaque-forming cells	No effect
1979	Dann et al.	Tuberal hypothalamus	Rat	Tissue	Skin graft	Stimulation of allograft rejection
1979	Dann et al.	Amygdala	Rat	Tissue	Skin graft	No effect
1980	Cross et al.	Anterior hypothalamus	Rat		Total cell number	Decrease thymus & spleen
1980	Keller et al.	Anterior hypothalamus	Guinea pig	Tuberculin	Skin-test	Suppression
1980	Keller et al.	Anterior hypothalamus	Guinea pig	(PHA)	Blastogenesis	Inhibition
1980	Warejcka & Levy	Hypothalamus	Rat	(PHA)	PHA response	Suppression
1982	Banet et al.	Hypothalamic preoptic area (cooling)	Rat	Sheep red blood cells	Antibody production	Increase
1982	Brooks et al.	Frontal cortex, ventromedial hypothalamus, amygdaloid complex, hippocampus anterior hypothalamus			Number of cells	No changes in thymus and spleen
1982	Cross et al.	Anterior hypothalamus	Rat		Thymus	Involution
1982	Cross et al.	Hippocampus	Rat		Thymus	Increased cellularity
1982	Roszman et al.	Preoptic and anterior hypothalamus	Rat	(Con A)	Blastogenesis	Impaired lymphocyte reactivity
1983	Renoux et al.	Cerebral cortex	Mouse		Thy-1 phenotype	Modulation
1984	Baçiu & Ivanov	Anterior hypothalamus	Rat	Salmonella enter. SRBC Myxovirus influ. A	Primary & secondary responses	No changes No changes Reduced
		Lateral hypothalamus	Rat	Salmonella enter. SRBC Myxovirus influ. A	Primary & secondary responses	No changes No changes Reduced
		Tuberal hypothalamus	Rat	Salmonella enter. SRBC Myxovirus influ. A	Primary & secondary responses	No changes No changes Suppressed
		Mammillary areas	Rat	Salmonella enter. SRBC Myxovirus influ. A.	Primary & secondary responses	No sign. change No sign. change Suppressed
1985	Baçiu et. al.	Tuber Cinereum of hypothalamus	Guinea pig	Staphylococcus	Phagacytosis	Decrease

(continued)

Table 1 (Continued)

BRAIN LESIONS (SAMPLING OF EXPERIMENTS)

Year	Authors	Lesion	Animal	Antigen/Treatment	Measure	Result
1985	Biziere et al.	Frontal, parietal or occipital cerebral cortex: unilateral	Mouse	SRBC	PFC(IgG) count	Left: decrease Right: increase
					Weight and number of T-cells in spleen and thymus	Left: decrease Right: increase
				(PHA or Con-A)	Thymidine incorporation	Left: decrease Right: increase
1985	Markesbery et al.	Anterior hypothalamus, preoptic area (AHT)	Rat: young and old	(Con-A)	Thymidine incorporation	Aged: no change Young: decrease
		Hippocampus, frontal cortex			NK activity	Aged: decrease Young: decrease
1985	Ovaida et al.	Anterior hypothalamus	Rat	Rat spinal cord	Clinical signs of EAE	Decrease
		Areas reached via lateral ventricles	Rat treated with reserpine (Norepinephrinr)	" "	" "	" "
		" "	Rat treated with 6-OHDA (Catecholamines)	" "	" "	" "
		" "	Rat treated with 5,7-DHT (Serotonin)	" "	" "	" "
1985	Cross et al.	Brain ventricles	Mouse	SRBC	IgM, IgG, PFC	Decrease
1985	Speplewski & Vogel	Brain ventricles	Rat treated with 5,6-DHT, (Serotonin)		Leucocyte count T-lymphocyte " NK activity	Increase Decrease Reduced
1985	Jankovic et al.	Epiphysis	Chick embryo		Histology	Bursa/Fabricius: size reduced
						Lymphocyte: count down
						Thymus: size reduced, number of pyroninophilic cells reduced
1985	Renoux et al.	Left neocortex Right neocortex	Mouse	SRBC	IgG-PFC	Left lesion- reduced (restored by imuthiol)
						Right lesion- increased
				Chick RBC	Cell-mediated cytotoxicity	No change
				Imuthiol	NK activity	Left lesion- reduction
1985	Wertman et al.	Anterior hypothalamus(AH) Hippocampus	Rat	Rat spinal cord Freund's Adj.	Ab to myelin basic protein (measure of EAE)	(AH) decreased
					Con A reactivity	(AH) increased

*Lesioned as newborns and tested as adults
In parenthesis: mitogens

The immune micromilieu is a multisystem (Janković, 1973, 1979) composed of components of the immune (lymphoepithelial), nervous and endocrine systems. Therefore, the immune response in vivo depends not only on lymphoid cells and their associates (e.g. macrophages, dendritic cells) but also on the function of nervous and endocrine systems. This generalization is especially applicable to the ontogeny of the entire immune complex, and implies that post-embryonic immune responses are rooted in the embryonic phase of dynamic interactions among constituents of the three systems. The nervous system and the immune system function simultaneously in the developing chick embryo (Romanoff, 1960). As for the nervous and endocrine system, the avian brain on the 12th day of incubation already possesses its essential features (Romanoff, 1960) whereas the hypophysis becomes active in the second half of incubation (Fugo, 1940). It has been postulated, therefore, that the brain exerts an early regulatory activity over the anterior hypophysis (Wingstrand, 1951). If the pituitary is the "master gland," then the brain (especially the hypothalamus) is the master of the master gland.

A basic question dealing with the neuroimmune relationship is: are there brain-related structural and functional changes of the immune system during embryogenesis? The answer to this question requires an adequate experimental approach. The surgical removal of the brain or of parts of the brain is a method of choice. Among other reasons: a large number of chemicals which influence the brain of the chick embryo have been found to exert, at the same time, toxic effects on a variety of tissues including the lymphoid ones (Romanoff and Romanoff, 1972). Earlier reports on destruction of the brain (Wolff, 1936) and surgical operations of the head (Schowing, 1959a, 1959b,1968a, 1968b) were concerned mainly with malformations in the development of skeletal elements of neurocranium of the avian embryo. The partial decapitation of the chick embryo which removes the forebrain and hypophysis usually was referred to as "embryonic hypophysectomy" (Fugo, 1940; Betz, 1967; Janković et al., 1978). Retardation in the development of non-lymphoid tissues of the chick embryo due to early hypophysectomy was reported (Fugo, 1940; Betz, 1967). In adult chickens, destruction of the paraventricular area and the anterior hypothalamus produced thymic atrophy (Kanematsu and Mikami, 1970).

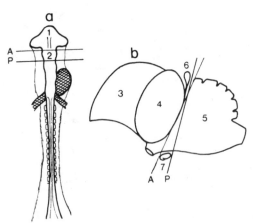

Fig. 7 Diagram of anterior and posterior decapitations performed on 33-hour-old chick embryos. Surgical procedures: A, anterior extirpation line (partial decapitation; Dx embryos), and P, posterior extirpation line (hypophysectom Hyx embryos). a. Embryo at the time of operation (about 33 h of incubatio 13 somites): 1. prosencephalon, and 2. mesencephalon. b. 17-day-old embryo (lateral view of the brain): 3. forebrain, 4. optic lobe, 5. cerebellum, 6. epiphysis, and 7. hypophysis. Missing parts are 3, 4, and 6 in correctly partially decapitated embryos, and 3,4,6 and 7 in hypophysectomized embryo (Modified from Janković et al., Develop. Comp. Immunol., 2:479, 1978.)

Experiments examining especially immuno-neuro-endocrine interactions in the developing chick embryo were performed by Janković and associates (Janković et al, 1977, 1978, 1979, 1981a, 1981b, 1982, 1983: Mićić et al., 1983). They developed a new procedure which enabled the removal of the forebrain and optic lobes while leaving the hypophysis intact (Figure 7) thus constituting a sound method for the study of neuroimmune interconnections in the chick embryo. The relationship between the brain, hypophysis and lymphoid organs (thymus and bursa of Fabricius) of the chick embryo is summarized in Table 2. Stereological analysis of the thymus epithelial cells situated in the cortex and medulla revealed an increase in the number of dense bodies and cysts. This implied that the secretory activity of thymic epithelial cells is under the influence of the brain and hypophysis. As for the bursa of Fabricius (a lymphoepithelial organ in birds), there was a pronounced retardation in the development of bursal follicles both in decapitated and hypophysectomized embryos (Figures 8-10). Operated embryos also showed a significant depletion of "light" and "dark" lymphocytes (Isaković et al., 1980) in the bursal follicles.

These studies provided evidence that the brain exerts both stimulatory and inhibitory effects on lymphoid tissues of the chick embryo and that communications between the nervous system and the immune system are functional during embryogenesis. The mechanisms by which brain hormones and neurally-active amines modulate the development and function of embryonic lymphocytes in general and in specific areas of the immune system remain to be elucidated. These mechanisms have been studied more in the adult animal, but only in some respects may be the same in the embryo.

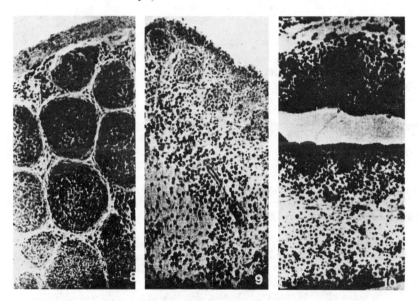

Fig. 8   Bursa of Fabricius of a 19-day-old sham-operated chick embryo Normal looking follicles (f). (X 320)

Fig. 9   Bursa of Fabricius of a 19-day-old decapitated (Dx) embryo (anterior decapitation which leaves intact the hypophysis.) Bursal follicles (f) are underdeveloped and plical mesenchyme (pm) contains large number of embryonic granulocytes. (X 320)

Fig. 10   Bursa of Fabricius of a 19-day-old hypophysectomized (Hyx) embryo (posterior decapitation which removes forebrain, optic lobes and hypophysis). Striking retardation in the development of the organ and follicles (f). (X 320)

All sections were stained with hematoxylin and eosin.

Table 2. Changes in the Thymus and Bursa of Fabricius of]7-Day Old
Chick Embryos Surgically Sham-Decapitated (SDx) , Decapitated (Dx)
or Hypophysectomized (Hyx) at 33-38 Hours of Incubation

		Thymus			Bursa of Fabricius		
		Stereological Analysis[a] of Epithelial Cells			Number of Follicles per 1 mm[2]	Number of Lymphocytes per Follicle	
		Density of Cells[b]	Numerical Density of				
Group	Region		Dense Bodies	Cysts		Light Cells	Dark Cells
SDx	Cortex	+	41.6	29.8	26.2	15.4	14.1
	Medulla	+	14.2	16.1			
Dx	Cortex	++	53.7[c]	69.4[c]	17.8[c]	7.9[c]	6.0[c]
	Medulla	++	19.3	32.8[c]			
Hyx	Cortex	+++	73.6[c]	109.2[c]	16.0[c]	5.1[c]	8.4[c]

[a]In analysis of electronmicrographs of the thymus stereological principles for morphometry were applied (Weibel, 1969).

[b]An arbitrary scale.

[c]Statistically significant difference determined by Student's t test by comparing values obtained from Dx and Hyx embryos to those from SDx control embryos.

All figures represent mean values of 14-35 embryos in group.

PINEALECTOMY AND IMMUNE RESPONSE

The epiphysis represents a part of the neuro-endocrine system (Thieblot, 1965). Although of brain origin, the pineal body receives autonomic peripheral innervation (Leeson and Leeson, 1976). In the rat, it seems that the pineal organ is innervated almost exclusively by orthosympathetic fibers originating in the superior cervical ganglia (Kappers, 1960).

The pineal's critical role in circadian and other biorhythms, in part via the superchiastmatic nucleus of the hypothalamus, is now well established, and there is beginning to accumulate a literature on the immunochronobiology of these structures.

The first reports on epiphysectomy are probably those of Exner and Boese (1910) and Foa (1912). The enhancement of transplantable tumor growth in animals without pineals has been repeatedly described (Rodin, 1963; Das Gupta and Terz, 1967; Lapin, 1974).

Jankovic et al. (1970) reported on the relationship between the pineal body and immune reactions in the rat. Neonatal epiphysectomy performed within 24 hours of birth did not exert any appreciable effect on Arthus reactivity and delayed hypersensitivity skin reactions to bovine serum albumin, anti-BSA antibody production, skin homograft rejection and incidence of experimental allergic encephalomyelitis in rats challenged at the age of 8 weeks. However, in rats pinealectomized at 6 weeks, Arthus and delayed skin reactions were reduced, and allergic encephalomyelitis was less expressed. Absolute lymphocyte and small lymphocyte counts were normal in rats pinealectomized at birth or at 6 weeks. The slight immunosuppressive effect of epiphysectomy in adult life was attributed to the lack of the secretory function of the pineal gland. Similarly, the removal of the epiphysis had little effect on skin homograft rejection, plaque-forming cells, haemagglutinin production and lipopolysaccharide (Rella and Lapin, 1976). The accelerated proliferation of immunocompetent cells in pinealectomized animals was attributed to the loss of the pineal antimitotic activity by the action of melatonin (Banerjee and Margulis, 1973).

It has been suggested that pinealectomy affects the function of T-suppressor lymphocytes and B-lymphocytes by reducing the formation and/or action of prostaglandin E_1 (Dunnane et al., 1979). Studies performed on chick embryos pinealectomized at 6 days of incubation revealed that the thymus and spleen of pineal-less embryos did not differ grossly and histologically from control embryos (Stalberg, 1965). It should be emphasized, however, that regeneration of pineal tissue occurred to some extent, even in completely pinealectomized birds, a fact which makes difficult the interpretation of the results.

Some data suggested the presence of lymphoid cells in the pineal gland of the avian central nervous system (Romieu and Jullien, 1942; Spiroff, 1958; Quay, 1965), whereas other studies failed to demonstrate lymphoid elements in the pineal body (Kappers, 1976). Lymphoid structures are present in the epiphysis of the mouse (Abe, et al., 1971). In the pineal region of the rat, the appearance and gradual increase of T-lymphocytes, beginning from the twentieth day after birth, has been reported (Uede et al., 1981). Studies of the pineal gland of 6-week-old chickens revealed that suspensions of pineal lymphocytes included 42% B-lymphocytes and 51% T-lymphocytes (Cogburn and Glick, 1983). Labeled bursal and thymic lymphocytes migrated to the pineal body, thus suggesting that both the thymus and bursa of Fabricius contributed to pineal lymphoid tissue. Moreover, injection of bovine serum albumin (BSA) into the carotid artery stimulated the production of anti-BSA antibodies in the lymphoid mass of the pineal gland. These studies indicated that the pineal gland is a functional part of the chicken lymphomyeloid system (Cogburn and Glick, 1983). Failure to identify immature forms of lymphocytes in the avian pineal body indicated that pineal lymphocytes are of extrapineal origin (Spiroff, 1958; Boya and Calvo, 1978). The invasion of the chicken epiphysis by lymphocytes was found to be much more massive at 1 month than at 4 months of age (Cogburn and Glick, 1981).

The ontogeny and function of lymphocytes in the pineal body remains unknown at present, and it appears that its T-lymphocytes are derived from T-lymphocyte-forming sites, such as the thymus. It has been reported recently (Janković et al., 1985) that early pinealectomy affects the thymus and bursa of Fabricius of the developing chick embryo, thus suggesting both a structural and a functional relationship between the pineal body and immune system during embryogenesis.

Because lymphocytes accumulate in the pineal capsular tissue, and because the choroid plexus of human, monkey, and rabbit contain receptors for the Fc fragment of immunoglobulin-G and for complement factor C3b (Breathen et al., 1979), it has been hypothesized that lymphocytes from the pineal body and the choroid plexus exert an immune function in the domain of the brain. Round aggregates of mononuclear cells resembling lymphoid follicles and germinal centers were described in the choroid plexus of chickens which developed experimental allergic encephalomyelitis following challenge with chicken or bovine spinal cord in complete Freund's adjuvant (Janković and Isvaneski, 1963).

RECEPTORS

The mechanisms of NIM at the cellular level began to emerge more clearly with the discovery of receptor site on the cells of the immune system for many neurotransmitters and neuromodulators. It seemed that whenever one looked for a receptor for a neurally-active polypeptide or a lymphocyte, it was almost always there! A representative sampling of these is shown on Table 3. Others, especially for endogenous opiates are discussed in more detail in Chapters 81, 263 of this book. There are receptors for a large number of intrinsic and extrinsic ligands on the surface membranes of immunocompetent cells (Cinander, 1977; Schulster and Levitzki, 1980).

Probably the first paper which called attention to the role of catecholamines in the immune response was that of Draškoci and Janković (1964): this described impaired delayed skin hypersensitivity reactions, antibody production and homograft rejection in rats treated with reserpine. Post mortem inspection of lymphoid tissues of reserpine-treated rats revealed pronounced changes in the cellular make-up of the thymus, spleen and lymph nodes. These changes were attributed, inter alia, to the lowering of catecholamine levels in different tissues caused by reserpine. Later investigations provided evidence that catecholamines can modulate cytotoxic activity mediated by T-lymphocytes (Henney et al., 1972), lymphocyte transformation induced by mitogens (Hadden, 1975), and antibody response to thymus-independent antigens (Miles et al., 1981).

We should note also the other side of the coin: production of lymphokines and immune-cell-type-products by cells of the central nervous system (e.g. Fontana, et al, 1985; Ovadia, et al 1985) as well as the production of neuroendocrine-like substances by lymphocytes (e.g. Johnson, et al., 1982; Smith and Blalock, 1985). These findings help us to visualize some of the means by which cells of the immune and nervous systems talk to each other.

Table 3
RECEPTORS FOR NEUROTRANSMITTERS, NEUROPEPTIDES,
MEDIATORS AND MODULATORS ON THE LYMPHOCYTE MEMBRANE:
DIRECT AND INDIRECT EVIDENCE
(A Partial List)

Receptor (for)	Cells	References
Catecholamines	Lymphocytes	Draškoci & Janković, 1964
Catecholamines	Lymphocytes	Henson et al., 1970
Noradrenaline	Lymphocytes	Hadden et al., 1970
Beta-adrenergic	Lymphocytes	Henney et al., 1972
Nicotinic cholinergic	Lymphocytes	Strom et al., 1972
Adrenaline	Lymphocytes	Sherman et al., 1973
Acetylcholine	Lymphocytes	Illiano et al., 1973
Adrenergic and cholinergic	Lymphocytes	Schreiner & Unanue, 1975
Adrenaline	Lymphocytes	Yu & Clements, 1976
Dopaminergic	Lymphocytes	Mitrova & Mayer, 1976
Beta-adrenergic	Lymphocytes	Williams et al., 1976
Cholinergic	Lymphocytes	Strom et al., 1977
Beta2-adrenergic	Thymocytes	Eskra et al., 1978
Dopaminergic	Lymphocytes	Ferguson et al., 1978
Muscarinic cholinergic	Lymphocytes	Gordon et al., 1978
Muscarinic cholinergic	T-cells	Lane & Strom, 1978
Menthionine-enkephalin	T-cells	Wybran et al., 1979
Morphine	T-cells	Wybran et al., 1979
Nicotinic cholinergic	Lymphocytes	Richman & Arnason, 1979
Beta-endorphin	Lymphocytes	Hazum et al., 1979
Beta-adrenergic	Thymocytes	Singh et al., 1979
Muscarinic cholinergic	T-cells	Shapiro & Strom, 1980
Beta-adrenergic	T and B cells	Bishopric et al., 1980
Dopaminergic	Lymphocytes	Le Fur et al., 1980
Substance P	Neutrophils	Marasco et al., 1981
Dopaminergic (D-1)	Spleen lymphocytes	Spetien et al., 1981
Dopaminergic	B cells	Le Fur et al., 1981
Beta-adrenergic	Lymphocytes	Brodde et al., 1981
Beta-endorphin	Spleen T cells, but not B cells	Gilman et al., 1982
Leucine-enkephalin	Lymphocytes	Plotnikoff, 1982
Adrenaline	Lymphocytes	Krall et al., 1982
Substance P	T-cells	Payan et al., 1983
Methionine-enkephalin	T-cells	Miller et al., 1983
Beta-endorphin	Natural killer cells	Mathews et al., 1983
Menthionine-enkephalin	Natural killer cells	Mathews et al., 1983
Enkephalins (met-and leu-enkephalin)	T-cells	Miller et al., 1984
Opioids	Natural killer cells	Shavit et al., 1984
Enkephalins	Natural killer cells	Faith et al, 1984
Somatostatin	T and B lymphocytes	Payan & Goetzl, 1986

PATHWAYS AND FEEDBACKS

The mechanisms by which brain lesions and brain stimulation alter immune repsonses are still not fully understood. Nonetheless, we do know that the central and peripheral nervous systems have two principal lines of communication with the organs, tissues and cells of the immune system: (1) endocrine-chemical, via the circulatory system, and (2) direct, "hard-wired" via nerve fibers, (principally the autonomic nervous system (Spector 1979, 1980, 1983). Feedback routes that modulate the modulation follow the same general pathways (Spector & Korneva, 1981).

It is now known also that leukocytes can produce certain neurally active polypeptides, which in turn act as lymphokines as well as neuromodulators (Blalock and Smith, 1985; see also page 119 in this volume): these, too, will undoubtedly be shown to be part of feedback cycles. In addition, other hormone-like polypeptides secreted by the thymus (thymosins) may also relay information, not only to the immune system, but to the brain. Hall and Goldstein (1985) have proposed the term "immunotransmitter" to describe the class of circulating substances that relay information back to the central nervous system.

Many circulatory connections are today fairly well recognized (e.g. steroids, catecholamines, neurally-active polypeptides, etc.) and need not be elaborated upon here. Other chapters in this book deal with the effects of opioids. The direct neural connections are less well recognized despite a long documentation of their existence. It is clear, also, that nerve endings exist in the parenchyma of these organs, in direct contact with the blast cells and with mature cells of the immune system. Table 4 provides partial lists, in chronological order of some of the studies describing the innervation of the thymus, the bone marrow, the lymph nodes and the spleen. Other tissues, in various species, related to the immune system are similarly innervated (Bulloch, 1985): we will not list all of them here, but we can mention briefly various elements of the reticuloendothelial system, Peyer's patches, appendix, tonsils, lacrimal glands (e.g. Harderian gland), jugular body and bursa of Fabricius.

Table 4

INNERVATION OF THE IMMUNE SYSTEM
(Partial List in Chronological Order)

I. THYMUS

1899	Bovera	1950	Tcheng
1911	Hallion and Morel	1955	Knoche
1912	Hallion and Morel	1966	Fujiwara
1915	Sjolander and Strandberg	1968	Solov'ev
1918	Crotti	1968	Shavlev
1923	Braeucker	1974	Serge'eva
1928	Terni	1980	Bulloch and Moore
1929	Pines and Majman	1980	Bulloch and Loy
1929	Terni	1980	Bulloch and Moore
1931	Cabanac	1980	Ghali et al.
1931	Terni	1981	Bulloch and Moore
1932	Hammar	1981	Williams and Felten
1933	Cordier	1981	Williams et al.
1933	Terni and Muratori	1982	Bulloch
1934	Koestowiecki	1983	Bulloch and Cullen
1935	Hammar	1983	Bulloch et al.
1938	Kostowiecki	1983	Cullen and Bulloch
1943	Bargmann	1985	Bulloch

(Continued)

Table 4 (Continued)
INNERVATION OF THE IMMUNE SYSTEM
(Partial List in Chronological Order)

II. BONE MARROW		III. SPLEEN		IV. LYMPH NODES	
1846	Gros	1928	Glaser	1899	Tonkoff
1880	Variot and Remy	1929	Riegele	1965	Volik
1902	Ottolenghi	1944	Harting	1979	Gordon et al.
1925	Castro	1948	Tischendorf	1980	Giron et al.
1928	Glaser	1952	Lentz	1980	Kiss
1929	Rossi	1955	Noerthen	1985	Bulloch
1929/30	Castro	1965	Dahlstrom		
1936	Takeyama	1966	Gillespie and Kirpekar	**REVIEW PAPERS: INNERVATION OF**	
1945	Kuntz	1970	Gersbach	**IMMUNE SYSTEM**	
1952	Fedoroff et al.	1970	Fillenz	1981	Jankovic et al.
1968	Calvo	1973	Zetterstrom et al.	1982	Bulloch
1970	Calvo	1976	Reilly, et al.	1983	Spector
1973	Miller and McCuskey	1979	Reilly et al.	1985	Bulloch
1981	Calvo	1979	Kudoh et al.		
1985	Bulloch	1981	Williams and Felten		
		1981	Williams et al.		
		1985	Bulloch		

BRAIN STIMULATION

Brain lesions are useful, but not perfect, tools for studying NIM. A lesion in one area may destroy a "center" (if indeed, one function can ever be relegated to only one center: see Spector, 1979 and 1980 for a discussion of this issue), interrupt a fiber pathway, change a circulatory route, interfere with a secretory process or effect any combination of these. Another difficulty is that no two lesions are ever precisely alike.

Brain stimulation techniques overcome some of these difficulties: if done correctly, a minimum of damage is done, and "normal" "physiologic" processes can be more nearly approximated. However, stimulation experiments have their difficulties also: stimulation spread to other nuclei and to other systems; rebound problems; puncture of the meninges and of brain tissue by the electrodes; the difficulties of finding optimal stimulaton wave form, amplitude and train parameters; and others.

Nonetheless, these experiments have had great value. In some cases (e.g. Korneva and Khai, 1967) stimulation produced the opposite effect from a lesion in the same area, indicating that there was a good chance that we were close to honing in on critical brain areas. In another instance, one of the earliest such experiments, an ingenious one (Baçiu, 1946) remains almost the only physiological (as opposed to anatomic or biochemical evidence) demonstration of a direct, "hard-

200

wired" functional connection between the brain and peripheral hemopoiesis; further experiments by the same group showed a similar neural connection between the brain and the host-defense system; i.e. electrical stimulation of the brain changed the rate of phagocytosis. More recently, Janković et al. (1983b) demonstrated that electrical stimulation of two areas: dorsomedial nucleus of the hypothalamus and of the sensorimotor cortex of the cerebrum in rats resulted in significant changes in Arthus skin reactions. Several investigators have measured changes in other immune reactions following electrical stimulation of various neclei of the hypothalamus. Table 5 outlines briefly, in chronological order, some experiments in NIM utilizing brain stimulation as a tool.

Table 5
BRAIN STIMULATION: (Partial List):

Date, Authors	Site of Stimulation	Animal	Antigen	Immune Response Assay	Results
1949, Benetato et al.	Hypothalamus	Dog		Phagocytosis	Increase
1957, Maslinski & Karszewski	Brain structures			Histamine shock	Reduction
1961, Halvorsen	Hypothalamus	Rabbit		Hematopoiesis	Increase
1961, Petrovski	Hypothalamic tubal region	Rabbit	Bacterial	Antibody production	Increase
1961, Petrovski	Mammillary bodies	Rabbit	Bacterial	Antibody production	Increase
1964, Binder	Anterior hypothalamus	Guinea pig	Horse serum	Anaphylaxis	Decrease
1967, Cipin & Malcev	Posterior hypothalamus	Rabbit		Natural agglutinins	Decrease
1967, Korneva & Khai	Various structures of mesencephalon	Rabbit	Horse serum	Antibody production	Increase
1969, Shiotani & Ban	Hypothalamus (b-sympathetic and c-sympathetic zones)	Rabbit		Thymus	Involution
1973, Abramchik & Shuvalova	Anterior and posterior hypothalamus	?	Spinal cord	Experimental allergic encephalomyelitis	Affected
1977, Plezitiy et al.	Dorsal hippocampus	Rabbit	Bovine serum	Arthus reaction	No effect
1979, Jankovic et al.	Hypothalamic dorsomedial nucleus	Rat	Bovine serum albumin	Arthus reaction Delayed skin reaction	Increase Increase
1981, Lambert et al.	Hypothalamic ventromedial area	Rat		Phagocytosis	Decrease
1983a, Jankovic et al.	Hypothalamic dorsomedial nucleus and sensorimotor cortex	Rat	Bovine serum albumin	Arthus and delayed skin hypersensitivity; antibody production	Increase
" " "	"	"	"	Thymus	Moderate increase in lymphoid cells
" " "	Hypothalamic ventromedial nucleus	"	"	Immune responses and thymus	No effect
" " "	Hypothalamic posterior nuclei	"	"	" "	Partial increase

POSSIBLE EXPLANATIONS OF THE EFFECTS EXERTED ON IMMUNE RESPONSES BY LESIONING AND STIMULATION: PATHWAYS AND MECHANISMS

Possible Pathways

Pathway One is: hypothalamus --→ pituitary --→ adrenals (glucocorticoids) and gonads (gonadal steroids) --→ thymus and lymphocytes.

Since the rat thymus contains high affinity androgen (Grossman et al., 1978; Stimson and McCruden, 1981) and estrogen (Grossman et al., 1979) receptors, it is possible that those receptors play a role in the determination of the thymus function. It is well established that the secretion of adrenal corticosteroids is under direct neural control (Mangilli et al., 1966), that there are steroid-sensitive neurons in the hypothalamus (Ruf and Steiner, 1967) and that steroids may play an essential role in the induction of immune response (Ambrose, 1970). The functional heterogeneity of lymhocytes appears to be a reflection of their sensitivity to corticosteroids (Claman, 1972; Fauci, 1976). Specific effects of steroid binding to the thymus (Munk et al., 1971) and variations in the number of glucocorticoid receptors on the lymphocyte membrane (Smith et al., 1977; Crabtree et al., 1980) are consistent with this immunoneuroendocrine pathway.

Pathway Two: hypothalamus --→ adenohypophysis --→ somatotropic hormone and/or thyroid hormones --→ lymphocytes.

Developmental hormones (Pierpaoli et al., 1970; Ahlqvist, 1976) and thyroid hormones (Leger and Masson, 1947; Nilzen, 1954) were shown to influence the immune machinery of the body. Thus, the presence of specific hormone receptors on the lymphocytes (Rimon et al., 1978; Harrison et al., 1979) (see also Table 3) would imply that specific regulation (lymphocytes, antibodies) and hormonally controlled non-specific regulation may work together (Besedovsky and Sorkin, 1977). Cyclic adenosine monophoshate (cAMP) is probably the most common mediator: hormones influence the formation of cAMP in the lymphocyte (MacManus et al., 1971).

Pathway Three: hypothalamus --→ fasciculus longitudinalis dorsalis (Schutz) postganglionic sympathetic fibres --→ (norepinephrine and other neurotransmitters) lymphocytes.

This interpretation, suggested in an earlier paper (Janković and Isaković, 1973), concerns the role of the sympathetic nervous system in the regulation of immune responses. The autonomic innervation of the thymus (Hammar, 1935; Gordon et al., 1979; Ghali et al., 1980; Bulloch, 1985) points to specific neuronal pathways. Indeed, the presence of adrenergic receptors on human lymphocytes (Hadden et al., 1970; see Table 3) and the general involvement of the sympathetic system in immune reactions (Korneva and Khai, 1961; Kozlov, 1973; Williams et al., 1981; Del Rey et al., 1981) have been reported. It is worthwhile mentioning here the presence of both nicotinic (Fuchs, 1979) and muscarinic (Maślinski et al., 1980) receptors for acetylcholine on the lymphocyte membrane. The increase of cyclic GMP level (Strom et al., 1974) in the lymphocyte induced by acetylcholine would indicate that this neurotransmitter may act as a regulatory ligand (Triggle, 1971) in immunity, suggesting the involvement of cholinergic mechanisms in immune phenomena. Pharmacological influences upon the immune response have been reviewed recently (Maestroni and Pierpaoli, 1981).

Pathway Four: hypothalamus (with hypothetical thymotropic hormone-releasing factor) --→ adenohypophysis --→ thymotropic hormone --→lymphocytes (Isakovic and Jankovic, 1973).

Since the first demonstration that the extract from the rat thymus restored immunological potential of rats thymectomized at birth (Janković et al., 1965), the humoral function of the thymus now is well documented (Luckey, 1973; Hall and Goldstein, 1985).

Pathway Five: hormones from different brain structures and centrally acting peptides (Hughes, 1978) --→ endocrine glands and lymphoepithelial system.

Several peptide and protein hormones, which are otherwise regarded to be of pituitary origin, are synthesized within the brain (Krieger and Liotta, 1979). These hormones of the brain may regulate not only the secretion of the anterior pituitary (Guillemin, 1978) but also the metabolic processes in the lymphocytes. Thus, it seems that low-molecular polypeptides from the calf cereral cortex were capable of altering the immune response in mice when injected into animals before immunization with sheep erythrocytes (Belokrylov and Sofronov, 1980). Experiments on mice with surgical lesions of the cerebral cortex suggested that the neocortex specifically modulates events mediated by T cells and not by B cells (Renoux, 1980; Renoux et al., 1983). Of particular interest are enkephalins which constitute a major neuroendocrine link between the central nervous system and the immune system (Plotnikoff and Miller, 1983). Their activity in "stress" processes are related to immune responses (Amir et al., 1980; see also pages 221 and 425 in this volume). It has been reported that human blood T-lymphocytes contain receptors for morphine and methionine-enkephalin (Wybran et al., 1979). In mice, met-enkephalin and leu-enkephalin were found to stimulate lymphoblastogenesis in the presence of PHA (Plotnikoff and Miller, 1983). In humans, enkephalins were found to increase significantly the formation of active T-cell rosettes (Miller et al., 1984). It appears that endogenous enkephalins have immunostimulatory activity in vitro (Plotnikoff and Miller, 1983; see also pages 35, 209 and 129, this volume.)

Pathway Six: follows the peripheral divisions of the diffuse neuroendocrine system (Pearse and Takor, 1979).

This system, which probably is the largest organ of the body, and has an excellent strategic position for participation in the neuroimmunomodulation, may exert an influence on lymphocytes and their related cells in the peripheral lymphoid organs.

Pathway Seven: In the case of pathology, as with artificial lesions in experiments animals, other pathways and other factors play a role. For example, any rupture of the meninges alters the blood-brain barriers. For discussion of such "abnormal" and experimental pathways, see Spector, 1979. Suffice it to mention here that in prehistoric times, man probably cured some diseases by trephining the skull (Guiard, 1930) and in "modern" times, i.e. in the 1920's and '30's, A.D. Speranskii (1934) and his colleagues claimed to have cured a host of diseases by "pumping" cerebrospinal fluid until it turned red!

The above-mentioned pathways of neuroimmunomodulation serve ultimately in the transmission of a variety of inhibitory and excitatory information (signals), different in nature and origin, to the intracellular machinery via the ligand-receptor-cAMP/cGMP system (Schulster and Levitzki, 1980) of the lymphoid and nonlymphoid cells of the immune micromilieu (Janković, 1973, 1979). Since the hypothalamus is associated with other brain structures by diffuse fibre systems (Nauta and Haymaker, 1969; Morgane and Panksepp, 1979) and peptidergic neural network (Renaud, 1978), the lesioning and stimulation of the hypothalamus and other brain regions may cause the propagation of impulses (signals, information) via neural fibres to the pituitary gland, adrenergic system, endocrine glands, diffuse neuroendocrine system, epithelial system, and lymphocytes and their associates, and thus modulate the immune response (briefly reviewed by Spector, 1983). The direct "hard-wired" pathways, afferent and efferent, must be considered along with circulatory pathways. In general, brain lesioning and stimulation upset the balance between the inhibitory and facilitatory factors (cellular, subcellular, humoral, molecular and ionic) which control the normal immune response: however, such experiments help greatly to delineate the "normal" physiologic pathways.

CONCLUSIONS AND SUMMARY

In this chapter, we have outlined part of the history of modern research on neuroimmunomodulation (NIM), emphasizing the contributions made to our knowledge by experiments utilizing partial ablations (lesions) of specific brain areas and by other experiments designed to stimulate many of these areas. Such experiments have demonstrated, in many species, the direct influences of the central nervous system upon many immune responses cellular and humoral, and upon many related host-defense mechanisms. While some of the conclusions based on this literature appear to be contradictory, we can say with certainty:

(1) That the nervous, immune and endocrine systems are inextricably linked via numerous feedback loops,

(2) that several nuclei in the hypothalamus, the corpora quadrigemina, the cerebral cortex, the reticular formation of the brainstem and the sympathetic nervous system in general, all play a role in immunity,

(3) that the two-way communicaton is carried out via circulatory and direct neural fiber routes, and

(4) that molecular links among the nervous, endocrine, and immune systems are apparent among the membrane receptor sites on cells of the immune system for neurally-active polypeptides, neurotransmitters and hormones; likewise receptors exist on cells of the nervous system for bioactive substances of the immune system,

(5) that links among the nervous, endocrine and immune systems develop even in the embryo.

Other mechanisms of NIM are explained in detail in many of the chapters in this book.

*POST-SCRIPT

In our introduction and in the table of experiments dealing with brain lesions and immunity, we restricted the list to an outline of "modern" experiments. It should be mentioned, however, that the earliest known experiments were those of Savchenko (1891) and London (1899) which showed that spinal section or removal of the cerebral hemispheres in pigeons made them susceptible to anthrax. Intact pigeons are not susceptible.

Savchenko, I. G. On the unsusceptibility to anthrax (in Russian). Vrach. 5: 132-134, 1891.

London, Ye.S. On the influence of the removal of various parts of the brain of pigeons on their immunity to anthax (in Russian) Arkh. Biol. Nauk 7:177-187, 1899.

The reference list at the end of this chapter should serve as a guide to the literature. In addition, a compilation of over a thousand abstracts covering a five year period in "Mind and Immunity" experiments appeared in 1984 (Locke, et al.), and a collection of important papers going back to the 1920's was published in 1985 (Locke, et al.). Neither of these volumes are comprehensive, but both contain important pieces of the big picture: other recent reviews are included in Ader (1983), Korneva et al. (1985), Guillemin, et al. (1985), Spector, (1979, 1983) and Janković (1985).

For those interested in historic roots, a very early book on NIM, one of great scientific importance and one well worth reading, is that of Metalnikov (1934).

REFERENCES

Abe, K., Matsushima, S. Kachi, T., and Ito, T. Lymphoid tissue in the pineal region of the mouse: a histological and histochemical study, Arch. Histol. Jap., 33:263, 1971.

Abinder, A.A., The effect of electric stimulation of the anterior portion of the hypothalamus on reconstitution of immune reaction of the body, Zh. Mikrobiol. Epidemiol. Immunobiol., 41:47, 1964.

Abramchik, G.V., and Shuvalova N.S. The role of the hypothalamus in the pathogenesis of experimental allergic encephalomyelitis, Zh.Nevropatol.Psikiatr., 73:988, 1973.

Ahlqvist, J. Endocrine Influence on Lymphatic Organs, Immune Responses, Inflammation and Autoimmunity. Almqvist and Wiksell Int. Stockholm, 1976.

Ambrose, C.T., The essential role of corticosteroids in the induction of the immune response in vitro, in Hormones and Immune Response, G.E.W. Wolstenholme and J. Knight, eds. Churchill, London, pp.100, 1970.

Amir, S. Brown, Z.W. and Zelman, A., The role of endorphins in stress: evidence and speculations. Neurosci. Biobehav.Rev., 4:77, 1980.

Baçiu, I., The role of the central nervous system in the inducement of the phagocytic reaction. Doctoral dissertation, Institute of Physiol. and Med. Physics, Univ. of Cluj, 1946. (Romanian: English translation available.)

Baçiu, I., and Ivanov, A. The role of hypothalamic centres in the immune specific response., Physiologie, 21(4):251,1984.

Baçiu, I., Olteanu, A., Prodan, T. Baiescu, M. and Vaida, A. Changes of phagocytic biological rhythm by reproduction of circadian times and by influences upon hypothalamus. Proc., First Int. Workshop on NIM, Bethesda, Md., November 1984, in press, 1985.

Banerjee S., and Margulis, L. Mitotic arrest by melatonin, Exp.Cell.Res., 78:314, 1973.

Banet, S., Brandt, S. and Hensel, H. The effect of continuously cooling the hypothalamic preoptic area on antibody titre in the rat, Experientia, 38:965, 1982.

Bargmann, W., Der Thymus, in Handbuch der Mikroskopischen Anatomie., Springer, Berlin. VI (4): 1-145, 1943.

Barone, R.M., and Das Gupta, T.K. Role of pinealectomy on the Walker 256 carcinoma in rats, J. Surg. Oncol., 2:3132, 1970.

Belokrylov, G.A. and Sofronov., B.N., Effect of thymic and cortical low-molecular polypeptides on different stages of immune response in mice. Immunologia, 4:66, 1980.(in Russian).

Benetato, G., Oprisiu, C. and Baciu, I. Sur le role du systeme nerveux central dans le declenchement de la reaction phagocytaire, Recuil d'Etudes Medicales, Ed. Inst. de Cultura Universala. Bucharest, 1949.

Besedovsky, H.O. and Sorkin, E., Network of immune-neuroendocrine interactions. Clin. Exp. Immunol., 27:1, 1977.

Betz, T.W., The effects of embryonic pars distalis grafts on the development of hypophysectomized chick embryos, Gen.Comp.Endocrinol., 9:172, 1967.

Bishopric, N.H., Cohen, H.J. and Lefkowitz, R.J. Beta-adrenergic receptors in lymphocyte subpopulations, J. Allergy Clin. Immunol., 65:29, 1980.

Bizière, K., Renoux, M. and Renoux, G. Modulation of the T-cell lineage by the cerebral neocortex, Proc., First Intl. Workshop on NIM, Bethesda, MD, Nov. 1984, in press, 1985.

Blalock. J.E., and Smith, E.M. Human leukocyte interferon: structural and biological relatedness to adrenocorticotropic hormone and endorphin, Proc. Natl.Acad. Sci. USA, 77:5972, 1980.

Bovera, A., Sui nervi della ghiandola di timo, Giron Acad. Med. Torino, 62:1, 1899.

Bowen, F.P., Immunological reactions after cortical lesions in rabbits, Arch. Neurol., 19:398, 1968.

Braeucker, W., Die Nerven des Thymus., Z. Anat. Entw., 69:309, 1923.

Breathen, L.R., Forre, O.T. Husby, G., and Williams, R.G., Jr. Evidence for Fc receptors in human choroid plexus, Clin. Immunolo. Immunopathol., 14:284, 1979.

Brodde, O.E., Engel, G. Hoyer, D., Bock, K.D., and Weber, F. The β-adrenergic receptor in human lymphocytes: Subclassification by the use of a new radio-ligand, ()-125 Iodacyanopindolol, Life Sci., 29:2189, 1981.

Brooks, W.H., Cross, R.J. Roszman, T.L., and Markesbery, W.R. Neuroimmunomodulation: neural anatomic basis for impairment and facilitation, Ann. Neurol., 12:56, 1982.

Bulloch, K., Neuroendocrine-immune circuitry pathways included with the induction and persistence of humoral immunity, University Microfilm International, Ann Arbor, MI, 727-1064 (Ph.D. dissertation, 1981, UCSD), 1982.

Bulloch, K., A light and ultrastructural analysis of innervation of the thymus gland during the perinatal period, Neurosc. Abst., 20: 572, 1982.

Bulloch, K., Neuroanatomy of lymphoid tissue: a review, in Neural Modulation of Immunity, Guillemin, R., Cohn,M. and Melnechuk, T.,eds. Raven Press, N.Y., pp. 111- 141, 1985.

Bulloch, K., and Cullen, M.R. An analysis of the thymic CNS relationship in the chick, Immunology, Fifth International Congress of Immunol. (Abst.), 1983.

Bulloch, K., Cullen, M.R. Davis, M.L. and Schwartz, R.H. Neuroimmunology of the thymus gland, Neurology, 33(4) Suppl. #2:194,pp 187 ff., 1983.

Bulloch, K., and Loy, R. The development of innervation in the thymus gland of wildtype and of the neuroimmune mutant Staggerer, Society for Neurosciences, Abstract. 26.5, 1980.

Bulloch, K., and Moore, R.Y. Central nervous system projections to the thymus gland. Possible pathways for the regulation of the immune response, Anat. Rec., 196:25A, 1980a.

Bulloch, K., and Moore, R.Y. Nucleus ambiguous projections to thymus gland -Possible pathways for regulation of the immune response and the neuroendocrine network, Am. Ass. Anat. (Abstr.), 25A, 1980b.

Bulloch, K. and Moore, R.Y. Thymus gland innervation by brainstem and spinal cord in mouse and rat, Am. J. Anat., 162:157, 1981.

Cabanac, J., Les nerfs du thymus, Bull. Assoc. Anat., 25:97, 1931.

Calvo, W., The innervation of the bone marrow in laboratory animals, Am. J.Anat., 123:315, 1968.

Calvo, W., Bone marrow hemopoiesis in the human fetus, in Adv. Physiol. Sci., Vol. 6 Genetics, Structure and Function of Blood Cells, S.R. Hollan, G. Gardos, B. Sardaki, eds., Akademiak Kiado, Budapest, 1981.

Calvo, W., and Forteza-Vila, J., Schwann cells of the bone marrow., Blood, 36: 186, 1970.

Castro, F. de, Technique pour la coloration du systeme nerveux quand il est porvu de ses etuis osseux, Trav. Lab. Rech. Biol. Univ. Madrid., 23:427, 1925.

Castro, F. de, Quelques observations sur l'intervention du système nerveux autonome dans l'ossification. innervation du tissu osseus de la moel osseuse, Trav. Labor. Rech. Biol. Univ. Madrid, 26:215, 1929.

Cinader, B. (ed.), Immunology of Receptors, Marcel Dekker, New York, 1977.

Cipin, A.B., and Malcev. V.N. Effect of hypothalamic stimulation on normal antibodies in the blood, Patol. Fiziol., 11:83 (in Russian), 1967.

Claman, N.H., Corticosteroids and lylmphoid cells. New Engl. J. Med., 287:388, 1972.

Cogburn, L.A., and Glick, B. Lymphopoiesis in the chicken pineal gland, Am.J.Anat., 162:131, 1981.

Cogburn, L.A., and Glick, B. Functional lymphocytes in the chicken pineal gland, J.Immunol., 130:2109, 1983.

Cordier, P. and Coulouma, P. Les nerfs du thymus, Ann. Anat. Path., 1104, 1933.

Crabtree, G.R., Munck, A. and Smith, K.A., Glucocorticoids and lymphocytes. I. Increased glucocorticoid receptor levels in antigen-stimulated lymphocytes. J. Immunol., 124:2430, 1980.

Cross, R.J., Brooks, W.H. and Roszman, T.L. Hypothalamic-immune interactions. I. The acute effect of anterior hypothalamic lesions on the immune response, Brain Res., 196:79, 1980.

Cross, R.J., Brooks, W.H. Roszman, T. L., and Markesbery, W.R. Hypothalamic-immune interactions. Effects of hypophysectomy on neuroimmunomodulation, J. Neurol. Sci., 53:557, 1982.

Cross, R.J., Jackson, J.C. Markesbery W.R., Brooks, W.H. and Roszman, T.L. Modulation of Immune Function by Electrolytic and Chemical Lesions of the Central Nervous System, Proc., First Intl. Workshop on NIM, Bethesda, Md. Nov. 1984, in press, 1985.

Cross, R.J., Markesbery, W.R., Brooks, W.H. and Roszman, T.L. Hypothalamic-immune interactions: Neuromodulation of natural killer activity by lesioning of the anterior hypothalamus. Immunology 51:399.

Crotti, A.,Thyroid and Thymus. Lea & Febiger, Philadelphia and New York, pp 536-559, 1918.

Cullen, M.R., and Bulloch, K. Innervation of thymus transplants in nude mice: An ultrastructural study, Society for Neuroscience, 9(1): 117, Abstract # 3410, 1983.

Cunnane, S.C., Manku, M.S. and Horrobin, D.F. The pineal and regulation of fibrosis: pinealectomy as a model of primary biliary cirrhosis: roles of melatonin and prostaglandins in fibrosis and regulation of T-lymphocytes, Med. Hypotheses, 5:403, 1979.

Dahlström, A.B., and Zetterstrom, B.E.M Noradrenaline stores in nerve terminals of the spleen: changes during hemorrhagic shock, Science, 147:1583, 1965.

Dann, J.A., Wachtel, S.S. and Rubin. A.L. Possible involvement of the central nervous system in graft rejection, Transplantation, 27:223, 1979.

Das Gupta, T.K., and Terz, J. Influence of pineal gland on the growth and spread of melanoma in the hamster, Cancer Res., 27:1306, 1967.

Del Rey, A., Besedovsky, H.O. Sorkin,E., DaPrada, M., and Arrenbrecht, S. Immunoregulation mediated by the sympathetic nervous system, Cell.Immunol., 63:329, 1981.

Draškoci, M., and Janković, B.D. Involution of thymus and suppression of immune response in rats treated with reserpine, Nature, 202:408, 1964.

Eskra, J.D., Stevens, J.S. and Carty, T.J. β2-adrenergic receptors in thymocytes, Fed.Proc., 37:687, 1978.

Exner, A., and Boese, J. Uber experimentelle Extirpation der Glandula pinealis, Dtsch.Z.Chir., 107:182, 1910.

Faith, R.E., Liang, H.J. Murgo, A.J., and Plotnikoff, N.P. Neuroimmunomodulation with enkephalins: enhancement of human natural killer cell activity in vitro, Clin., Immunol. Immunopathol., 31:412, 1984.

Fauci, A.S., Mechanisms of corticosteroid action on lymphocyte subpopulations. Clin. Exp. Immunol., 24:54, 1976.

Federoff, N.A., Terentyeva, E.I. Garfunkel, M.L., Tsesarskaya, T.P. and Rozanova, N.S. The bone marrow after damage to the sacral plexus and the sympathetic innervation, Arch. Pat., 14:25 (in Russian), 1952.

Ferguson, R.M., Schmidtke, J.R. and Simmons, R.L. Effects of psychoactive drugs on in vitro lymphocyte activation, Birth Defects: Original Article Series, 14:379, 1978.

Filipp, G., and Szentivanyi, A. Anaphylaxis and the nervous system, III, Ann. Allergy, 16:306, 1958.

Fillenz, M.,The innervation of the cat spleen, Proc. Roy Soc. B London, 174:459-468, 1970.

Foa, C., Hypertrophie des testicles et de la crête après l'extirpation de la glande pineale chez le coq, Arch. Ital. Biol., 57:233, 1912.

Freedman, D.X., and Fenichel, G. Effect of midbrain lesion on experimental allergy, Arch. Neurol. Psychiat., 79:164, 1958.

Fuchs, S., Immunology of the nicotinic acetylcholine receptor, Curr. Topics Microbiol. Immunol., 85:1, 1979.

Fugo, N.W., Effects of hypophysectomy in the chick embryo, J. Exp.Zool., 85:271, 1940.

Fujiwara, M., Muryobayashi, T. and Shimamoto, K.
Histochemical demonstration of monoamines in the
thymus of rats, Japan J. Pharmocol., 16:493, 1966.

Gersbach, P., Contribution to the study of the innervation
of the spleen. Comparative anatomical study, Arch.
Anat. Histol. Embryol. (Strasbourg), 53(5):397,
1970.

Ghali, W.M., Abdel-Rahman, S. Nagib, M. and Mahran, Z.Y.
Intrinsic innervation and vasculature of pre-and
post-natal human thymus, Acta anat., 108:115, 1980.

Gillespie, J.S., and Kirpekar, S.M. The histological
localization of noradrenaline in the cat spleen,
J.Physiol, 187:69, 1966.

Gilman, S.C., Schwartz, J.M. Milner, R.J., Bloom, F.E. and
Feldman, J.D. Beta-endorphin enhances lymphocyte
proliferative responses, Proc. Natl.Acad. Sci. USA,
79:4226, 1982.

Giron, L.T., Crutacher, K.A. and Davis, J.N. Lymph nodes-A
possible site for sympathetic neuronal regulation of
immune responses, Ann. Neurol., 8:520, 1980.

Glaser, W., Über die motorische Innervation der Blutgefásse
der Milz nebst einigen Bemerkungen der intramuralen
Nervenversorgung der Blutgefasse Knochenmark, Z.
Anat., 87:741, 1928.

Goldstein, M.M., The effect of bilateral destruction of the
medial hypothalamic structures on the course of
anaphylactic shock, Bull. Exp. Biol. Med., 82:977,
1976.

Goldstein, M.M., Antibody-forming cells of the rat spleen
after the injury to the midbrain, Bull. Exp. Biol.
Med., 85:185, 1978.

Gordon, D.S., Serge'eva, V.E. and Zelenova, I.G. Functional
morphologyof adrenergic innervation and adreno-
containing structures in lymphoid organs, Arkh.
Anat. Gistol. Embriol., 77:13 (in Russian), 1979.

Gordon, M.A., Cohen, J.J. and Wilson, I. B. Muscarinic
cholinergic receptors in murine lymphocytes:
Demonstration by direct binding, Proc. Nat.Acad.Sci.
USA, 75:2902, 1978.

Gros, M., Note sur les nerfs des os, C.R. Acad. Sci.,
(Paris), 71:1106, 1846.

Grossman C.J., Nathan, P. and Sholiton, L.J. Specific
androgen receptor in the thymus of the castrated
male rat, Biol. Reprod., 18:48A, 1978.

Grossman C.J., Sholitan, L.J. Blaja, G.C., and Nathan, P.
Rat thymic estrogen receptor: II. Physicochemical
properties, J.Steroid. Chem., 11:1241, 1979.

Guiard, E., La Trépanation Cranienne: Chez les Neolithiques
et Chez les Primitifs Modernes, Masson, Paris, 1930.

Guillemin,R., The brain as an endocrine organ. Neurosci.
Res. Prog. Bull. (Suppl.), 16:1, 1978.

Hadden, J.W., Cyclic nucleotides in lymphocyte function,
Ann. N.Y. Acad. Sci., 256:352, 1975.

Hadden, J.W., Hadden, E.M., and Middleton, E., Jr.
Lymphocyte blast transformation. 1. Demonstration of
adrenergic receptors in human peripheral
lymphocytes, Cell. Immunol., 1:583, 1970.

Hall, N. R. McGillis, J.P. Spangelo, B.L., Healy, D.L. and
Goldstein, A. Immunoreactive peptides and the
central nervous system. Springer Seminar
Imunopathol. 8:153, 1985.

Hallion, L., and Morel, L. L'innervation vaso-motrice du
      thymus, C.R. Soc. Biol. (Paris), 71:382, 1911.
Hallion, L., and Morel, L. L'innervation vaso-motrice du
      thymus, J. Physiol. Path. Gen., 14:1, 1912.
Halvorsen, S., Plasma erythropoietin levels following
      hypothalamic stimulation in the rabbit, Scan. J.
      Clin. Investig., 13:564, 1961.
Hammar, J.A., Glasrekonstruktionen zur Beleuchtung der
      fruhen embryonalen Enlwicklung der thymus-
      innervation, Vers. Verh. Anat. Ges., 41:234,
      1932.
Hammar, J.A., Innervations-verhältnisse der Krelorgane der
      Thymus bis in den 4 Fetalmonat, Z.Mikroskanst.
      Forsch., 8:253, 1935.
Harrison, L.C., Flier, J., Itin, A., Kahn, C.R. and Roth,
      J., Radioimmunoassay of the insulin receptor: a new
      probe of receptor structure and function. Science,
      203:544-547, 1979.
Harting, K., Vergleichende Untersuchungen über die
      mikroskopische Innervation der Milz des Menschen und
      einigen Säugetiere., Erg. Anat., 34:1, 1944.
Hazum, E., Chang, K.-J. and Cuatrecasas, P. Specific
      nonopiate receptors for beta-endorphin, Science,
      205:1033, 1979.
Henney, C.S., Bourne, H.R. and Lichtenstein, L.M. The role
      of 3',5'-adenosine monophosphate in the specific
      cytolytic activity of lymphocytes, J.Immunol.,
      108:1526, 1972.
Henson, E.C., Brunson, J.G., and Everes, C.G. Prevention of
      the Arthus reaction in rats and mice by combination
      of epinephrine and a phenothiazine derivate,
      propiomazine, Int. Arch. Allergy Appl. Immunol.,
      37:458, 1970.
Hughes, J., Centrally Acting Peptides, MacMillan Press
      London, 1978.
Illiano, G., Tell, G.P.E., Siegel, M.I. and Cuatrecasas, P.
      Guanosine 3',5'-cyclic monophosphate and the action
      of insulin and acetylcholine, Proc. Nat. Acad. Sci.
      USA, 70:2443, 1973.
Isaković, K., and Janković, B.D. Neuro-endocrine correlates
      of immune response. II. Changes in the lymphatic
      organs of brain-lesioned rats, Int. Arch. Allergy
      Appl. Immunol., 45:373, 1973.
Isaković, K., Janković, B.D., Mićić, M., and Knežević, Z.
      Thymus-bursa relationship in the developing chick
      embryo, in Aspects of Developmental and Comparative
      Immunology, I. J. B. Solomon, ed., pp. 217-220,
      Pergamon Press, Oxford, 1980.
Janković, B.D., Structural correlates of immune
      microenvironment, in Microenvironmental Aspects of
      Immunity, B.D. Janković and K. Isaković, eds., pp.1-
      4, Plenum Press, New York., 1973.
Jankovic B.D., The immune microenvironment is a multisystem,
      Immunol.Lett., 1:145, 1979.
Janković, B.D., From immunoneurology to immunopsychiatry:
      neuromodulating activity of antibrain antibodies,
      Int. Rev. Neurobiol., 26:249-314, 1985.

Janković, B.D., and Isaković, K. Neuro-endocrine correlates
of immune response. I. Effects of brain lesions on
antibody production, Arthus reactivity and delayed
hypersensitivity in the rat, Int. Arch. Allergy
Appl. Immunol., 45:360, 1973.
Janković, B.D., Isaković, K. and Horvat, J. Effect of a
lipid fraction from rat thymus on delayed
hypersensitivity reactions of neonatally
thymectomized rats, Nature, 208:356, 1965.
Janković, B.D., Isaković, K. and Knežević, Z. Ontogeny of
the immuno-neuro- endocrine relationship. Changes
in lymphoid tissues of chick embryos surgically
decapitated at 33-38 hours of incubation,
Develop.Comp. Immunol., 2:479, 1978.
Janković, B.D., Isaković, K. and Knežević, Z. Ontogeny of
the immuno-neuro- endocrine relationship. Early
thymectomy of the chick embryo, Immunol. Lett., 1:7,
1979.
Janković, B.D., Isaković, K. Marković, B.M. and Rajčević, M.
Immunological capacity of the chicken embryo. II.
Humoral immune responses in embryos and young
chickens bursectomized and sham-bursectomized at 52-
64 h of incubation, Immunology, 32:689, 1977.
Janković, B.D., Isaković, K., Mićić, M., and Knežević, Z.
Thymus-bursa-hypophysis interactions in the
developing chick embryo,in, Aspects of Developmental
and Comparative Immunology I. J. B. Solomon, ed., pp
529-532, Pergamon Press, Oxford, 1981a.
Janković, B.D., Isaković, K., Mićić, M., and Knežević, Z.,
The embryonic lympho-neuro-endocrine relationship,
Clin. Immunol Immunopathol., 18:108, 1981b.
Janković, B.D., Isaković, K. and Mićić, M. The thymus-
hypophysis interaction in the developing chick
embryo. Thymic epithelial cells in
hypopohysectomized embryos, in In Vivo Immunology,
P. Nieuwenhuis, A.A. van den Broek and G. Hanna,
Jr., eds., pp. 343-348, Plenum Press, N.Y., 1982.
Janković, B.D., Isaković, K. and Petrović, S. Effect of
pinealectomy on immune reactions in the rat,
Immunology, 18:1, 1970.
Janković B.D., and Išvaneski, M. Experimental allergic
encephalomyelitis in thymectomized, bursectomized
and normal chickens, Int. Arch. Allergy Appl.
Immunol., 23:188, 1963.
Janković, B.D., Janković, D.Lj. and Savovski, Lj. Effect of
early epiphysectomy on the immune system of the
chick embryo, Proc., First Int. Workshop on NIM,
Bethesda, Md., November, 1984 in press, 1985.
Janković, B.D., Jovanova, K. and Marković, B.M. Effect of
hypothalamic stimulation on the immune reactions in
the rat, Period. Biol., 81:211, 1979.
Janković, B.D., Mićić, M., Janković, D. Lj. and Isaković, K.
The brain-thymus-hypophysis interconnection during
embryogenesis, Immunobiology, 165:285, 1983.
Janković, B.D., Nešic, K. and Marković, B.M.
Neuroimmunomodulation: electrical stimulations of
the hypothalamus and cortex potentiate the immune
response, Neurosci. Lett., 14:S180, 1983a.

Johnson, H.M., Smith, E.M., Torres, B.A. and Blalock, J.E.
Regulation of the in vitro antibody response by
neuroendocrine hormones, Proc. Nat. Acad. Sci USA,
79:4171, 1982.

Kanematsu, S., and Mikami, S.I.   Effects of hypothalamic
lesions on protein-bound ^{131}Iodine and thyroidal
^{131}I uptake in the chicken, Gen. Comp. Endocrinol.,
14:25, 1970.

Kappers, J.A., The development, topographical relations and
innervation of the epiphysis cerebri in the albino
rat, Z. Zellforsch., 52:163, 1960.

Kappers, J.A., The mammalian pineal gland, a survey, Acta
Neurochirurgica, 34:109, 1976.

Keller, S.E., Stein, M., Camerino, M.S., Schleifer, S.J.,
and Sherman, J.   Suppression of lymphocyte
stimulation by anterior hypothalamic lesions in the
guinea pig, Cell. Immunol, 52:334, 1980.

Khai, L.M., Kovalenkova, M.V. Korneva, E.A., and Seranova,
A.E., Further study on the role of the hypothalamic
region in the regulation of immunogenesis, Zh.
Mikrobiol. Epidemiol. Immunobiol., 41:7, 1964.

Kiss, F., Topographic relationship between the nerve
plexuses and lymph nodes of the abdomen, Arch.
Surgery, 21:405, 1980.

Klimenko, V.M., The study of some neuronal mechanisms of
hypothalamic regulation of immune reactions in
rabbits, Avtoref. Kand. diss. Inst. for Exper. Med.
Leningrad (Russian), 1972.

Knoche, H., Zur feineren Innervation des Thymus von
Menschen, Z.Zellforsch., 41:556, 1955.

Kopeloff, L.M., Barrera, S.E. and Kopeloff, N. Recurrent
convulsive seizures in animals produced by
immunologic and chemical means, Am.J. Psychiat.,
98:881, 1942.

Korneva, E.A., and Khai, L.M.   Role of the sympatho-adrenal
system in the control of immunogenesis, Fiziol.
Zh.SSSR, 47:1298   (in Russian), 1961.

Korneva, E.A. and Khai, L.M.   Effect of destruction of areas
within the hypothalamic region on the process of
immunogenesis, Fiziologicheskii Zh. SSSR. 49(1):42
(in Russian), (English translation in Fed. Proc.
Translations Suppl. 23(1): T88, 1964.

Korneva, E.A., and Khai, L.M.   Effect of stimulation of
various structures of the mesencephalon on the
course of immunological reactions, Fiziol. Zh. SSSR
I.M. Sechenova, 53:42 (in Russian), 1967.

Korneva, E.A., and Klimenko, V.M., Neuronale
hypothalamusakivitat and homoostatische reactionen,
Ergeb. exp. Med., 23:373-382, 1976.

Kostowiecki, M., Untersuchungen über Nervenendigungen in
den Thymus menschlicher Feten., Vorl. Mitteil.
Anat. Anza Bd., 80:231, 1934.

Kostowiecki, M., Uber die Nervenfasern und Nervenendigung
in der Thymus wahrend der Fetalperiode, Zool. Pol.,
3:23, 1938.

Kozlov, V.A., Anaphylaxis and the vegetative nervous
system, Meditzina, Moscow, 1973.

Krall, J.F., Connelly, M. and Tuck, M.L. In vitro
desensitization of human lymphocytes by
epinephrine, Biochem. Pharmacol., 31:117, 1982.

Krieger, D.T. and Liotta, A.S., Pituitary hormones in
      brain:where, how and why? Science, 205:366,1979.
Kudoh, G., Hoshi, K. and Murakami,T. Fluorescence
      microscopic and enzyme histochemical studies of the
      innervation of the human spleen, Arch. Histol. Jap.,
      42(2):169-180, 1979.
Kuntz, A. and Richins, C.A. Innervation of the bone marrow,
      J. Comp. Neurol., 83:213-222, 1945.
Lambert, P.L., Harrell, E.H., and Achterberg,J. Medial
      hypothalamic stimulation decreases the phagocytic
      activity of the reticuloendothelial system, Physiol.
      Psychol, 9:193, 1981.
Lane, M.A., and Strom, T.B. The muscarinic cholinergic
      receptor: the effect of T cell activation, Fed.
      Proc., 37:1788, 1978.
Lapin, V., Influence of simultaneous pinealectomy and
      thymectomy on growth and formation of the Yoshida
      sarcoma in rats, Exp. Pathol., 9:108, 1974.
Le Fur, G., Phan, T. Canton, T., Tur, C. and Uzan, A.
      Evidence for a coupling between doipaminergic
      receptors and phospholipid methylation in mouse B-
      lymphocytes, Life Sci., 29:2737, 1981.
Le Fur, G., Phan, T. and Uzan, A. Identification of
      stereospecific (3H) spiroperidol binding sites in
      mammalian lymphocytes, Life Sci., 26:1139, 1980.
Leeson, C.R., and Leeson, T.S., in Histology, C.R. Leeson
      and T.S. Leeson, eds., p. 475, W.B. Saunders,
      Philadelphia, 1976.
Leger, J., and Masson, G. Factors influencing an
      anaphylactic reaction in the rat, Fed. Proc., 6:150,
      1947.
Lentz, H., Die Nervencersorgung der Kanichen-Milz,
      Z.Zellforsch., 37:494, 1952.
Luckey, T.D., Thymic Hormones, Univ. Park Press, Baltimore,
      1973.
Luparello, T.J., Stein, M. and Park, C.D. Effect of
      hypothalamic lesions on rat anaphylaxis, Am. J.
      Physiol., 207:911, 1964.
MacManus, J.P. Whitfield, J.F. and Youdale, T., Stimulation
      by epinephrine of adenylcyclase activity, cyclic AMP
      formation, DNA synthesis and cell proliferation in
      populatiions of rat thymic lymphocytes, J. Cell
      Comp. Physiol., 77:103, 1971.
Macris, N.T., Schiavi, R.C. Camerino, M.S. and Stein, M.
      Effect of hypothalamic lesions on immune processes
      in the guinea pig, Am.J. Physiol., 219:1209, 1970.
Macris, N.T., Schiavi, R.C., Camerino, M.S. and Stein, M.
      Effect of hypothalamic lesions on passive
      anaphylaxis in the guinea pig, Am. J. Physiol.,
      222:1054, 1972.
Maestroni, G.J.M. and Pierpaoli, W., Pharmacological control
      of the hormonally mediated immune response, in
      Psychoneuroimmunology, pp. 405-428, R. Ader, Ed.
      Academic press, New York, 1981.
Mangilli, G., Motta, M. and Martini, L. Control of
      adrenocorticotropic hormone secretion, in
      Neuroendocrinology,, L. Martini and W.F. Ganong,
      eds. pp.298-360, Academic Press, N.Y., 1966.
Markesbery, W.R., Cross, R.J., Roszman, T.L. and Brooks,
      W.H. Aging changes in Neuroimmunomodulation in the
      Fischer 344 Rat, Proc. First Int. Workshop on NIM,
      Bethesda, Md. November 1984, in press, 1985.

Maślinśki, C., and Karszewski, W. The protective influence of brain stimulation by electric currents on histamine shock in guinea pigs, Bull. Acad. Pol. Sci.l, 5:57, 1957.

Maślinśki, W., Grabszewska, E. and Ryzewski, J., Acetylcholine receptors on rat lymphocytes. Biochim. Biophys. Acta, 633:269, 1980.

Mathews, P.M., Froelich, C.J., Sibbitt, W. L., Jr. and Bankhurst, A. D. Enhancement of natural cytotoxicity by beta-endorphin, J. Immunol., 130:1658, 1983.

Mićić, M., Janković, D. Lj., Isaković, K. and Janković, B.D. Forebrain and hypophysis affect development of the bursa of Fabricius in the chick embryo, Period. Biol., 85(Suppl 3):9, 1983.

Miles, K., Quintans, J., Chelmicka-Schorr, E. and Arnason, B.G.W. The sympathetic nervous system modulates antibody response to thymus-independent antigens, J. Neuroimmunol., 1:101, 1981.

Miller, G.C., Murgo, A.J. and Plotnikoff, N.P. Enkephalins-Enhancement of active T-cell rosettes from lymphoma patients, Clin. Immunol. Immunopathol., 26:446, 1983.

Miller, G.C., Murgo, A.J. and Plotnikoff, N.P. Enkephalins-Enhancement of active T-cell rosettes from normal volunteers, Clin. Immunol. Immunopathol., 31:132, 1984.

Miller, M., and McCuskey, R. Innervation of bone marrow in the rabbit., Scand. J. Haemat., 10:17, 1973.

Mitrova E. and Mayer, V. Phenotiatine-induced alterations of immune response in experimental tick-borne encephalitis: morphological model analysis of events, Acta. Virol., 20:479, 1976.

Morgane, P.J., Panksepp, J. Editors. Handbook of the Hypothalamus. Vol I. Anatomy, Dekker, N.Y., 1979.

Munck, A., Young, D.A., Mosher, K.M. and Wira, C.R., Specific metabolic and physiocochemical interactions of glucocorticosteroids with rat thymus cells, in Hormones in Development, pp. 191-201, M. Hamburgh and E.J.W. Barrington, Eds., Appleton Century Crofts, New York, 1971.

Nauta, W.J.H., and Haymaker, W. Hypothalamic nuclei and fiber connections, in: The Hypothalamus, pp. 139-209, W. Haymaker, E. Anderson and W.J.H. Nauta, Eds., Thomas, Springfield, 1969.

Nilzen, A., The influence of the thyroid gland on hypersensitivity reactions in animals. I., Acta. Allerg., 7:231, 1954.

Noerthen, K., Die Nervenversorgung der Katzenmilz., Morph. Jb., 95:55, 1955.

Ottolenghi, D., Sur les nerfs de la moelle des os, Arch. Ital. Biol, 37:73-80, 1902.

Paunović, V.R., Petrović, S. and Janković, B.D. Influence of early postnatal hypothalamic lesions on the immune response in adult rats, Period. Biol.,(Suppl.) 78:50, 1976.

Payan, D.G., Brewster, D.R. and Goetzl, E.J. Specific stimulation of human T- lymphocytes by substance P, J. Immunol., 131:1613, 1983.

Payan, D.G., and Goetzl, E.J. Neuropeptide regulation of immediate and delayed hypersensitivity, in Neuroimmunomodulation II, ed. N.H. Spector et al. Gordon and Breach, N.Y., in press, 1986.

Pearse, A.G.E., and Takor, T.T. Embryology of the diffuse neuroendocrine system and its relationship to the common peptides, Fed. Proc., 38:2288, 1979.

Petrovski, I.N., Effect of stimulation of different brain regions on agglutinin titers, Zh. Mikrobiol. Epidemiol. Immunobiol., 32:103 (in Russian), 1961.

Pierpaoli, W., Fabris, N. and Sorkin , E. Developmental hormones and immunological maturation, in Hormones and the Immune Response, G. E. W. Wolstenholme and J. Knight, eds. pp. 126-143, Churchill, London, 1970.

Pines, L., and Majman, R. The innervation of the thymus, J. Nerv. Dis., 69:361, 1929.

Plezitiy, K.D., Magaeava, S.V. and Evseev, V.A. Effect of lesions and stimulations of dorsal hippocampus on Arthus reaction, in Physiology of Immune Homeostasis,II Symposium, pp. 34-35, Rostov-on-Don, (in Russian), 1977.

Plotnikoff, N.P., and Miller, G.C. Enkephalins as immunomodulators, Int.J. Immunopharmacol., 5:437, 1983.

Polyak, A.I., Rumbeshet, L.M. and Sinichkin, A.A. Antibody synthesis following electrocoagulation of the posterior hypothalamic nucleus, Zh. Mikrobiol. Epidemiol. Immunobiol., 46:52 (in Russian), 1969.

Quay, W.B., Histological structure and cytology of the pineal organ in birds and mammals, Prog. Brain Res., 10:49, 1965.

Reilly, F.D., McCluskey, P.A., Miller, M.L., McCluskey, R. S., and Meineke,H.A. Innervation of the periarteriolar lymphatic sheath of the spleen, Tissue & Cell, 11:121, 1979.

Reilly, F. D., McCluskey, R.S. and Meineke, H.A. Studies of the hematopoietic microenvironment. VIII. Adrenergic and cholinergic innervation of the murine spleen, Anat. Rec., 185:109, 1976.

Rella, W., and Lapin, V. Immunocompetence of pinealectomized and simultaneously pinealectomized and thymectomized rats, Oncology, 33:3, 1976.

Renaud, L.P. Neurophysiological organization of the endocrine hypothalamus, in The Hypothalamus, pp. 269-301, S. Reichlin, R.J. Baldessarini and J.B. Martin, Eds., Raven Press, New York, 1978.

Renoux, G. Differentiation of T-cell lineage by sodium diethyldithiocarbamate (DTC). Influence of the neocortex, in New Trends in Human Immunology and Cancer Immunotherapy, pp. 966-994, Serrou, B. and Rosenfeld, C., Eds, Doin, Paris, 1980.

Renoux, G., Bizière, K., Renoux, M. and Guillaumin, J.M., The production of T-cell inducing factors in mice is controlled by the brain neocortex. Scand. J. Immunol., 17:45, 1983.

Renoux, G., Bizière, K., and Renoux, M. Imuthiol reveals brain cortical asymmetry in the regulation of T-cell activities, Proc., First Int. Workshop on NIM, Bethesda, Md. November, 1984, in press, 1985.

Richman, D.P., and Arnason, B.G.W. Nicotinic acetylcholine
    receptor: Evidence for a functionally distinct
    receptor on human lymphocytes, Proc. Natl. Acad.
    Sci. USA, 76:4632, 1979.
Rimon, G., Hanski, E, Braun, S. and Levitzki, A., Mode of
    coupling between hormone receptors and adenylate
    cyclase elucidated by modulation of membrane
    fluidity, Nature, 276:394, 1978.
Riegele, L., Uber die mikroskopische Innervation der
    Milz., Z. Zellforsch., 9:511, 1929.
Rodin, A.E., The growth and spread of Walker 256 carcinoma
    in pinealectomized rats, Cancer Res., 27:1545, 1963.
Romanoff, A.L., The Avian Embryo, MacMillan, New York,
    1960.
Romanoff, A.L. and Romanoff, A.J. Pathogenesis of the Avian
    Embryo, Wiley-Interscience, New York, 1972.
Romieu, M. and Jullien, G. Sur l'existence d'une formation
    lymphoid dans l'epiphyse de Gallinaces, C.R. Soc.
    Biol., 136:626, 1942.
Rossi, F., La distribuzione di fibre nervose nell 'uomo e
    particolarmente nel midollo osseo, studieta con
    metodi specifici delle neurofibrille., Boll. Soc.
    Ital. Biol. Sper., 3:863, 1929.
Roszman, T.L., Cross, R.J. Brooks, W.H., and Markesbery,
    W.R. Hypothalamic-immune interactions. II. The
    effect of hypothalamic lesioins on the ability of
    adherent spleen cells to limit lymphocyte
    blastogenesis, Immunology, 45:737, 1982.
Ruf, K., and Steiner, F.A. Steroid-sensitive neurons in rat
    hypothalamus and mid-brain:identification by
    microelectrophoresis, Science, 156:667-669, 1967.
Schiavi, R.C., Adams, J. and Stein, M. Effect of
    hypothalamic lesions on histamine toxicity in the
    guinea pig, Am. J. Physiol., 211:1269, 1966.
Schiavi, R.C., Macris, N.T. Camerino, M.S. and Stein, M.
    Effect of hypothalamic lesions on immediate
    hypersensitivity, Am. J. Physiol., 228:596, 1975.
Schowing, J., Influence de l'excision du rhombencéphale et
    du mesencéphale sur la morphogenese du crane chez
    l'embryon de Poulet, Compt. Rend. Acad. Sci., Paris,
    248:2391, 1959a.
Schowing, J., Influence de l'excision du mesencéphale et du
    prosencephale sur la morphogenese du crâne chez
    l'embryon du Poulet. Compt. Rend. Acad. Sci.,
    Paris.- 249:170, 1959b.
Schowing, J., Influence inducrice de l'encéphale
    embryonnaire sur le développement du crâne chez le
    Poulet. I. Influence de l'excision des territoires
    nerveux anterieurs sur le dévelopment cranien. J.
    Embryol. Exp. Morph., 19:9, 1968a.
Schowing, J., Influence inducrice de l'encéphale
    embryonnaire sur le dévelopment du crâne chez le
    Poulet. II. Influence de l'excision de la chorde et
    des territoires encéphaliques moyen et posterieur
    sur le development cranien. J. Embryol. Exp.
    Morphol., 19:23, 1968b.
Schreiner, G.F., and Unanue, E.R. The modulation of
    spontaneous and anti-Ig-stimulated motility of
    lymphocytes by cyclic nucleotides and adrenergic and
    cholinergic agents, J.Immunol, 114:802, 1975.

Schulster, D., and Levitzki, A. _Cellular Receptors for Hormones and Neurotransmitters_, John Wiley & Sons, Chichester, 1980.

Serge'eva, V.E., Histotopography of catecholamines in the mammalian thymus., _Bull. Exp. Biol. Med._, 77:456, (in Russian), 1974.

Shapiro, H.M., and Strom, T.B. Electophysiology of T-lymphocyte cholinergic receptors, _Proc. Nat. Acad. Sci. USA_, 77:4317, 1980.

Shavit, Y., Lewis, J.W. Terman, G.W., Gale, R.P., and Liebeskind, J.C., Opoid peptides mediate the suppressive effect of stress on natural killer cell cytotoxicity, _Science_, 223:188, 1984.

Shavlev, V.N., On the innervation of lymph nodes., _Arkh. Anat. Giol. Embriol._, 54(2):96 (in Russian), 1968.

Sherman, N.A., Smith, R.S. and Middleton, E. Jr. Effect of adrenergic compounds, aminophylline and hydrocortisone on _in vitro_ immunoglobulin synthesis by normal human peripheral lymphocytes, _J. Allergy Clin. Immunol._, 52:13, 1973.

Shiotani, Y., and Ban. T. Effect of long-term electrical stimulation of the hypothalamus on pituitary-target gland system in rabbits, _Med. J. Osaka Univ._, 20:119, 1969.

Singh, U., Millson, D.S. Smith, P.A., and Owen, J.J.T. Identification of beta-adrenoreceptors during thymocyte ontogeny in mice, _Eur. J. Immunol._, 9:31, 1979.

Sjolander, A., and Strandberg, A. Über die zur Thymusdrüse tretenden Nerven, _Upsala, Lak forh Forkh._, 20:243, 1915.

Smith, E., and Blalock, J.E. Lymphocyte production of neurally active pituitary hormone-like molecules, _Proc., First Int. Workshop on NIM_, in press, 1985.

Smith, K.A., Crabtree, G.R., Kennedy, S.J. and Munck, A., Glucocorticoid receptors and glucocorticoid sensitivity of mitogen stimulated and unstimulated human lymphocytes, _Nature_, 267:523, 1977.

Solov'ev V.N., On the sources of innervation of the thymus gland., _Arkh. Anat. Gistol. Embriol._, 51:76-82 (in Russian), 1966.

Spector, N.H. Can hypothalamaic lesions change circulating antibody responses to antigens? _Current Problems in Experimental and Clinical Allergy_ (V.I. Pytskii, ed.),pp. 21-37, Moscow, (Russian), 1979.

Spector, N.H. The "central state" of the hypothalamus in health and disease:old and new concepts. _Physiology of the Hypothalamus_, P, Morgane and J. Panksepp, eds., Dekker, N.Y., pp. 453-517, 1980.

Spector, N.H., Anatomical and physiological connections between the central nervous and the immune systems (neuroimmunomodulation), in _Immunoregulation_ , pp. 231-258, N. Fabris, E. Garaci, J. Hadden, and N.A. Mitchison, eds. Plenum Press, New York, 1983.

Spector, N.H. Information explosions in an old-new research domain. in _The Year in Immunology 1984-85_, pp. 202-207 J.M. Cruse and R.E. Lewis, Jr. eds. Karger Basel, 1985.

Spector, N.H., Cannon, L.T. Diggs, C.L., Morrison, J.E., and Koob,G.F. Hypothalamic lesions: effects on immunological responses, Physiologist, 18:401, 1975.

Spector, N.H., Koob, G.F. and Baron,S. Hypothalamic influence upon interferon and antibody responses to Newcastle Disease. Virus infection: preliminary report. Proc. Internatl. Union Physiol. Sci. 13:711 (Abstr.)

Spector, N.H. and E. Korneva Neurophysiology and Neuroimmunomodulation in Psychoneuroimmunology R. Ader, ed., Academic Press, N.Y., pp. 449-473, 1981.

Spector, N.H., Martin, L.K., Diggs, C.L. and Koob, G.F. Hypothalamic lesions: effects upon malaria and antibody production in rats. Proceedings of the 26th International Congress, New Delhi, India. Proc. Inter. Union Physiol. Sci (Abstr.), 1974.

Speplewski, C. and Vogel, W. Changes in brain serotonin affect leucocytes, T-cells and natural killer cell activity in rats, in preparation for press, 1985.

Speranskii, A.D., A Basis for the Theory of Medicine (first Russian Ed.) (English translation, International Publisher, N.Y. 1943), 1934.

Spetien, H., Kunert-Radek, J. Karasek, E., and Pawlikowski, M. Dopamine increases cyclic AMP concentration in the rat spleen lymphocytes in vitro, Biochem.Biophys. Res. Commun., 10:1057, 1981.

Spiroff, B.E.N., Embryonic and post-embryonic development of the pineal body of the domestic fowl, Am. J. Anat., 103:375, 1958.

Stalberg, H., Effects of extirpation of the epiphysis cerebri in 6-day chick embryos, Dissertation, Olaf Norlis Forlag, Oslo.,1965.

Stimson, W.H., and McCruden, A.B. Androgen binding cytosol receptors in the rat thymus: physicochemical properties, specificity, and localization, Thymus, 3:105, 1981.

Strom, T.B., Diesseroth, A. Morganroth,J. Carpenter, C.B., and Merrill, J.P. Alteration of the cytotoxic action of sensitized lymphocytes by cholinergic agents and activators of adenylate cyclase, Proc.Natl. Acad. Sci. USA, 69:2995, 1972.

Strom, T.B., Lundin, A.P. and Carpenter, C.B. The role of cyclic nucleotides in lymphocyte activation and function, Prog. Clin. Immunol., 3:115, 1977.

Strom, T.B., Sytkowski, A.J., Carptenter, C.B., and Merrill, J.P., Cholinergic augmentation of lymphocyte-medicated cytotoxicity, A study of the cholinergic receptor of cytotoxic T-lymphocytes. Proc. Natl. Acad. Sci, USA, 71:1330, 1974.

Szentivanyi, A., and Filipp, G. Anaphylaxis and the nervous system, II., Ann. Allergy, 16:143, 1958.

Szentivanyi, A., and Szekely, J. Anaphylaxis and the nervous system, IV., Ann. Allergy, 16:389, 1958.

Takeyama, K., Morphologische Beobachtungen über diesich im Knochenmark verteilenden, peripheren Nerven, Mitt. med. Akad. Kioto, 16:895, 1936.

Tcheng, K.T., Fibres nerveuses momifiées dans les corpuscules de Hassall chez le chat, Bull. Histol. Appl., 27:100, 1950.

Terni, T., Les cellules myoides du thymus des sauropsides et leur innervation., Bull. Ass. Anat., Paris, 3:448, 1928.

Terni, T., Ricerche istologiche sull innervazione del timo dei Sauropsidi, Z. Zellforsch, 9:377, 1929.

Terni, T., L'innervazione del timo, Arch.Zool. Ital., 16:714, 1931.

Terni, T., and Muratori, G. Sulla innervazione del timo e del corporvultim onbranchiale dopo estirpazione del ganglio nodoso del vago, Monit. Zool. Ital., 43: Suppl., 85, 1933.

Thakur, P.K., and Manchanda, S.K. Hypothalamic influence on the activity of reticuloendothelial system in cat, Indian J.Physiol. Pharmacol., 13:11, 1969.

Thiéblot, L., Structure and function of the epiphysis cerebri, Prog. Brain Res., 10:479, 1965.

Thrasher, S.G., Bernardis, L.L. and Cohen,S. The immune response in hypothalamic-lesioned and hypophysectomized rats, Int.Arch. Allergy Appl. Immunol., 41:813, 1971.

Tischendorf, F., Beobachtungen über die feinere Innervation der Milz, Kölner Univ. Verlag, Köln , 1948.

Tonkoff, W., Zur Kenntnis der Neervender Lymphdrüsen, Anat. Anzeiger, 16: 456, 1899.

Triggle, D.J., Neurotransmitter-Receptor Interactions, Academic Press, London, 1971.

Tyrey, L., and Nalbandov. A.V. Influence of anterior hypothalamic lesions on circulating antibody titers in the rat, Am. J. Physiol., 222:179, 1972.

Uede, T., Ishii, Y. Matsuura, A. Shimogawara, I. and Kikuchi, K. Immunohistochemical study of lymphocytes in rat pineal gland: selective accumulation of T-lymphocytes, Anat. Rec., 199:239, 1981.

Variot, P., and Remy, C. Sur les nerfs de la moelle des os., J. Anat. Physiol., 6:273, 1880.

Volik, V.Ia, Development of the neural apparatus of inguinal lymph nodes in man, Arkh. Anat. Gistol. Embriol., 45:(5):34 (in Russian), 1965.

Warejcka, D.J., and Levy, N.L. Central nervous system (CNS) control of the immune response: effect of hypothalamic lesions on PHA responsiveness in rats, Fed. Proc., 39:914, 1980.

Weber, R.J., and Pert, C.B. Opiatergic modulation of the immune system, in Central and Peripheral Endorphins: Basic and Clinical Aspects, E.E. Muller and A.R. Genazzani,eds, pp.35-42, Raven Press, New York, 1984.

Weibel, E.R., Stereological principles for morphometry in electron microscopic cytology, Int. Rev. Cytol., 26:235, 1969.

Wertman, E., Ovadia, H., Feldman, S., and Abramsky, O. Prevention of experimental autoimmune disease by anterior hypothalamus lesion in rat, Proceedings First Int. Workshop on NIM, Bethesda, Maryland, November 1984, in press, 1985.

Williams, J.M., and Felten, D.L. Sympathetic innervation of murine thymus and spleen: A comparative histofluorescence study, Anat. Rec., 199:531, 1981.

Williams J.M., Peterson, R.G. Shea, P.A., Schmedtje, J.F.,
     Bauer, D.C. and Felten, D.L. Sympathetic innervation
     of murine thymus and spleen: Evidence for a
     functional link between the nervous and immune
     systems., Brain Res. Bull., 6:83, 1981.
Williams, L.T., Snyderman, R. and Lefkowitz, R.J.
     Identification of beta-adrenergic receptors in human
     lymphocytes by (-) [3H] alprenolol binding, J. Clin.
     Invest., 57:49, 1976.
Wingstrand, K.O., The Structure and Development of the Avian
     Pituitary, Gleerup, Lund, 1951.
Wolff, E., Les bases de la teratogenese expérimentale des
     vertèbres amniotes d'après les resultats des
     methodes directes, Arch.Anat. Histol.Embryol. 22:1,
     1936.
Wybran, J., Appelboom, T. Famaly, J.P. and Govaerts, A.
     Suggestive evidence for receptors for morphine and
     methionine-enkephalin on normal human blood T-
     lymphocytes, J. Immunol., 123:1068, 1979.
Yu, D.T.Y., and Clements, P.J. Human lymphocyte
     subpopulations: effect of epinephrine, Clin. Exp.
     Immunol., 25:472, 1976.
Zetterstrom, B.E., Høkfelt, M.T. Norbert, K.A., and
     Olsson,P. Possibilities of a direct adrenergic
     influence on blood elements of the dog spleen, Acta.
     Chir. Scand., 139:17, 1973.

ENKEPHALINS: MEDIATORS OF STRESS-INDUCED IMMUNOMODULATION

Anthony J. Murgo[a], Robert E. Faith[b], and
Nicholas P. Plotnikoff[c]

[a]West Virginia University Medical Center, Morgantown, WV;
[b]University of Houston, Houston, TX;
[c]Oral Roberts University School of Medicine, Tulsa, OK

INTRODUCTION

It is well known that environmental stress can influence the immune
response and tumor growth (1). Although stress has usually   been
associated with detrimental effects on the host, under certain
experimental conditions of timing and duration of stressful stimuli,
immunoenhancement and inhibition of tumor growth can result (1,2,3,4). In
addition, stress brings about numerous biochemical changes including the
release of neurotransmitters, corticosteroids, and other hormones that can
have various effects on the immune system and which may be benificial or
detrimental to the host (5,6,7).

Among the potential mediators of stress-induced immunomodulation are
the endogenous opioids, including beta-endorphin and the enkephalins.
These peptides are found within the central nervous system, pituitary, and
other tissues including the adrenals and sympathetic neurons and can be
released in response to stressful stimuli (8,9,10,11). This chapter will
review in some detail the various effects of the opioids on the immune
system and tumor growth.

OPIOID RECEPTORS ON IMMUNE SYSTEM COMPONENTS

The various pharmacological and physiological effects of the opioids
on the nervous system such as analgesia, euphoria, and thermoregulation
are mediated through interactions with specific membrane receptors (12).
Cells vary as to the types and subtypes of opioid receptors they bear and
opioids differ in their binding affinities for these receptors. Briefly,
[Met]enkephalin and [Leu]enkephalin have relatively high affinities for
delta receptors whereas beta-endorphin appears to bind preferentially to
epsilon receptors. Morphine has a high affinity for mu and Kappa
receptors. Naloxone and naltrexone are pure opioid antagonists which have
high affinity binding to mu and Kappa type receptors and lower affinity
for delta and epsilon receptors. Since the opioids can directly influence
the function of immune cells it is not surprising that these cells possess
specific opioid receptors.

Lymphocytes

Indirect evidence: Wybran et al (13) were the first to suggest that
lymphocytes possess opioid receptors. This conclusion is based mainly
upon the indirect evidence that opioids can influence the binding
characteristics of human thymus-derived lymphocytes to sheep erythrocytes.
Pheripheral blood lymphocytes treated with 10^{-10} M to 10^{-7} M morphine
and 10^{-9} M to 10^{-7}M, dextromoramide inhibit the formation of active
(high-affinity) rosettes. T cells forming active rosettes are felt to
represent a subpopulation of lymphocytes that may be decreased in certain
states of cellular immune deficiency (14). Morphine but not
dextromoramide also inhibits total T cell rosettes. In contrast, 10^{-7} M
to 10^{-4} M [Met]enkephalin enhances active T cell rosettes and does not
affect total T cell rosettes. Similar to mechanisms in the nervous
system, the effects of the opioids on the immune system appear to be
mediated by interactions with specific receptor types. In the case of
active T cell rosette formation specific ligand binding to the mu receptor
(morphine) is inhibitory and to the delta receptor ([Met]enkephalin) is
stimulatory. Further support for specific opioid receptors on lymphocytes
is provided by effects observed with naloxone on the active T cell rosette
assay (13). Naloxone, which alone has no effect, very effectively blocks
the inhibitory effects of morphine. In contrast, much higher molar
concentrations (10 to 100 fold) are needed to block the enhancing effects
of [Met]enkephalin.

[Leu]enkephalin as well as [Met]enkephalin can influence the formation
of active T cell rosettes. However, in the study by Miller et al (15)
only 76 to 77% of the samples tested showed enhancement by the enkephalins
and the remainder were either not effected or inhibited. The reason for
this variability is not clear but similar inconsistent results with the
enkephalins has been noted with other immunological assays (16,17,18).
One explanation may be that the binding of opioids may be influenced by
endogenous factors and the state of the cell at the time of the assay.
For example, enhancement of active T cell rosettes by enkephalin appears
to be greater and more consistently found when the lymphocyte samples are
obtained from immunosuppressed lymphoma patients (19). In this situation
[Met]enkephalin is active over a broader concentration range (10^{-14} to
10^{-2} mg/ml) than [Leu]enkephalin which is only active at a very low
concentration (10^{-14} mg/ml) and inactive at higher concentrations
(10^{-10} to 10^{-2} mg/ml). This difference in activity between these two
endogenous enkephalins may be due to dissimilar binding affinities to the
human lymphocyte but this is yet to be determined. Plotnikoff has
proposed that the delta [Met]enkephalin receptor and also the delta
[Leu]enkephalin receptor are subpopulations of delta (20). Other factors
may influence the binding of enkephalins to lymphocytes. Metal ions have
been shown to influence the binding of enkephalins to brain receptors
(21). Similarly, zinc ions may influence the binding of enkephalin to
human T lymphocytes. For example the enhancement of active T cell rosette
formation by [Met]enkephalin in the presence of $ZnCl_2$ is greater than
the effects of either of these agents alone (22). Furthermore, the
enhancement of active T cell rosettes with [Met]enkephalin plus $ZnCl_2$ is
not blocked by equimolar concentrations of naloxone but is inhibited by
the zinc-chelator 1,10-phenanthroline. Zinc is important for normal
lymphocyte function (23) and is essential for the biological activity of
serum thymic factor, an immunomodulatory polypeptide (24). Perhaps zinc
is an important modulator of enkephalin binding and function in the immune
system as well as the nervous system.

There is also indirect in vivo evidence supporting the existence of
opioid binding to receptors on human lymphocytes (25). The total number
of T cell rosettes is markedly decreased and the number of null cells

markedly increased in the peripheral blood of morphine addicts (25).
These effects are reversed with incubation in vitro with naloxone (25).

Direct evidence: Direct evidence for specific opioid receptors on
lymphocytes has been obtained by several groups of investigators.
Mehrishi and Mills (26) studied the binding characteristics of
[³H]naloxone to fresh human peripheral blood lymphocytes and platelets.
This radioligand is displaced by morphine to the extent of 43 to 57%.
This suggests that at least some, but not all, of the binding sites on
lymphocytes are specific opioid receptors of the mu type. Displacement
studies using opioids with other specific affinities, such as for delta or
epsilon, were not reported. In the presence of Na⁺ ions the decrease in
binding of [³H]naloxone by morphine is not observed. It appears that
opioid receptor sites on lymphocytes and platelets may be similar to those
on nerve cell membranes.

Hazum et al (27) studied the binding characteristics of iodinated
beta$_H$-[2-D-alanine]endorphin to cultured human lymphocytes. This
binding appears to be completely inhibited by beta-endorphin, partially
inhibited by [Leu] and [Met]enkephalin but not by opiate agonists,
enkephalin analogues, or opioid antagonists. Since alpha-endorphin is not
active, the carboxy-terminal region of beta-endorphin is essential for the
binding activity. This suggests the existence of a specific
beta-endorphin receptor on lymphocytes which is different from
beta-endorphin receptors on nerve cells.

Johnson et al (28) reported specific binding sites for ACTH and
[Met]enkephalin on mouse spleen cells. Schatchard analysis of
^{125}I-labeled ACTH demonstrated the presence of both high-affinity
(Kd=1x10^{-10} M) and low affinity (Kd=4.8x10^9 M) binding sites
suggesting the possibility of at least two different receptor sites for
this peptide. At least one type of binding site for [³H][Met]enkephalin
exists with a Kd=5.9x10^{-10} M.

The function of the various types of opioid receptors on lymphocytes
is yet to be determined. The adrenals release many prohormone fragments
with preferential binding to different opioid receptors (29). Plotnikoff
has proposed (20) the "Ying-Yang" hypothesis which suggests that the final
outcome of immunomodulation by stress (suppression versus enhancement) is
by virtue of adrenal prohormone fragments binding to mu and kappa
receptors (downregulators) and/or delta and epsilon receptors
(upregulators).

Phagocytic Leukocytes

[³H]dihydromorphine stereospecifically binds to human granulocytes
and monocytes indicating that these bone marrow derived cells possess
opioid receptors (30). The calculated Kd for granulocytes is 1x10^{-8} M
and for monocytes 8x10^{-9} M. The estimated number of binding sites per
cell is 3000 and 4000 for granulocytes and monocytes, respectively.

Complement

Beta-endorphin binds specifically to the terminal (C5b-9) and
preterminal (C5b-7 and C5b-8) complexes of complement (31,32). Similar to
the binding of beta-endorphin to lymphocytes (27), binding to complement
is dependent upon the carboxy-terminus of beta-endorphin rather than the
amino-terminus and is not blocked by naloxone (32). This implies that the
binding site for beta-endorphin on complement is specific but differs from
the brain opioid receptor.

Other Blood Components

As noted above naloxone binds specifically to normal human platelets (26). However, other studies using human platelet lysate preparations failed to demonstrate specific binding of [3H]etorphine (33).

Abood et al (34) studied the binding of dihydromorphine to human erythrocyte membranes. Since naloxone is not competitive in this situation, erythrocyte receptors are distinctly different from brain receptors for dihydromorphine. In addition, it is interesting that the binding is significantly increased when erythrocytes are obtained from heroin addicts (34). This provides further evidence that the in vivo mileau can effect the binding characteristics of opioids to cellular elements in vitro.

Yamasaki and Way (35) studied the effects of various opioids on the Ca^{++} flux of rat erythrocyte membranes and it appears that erythrocytes bear Kappa type opioid receptors which inhibit the Ca^{++} pump mechanism.

Table 1 outlines some of the data concerning opioid receptors on immunocompetent cells and other blood components. It would be important to extend this information to a larger number of ligands and receptors and to more primitive cells such as those which differentiate in the bone marrow and thymus. Such data would further identify potential target cells which may be influenced by the enkephalins and other opioids.

TABLE 1. Binding Studies To Immune and Blood Components

Target	Ligand	Naloxone Reversible	Possible Receptor(Kd)	Ref.
Transformed Human Lymphocytes	$Beta_H$-[125I] [D-Ala2]endorphin	No	Beta-endorphin (c-term)specific	27
Human Peripheral Blood Lymphocytes	[3H]naloxone	Partial	Mu and non-mu	26
Mouse Spleen Cells	[3H[Met]enkephalin	NR	Delta $(5.9x10^{-10}M)$	28
Human Monocytes	[3H]dihydromorphin	NR	$Mu(8x10^{-9}$ M)	30
Human Granulocytes	[3H]dihydromorphin	NR	$Mu(1x10^{-8}$ M)	30
Human Platelets	[3H]naloxone	Partial	Mu and non-mu	26
Human Erythrocytes	[3H]dihydromorphin	No	Non-mu $(9x10^{-9}M)$	34
Complement	$Beta_H$[125I] endorphin	No	Beta-end(C-term) specific	32

NR = not reported

EFFECTS ON LYMPHOCYTE PROLIFERATION

Murine Studies

Both [Leu]enkephalin and [Met]enkephalin enhance the in vitro
blastogenic response of mouse spleen cells to phytohemagglutinin (PHA), a
predominantly T cell mitogen (36). With suboptimal PHA concentrations
[Met]enkephalin is active over a broad concentration range $(10^{-12}-10^{-3}$
M) whereas [Leu]enkephalin is only active at relatively low concentrations
$(10^{-12}-10^{-8}$ M). The reason for this apparent difference in activity
between these two enkephalins is not clear but is similar to that noted
above for the enhancement of active T cell rosette formation (19). At
optimal concentrations of PHA both [Met]enkephalin and [Leu]enkephalin are
active only at relatively high concentrations $(10^{-8}-10^{-3}$ M).

Gilman et al (16) studied the effects of various opioid peptides on
the proliferative response of rat splenic lymphocytes. Beta-endorphin in
nM concentrations enhances the proliferative response to PHA and another T
cell mitogen, concanavalin A (ConA). It is interesting to note that in
this study significant enhancement with beta-endorphin was observed in
only 10 of 18 experiments using Lewis rats and 2 of 5 experiments with
Brown Norway rats. One explanation for the inconsistency in the results is
relative insensitivity of some of the samples (rats) to beta-endorphin
rather than due to other variables of the experiments (16). Such
inconsistency has been noted above in the active T cell rosette assay with
the enkephalins using normal human peripheral blood leukocytes (15). In
contrast to beta-endorphin, alpha-endorphin and [D-Ala^2, Met^5]enk do
not effect the proliferative response of rat spleen cells to T cell
mitogens and none of these agents affect B mitogen-induced or unstimulated
blastogenesis (16). The enhanced response to a T cell mitogen with 3.3 mM
of beta-endorphin is not inhibited with as much as 10 uM naloxone (16).
This would indicate that the enhancement is mediated through
beta-endorphin specific but not typical opioid receptors. These receptors
may be similar to those identified on human cultured (transformed)
lymphocytes by Hazum et al (27) and discussed above.

Human Studies

In contrast to the enhancing effect on rat spleen cell proliferation
(16), beta-endorphin appears to be a potent inhibitor of PHA induced human
lymphocyte proliferation (37). This suppressive effect, however, appears
to be most marked (75% reduction) with a relatively high concentration
$(10^{-7}$ M) of beta-endorphin: much higher than that expected to occur in
vivo (37). A lower concentration of beta-endorphin $(10^{-9}$ M) is also
suppressive but to a lesser degree (30% reduction) and only does so at
high intensity PHA stimulation (37). These are the only two
concentrations of beta-endorphin reported by McCain et al (37) and no
indication was given as to how many different donors were studied; this
would be important since the response to opioid peptides in vitro is
usually concentration dependent and may vary among the individuals studied
as discussed above. Similarly to observations with rat spleen cells (16),
the inhibition of human lymphocyte blastogenesis with beta-endorphin is
not blocked by naloxone (37). This would indicate that the suppressive
effect of beta-endorphin on human lymphocyte proliferation may not be
mediated through Mu receptors but possibly through the specific receptors
for beta-endorphin previously described by Hazum et al (27) on cultured
lymphocytes. Whether this binding is at the epsilon receptor, which is
not naloxone sensitive, is yet to be determined.

Wybran (38) studied the effects of morphine and various enkephalins on
PHA and pokeweed (a mixed T and B cell mitogen) induced blastogenic

responses of human peripheral blood leukocytes. The results were negative with the exception of [Leu]enkephalin, which is active at a very narrow concentration range (10^{-5}M). At suboptimal concentrations of PHA the response is enhanced but with optimal PHA stimulation [Leu]enkephalin suppresses the response. [Leu]enkephalin does not effect the response to pokeweed mitogen (38). In contrast to these results, Bocchini et al. (39) found that both naloxone and morphine effect the PHA response of peripheral blood lymphocytes (i.e. nonadherent mononuclear cells) from 6 healthy donors. Both naloxone (10^{-15} - 10^{-7}M) and morphine (10^{-14} - 10^{-6}M) increased the response whereas a higher concentration of naloxone (10^{-4}M) and morphine (10^{-3}M) inhibited the response in each of the 6 donors tested. Both naloxone (10^{-8}M) and morphine (10^{-7}M) increase the percentage of total T cells and decrease the percentage of null cells (39). It appears that opioids may have opposing effects on different cell types and this may depend upon the specific receptors that they bear. If the in vitro assay system contains several different cell types, the net effect of a particular opioid may be different than that obtained when only one type of target and effector cell is present. This may account for some of the inconsistent results in the literature.

Table 2 summarizes the effects of various opioids on the proliferative response of mitogen stimulated lymphocytes. In general, murine lymphocytes appear to be stimulated by [Met]enkephalin, [Leu]enkephalin, and beta-endorphin but alpha-endorphin and [D-Ala^2, Met^5]enkephalin are inactive. In man the effects appear to be more variable and the results are not definitive. However, beta-endorphin thus far has proven to be depressive. Morphine and naloxone seem to enhance at low concentrations but inhibit at high concentrations.

ENHANCEMENT OF NATURAL KILLER (NK) CELL ACTIVITY

Spontaneous cytotoxicity by NK cells may represent a potential immunosurveillance mechanism against tumors but the role of these cells in vivo remains contraversial (40, 41). Numerous endogenous and exogenous factors may influence NK cell activity (42). Pertinent to this discussion is that murine animal models have shown that these changes in NK cell activity can occur with hypothalamic lesioning (43) and stressful stimuli (44).

Several groups have studied the effects of various opioids on the NK cell activity of human peripheral blood mononuclear cells in vitro and the results are summarized in Table 3. Beta-endorphin and [Met]enkephalin can enhance NK cell activity over a broad concentration range including amounts considered to be physiological (18, 45-47). The increased cytotoxicity can be attributed to both enhanced effector-tumor cell conjugate formation and accelerated kinetics of lysis (45). The enhancing effects of [Met]enkephalin and beta-endorphin can be blocked by naloxone. However Mathews et al., (45) have shown that relatively high concentrations of the antagonist was required for this effect; also the enhancing effect of [Met]enkephalin and beta-endorphin was not blocked by equimolar concentrations of naloxone. Kay et al. (47), however, showed that the enhancing effect of beta-endorphin can be blocked by high concentrations of naloxone. In contrast, Wybran (38) reported that enhancement with 10^6 [Met]enkephalin and beta-endorphin could be completely inhibited with 10^6M naloxone. The reasons for this conflicting data is as yet unclear. It does appear however, that the enhancement of NK cell activity by beta-endorphin and [Met]enkephalin are mediated through opioid receptors but the specific type is yet to be determined. It is not known whether these receptors are similar to those

Table 2. Effect of Opioids in Mitogen-Induced Lymphocyte Prolieration

Ligand	Concentration	Lymphocyte Species	Mitogen	Effect	Reference
[Leu]enk	10^{-12}-10^{-8}M	Mouse	PHA	I	36
	10^{-5}M	Human	Subopt. PHA	I	38
	10^{-5}M	Human	opt. PHA	D	38
	10^{-5}M	Human	Pokeweed	NE	38
[Met]enk	10^{-12}-10^{-3}M	Mouse	PHA	I	36
Beta-end	10^{-9}M	Rat	PHA	I	16
			Con A	I	16
	10^{-9}, 10^{-7}M	Human	PHA	D	37
Alpha-end	10^{-9}M	Rat	PHA	NE	16
			Con A	NE	16
[D-Ala^2, Met^5]enk	10^{-9}M	Rat	Con A	NE	16
Morphine		Human	PHA	NE	38
			Pokeweed	NE	38
	10^{-14}-10^{-6}M	Human	PHA	I	39
	10^{-3}M	Human	PHA	D	39
Naloxone	10^{-15}-10^{-7}M	Human	PHA	I	39
	10^{-4}M	Human	PHA	D	39

I = enhancement
D = suppression
NE = no effect

described by Hazum et al. (27) on cultured lymphocytes or whether they are delta and/or epsilon which are relatively insensitive to naloxone.

As shown in Table 3, various other opioids can enhance NK activity. These include beta[D-Ala^2, Met^5]enkephalin (18, 38, 46, 47). Alpha-endorphin has little or no activity (45, 47). Beta-lipotropin, a pituitary hormone which contains beta-endorphin as part of its structure, is also active (47). Interestingly, Wybran (38) has reported that morphine is as active in enhancing NK cell activity as the other opioid peptides studied; however, at least two other groups failed to show an effect with this agent (45, 47).

Peripheral blood mononuclear NK cell activity may vary in the response to opioids depending on the individual donor. Enhancement of NK cell activity may not occur in every subject tested (47). In those who do respond, the degree of enhancement may vary considerably. Mononuclear cells obtained from individuals with low control (baseline) activity appear to be enhanced to a greater degree with enkephalin treatment than those obtained from individuals with relatively high baseline activity; this occurs with both normal individuals and cancer patients (18, 48). In vivo studies in humans treated with [Met]enkephalin have resulted in variable effects on NK cell activity with both increases and decreases (49).

Table 3. Enhancement of Human NK Cell Activity In Vitro by Various Opioids

Opioid	Kay et al	Wybran	Faith et al	Mathews et al	Froelich & Bankhurst
Beta-end	15*			30-55	
Beta-[D-Ala^2]end					23
Alpha-end	5			NE	
Gamma-end	25				
Morphine	NE	35		NE	
[Met]enk		31	40	10-45	
[D-Ala^2,Met^5]enk		23			
[Leu]enkephalin	4	29	70	NE	
Beta-lipotropin	16				

* percent increase in activity; NE, no effect

EFFECTS ON PHAGOCYTIC CELL FUNCTIONS

It has previously been shown that morphine and similar opiate alkyloids inhibit phagocytosis and can impair the ability of the host to eradicate infections with bacterial organisms (50, 51). In contrast there is more recent evidence that the endogenous opioids stimulate phagocyte function and, therefore, may increase resistance to infections (52-58).

Van Epps and Saland (54) studied the effects of beta-endorphin and [Met]enkephalin on human peripheral blood leukocyte chemotaxis using various in vitro assays including the "leading front technique". Both of these opioid peptides stimulate mononuclear cell chemotaxis and, to a lesser degree, neutrophil chemotaxis. The response with mononuclear cells is approximately 80% of that obtained with formyl-methionyl-leucyl-phenylalanine (f-MLP), a potent chemoattractant. The response with neutrophils, however, is only less than 30% of that of f-MLP. It is interesting that the chemotactic response of mononuclear cells to beta-endorphin and [Met]enkephalin is bimodal with peak activities occurring at 10^{-12}M and 10^{-8}M concentrations. One can speculate that the biomodal chemotactic response of cells to these agents reflects the existence of multiple receptor types on the cell or subpopulations of functionally distinct cells bearing receptors with different binding affinites. It is also interesting that a positive chemotactic response to beta-endorphin or [Met]enkephalin is only obtained in about 70-75% of cases compared to a universal response to f-MLP (53). As discussed above, the lack of universal responsiveness to the opioid peptides in vitro has been noted repeatedly with other immunological assays with human (15, 47) and murine (16) cells. Perhaps this variability in the response observed in vitro is related to the in vivo influence of endogenous opioids, the levels of which fluctuate with various physiological and pathological conditions (52).

The stimulation of chemotaxis by beta-endorphin and [Met]eskephalin is more than 89% inhibited by equimolar concentrations of naloxone indicating that the effect is mediated by opioid receptors (53). The administration of beta-endorphin into the cerebral ventricles of the rat results in the migration of macrophage-like cells which is consistent with the chemoattractant response observed in vitro (54).

In addition to its chemoattractant properties, beta-endorphin enhances the migration of f-MLP (55). This effect which is observed with 10^{-9} to 10^{-10}M beta-endorphin, can be blocked by 10^{-6}M naloxone suggesting that the activity is dependent upon the interaction with specific opioid receptors (55).

Opioid peptides may also cause morphological changes in phagocytic leukocytes (56). Treatment with 10^{-9} to 10^{-8}M beta-endorphin, [Met]enkephalin, and opiates, but not with antagonists, causes visible flattening of human neutrophilic granulocytes in vitro. This specific change in shape is felt to reflect an adherence phenomenon similar to that which occurs with other known chemoattractants, such as f-MLP. Since the flattening caused by the opioids can be blocked by equimolar concentrations of opioid antagonist, this effect appears to be mediated through specific opioid receptors (56).

Effects of opioids on various macrophage functions in vitro have also been noted (57). At relatively low concentrations (10^{-9} to 10^{-7}M) [Met]enkephalin stimulates IgG2a-mediated antibody dependent cytotoxicity (ADCC) of rat peritoneal macrophages and this appears to occur through naloxone-sensitive receptors (57). Similar concentrations of [Met]enkephalin suppress phagocytosis of (IgG2a-coated sheep erythrocytes and induces a significant increase in the generation of luminol dependent chemoluminescence (LDCL) of rat macrophages (57). At relatively high concentrations (10^{-6} to 10^{-5}M) [Met]enkephalin results in an enhancement of phagocytosis and an inhibition of LDCL. The involvement of cyclic nucleotides in [Met]enkephalin induced functional alterations of macrophages is suspected because cGMP accumulation is augmented in the treated cells (57). Also, calmodulin is felt to play a role since the effects of [Met]enkephalin on ADCC is abolished by trifluoroperazine, a calmodulin inhibitor (57).

In regard to LDCL, the response of neutrophils obtained from normal individuals and cancer patients may be influenced by [Leu]enkephalin and [Met]enkephalin in vitro (59). The responses obtained may be either increased, decreased, or not significantly changed, depending upon the type of enkephalin, concentration, and the individual being studied. However, an observed increase in activity for LDCL with enkephalin occured only with the cells obtained from cancer patients (59).

As noted in Table 4 the endogenous opioid peptides have numberous effects on phagocyte function. In vitro and possibly in vivo they behave as chemoattractants and stimulate cellular adhesion and migration of neutrophilic granulocytes. Effects on ADCC, chemoluminesence, and macrophage phagocytosis are more variable, depending on the concentration of opioid and the population studied. Stimulation of cGMP accumulation may be responsible for some of the effects.

229

Table 4. Phagocyte Functions Effected by Endogenous Opioid Peptides

Function	Effect
Chemotaxis	Stimulated
Adhesion	Stimulated
Antibody Dependent Cytotoxicity	Stimulated
Phagocytosis	Stimulated or Depressed
Chemoluminesence	Stimulated or Depressed
cGMP accumulation	Stimulated

EFFECTS ON HUMORAL IMMUNITY

In Vitro Studies

Johnson et al. (28) studied the effect of various neuropeptides including ACTH, endorphins, and enkephalins on the in vitro antibody response of mouse spleen cells to a T cell dependent (sheep erythrocytes) and T cell independent (DNP-Ficoll) antigen. ACTH in uM concentrations markedly inhibits the response to both of these antigens. The inhibitory effect of ACTH does not occur in the presence of the thiol reducing agent 2-mercaptopurine, a property shared with alpha-interferon. Alpha-endorphin (0.5 uM) is also active and causes a 76 to 92% reduction in the response to sheep erythrocytes. [Leu]enkephalin and [Met]enkephalin are somewhat less active than alpha-endorphin resulting in a 64% and 73% reduction, respectively. Beta-endorphin and gamma-endorphin are very weak or inactive as antibody response inhibitors. The suppression in antibody formation caused by 0.5 uM alpha-endorphin is blocked by the addition of 3 uM naloxone and also diminished when combined with 12 uM beta-endorphin. These results imply that the agonistic binding to the endorphin receptor does not necessarily activate immunosuppressive events (28). These results, however, convincingly show that neuroendocrine peptide hormones can regulate the antibody response in vitro.

Opioids have also been shown to modulate IgE-mediated ^{14}C-serotonin release from rat mast cells (60). The opioids apparently do not have a direct effect but are capable of reversing the inhibition of serotonin release by PGE$_1$. Levorphanol appears to be most potent in this regard with 10^{-6}M resulting in a 35% reversal of PGE$_1$ effects (60). In contrast as much as 3×10^{-5}M morphine, 10^{-5}M beta-endorphin and 10^{-4}M [Met]enkephalin are required to give an equivalent response. Dextrorphan, an enantiomer of levorphanol, is completely inactive. The effects of the opioids on PGE$_1$ inhibition of serotonin release are blocked by naloxone (60). These results suggest that opioids can modulate IgE-mediated release from rat mast cells through opioid receptors; however, the types of binding sites on mast cells remains to be defined.

In Vivo Studies

The effect of various neuropeptides including [Met]enkephalin and [Leu]enkephalin on the antibody response of mice to sheep erythrocytes has been studied (61). The antibody response is enhanced by 20 mg/kg of

[Leu]enkephalin when given as a single intravenous dose 3 days prior to antigen. However, the response is inhibited by a higher dose (100 mg/kg) of [Leu]enkephalin (61). [Met]enkephalin has not been shown to effect the _in vivo_ antibody response of mice to sheep erythrocytes (61). Similarly, we have treated 4 week old male C57BL/6J mice with 3 mg/kg of [Met]enkephalin subcutaneously daily for seven days and then injected 4×10^6 or 2×10^8 sheep erythrocytes subcutaneously on day 8 and found no significant effect on the hemagglutinin response (unpublished data).

In summary, the opioids can modulate the antibody response to T cell dependent and T cell independent antigens and the immunologically mediated release mechanism of mast cells. These effects are dependent upon the specific opioid peptide and its concentration.

EFFECTS ON LYMPHOID TISSUE

Preliminary evidence suggests that the endogenous opioids not only modulate immune function but may also play a role in the growth and development of lymphoid tissue. Rodents injected with enkephalins develop marked changes in thymus and spleen size. The subcutaneous administration of 10 mg/kg of [Met]enkephalin and 30 mg/kg of [Leu]enkephalin daily for 7 days into young adult female BDF_1 mice causes a significant increase in thymus weight (62). Similarly, thymic enlargement occurs in young adult C57BL/6 male mice (Murgo, unpublished observations) and in rats treated with [Met]enkephalin (63). Histological studies in mice treated with enkephalin shows that the thymic cortex is enlarged to a greater degree than the medulla (62). In contrast to the hypertrophy that occurs with a dose of 30 mg/kg of [Leu]enkephalin, 10 mg/kg of this enkephalin results in a significant decrease in thymus weight in mice and both [Met]enkephalin and [Leu]enkephalin result in a decrease in spleen weight (62). In rats, spleen size may actually be increased with [Leu]enkephalin (63).

The mechanism by which the enkephalins can cause changes in lymphoid tissue weight is not known. The fact that endogenous opioids can cause thymic enlargement is particularly interesting since this effect is opposite that reported to occur with stress, corticosteroids, and aging (1). The results with enkephalins provide further support for the role of endogenous opioids as modulators between the neuroendocrine and immune systems. Both of these systems appear to be sources as well as targets for the endogenous opioids. Immunoreactive ACTH and endorphins may be produced concomitantly with alpha-interferon in human leukocytes (64) and in adherent mouse spleen cells (65). In addition, the enkephalins have been identified immunohistochemically within thymic epithelial cells (66). The discovery of the enkephalins in this specific location supports their potential role in T cell growth and differentiation. In addition, preliminary human _in vivo_ studies have shown that treatment with [Met]enkephalin increases peripheral blood OKT3, OKT4, and OKT11 subsets (49).

OPIOID MODULATION OF TUMOR GROWTH

It is well known that environmental stress can influence the immune response and neoplastic growth (1). Although there is mounting evidence that a number of substances may play a role in mediating these stress induced changes, early investigations have focused on the adrenal corticosteroids which are generally considered to be immunosuppressive (1). However, under certain experimental conditions of duration and timing of stressful stimuli, immunoenhancement and inhibition of tumor growth can result (1-4). These results support the existence of stress hormones with immunostimulatory and tumor inhibitory properties. The endogenous opioids should be considered in this regard since they are released from the pituitary and the adrenals with stress (8,9,11); however there are conflicting opinions as to whether these neuropeptides are detrimental or beneficial to the tumor-bearing host (20,44,63).

Paradoxically, heroin which is felt to directly contribute to the increased risk of infection and immunological abnormalities that occur in addicts (67, 68) has been found to inhibit tumor growth in mice (69). The administration of heroin at a dose of 3-15 mg/kg daily for 2 weeks prior to or 6 mg/kg daily one week after the inoculation of S20Y neuroblastoma cells results in prolonged survival times and tumor growth retardation (69). Since neuroblastoma cells bear opioid receptors, it is not known whether the effects of heroin are related to direct toxicity against the tumor cells or to immunomodulation.

Opioid antagonists have also been found to influence tumor growth (70-73). Mice treated daily with 5-20 mg/kg of naloxone either 14 days before or 7 days after the inoculation of neuroblastoma cells have a prolonged survival compared to untreated mice; however, the effect is greatest in mice pretreated with naloxone (70). In contrast to the results with naloxone, naltrexone which is a longer acting and more potent opioid antagonist has both stimulatory and inhibitory effects on the growth of neuroblastoma depending upon the dose used (71). Daily injections of 0.1 mg/kg results in a decrease in tumor incidence, delay in tumor appearance, and increase in survival time. In contrast a higher dose (10 mg/kg) shortens the time to tumor appearance and decreases survival. Later studies have implicated the duration of opioid receptor blockade rather than the dosage of the antagonist to be responsible for the variable effects on tumor growth (72).

Opioid antagonists have also been shown to effect the growth of animal tumors other than neuroblastoma. Both naloxone and naltrexone have been shown to inhibit the growth of carcinogen-induced mammary carcinoma in rats (73). The inhibition of mammary tumor growth by these agents may be related to a reduction in prolactin and growth hormone which tend to stimulate mammary tumor growth rather than to immunomodulation (73).

The effects of certain patterns of experimental stress are presumed to be mediated by endogenous opioids (74). Intermittent inescapable footshock stress applied to rats for 4 consecutive days prior to mammary ascites tumor inoculation results in reduced survival compared to nonstressed controls (74). A role for endogenous opioid systems in this process is further implicated since the tumor enhancing effect of this stress is prevented by naltrexone (74). Also, high doses of morphine affects the survival of rats with these tumors but the result depends somewhat upon the schedule of drug administration (75). Animals given 4 daily injections of morphine (50 mg/kg) either before or after tumor inoculation, and those given 14 injections of morphine, but only after tumor inoculation, have a significant decrease in survival comparable to that caused by footshock stress (75). Survival of animals given morphine for 14 days prior to tumor inoculation did not differ from controls, suggesting that tolerance can develop to this morphine effect (75).

The fact that stress can result in the release of numberous hormones including different types of opioid precursers and derivatives makes it difficult to attribute the effects of stress on tumor growth to a specific opioid. This is also true with interpreting the results of naloxone or naltrexone treatment. For example, these agents have a much higher affinity for mu than for delta receptors (12) and not all of the effects of these agents are necessarily related to the antagonism of endogenous opioids (76).

A more direct approach to determining the role endogenous opioids play
in tumor growth is to study the effects of these substances when
administered to tumor-bearing animals. Systemically administered
enkephalins do have activity as tranquilizers, antidepressants and
anticonvulsants (77). As discussed above, enkephalins administered
subcutaneously to rodents can also cause marked changes in lymphoid tissue
weight. In addition, both [Met]enkephalin and [Leu]enkephalin can have
beneficial effects on the tumor-bearing host (36,78,79). The daily
subcutaneous administration of [Leu]enkephalin (10 mg/kg) increases the
survival of BDF, female mice inoculated intraperitoneally with $1x10^2$
L1210 leukemia cells. This protective effect is also seen with
[Met]enkephalin at a dose of 30 mg/kg daily in mice inoculated with
$1x10^4$ L1210 cells (36).

The enkephalins have also been shown to be beneficial to mice bearing
solid tumors. The treatment of C57B1/6J mice with 3 mg/kg of
[Met]enkephalin daily for 7 or 14 days beginning the day after the
subcutaneous inoculation of 10^5 B16 melanoma cells inhibits local tumor
(78,79). This antitumor effect occurs only in mice treated following
tumor inoculation, since pretreatment with [Met]enkephalin for 7 days
prior to tumor inoculation does not inhibit local tumor growth and may
increase the number of metastatic lesions (78).

The mechanism of antitumor effect of the endogenous opioids is not
clearly known but immunomodulation is felt to be an important factor
(36). Direct cytotoxicity is probably not a major factor since the
treatment of various tumor cell lines (including L1210 and B16 melanoma)
results in either minimal stimulation, minimal inhibitiion, or no effect
on growth in vitro (80;Plotnikoff, unpublished data; Murgo, unpublished
data).

Studies with genetically obese (C57BL/6J, ob/ob) mice provides further
supportive evidence that the endogenous opioids can be beneficial to the
tumor-bearing host. The proliferative response of splenocytes to a T cell
mitogen is markedly increased and the frequency of lung metastases from
B16 melanoma is greatly reduced in obese mice compared to lean littermates
(81,82). Higher levels of beta-endorphin which is known to exist in the
obese mice may be responsible for the enhanced level of immunocompetence
and relative tumor resistance (82).

There is preliminary evidence that the enkephalins may potentiate the
antitumor effects of cytotoxic chemotherapeutic drugs. [Met]enkephalin
potentiates the protective effect of cis-platinum in mice inoculated with
L1210 leukemia (83). In contrast, morphine administration reduces the
survival of tumor-bearing mice treated with cis-platinum (83).

In summary, the opioid peptides are potential mediators of some of the
effects of stress on tumor growth. The overall picture, however, is
complicated by the fact that stress can result in the release of many
different opioid peptides and precursors which differ in their receptor
binding affinities and effects on target cells (29). Therefore, the
ultimate effect on the immune system and tumor growth may vary depending
upon the predominance of a particular ligand and its receptor affinities.

MODULATION OF LYMPHOKINES

The production of endorphin by lymphocytes suggests that the opioids
function as lymphokines and in the regulatory loop between the immune and
neuroendocrine systems (64). There is also preliminary data which
indicates that the endogenous opioids may modulate the production and
efects of other lymphokines. Hung et al (84) have reported on the

inhibition of interferon by narcotic analgesics. More recently, Brown and Van Epps (85) have shown that beta-endorphin and [Met]enkephalin modulate the production of gamma-interferon in vitro. In addition, the administration of [Met]enkephalin to humans increases interleukin II receptors as measured with monoclonal antibodies (49). The modulation of lymphokines by opioids is discussed in greater detail in other chapters of this book.

CONCLUSION

It is clear that opioids can effect various aspects of the immune system. We feel that part of the function of the endogenous opioids is to participate in immune regulatory pathways, particularly during periods of stress when the levels of these neuropeptides are very high. The apparent divergent activities of the various opioids probably is due to differences in affinities for receptors on a variety of cells. Although the opioids have been associated with both immunoenhancement and immunodepression, the enkephalins appear to enhance cellular immune mechanisms and inhibit tumor growth.

ACKNOWLEDGEMENT

The authors thank Ms. Annorah Cale for her excellent assistance in preparing the manuscript.

REFERENCES

1. V. Riley, Pyschoneuroendocrine influences on immunocompetence and neoplasia, Science 212:1100 (1981).

2. A.A. Monjan and M.I. Collector, Stress induced modulation of the immune response, Science 196:307 (1977).

3. H.A. Rashkis, Systemic stress as an inhibitor of experimental tumors in Swiss mice, Science 116:169 (1952).

4. A. AmKraut and G.F. Solomon, Stress and murine sarcoma virus (Moloney)-induced tumors, Cancer Res. 32:1428 (1972).

5. A.W. Coquelin and R.A. Gorski, Neuroendocrine control, stress, and immunity, in: "Stress, Immunity, and Aging," E.L. Cooper, ed., Dekker, New York (1984).

6. J. Ahlqvist, Hormonal influences on immunologic and related phenomena, in: "Psychoneuroimmunology," R. Ader, ed., Academic Press, New York (1981).

7. N.R. Hall and A.L. Goldstein, Neurotransmitters and the immune system, in, "Psychoneuroimmunology," R. Ader, ed., Academic Press, New York (1981).

8. R. Guillemin, T. Vargo, J. Rossier, S. Minick, N. Ling, C. Rivier, W. Vale, and F. Bloom, Beta-endorphin and adrenocorticotropin are secreted concomitantly by the pituitary gland, Science 197:1367 (1977).

9. S. Amir, Z.W. Brown, and Z. Amit, The role of endorphins in stress: Evidence and speculations, Neurosci. Biobehav. Rev. 4:77 (1980)

10. G.W. Terman, Y. Shavit, J.W. Lewis, J.T. Cannon, and J.C. Liebeskind, Intrinsic mechanisms of pain inhibition: activation by stress,

Science 226:1270 (1984).

11. O.H. Viveros, E.J. Diliberto, E. Hazum, and K-J. Chang, Opiate-like materials in the adrenal medulla: evidence for storage and secretion with catecholamines, Mol. Pharmacol. 16:1101 (1979).

12. W.R. Martin, Pharmacology of Opioids, Pharmacol. Rev. 35:283 (1984).

13. J. Wybran, T. Appelboom, J-P. Famaey, and A. Govaerts, Suggestive evidence for receptors for morphine and methionine-enkephalin on normal human blood T lymphocytes, J. Immunol. 123:1068 (1979).

14. H.H. Fudenberg, J. Wybran, and D. Robbins, T-rosette-forming cells, cellular immunity and cancer, N. Engl. J. Med. 292:475 (1975).

15. G.C. Miller, A.J. Murgo, and N.P. Plotnikoff, Enkephalins:enhancement of active T-cell rosettes from normal volunteers, Clin. Immunol. Immunopathol. 31:132 (1984).

16. S.C. Gilman, J.M. Schwartz, R.J. Milner, F.E. Bloom, and J.D. Feldman, Beta-endorphin enhances lymphocyte proliferative responses, Proc. Natl. Acad. Sci. (USA) 79:4226 (1982).

17. D.E. Van Epps and L. Saland, Beta-endorphin and met-enkephalin stimulate human peripheral blood mononuclear cell chemotaxis, J. Immunol. 132:3046 (1984).

18. R.E. Faith, H.J. Liang, A.J. Murgo, and N.P. Plotnikoff, Neuro-immunomodulation with enkepahlins: enhancement of human natural killer (NK) cell activity in vitro, Clin. Immunol. Immunopathol. 31:412 (1984).

19. G.C. Miller, A.J. Murgo, and N.P. Plotnikoff, Enkephalins: enhancement of active T-cell rosettes from lymphoma patients, Clin. Immunol. Immunopathol. 26:446 (1983).

20. N.P. Plotnikoff. Enkephalins-Endorphins: Emotional stress, depression and immune system, Pyschpharmacol. Bull. in press (1985).

21. K. Stengaard-Pedersen, Inhibition of enkepahlin binding to opiate receptors by zinc ions: possible physiological importance in the brain, Acta. pharmacol. et toxicol. 50:213 (1982).

22. A.J. Murgo, N.P. Plotnikoff and R.E. Faith, Effect of methionine-enkephalin plus Zn-Cl$_2$ on active T cell rosettes, Neuropeptides 5:367 (1985).

23. R.O. Williams and L.A. Loeb, Zinc requirement for DNA replication in stimulated human lymphocytes, J. Cell Biol. 58:594 (1973).

24. M. Dardenne, J-M, Pleau, B. Nabarra, P. Lefrancier, M. Derrien, J. Choay,and J-F, Bach, Contribution of zinc and other metals to the biological activity of the serum thymic factor, Proc. Natl. Acad. Sci. (USA) 79:5370 (1982).

25. R.J. McDonough, J.J. Madden, A. Falek, D.A. Shafer, M. Pline, D. Gordon, P. Bokos, J.C. Kuehnle, and J. Mendelson, Alteration of T and null lymphocyte frequencies in the peripheral blood of human opiate addicts in vivo evidence for opiate receptor sites on T lymphocytes, J. Immunol. 125:2539 (1980).

26. J.N. Mehrishi and I.H. Mills, Opiate receptors on lymphocytes and platelets in man, Clin. Immunol. Immunopathol. 27:240 (1983).

27. E. Hazum, K-J Chang, and P. Cuatrecasas, Specific nonopiate receptors for beta-endorphin, Science 205:1033 (1979).

28. H.M. Johnson, E.M. Smith, B.A. Torres, and J.E. Blalock, Regulation of the in vivo antibody response by neuroendocrine hormones, Proc. Natl. Acad. Sci. (USA) 79:4171 (1982).

29. A. Herz, Multiple endorphins and natural ligands of multiple opioid receptors, in, "Central and Peripheral endorphins: Basic and Clinical Aspects," E.E. Miller and A.R. Genazzini, ed., Raven Press, New York (1984).

30. A. Lopker, L.G. Abood,W. Hoss, and F.J. Lionetti, Stereoselective muscarinic acetylcholine and opiate receptors in human phagocytic leukocytes, Biochem. Pharmacol. 29:1361 (1980).

31. L. Schweigerer, H. Teschemacher, and S. Bhakdi, Interaction of human beta-endorphin with the terminal SC56-9 and "preterminal" SC56-7 and SC5b-8 complexes of human complement, Life Sci. 31:2275 (1982).

32. L. Schweigerer, S. Bhakdi, and H. Teschemacher, Specific non-opiate binding sites for human beta-endorphin on the terminal complex of human complement, Nature 296:5857 (1982).

33. A. Reches, A. Eldor, Z. Vogel, and Y. Salomon, Do human platelets have opiate receptors?, Nature 288:382 (1980).

34. L.G. Abood, H.G. Atkinson, and M. MacNeil, Stereospecific opiate binding in human erythrocyte membranes and changes in heroin addicts, J. Neurosci. Res. 2:427 (1976).

35. Y. Yamasaki and E.L. Way, Possible inhibition of CA^{++} pump of rat erythrocyte ghosts by opioid K agonists, Life Sci. 33:723 (Sup. I, 1983).

36. N.P. Plotnikoff and G.C. Miller, Enkephalins as immunomodulators, Int. J. Immunopharmacol. 5:437 (1983).

37. H.W. McCain, I.B. Lamster, J.M. Bozzone, and J.T. Grbic, Beta-endorphin modulates human immune activity via non-opiate receptor mechanisms, Life Sci. 31:1619 (1982).

38. J. Wybran, Enkephalins and endorphins as modifiers of the immune system: present and future, Fed. Proc. 44:92 (1985).

39. G. Bocchini, G. Bonanno, and A. Canevari, Influence of morphine and naloxone on human peripheral blood T-lymphocytes, Drug Alcohol Depend. 11:233 (1983).

40. N. Hanna, Role of natural killer cells in host defense against cancer metastasis, in, "Cancer Invasion and Metastatic Biologic and Therapeutic Aspects," G.L. Nicolson and L. Milas, ed., Raven Press, New York (1984).

41. O. Fodstad, C.T. Hansen, G.B. Cannon, C.N. Statham, G.R. Lichtenstein, and N.R. Boyd, Lack of correlation between natural killer activity and tumor growth control in nude mice with different immune defects, Cancer Res. 44:4403 (1984).

42. R.B. Herberman and H.T. Holden, Natural cell-mediated immunity, _Adv. Cancer Res._ 27:305 (1978).

43. R.J. Cross, W.R. Markesbery, W.H. Brooks, and T.L. Roszman, Hypothalamic-immune interactions: neuromodulation of natural killer activity by lesioning of the anterior hypothalamus, _Immunol._ 51:399 (1984).

44. Y. Shavit, J.W. Lewis, G.W. Terman, R.P. Gale, and J.C. Liebeskind, Opioid peptides mediate the suppressive effect of stress on natural killer cell cytotoxicity, _Science_ 223:188 (1984).

45. P.M. Mathews, C.J. Froelich, W.L. Sibbitt, and A.D. Bankhurst, Enhancement of natural cytotoxicity by beta-endorphin, _J. Immunol._ 130:1658 (1983).

46. C.J. Froelich and A.D. Bankhurst, The effect of beta-endorphin on natural cytotoxicity and antibody dependent cellular cytotoxicity, _Life Sci._ 35:261 (1984).

47. N. Kay, J. Allen, and J.E. Morley, Endorphins stimulate normal human peripheral blood lymphocyte natural killer activity, _Life Sci._ 35:53 (1984).

48. R.E. Faith, H.J. Liang, N.P. Plotnikoff, A.J. Murgo, and N.F. Nimeh, Neuroimmunomodulation with enkephalins: _in vitro_ enhancement of natural killer (NK) cell activity in peripheral blood lymphocytes from cancer patients, Nat. Imm. Cell Growth Reg. in press.

49. N.P. Plotnikoff, et al, this book.

50. D. Zucker-Franklin, P. Elsbach, and E.J. Simon, The effect of the morphine analog levorphanol on phagocytosing leukocytes: a morphologic study, _Lab Invest._ 25:415 (1971).

51. E. Tubaro, G. Borelli, C. Croce, G. Cavallo, and C. Santiangeli, Effect of morphine on resistance to infection, _J. Infect. Dis._ 148:656 (1983).

52. A.E. Panerai, A. Martini, A. DeRosa, F. Salerno, A.M. DiGiulio, and P. Mantegazza, Plasma beta-endorphin and met-enkephalin in physiological and pathological conditions, _in_, "Regulatory Peptides: From molecular biology to function," E. Costa and M. Trabucchi, ed., Raven Press, New York (1982).

53. D.E. VanEpps and L. Saland, Beta-endorphin and met-enkephalin stimulate human peripheral blood mononuclear cell chemotaxis, _J. Immunol._ 132:3046 (1984).

54. L.C. Saland, D.E. VanEpps, E. Ortiz, and A. Samora, Acute injections of opiate peptides into the rat cerebral ventricle: a macrophage-like cellular response, _Brain Res. Bull._ 10:523 (1983).

55. C.O. Simpkins, C.A. Dickey, and M.P. Fink, Human neutrophil migration is enhanced by beta-endorphin, _Life Sci._ 34:2251 (1984).

56. E.G. Fischer and N.E. Falke, Beta-endorphin modulates immune functions: a review, _Psychother. Psychosom._ 42:195 (1984).

57. G. Foris, G.A. Medgyesi, E. Gyimesi, and M. Hauck, Met-enkephalin induced alterations of macrophage functions, _Mol. Immunol._ 21:747 (1984).

58. M.R. Ruff and C.B. Pert, Neuropeptides as chemoattractants for human macrophages, Proc First International Workshop on Neuroimmunomodulation, in press (1985).

59. G.C. Miller, A.J. Murgo, and N.P. Plotnikoff, The influence of leucine and methionine enkephalin on immune mechanisms, Int. J. Immunopharmacol. 4:367 (1982).

60. Y. Yamasaki, O. Shimamura, A. Kizu, M. Nakagawa, and H. Ijichi, IgE-mediated ^{14}C-serotonin release from rat mast cells modulated by morphine and endorphins, Life Sci. 31:471 (1982).

61. E.M. Kukain, R.K. Muceniece, and V.E. Klusha, Comparison of neuro- and immunomodulator properties of low-molecular-weight neuropeptides, Bull. Exp. Biol. Med. 94:1105 (1982).

62. N.P. Plotnikoff, A.J. Murgo, and R.E. Faith, Neuroimmunomodulation with enkephalins: effects on thymus and spleen weights in mice, Clin. Immunol. Immunopathol. 32:52 (1984).

63. N.P. Plotnikoff, A.J. Murgo, G.C. Miller, C.N. Corder, and R.E. Faith, Enkephalins: immunomodulators, Fed. Proc. 44:118 (1985).

64. J.E. Blalock and E.M. Smith, A complete regulatory loop between the immune and neuroendocrine systems, Fed. Proc. 44:108 (1985).

65. S.J. Lolait, A.T.W. Lim, B.H. Toh, and J.W. Funder, Immunoreactive beta-endorphin in a subpopulation of mouse spleen macrophages, J. Clin. Invest. 73:277 (1984).

66. W. Savino and M. Dardenne, Enkephalin immunohistochemical detection in human thymic epithelial cells, Proc. First Internat. Workshop on Neuroimmunomodulation, in press (1985).

67. S.M. Brown, B. Stimmel, R.N. Taub, S. Kochwa, and R.E. Rosenfield, Immunologic dysfunction in heroin addicts, Arch. Intern. Med. 134: 1001 (1974).

68. R.E. Faith, N.P. Plotnikoff, and A.J. Murgo, Effects of opiates and Neuropeptides on immune functions, in: "Mechanisms of Tolerance and Dependence, C.W. Sharp, ed., NIDA Research Monograph 54, Rockville, MD (1984).

69. I.S. Zagon and P.J. McLaughlin, Heroin prolongs survival time and retards tumor growth in mice with neuroblastoma, Brain Res. Bull. 7:25 (1981).

70. I.S. Zagon and P.J. McLaughlin, Naloxone prolongs the survival time of mice treated with neuroblastoma, Life Sci. 28:1095 (1981).

71. I.S. Zagon and P.J. McLaughlin, Naltrexone modulates tumor response in mice with neuroblastoma, Science 221:671 (1983).

72. I.S. Zagon and P.J. McLaughlin, Duration of opiate receptor blockade determines tumorigenic response in mice with neuroblastoma: a role for endogenous opioid systems in cancer, Life Sci. 35:409 (1984).

73. C.F. Aylsworth, C.A. Hodson, and J. Meites, Opiate antagonists can inhibit mammary tumor in rats, Proc. Soc. Exp. Biol. Med. 161:18 (1979).

74. J.W. Lewis, Y. Sharit, G.W. Terman, L.R. Nelson, R.P. Gale, and J.C. Liebeskind, Apparent involvement of opioid peptides in stress-induced enhancement of tumor growth, Peptides 4:635 (1983).

75. J.W. Lewis, Y. Shavit, G.W. Terman, R.P. Gale, and J.C. Liebeskind, Stress and morphine affect survival of rats challenged with a mammary ascites tumor (MAT 13762B), Nat. Immun. Cell Growth Regul. 3:43 (1983/84).

76. A.A-B Badawy, M. Evans, N.F. Punjani, and C.J. Morgan, Does naloxone always act as an opiate antagonist? Life Sci. 33:739 (Sup. I, 1983).

77. N.P. Plotnikoff, Abba J. Kastin, D.H. Coy, C.W. Christensen, A.V. Schally, and M.A.Spirtes, Neuropharmacological actions of enkephalin after systemic administration, Life Sci. 19:1283 (1976).

78. A.J. Murgo, Modualtion of tumor growth in mice treated with methionine-enkephalin and corticosterone, Proc. First Internat. Workshop on Neuroimmunomodulation, in press (1985).

79. A.J. Murgo, Inhibition of B16 melanoma growth in mice by methionine-enkephalin, J. Natl. Cancer Instit. in press (1985).

80. D.D. Von Hoff and B. Forseth, Modulation of growth of human and murine tumors by human beta-endorphin, Proc. Amer. Assoc. Cancer Res. 23:236 (1982).

81. C.I. Thompson, J.W. Kreider, P.L. Black, T.J. Schmidt, and D.L. Margules, Genetically obese mice: resistance to metastasis of B16 melanoma and enhanced T-lymphocyte mitogenic responses, Science 220:1183 (1983).

82. P.L. Black, M. Holly, C.I. Thompson, and D.L. Margules, Enhanced tumor resistance and immunocompetence in obese (ob/ob) mice, Life Sci. 33:715 (Sup. I, 1983).

83. N.P. Plotnikoff, R.E. Faith, A.J. Murgo, and G.C. Miller, Enkephalins: immunomodulators and antitumor activities, Proc. First Internat. Workshop on Neuroimmunomodulation in press (1985).

84. C.Y. Hung, S.S. Lefkowitz, and W.F. Geber, Interferon inhibition by narcotic analgesics, Pro. Soc. Exp. Biol. Med. 142:106 (1973).

85. S.L. Brown and D.E. VanEpps, Beta-endorphin, [Met]enkephalin and corticotrophin modulate the production of gamma interferon in vitro, Fed. Proceed. (abst.), 44:949 (1985).

RELATIONSHIP BETWEEN LYMPHOKINE AND OPIATERGIC MODULATION OF LYMPHOCYTE PROLIFERATION

William L. Farrar

Laboratory of Molecular Immunoregulation, Biological
Response Modifiers Program, National Cancer Institute-FCRF
Frederick, MD 21701 USA

INTRODUCTION

T lymphocytes are primary effector cells of cell-mediated immunity
as well as regulators of growth (clonal expansion) and differentiation of
the immune system. Until less than a decade ago, their regulatory activity
was presumed to be attributed to predominantly cellular interactions
mediated by membrane-bound recognitive elements often associated with the
major histocompatibility (H2 or HLA) complex. Recently, in the historical
context of the development of immunological models, many regulatory
functions of T lymphocytes appear to be mediated by molecules secreted by
various functionally distinct subpopulations of lymphoid and nonlymphoid
cells. Indeed, the principle regulatory cells of the immune system, T
lymphocytes, are also under the regulatory influence of specific monocyte/
macrophage derived cytokines referred to as monokines. In addition to
regulating lymphocyte activities, there is considerable evidence that
lymphocyte-derived molecules, lymphokines, influence the differentiation
of hematopoietic cells, mast cells, fibroblasts, and osteoclasts[1-6].
This suggests that the regulatory cytokines produced by specific antigen
may also effect hematopoietic homeostasis as well as inflammatory cells
involved in immediate hypersensitivities. Lymphokines are considered to
be actively synthesized (transcription of DNA) and secreted by either
native lymphoid cells or their malignant cell line counterparts (macrophage
or lymphocyte). While normal lymphoid tissues or cells must be activated
by antigen or polyclonal stimulation to produce lymphokines, some long-
term cell lines have been fortuitously shown to constitutively secrete
lymphokines. Indeed, such cell lines have been critical for providing
the genetic library for the recombinant DNA cloning of several lymphokines.
Lymphokines provide nonspecific augmentation to antigen-specific responses.
Lymphokines can generally be readily separated by conventional biochemical
chromatography, but standard 280 nm absorbance and protein stains have
been of little value since they are usually present in culture media in
nanomolar concentrations. Finally, with the introduction of monoclonal
antibodies, several lymphokines may be neutralized and quantitated in
vitro by specific antibody.

Although soluble factors were reported to influence (in a nonspecific
fashion) antigen specific immune responses[7], it wasn't until 1978 when
chromatographic separation was used to try to discriminate individual
lymphokine molecules and their effects on discrete immune responses[8,9].

An apparent enigma from these studies was the observation that biochemically distinct factors derived from cells of different functional phenotypes (i.e., macrophages and T cells) produced identical biological effects. For example, interleukin 1 (IL 1), a soluble factor of 15,000 dalton molecular weight derived from endotoxin-stimulated macrophages, enhanced both antibody producing cell responses to sheep erythrocytes in nude mice, stimulated thymocyte proliferation[9,10] and augmented the production of cytotoxic lymphocytes in macrophage-depleted cultures[11] . The issues were complicated by the observation that three apparently different biological activities mentioned above could be ascribed to a single macrophage-derived molecule (IL 1) and that interleukin 2 (IL 2), derived from T helper lymphocytes (molecular weight 15-21,000 daltons), also exhibited the same three immunobiological activities [9,12,13]. Not only did IL 2 enhance the primary plaque-forming responses of nude mouse spleen cells to sheep erythrocytes and stimulate thymocyte proliferation and cytotoxic T cell responses, but IL 2 could also maintain the selective indefinite growth of cytotoxic T cell clones[12,14]. Although IL 1 and IL 2 were apparently biochemically distinct and were derived from macrophages and T lymphocytes respectively or their corresponding tumor cell lines[15,16], both molecules elicited or enhanced similar immuno-biological phenomena. Based on these observations, our laboratory chose to investigate several possible explanations to resolve whether IL 1 and IL 2 acted on the same populations of cells or alternatively were involved in a sequence of factor-cell interactions with a degree of linearity which resulted in the manifestation of similar biological expression (i.e., the development of antibody-forming cells or cytotoxic T cells).

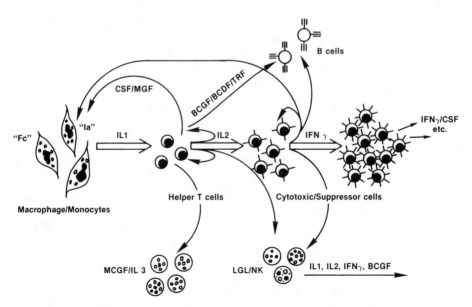

Figure 1: The Lymphokine Regulatory Network

The Lymphokine Regulatory Network

IL 1 Induction of IL 2. Although the similarity of IL 1 and IL 2 bioactivities was striking, data began to accumulate to argue against the possibility that both IL 1 and IL 2 exerted activity on the same target cell populations. The inability of supernatants from activated macrophages to support the growth of long-term T cells[14] and the ability of such supernatants to stimulate production of IL 2 from purified T cells[11] suggested that indeed macrophage-derived soluble mediators did not act on the same target population as did T cell-derived IL 2[17]. Confirmation that IL 1 stimulates T cells to produce IL 2 was demonstrated later by the studies of Smith and colleagues[18] and Larsson et al.[19]. The finding that macrophage-derived factors were required for T cells to produce immunoregulatory factors was further supported by the observation of Moore et al.[20] who showed that the T cell product, colony stimulating factor (CSF), activated macrophages to produce IL 1, thus completing at least one regulatory circuit (Figure 1). CSF was also shown to enhance the production of prostaglandins and interferon from macrophages[21]. It was apparent from these studies that lymphokines operated in a sequential fashion, with possible feedback loops, which result in a sophisticated system of intercellular communication.

IL 2 Induction of IFN γ. The discovery that IL 2 not only regulated the growth of cytotoxic cells, but also the production of another lymphokine, gamma interferon, (IFN γ) further reinforced the notion that a linear series of factor-cellular interactions was involved in the amplification of cytotoxic T lymphocyte responses (Figure 1)[22]. Because of the "cascading" appearance of these interactions the term "lymphokine cascade" was applied when referring to the interdependent interactions of cells and lymphokines[13]. During the original investigation demonstrating IL 2 regulation of IFN γ, it was shown that antisera directed to gamma interferon inhibited the development of cytotoxic T lymphocytes[22].

In a parallel system, IL 2 has been shown to augment cytotoxic responses of natural killer (NK) cells[23], as well as promote the growth of NK cells[24]. The ability of IL 2 to enhance the cytotoxic responses of NK cells apparently is independent of IL 2 growth promotion and is also neutralized by antisera directed against IFN γ in response to IL 2 and since IFN γ has been described to enhance NK cytolytic activity, it was concluded that IL 2 augments NK activity via the production of IFN 25.

Possible Role of Gamma Interferon in Immunity. Data from a variety of studies have recently demonstrated rather pleotypic differentiating effects of gamma interferon. With regards to the effects observed with NK and cytotoxic T lymphocytes, recent work has suggested that IFN γ may act on T cells by enhancing the expression of IL 2 receptors[26]. Further support for the differentiation signal activity of IFN γ was demonstrated by Steeg et al. who showed that IFN γ induced Ia antigen expression on macrophages[27]. Other investigators have shown that IFN γ increased HLA expression on human lymphocytes, Fc receptor expression on macrophages, immunoglobulin synthesis by B cells, and the activation of macrophages and NK cells for tumor cytolysis[28-31]. The evidence remains overwhelming implicating IFN γ as a major differentiating signal required for cellular immunity.

T Cell-Derived Lymphokines and B Cell Responses. The existance of a T cell-derived B cell growth factor (BCGF) was previously implied by the observation that activated mouse B lymphocytes could be grown in vitro by the addition of Con A-conditioned medium or with PMA-induced EL4 cell line supernatant[32]. BCGF has been shown to be produced by helper T

lymphocytes and is biochemically separable from IL 2. T cell replacing
factor (TRF) is functionally distinct from BCGF in that it is most active
in promoting B cell differentiation when added late (day 2 or 3) to
cultures of spleen cell cultures undergoing primary immunization in vitro[33].
Although IL 2, BCGF and TRF are biochemically separable, it is not
clear whether TRF and B cell differentiation factor (BCDF), a factor
which induces B cells to secrete immunoglobulin, are the same or similar
molecules.

T Cell Regulation of Other Peripheral Cells. It was mentioned
earlier that IL 2 is also known to regulate the growth of NK cells[24].
Subsets of large granulocyte lymphocytes with NK activity have been
shown to produce IL 2, IFN and CSF and may also possibly produce IL 1 and
BCGF (Scala and Ortaldo, personal communication)[34]. The findings that
NK cell subsets produce a variety of immunomodulatory signals may broaden
their potential role as central regulatory cells that influence antigen-
specific humoral and cellular immunities.

Murine T lymphocytes have been suggested to also produce a unique
class of colony stimulating factor(s) referred to as IL 3[35]. Although
originally believed to be active on pre-helper T cells, it is now well
established that IL 3 does not act on helper T cell precursors and is
biochemically identical to burst-promoting activity (BPA), P cell
stimulating factor, mast cell growth factor, and multi-colony stimulating factor. The human equivalent has not been well characterized, but
it is believed to act as a growth signal for pluripotent stem cells[36].

RELATIONSHIP OF β-ENDORPHIN WITH IL 2 REGULATION OF PROLIFERATION

Among the hormonal consequences of acute stress is the release of
corticotropin (ACTH) and β-endorphin by the pituitary. The peripheral
effects of β-endorphin and its hormonal relationships to stress remains
obscure. Recently immunoenhancing effects of β-endorphin have been
reported. β-endorphin has been shown to specifically bind to the human
B-cell line RPMI 6237[37], as well as increase the proliferative response
of rat splenocytes to T-cell lectins[30]. Additionally, β-endorphin
has been shown to increase natural killer (NK) cytotoxic activity[39].

Based on the observations that β-endorphin enhances immunological
activities (i.e., lymphocyte proliferation and NK cytotoxicity) that are
under the specific regulatory control of interleukin 2 (IL 2), a growth
and regulatory peptide of the immune system, our laboratory examined
whether β-endorphin may specifically modulate IL 2-dependent proliferative
events. Since it was reported by Hazum et al.[37] that cultured transformed RPMI 6237 cells had specific receptors for β-endorphin, we examined
whether discrete polulatons of highly purified human T lymphocytes demonstrate any specific binding of ³H-etorphine. The availability of purified
lymphocytotropic growth factors such as BCGF and IL 2 have allowed us to
selectively expand specific lineages of lymphoid cells. Table 1 shows
data obtained from binding studies with subpopulations of lymphocytes
expanded in either B-cell growth factor (B cells) or IL 2 (T and LGL).
Both T lymphocytes and large granulocyte lymphocytes, which express
natural killer cell (NK) activity, demonstrate a similar class of receptors
suggesting broad specificity since diprenorphine and β-endorphin effectively displaced ³H-etorphine. B lymphocytes, however, demonstrated
competitive displacement of ³H-etorphine, binding of a different pattern

TABLE 1

HUMAN LYMPHOCYTE OPIATE RECEPTOR ANALYSIS

Specificity	Compound [M]	%Inhibition Total Binding*		
		B**	T	LGL (NK)
Broad	Diprenorphine [10⁻⁵]	35%	33%	41%
Delta	DADle [10⁻⁶]	<1%	<1%	13%
Delta	DSTle [10⁻⁶]	<1%	<1%	<1%
Kappa	EKC [10⁻⁶]	<1%	22%	20%
Kappa	Bremazocine [10⁻⁶]	<1%	14%	13%
Broad	β-endorphin [10⁻⁶]	<1%	25%	44%
f-m Specific binding/10⁶ cells		67	93	59

*Percentages represent the decrease in total binding of ^{3}H-etorphine at 40 nM.

**Factor-dependent cell lines BD-7 (B cell), TD-1 (T cell) and IL 2 dependent LGL were washed free of conditioned media, resuspended to 20 x 10⁶ cells/assay tube. Assay was run at 37°C for 30 min in presence of 50 ul ^{3}H-ligand, 50 ul cold ligand, 50 ul Hanks BSS and 400 ul. Data is result of the mean of triplicate samples. Data courtesy of Dr. Richard Weber, NIH, Bethesda, MD.

suggesting a fundamental difference in the nature of opiate receptor between antibody-producing cell lineage and IL 2 promoted lymphocytes.

Since there is parallel receptor appearance for IL 2 and β-endorphin and similar biological enhancements, we tested whether homogenous IL 2 prepared from the gibbon T lymphoid MLA-144 cell line can possibly compete with β-endorphin bind on brain caudate sections. The results suggest that even when 10⁶ M excess concentrations of pure IL 2 are used, absolutely no competition with β-endorphin binding to brain caudate sections occurs (data not shown). Therefore, based on the facts that no primary amino acid sequence homology exists between IL 2 and β-endorphin (or other neuroendocrine hormones; Farrar, unpublished data), and no competition of IL 2 for the opiate receptor was observed, we conclude that β-endorphin enhancement of immune responses does not occur via common structural receptor elements shared with the IL 2 receptor. Additional support for this conclusion comes from our observation that monoclonal anti-TAC antibody, directed against the IL 2 receptor, does not bind to brain sections, further substantiating the possibility that opiate receptors do not immunologically cross-react with IL 2 receptors (Pert, C. and Farrar, W., unpublished data).

β-endorphin Modulation of IL 2 Induced Proliferation. Experiments compared the effects of β-endorphin on the proliferative responses of cloned IL 2 dependent (CT6) murine cytotoxic T cells and peripheral blood lymphocytes (PBL) to PHA. The data in Figure 2 demonstrated that β-endorphin had no modulating activity on the CT6 response to IL 2, however, β-endorphin (10⁻⁹M) enhanced the proliferative response of PBL to PHA 30-40%. It was apparent from these experiments that β-endorphin does not have direct modulatory activity on IL 2-mediated events but still maintains a profound influence on the proliferation of mitogen-stimulated T lymphocytes when present in mixed cellular populations. Although both systems represent a proliferative response to IL 2, PBL responses to mitogen are under the exquisite regulatory control of macrophages partially through cellular contact but predominantly through the participation of soluble mediators.

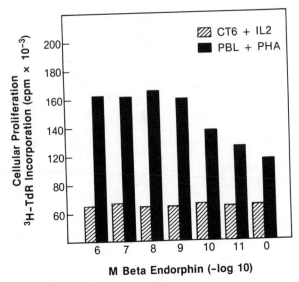

Fig. 2 Effects of β-endorphin on the proliferative responses of IL 2-dependent T cells and PBL mitogen-induced proliferation.

Among the peripheral effects of the endorphins is the observation that β-endorphin can modulate the effects of prostaglandins on mast cells and rat brain cells[40-42]. Since prostaglandins are considered to be produced by macrophages and exert a negative regulatory influence on T-cell proliferaton as well as IL 2 responsiveness[43,44], we test the ability of β-endorphin to influence the effects of prostaglandin E_2 (PGE_2) on CT 6 proliferation to IL 2 as well as purified human T-lymphocyte PHA responses (Figure 3).

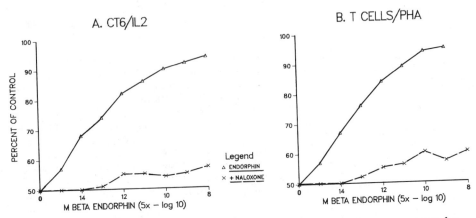

Fig. 3 Reversal of PGE_2 inhibition of proliferative responses by β-endorphin.

From the data, it can be seen that exogenous addition of 10^{-7}M PGE$_2$ to either CT6 plus 10 units IL 2 or to purified T cells plus PHA results in at least 50% inhibition of proliferation. If either cell population were preincubated with β-endorphin, the inhibitory activity of PGE$_2$ on proliferative responses is reversed in a dose-dependent manner. This suggests that the enhancement of proliferation of PBL seen in earlier experiments may be due to β-endorphin's ability to reduce the effects of endogenous PGE$_2$. Similar data are seen when PBL are treated with indomethacin to prevent endogenous production of PGE$_2$.

When CT6 cells or human T lymphocytes were preincubated with the opiate antagonist naloxone (10^{-6}M), β-endorphin reversal of PGE$_2$ inhibition of IL 2 responsiveness was not seen, indicating that the effects of β-endorphin observed were the results of specific opiate receptor interaction.

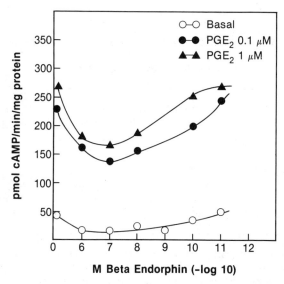

Fig. 4   T lymphocyte adenylate cyclase activity.

Effect of β-endorphin on T Lymphocyte Adenylate Cyclase Activity. Since the data suggested that β-endorphin could modulate the inhibitory effects of PGE$_2$ on either IL 2 stimulated CT6 proliferation or mitogen induced human T lymphocyte responsiveness, we tested whether β-endorphin had any effects on hormone stimulated membrane-associated adenylate cyclase activity. CT6 cells were pretreated with the indicated doseages of β-endorphin for 10 mins at 37°C. The cells were then centrifuged, lysed and particulate membrane fractions prepared. From the data in Figure 4 it can be seen that β-endorphin pretreatment of CT6 cells decreased the basal activity of adenylate cyclase activity by at least 50%. Unstimulated CT6 membranes exhibited a basal activity of 45 pmoles/min/mg and PGE$_2$ stimulated particulate membranes increased adenylate cyclase activity to 230 (.1uM) and 266 (1 uM) pmoles/min/mg respectively. The pretreatment of intact CT6 cells with β-endorphin for 10 mins was sufficient to decrease basal adenylate cyclase (AC) activity by at least 50% and PGE$_2$ induced activity from 30-50% compared to untreated cells. β-endorphin treatment of isolated CT6 membranes reduced basal AC activity by 15-20% and PGE$_2$ induced AC activity by 22-35% (data not shown). These experiments provided biochemical support for the hypothesis suggested by the cellular studies (Fig. 3) that β—endorphin could mitigate the negative influence of prostaglandins on the T lymphocyte proliferative response.

Effects of Interleukins on Pituitary Function. Coincident with peak antibody responses in sheep erythrocyte immunized mice are elevations of serum cortisol levels. This observation suggested a casual relationship between the development of immunity and pituitary-adrenal activity[45]. Utilizing a murine pituitary cell line AtT20, we tested whether purified interleukins 1 or 2 had any effects on AtT20 pituitary ACTH or β—endorphin secretion (Table II).

Although AtT20 cells constituatively secrete ACTH and β—endorphin, interleukin 1 and 2 both stimulated 2-3 fold increases in synthesis of the neuropeptides. Gamma interferon had no effect on the secretory activity of AtT20, IL 1 generally stimulated a 60-80% increase in neuropeptide secretion whereas IL 2 stimulated almost 3-fold over background synthesis.

TABLE II

EFFECTS OF LYMPHOKINES ON PITUITARY CELL LINE AtT20 SECRETION OF

β—ENDORPHIN AND ACTH

| Stimulant | ng BEP/10^6 cells* | | ng ACTH/10^6 | |
	24 hr	48 hr	24 hr	48 hr
Media	610	1150	720	1440
Lectin-free**				
conditioned (5%) media	1240	1650	1490	2360
IL 2 (100 U)***	1870	2115	2670	3318
IFN γ (100 U)	575	1010	698	1384
IL 1 (50 U)	1130	1500	1375	1890

  *RIA was performed on duplicate culture supernatants for β—endorphin and ACTH. Supernatants were harvested at 24 and 48 hr filtered and frozen at −70ºC until extraction. Data is presented as ng/10^6 cells.
  **Lectin-free conditioned media from human PBL was purchased from Cellular Products, Inc.
  ***Recombinant human IL 2, IFN γ and partially purified human IL 1 was used at the dosages indicated.

DISCUSSION AND SUMMARY

The biochemical resolution of the lymphokines and the recent ability to initiate and maintain antigen-specific lymphoid cells with lymphocytotropi growth factors established the investigative elements for the examination of physiological and molecular events which regulate immunity. Cellular immunologist are no longer burdened with the "black box" of murine spleen cells as the mechanism of investigative research. The clonal expansion and propagation of lineage specific cells allows the development of homogeneous populations of cells which may respond uniformly to a defined growth progession signal, such as IL 2 or a differentiation signal i.e., IFN γ . Utilizing this approach we have been able to expand specific lineages of cells and examine opiate receptor expression and the effects of the opiatergic ligands on the cellular response to the lymphocytotropic hormones of immunity, the interleukins.

Within these studies the data shows an increase in opiate receptors on activated T lymphocytes and large granulocyte lymphocytes, both cell types which have cytolytic activity against tumor cells. B lymphocytes, however, exhibited opiate-like receptors which differ from those found on T lymphocytes (Table 1). Associated with receptor appearance is the ability of β-endorphin to modulate (uncouple) T-lymphocyte responses to prostanglandins (Figure 3,4). The mechanism of β-endorphin activity is mediated through specific naloxone reversible opiate receptors and does not directly involve IL 2 receptors or IL 2 growth-promoting activity. Both T lymphocyte proliferation and natural cytotoxicity are suppressed by the endogenous production or exogenous addition of PGE_2. β-endorphin has been shown to modulate PGE_1 inhibition of serotonin release from mast cells as well as abrogate prostaglandin induced elevation of cyclic AMP in neurocytoma cells[40,41]. The experiments present here (Figure 4) indicate that β-endorphins may also modulate the basal and hormonal induced membrane adenylate cyclase activity of T lymphocytes. Based on these data, it is reasonable to suggest that the enhancement activity reported for IL 2-mediated phenomenon[38,39] by β-endorphin may be attributed to the ability of β-endorphin to mitigate the intrinsic effects of PGE_2 produced in PBL cultures.

This data contributes to a growing body of evidence suggesting a reciprocity of regulatory functions between neuroendocrine hormone systems and peripheral physiologies such as the immune system. Since endorphin release has been associated with acute stress (exercise, sexual activity, etc.), we may be able to extrapolate the notion that endorphins may mitigate some of the effects of chronic inflammation and other deleterious consequences of aberrant prostaglandin production. Of singular significance is the observation of Thomas et al.[46] that the ob/ob obese mouse strain has three- to four-fold greater resistance to metastatic melanoma, heightened T-cell mitogen responsiveness, and elevated serum levels of β-endorphin. This suggests a possible role of β-endorphin in the in vivo maintenance or enhancement of natural immunities.

Following sensitization for T-dependent antigens, rodents exhibit a significant increase in serum corticosterone[45]. This elevation coincides temporarily with peak antibody titers and has been suggested to be under the regulatory control of the immune system . Recent investigators have proposed that either lymphokines or thymic hormones may have activity on the anterior hypothalmus thus regulating corticosterone release[45]. Data from our laboratory using purified lymphokines (Table II) demonstrated a direct effect on ACTH and β-endorphin release by pituitary tumor cells. The findings that IL 2 may have low affinity receptors on pituitary cells and that lymphocytes possess receptors for neuroendocrine hormones further substantiate the possibility of bi-directional peptide-mediated regulation between the chemical regulators of antigen-stimulated immune responses and the pituitary-adrenal axis. The potential effects of β-endorphin interaction with the immune system have been discussed. Corticosterone (CS) production as a consequence of ACTH release, however, may have many negative regulatory effects on the immune system. Corticosterone has been previously shown to inhibit IL 2 production. It is therefore possible that the binding of CS to receptors may be viewed as a possible mechanism for signaling the switching off of lymphokine production which may in turn result in the cessation of the CS response seen during the later stages of development of the immune response (Figure 5).

Hormonal Regulation of the Immune - Pituitary/Adrenal Axis

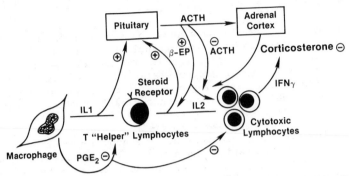

These data suggest that a regulatory circuit of negative-feedback reciprocity between the immune system and the pituitary-adrenal axis exists in response to antigen stimulation and that specific lymphokines such as IL 1 and IL 2 may be involved directly on pituitary function.

REFERENCES

1. R. W. Ruscetti, R. H. Cypess, and P. S. Chervenick, Blood 47:757 (1976).
2. J. J. Oppenheim and I. Gery, Immunology Today 3:113 (1982).
3. K. Tadokoro, B. M. Stadler and A. L. DeWeck, J. Exp. Med. 158:857 (1983).
4. J. W. Adamson, W. J. Dopovic and J. E. Brown, in: "Hematopoitetic Cell Differentiation," D. W. Golde, M. J. Cline, D. Metcalf, C. F. Fox, eds., Academic Press, New York (1978).
5. A. W. Burgess, D. Metcalf, N. A. Nicola and S.H.M. Russel, in: "Hematopoietic Cell Differentiation," D. W. Golde, M. J. Cline, D. Metcalf, C. F. Fox, eds., Academic Press, New York (1978).
6. Y. P. Yung, R. Eger, G. Tertian and M.A.S. Moore, J. Immunol. 127:794 (1981).
7. J. J. Farrar and J. Fuller-Bonar, J. Immunol. 117:274 (1976).
8. J. J. Farrar, W. J. Koopman and J. Fuller-Bonar, J. Immunol. 114:47 (1977).
9. J. J. Farrar, P. L. Simon, W. J. Koopman and J. F. Bonar, J. Immunol. 121:1353 (1978).
10. D. D. Wood, J. Immunol. 123:2400 (1979).
11. W. L. Farrar, S. B. Mizel and J. J. Farrar, J. Immunol. 124:1371 (1980).
12. S. Gillis, P. E. Baker, F. W. Ruscetti and K. A. Smith, J. Exp. Med. 154:983 (1978).
13. J. J. Farrar, W. R. Benjamin, M. L. Hilfker, M. Howard, W. L. Farrar and J. Fuller-Farrar, Immunol. Rev. 63:129 (1982).
14. R. W. Ruscetti, D. A. Morgan and R. C. Gallo, J. Immunol. 122:2527 (1979).

15. S. B. Mizel and D. L. Rosenstreich, J. Immunol. 122:2173 (1979).
16. J. J. Farrar, J. Fuller-Farrar, P. L. Simon, M. L. Hilfiker, B. M. Stadler and W. L. Farrar, J. Immunol. 125:2555 (1980a).
17. J. J. Farrar, S. B. Mizel, J. Fuller-Bonar, M. L. HIlfiker and W. L. Farrar, Microbiol. 36:39 (1980b).
18. K. A. Smith, L. B. Lachman, J. J. Oppenheim and M. F. Favata, J. Exp. Med. 151:1551 (1980).
19. E. L. Larsson, N. N. Iscove and A. Coutinho, Nature 283:664 (1980).
20. R. N. Moore, J. J. Oppenheim, J. J. Farrar, C. S. Carter, A. Waheed and R. K. Shadduck, J. Immunol. 3:119 (1980).
21. R. N. Moore, J. T. Haffeld, J. J. Farrar, S. E. Mergenhagen, J. J. Oppenheim and R. K. Shadduck, Lymphokines 3:119 (1981).
22. W. L. Farrar, H. M. Johnson and J. J. Farrar, J. Immunol. 126:1120 (1981).
23. C. S. Henney, K. Kuribaysashi, D. E. Kern and S. Gillis, Nature 291:335 (1981).
24. W. Domzig, B. M. Stadler and R. B. Herberman, J. Immunol. 130:1970 (1983).
25. D. A. Weignet, G. J. Stanton and H. M. Johnson, Infect. Immun. 41:992 (1983).
26. H. M. Johnson and W. L. Farrar, Cell. Immunol. 75:154 (1983).
27. P. S. Steeg, R. N. Moore, H. M. Johnson and J. J. Oppenheim, J. Exp. Med. 156:1780 (1983).
28. T. Y. Basham and T. C. Merigan, J. Immunol. 130:1492 (1983).
29. B. Harfest, J. R. Huddleston, P. Casali, T. C. Merigun and M.B.A. Olstone, J. Immunol. 127:2146 (1981).
30. D. N. Mannel and W. Falk, Cell. Immunol. 79:396 (1983).
31. J. R. Ortaldo, A. Mantovani, D. Hobbs, M. Rubinstein, S. Pestica and R. B. Herberman, Int. J. Cancer 31:285 (1983).
32. M. C. Howard, J. Farrar, M. Hilfiker, B. Johnson, T. Takatsu and W. L. Paul, J. Exp. Med. 155:914 (1982).
33. A. Schimpl and W. Wicker, Nature 237:15 (1972).
34. T. Kasahara, J. Y. Djeu, S. F. Dougherty and J. J. Oppenheim, J. Immunol. 131:2379 (1983).
35. A. Hapel, J. C. Lee, W. L. Farrar and J. W. Ihle, Cell 25:179 (1981).
36. J. W. Schrader and I. Clark-Lewis, J. Immunol. 129:30 (1982).
37. E. Hazum, K-J. Chang and P. Cuatrecasas, Science 205:1033 (1979).
38. S. C. Gilman, J. M. Schwartz, R. J. Milner, F. E. Bloom and J. D. Feldman, PNAS 79:4226 (1982).
39. P. M. Mathews, C. J. Froelich, W. L. Sibbitt and A. D. Bankhurst, J. Immunol. 130:1658 (1983).
40. Y. Yamasaki, K. Shimamura, A. Kizu, M. Nakagawa and H. Ijichi, Life Sciences 31:471 (1982).
41. H.O.J. Callier and A. C. Roy, Nature 248:24 (1974).
42. R. S. Childers, S. M. Lambert and G. LaRiviere, Life Sciences 33:215 (1983).
43. R. D. Maca, Immunopharmacol. 6:267 (1983).
44. P. E. Baker, J. V. Fahey and A. Munck, J. Exp. Med. 61:52 (1981).
45. P. N. Shek and B. H. Sabiston, Int. J. Immunopharmacol. 5:23 (1983).
46. C. I. Thompson, J. W. Kreider, P. L. Black, T. J. Schmidt and D. L. Margules, Science 220:1183 (1983).

ENKEPHALINS AS MOLECULES OF LYMPHOCYTE ACTIVATION AND MODIFIERS OF THE BIOLOGICAL RESPONSE

Joseph Wybran

Department of Immunology, Hematology and Transfusion
Erasme Hospital, Université Libre de Bruxelles, 1070
Brussels, Belgium

INTRODUCTION

In these recent years, a new stream of investigation has emerged which tightens narrowly the relations existing between the central nervous system, the endocrine system and the immune system through the action of endogenous opioid peptides like enkephalins and endorphins. In the present review, we will attempt to summarize the data related only to the actions of enkephalins upon the immune system.

Enkephalins are small peptides composed of five amino acids whereas endorphins are composed of 16 to 31 amino acids. The first five amino acids of the endorphins are similar and in the same sequence as Methionine-Enkephalin namely Tyr-Gly-Gly-Phe-Met. In contrast, Leucine-Enkephalin is composed by the following sequence Tyr-Gly-Gly-Phe-Leu. A synthetic enkephalin D-Ala^2 Met^5 composed by Tyr-D-Ala-Gly-Phe-Met has been produced. Physiologically the enkephalins are rapidly destroyed by serum enkephalinases.

Enkephalins are synthetized in the adrenals and their main action is upon the nervous system. It is also usually accepted that naloxone is a specific antagonist of the opioid activities of enkephalins. Therefore, any inhibition by naloxone of some immunological function induced by an opioid peptide is accepted as evidence that the immunological activity has been specifically induced by a naloxone sensitive opioid dependent mechanism.

LYMPHOCYTE ENKEPHALIN RECEPTORS

The first demonstration that human T lymphocytes bear a surface receptor for Met-Enk stems from the work of Wybran et al in 1979 (1). Interestingly, at the same time, Hazum et al showed the presence of β endorphin receptors on human lymphoblastoid cell lines (2).

The method for detecting the receptors on human T cells was based on a rosette assay between human T lymphocytes and sheep red blood cells. In this test, termed the active T rosette assay, the technical conditions for performing the rosette assay are not optimal (low ratio of sheep red blood cells to lymphocytes, short incubation time, and temperature of 37 C), so that the active rosette assay is very sensitive to multiple factors (3).

ipheral blood lymphocytes with morphine or Met-Enk, the
tive T rosettes was modified : morphine decreased the
as Met-Enk increased it. Nonspecificity was ruled out
restored a normal percentage of active rosettes in the
phine or Met-Enk. On the basis of these results, it was
human blood T cells possess surface receptorlike structures
nd Met-Enk.

and relevant to the receptor problem, Mehrishi et al have
recently c..firmed the presence of morphine receptors on human blood lymphocytes by direct radioligand techniques. They also showed the presence
of such receptors for naloxone and morphine on human blood platelets (4).
Also, Johnson et al have shown, by direct labeling, that Met-Enk binds to
mice spleen cells (5) allowing the conclusion that enkephalin receptors
are present both on human and animal lymphocytes.

The property of Met-Enk to increase,in vitro, active T cell rosettes
of normal individuals has been confirmed (6). Furthermore, Leu-Enk can
also increase, in vitro, the active T cell rosettes of normal subjects at
concentrations lower to the ones which are active for Met-Enk (between
10^{-11} and 10^{-5}M). Interestingly enough, both Met- and Leu-Enk can also,
in vitro, enhance the percentage of active T cell rosettes of lymphoma patient
(7).

Finally, $ZnCl_2$ appears synergystic with Met-Enk in the active rosette
enhancement. This can be blocked by the zinc chelator phenathroline but
not by naloxone. These data suggest some type of relationship between
zinc may help binding of Met-Enk to the lymphocytes (8).

All the data related to the findings using the active T rosette assay
can lead to two possible explanations : one which is purely related to a
steric hindrance mechanism which postulates the presence of enkephalin
receptor close (or even similar) to the sheep red blood cell (E) receptor
on human T lymphocytes and another one related to the functional meaning
of the active rosette test (3). Indeed, it has been shown that both
specific antigen and drugs (or molecules) able to increase T cell functions
(e.g. isoprinosine, thymosin) (9, 10) also enhance, in vitro, the active
T cell assay. Therefore, one can also postulate that both Met-Enk and
Leu-Enk which increase the active T rosettes assay possess enhancing T
cell properties both in normal subjects and in lymphoma patients.

THE TWO-HIT OPIOID PEPTIDE LYMPHOCYTE RECEPTOR HYPOTHESIS

The above findings have allowed the proposal of the two-hit opioid
peptide lymphocyte hypothesis in which it is suggested that opioid peptides
recognize T and B cells by two different determinants of their molecule,
one naloxone sensitive and the other one non naloxone sensitive (indeed,
the β endorphin receptor is not inhibited by naloxone). This double recognition of one molecule by two different types of lymphocytes (indeed,
human lymphoid cell lines are usually of B cell origin) may provide some
type of chemical bridge between T and B cells and therefore allowing T
and B cell cooperation (11). Because T and B cell cooperation is of
utmost importance in mounting the immune response, the two-hit hypothesis
suggests that opioid peptides are a physiological regulator of the immune
response and that their modification (in quantity or quality) may influence
the immune response.

LYMPHOCYTE PROLIFERATION ASSAYS

The data obtained with enkephalins using lymphocyte stimulation in presence of various mitogens are conflicting. In animals, Gilman et al showed that D-Ala^2 Met^5 Enk does not modify the proliferative response to mitogens (12). In contrast, Plotnikoff et al showed that Met-Enk, and to a lesser extent Leu-Enk, increases the response of mouse spleen cells to phytohemagglutinin. Usually, the results obtained were twice higher than the stimulation performed without enkephalins (13).

In humans, Wybran could usually not show any significant effect of enkephalins using human blood lymphocytes (14). In a series of experiments, the effect of various enkephalins on spontaneous thymidine uptake, the PHA response, and the pokeweed mitogen response was studied (unpublished observations). The results were basically negative. No effect on thymidine uptake was observed except in the case of Leu-Enk at a very narrow concentration range (10^{-5} M). At this concentration, Leu-Enk increased the PHA response when PHA was present at a suboptimal concentration whereas it decreased the optimal PHA response. These results suggest that, in humans, these drugs do not modify nonspecific proliferation assays.

ANTIBODY SYNTHETIS

Johnson et al have studied the in vitro regulation of the antibody response to sheep red blood cells, a T cell dependent antigen (5). They could show that the number of plaque forming cells (antibody producing cells) were moderatly inhibited (around 60 %) by Met-Enk and Leu-Enk.

NATURAL KILLER ACTIVITY

This in vitro assay investigates the spontaneous cytotoxic effect of mononuclear cells (natural killer cells - NK cells) against various target cells which are normally of leukemic or lymphomatous origin. It is thought that NK cells are of importance in controlling the metastasization of tumor cells as well as in various viral and parasitic diseases. Therefore, any agent able to increase NK activity may be considered as potentially useful in the treatment of cancer, viral and parasitic diseases. Interferon, for instance, is known to be able to enhance NK activity and is clinically tried in various malignancies. Mathews et al have published data for humans that show that β-endorphin and Met-Enk could significantly (± 30 %) increase the spontaneous cytotoxicity induced by NK cells against radiolabeled K562 leukemic cells (15). The increased NK activity was dose dependent. Naloxone inhibited the NK augmentation of activity. However, they could not show any modification of NK activity with Leu-Enk.

We have ourselves, in a series of experiments, attempted to see whether morphine and several enkephalins could modify the human NK activity of peripheral blood mononuclear cells against ^{51}Cr radiolabeled K562 cells (14). The effector cells were incubated for 1 h at 37 C, washed, and then mixed at a ratio of 80:1 (effector/target) with K562 cells for 4 h. Several concentrations of drugs (10^{-5}-10^{-8} M) were used. The results can be summarized as follows : morphine, Leu-Enk and Met-Enk increase NK activity by approximately 30 % and usually at a concentration between 10^{-8} and 10^{-5}M. However, D-Ala^2-Met^5 enkephalin increased NK activity less (around 20 %) and in a smaller range of concentrations. Finally, all the NK increments could be abolished by incubation of the effector cells with equimolar naloxone. These results demontrate that NK activity can be enhanced by enkephalins probably acting through opiate-specific (receptors?) mechanisms. Similar results have been obtained with enkephalins by Faith et al (16).

In order to further unravel the possible mechanism by which the NK activity is increased by the opioids, we have investigated whether this effec can be obtained by the supernatant of blood mononuclear cells incubated with opioids (17). The experiments were performed as follows : various concentrations of opioid peptides (10^{-7} M to 10^{-10} M) are incubated at 37 C with blood mononuclear cells of a donor A. After incubation, the cells are washed with culture medium and left overnight at 37 C in culture medium alone. This supernatant is removed by cell centrifugation. Blood mononuclear cells of a donor B are mixed with K562 radiolabeled cells in the presence of the supernatant and NK activity is measured by ^{51}Cr release. A representative experiment is reported hereunder :

NK Cytotoxicity and Supernatants of Enkephalins treated Lymphocytes

Control	Met–Enk (M)				Leu–Enk (M)			
	10^{-7}	10^{-8}	10^{-9}	10^{-10}	10^{-7}	10^{-8}	10^{-9}	10^{-10}
48.2 %	47.3 %	48 %	57.5 %	52.2 %	49.2 %	49 %	57 %	53.3 %

As it can be observed, the supernatant of mononuclear cells incubated with Leu- or Met-enkephalin will increase the NK activity of "naive" blood mononuclear cells of another donor. This suggests that the supernatant contains factor(s) enhancing natural killing. We are currently attempting to identify this (these) factor(s).

Premiminary results suggest that, at least, interleukin 2 might play some role in the enhancement of NK activity by the supernatant.

Finally, we have studied the effect of Met-Enk and Leu-Enk as well as the supernatant of enkephalin treated blood mononuclear cells upon the expression of the Leu 11 phenotype which is associated with NK cells. Clearly, the percentages of Leu 11 cells increase under these conditions which further indicate that enkephalins can enhance natural killer acti- vity (18).

These studies have to be discussed in relation to immunological studies performed in animals during stress. It is generally accepted that stress can influence the immune system either suppressing it or enhancing it, depending mainly on the type of stress as well as the immune mecha- nisms investigated.

Interestingly, Shavit et al have reported that in rats subjected to one of two inescapable footshock stress paradigms, analgesia can be indu- ced by both, but only one via activation of opioid mechanisms (19). Splenic natural killer cell activity was suppressed by the opioid, but not the nonopioid form of stress. This suppression was blocked by the opioid antagonist naltrexone. These results suggest that some endogenous opioid peptides released during the stress mediate mechanisms regulating the natural killer cytotoxicity of certain forms of stress.

EARLY MARKERS OF ACTIVATION

____Lymphocytes in presence of specific antigens or mitogens will undergo a series of events before division. The appearance of some cell surface markers is one of the event of lymphocyte activation (18). In preliminary studies, we have now shown that enkephalins may enhance markers linked to lymphocyte activation like the active T rosette, the OKT10, the Tac and the Ia receptors. Furthermore, naloxone will block this marker enhancement.

These data suggest that enkephalins may be considered as molecules of lymphocyte activation and may play a physiological role in the immune response (e.g., the increased Tac antigen (IL2 receptor) is certainly a regulation mechanism of the immune response).

EFFECT ON TUMOR

In BDF$_1$ mice challenged with the L1210 murine leukemia line, Plotnikoff and Miller have observed a significant increased survival rate in mice treated with 30 mg/kg s.c. of Met-Enk. A similar improvement in survival was also observed using 10 mg/kg s.c. of Leu-Enk (13). The role of opiates, in general, in the control of tumor growth appears complex. For instance, a high dose of morphine reduces the survival of rats injected with a mammary ascites tumor (20). In contrast, heroin inhibits tumor growth in mice transplanted with neuroblastoma (21). Interestingly, naltrexone has dose-dependent stimulatory or inhibitory effects on neuroblastoma growth in mice (22).

All these experiments are difficult to interpret but would, at least, support the hypothesis according to which opioid peptides and especially enkephalins are able to modulate tumor growth perhaps through immune mechanisms and as such are thus immunomodulators.

HUMAN MONOCYTES AND NEUTROPHILS

Met-Enk has, in vitro, a bimodal stimulating activity on human monocytes chemotaxis with peak activities occuring at 10^{-12} M and 10^{-8} M (23). The distance migrated in response to optimal concentrations of Met-Enk was approximatively 80 % of that obtained with a classical stimulator (f-MLP) and was blocked by 10^{-8} M naloxone.

Human neutrophils showed some migration in response to Met-Enk although the average optimal migration was inferior to 30 % of that observed with f-MLP. All these studies suggest that Met-Enk possesses a chemotactic effect.

Met-Enk, between 10^{-9} M and 10^{-7} M, was found to stimulate IgG2a mediated antibody dependent cytotoxicity of thyroglycollate treated rat peritoneal macrophages through naloxone sensitive mechanisms (24). In contrast to this extracellular phenomenon, phagocytosis of the sensitized sheep red blood cells was suppressed by Met-Enk in the same dose range. Furthermore, cyclic GMP concentration was augmented by Met-Enk treated peritoneal macrophages.

All these data are probably to be related to the finding of receptors for dihydromorphine on human monocytes and neutrophils (25).

HUMAN MAST CELL DEGRANULATION

D-Ala^2-D-Leu^5 enkephalin is able to elicit immediate skin reactivity as judged by a wheal and fare phenomenon. This appears to be related to mast cell degranulation (26). The activity of the synthetic enkephalin appears less potent than other opioids like dymorphin or β-endorphin. The possibility that endogenous opioids may regulate mast cell function can eventually lead to the understanding of nonimmunologic mediator release in normal and diseased states.

PLATELETS

Receptors for naloxone have been identified on human lymphocytes and platelets using as assay the binding of (H^3) naloxone to these cells (4). Since morphine appears able to decrease by half the binding of the radio-labeled naloxone, it appears that some receptors are of the μ type. The possible inhibitory effect of enkephalins upon the binding was not studied.

ENKEPHALINS AND LYMPHOID WEIGHT

The subcutaneous injection of either Met-Enk or Leu-Enk in BDF_1 mice results in increase in thymus weight and decrease in spleen weight (27). These studies are also indirect evidence of the effect of enkephalins upon the immune system.

SURFACE SIMILARITIES AND REGULATION BETWEEN NERVOUS CELLS AND IMMUNE CELLS

One clue to the action of the enkephalins upon the immune cells lies certainly in the presence of specific surface receptors. Therefore, it appears very attractive to know that surface antigens present on immune cells can also be found on nervous cells. For instance, the HNK1 monoclonal antibody detects all the NK cells (through the Leu 7 surface antigen). It has recently been shown that the HNK1 antiserum will also recognize cells of neuroectodermal origin (28). Furthermore, HNK1 also recognizes a common carbohydrate moiety found on neural cell adhesion molecules and myelin-associated glycoprotein (29).

The Thy-1 antigen is expressed on T lymphocytes as well as on the surface of many neurons like in the inner retina. Monoclonal antibodies directed against Thy-1 can selectively enhance the growth of retinal ganglion cells (30).

Using neuroblastoma cell lines, it has also been shown that HLA A, B, C (class I molecules) and β_2 microglobulin can be induced by interferon which, itself, can be a product of immune mechanisms (31). The possibility that neuronal HLA A, B, C expression may be under regulatory control by interferon is interesting in the concept of immunosurveillance.

Conversely, the elimination of limited areas of the cephalic crest in stage 9 or 10 chick embryos markedly reduces the size of the thymus gland or results in its absence (32).

CONCLUDING REMARKS

In this chapter, the author has reviewed the data related to the influence of enkephalins upon the immune system.

Clearly, enkephalins possess immunological properties which are best demontrated by their action upon natural killer activity and in lymphocyte activation. The concentrations necessary to trigger these mechanisms are very low, usually between 10^{-9} M and 10^{-11} M, indicating that these levels can easily be reached in physiological states as well as in, for instance, stress.

The interpretation of these data remains conje
relevant in vivo studies are not performed.

Nevertheless, one can hypothesize the following
way : antigenic challenge leads to lymphocyte activa
amplified by serum enkephalins (perhaps even, enkeph
during antigenic challenge). The production of lymp
by the enkephalins which also increase the nonspecif
of immune mechanisms. One particular system appeari
target of the enkephalins, is   the natural killer
explain the enhanced survival observed in mice inocul
cells and treated with enkephalins.

REFERENCES

1. Wybra
evi

The control of tumor growth may perhaps also be direct since malignant cells, like neuroblastoma, appear also to possess opiate receptors.
The relevance of these receptors to tumor growth and metastasization is
unclear.

Another hypothesis to be proposed is related to AIDS. Indeed, it
has been clinically observed that Kaposi sarcoma is more prevalent in the
homosexual group rather than in the addicted group of AIDS patients. We
suggest that drug addiction (through opiates) has led to enhanced NK
activity and thus provided a better resistance to malignancies like Kaposi
sarcoma.

Speculation about the role of enkephalins is also interesting in stress.
Indeed, during stress, many hormones are released. Among them, corticosteroids and endogenous opioid peptides. Corticosteroids are known for
their immunosuppressive properties whereas enkephalins, as well as endorphins, appear to have immunoenhancing activities. Thus, one can hypothesize that multiple innappropriate stress can lead to some type of
immunological unbalance (the global effect of corticosteroids and opioids).
This unbalance will disrupt the normal immunosurveillance mechanisms and
perhaps lead to somatic diseases like autoimmune diseases (known to be
triggered by stress), cancer, or recurrent infections (e.g. tuberculosis
is also known to be stress related). This hypothesis can be experimentally
tested.

The action of enkephalins appears also to be rather wide since they
affect also monocyte and neutrophil chemotaxis as well as mast cell
degranulation suggesting a potential role in infections and allergic
diseases.

Finally, in view of the in vitro data, it is very tempting to
postulate that enkephalins are also modifiers of the biological response.

This hypothesis is under current investigation by injecting enkephalins
to normal volunteers as well as patients with various diseases like cancer
and AIDS. The preliminary data suggest that enkephalin will also in vivo
and in man enhance T cell function and perhaps NK function (33, 34).

In summary, all current evidences indicate that enkephalins are agents
of lymphocyte activation as well as modifiers of the biological response.
As such, they may play a role in the pathogenesis of stress related
diseases and may also become useful agents in the treatment of a variety
of disorders associated with immunological deficiencies.

n, J., Appelboom, T., Famaey, J.P. Govaerts, A. (1979). Suggestive
dence for morphine and methionine–enkephalin receptors–like on
ormal blood T lymphocytes. J. Immunol. 123, 1068–1070.

2. Hazum, E., Chang, K.J., Cautrecasas, P. (1979). Specific nonopiate
   receptors for β–endorphins. Science 205, 1033–1035.

3. Wybran J., Dupont E. (1982). The active T rosette : an early marker
   for T–cell activation. Ann. Immunol. (Paris) 133, 211–218.

4. Mehrishi J.N., Mills, I.H. (1983). Opiate receptors on lymphocytes
   and platelets in man. Clin. Immmunol. Immunopathol. 27, 240–249.

5. Johnson, H.M., Smith, E.M., Torres, B.A., Blalock, J.E. (1983).
   Regulation of the in vitro antibody response by neuroendocrine hormones.
   Proceedings of the National Academy of Sciences. 79, 4171–4174.

6. Miller G.C., Murgo, A.J., Plotnikoff, N.P. (1984). Enkephalins :
   enhancement of active T cell rosettes from normal volunteers. Clin.
   Immunol. Immunopathol. 31, 132–137.

7. Miller, G.C., Murgo, A.J., Plotnikoff, N.P. (1983). Enkephalins–
   enhancement of active T–cell rosettes from lymphoma patients. Clin.
   Immunol. Immunopathol. 26, 446–451.

8. Murgo, A.J., Plotnikoff, N.P., Faith, R.E. (1985). Effect of Methionine–Enkephalin plus ZnCl$_2$ on active T cell rosettes. Neuropeptides,
   5, 367–370.

9. Wybran, J., Appelboom, T., Govaerts, A. (1978). Inosiplex, a stimulating agent for normal human T cells and human leucocytes.
   J. Immunol. 121, 1184–1187.

10. Wybran, J., Levin, A.S., Fudenberg, H.H., Goldstein, A.L. (1975).
    Thymosin : effects on normal human blood T cells. Ann. N.Y. Acad.
    Sci. 249, 300–307.

11. Wybran, J., Appelboom, T., Famaey, J.P., Govaerts, A. (1980).
    Receptors for morphine and methionin–enkephalin on human T lymphocytes:
    the two hits opioid lymphocyte receptor hypothesis. Serrou, B.,
    Rosenfeld, C., eds. New Trends in Human Immunology and Cancer
    Immunotherapy. Paris, Doin Publishers, 48–55.

12. Gilman, S.C., Schwartz, J.M., Milner, R.J., Bloom, F.E., Feldman, J.D.
    (1982). β–Endorphin enhances lymphocyte proliferative responses.
    Proceedings of the National Academy of Sciences 79, 4226–4230.

13. Plotnikoff, N.P., Miller, G.C. (1983). Enkephalins as immunomodulators.
    Int. J. Immunopharmacol. 5, 437–441.

14. Wybran, J. (1985). Enkephalins and endorphins as modifiers of the immune
    system : present and future. Fed. Proc. 44, 92–94.

15. Mathews, P.M., Froelich, C.J., Sibbitt, W.L.,Jr., Bankhurst, A.D.
    (1983). Enhancement of natural cytotoxicity by β–endorphin. J.
    Immunol. 130, 1658–1662.

16. Wybran, J. (1985). Enkephalins and endorphins : activation molecules
    for the immune system and natural killer activity? Neuropeptides.
    5, 371–374.

17. Faith, R.E., Liang, J.H., Murgo, A.J., Plotnikoff, N.P. (1984). Neuroimmunomodulator with enkephalins : enhancement of human natural killer (NK) cell activity in vitro. Clin. Immunol. Immunopathol. 31, 412-418.

18. Wybran, J., Schandené, L. : in preparation.

19. Shavit, Y., Lewis, J.W., Terman, G.W., Gale, R.P., Liebeskind, J.C. (1984). Opioid peptides mediate the suppressive effect of stress on natural killer cytotoxicity. Science. 223, 188-190.

20. Lewis, J.W., Shavit, Y., Terman, G.W., Gale, R.P., Liebeskind, J.C. Stress and morphine affect survival of rats challenged with a mammary ascites tumor (MAT 13762B). Nat. Immunol. Cell. Reg. (in press).

21. Zagon, I.S., McLaughin, P.J. (1981). Heroin prolong survival time and retard tumor growth in mice with neuroblastoma. Brain Res. Bull. 7, 25-32.

22. Zagon, I.S., McLaughin, P.J. (1983). Naltrexone modulates tumor response in mice with neuroblastoma. Science. 221, 671-673.

23. Van Epps, D.E., Saland, L. (1984). β-endorphin and Met-Enkephalin stimulate human peripheral blood mononuclear cell chemotaxis. J. Immunol. 132, 3046-3053.

24. Foris, G., Medgyesi, G.A., Gyimesi, E., Hauck M. (1984). Met-Enkephalin induced alterations of macrophage function. Molecul. Immunol. 21, 747-750.

25. Lopker, A.L., Abood, G., Hass, W., Lionetti, F. (1980). Stereoselective muscarine acetylcholine and opiate receptors in human phagocytic leucocytes. Biochem. Pharmacol. 29, 1361-1365.

26. Casale, T.B., Bowman, S., Kaliner, M. (1984). Induction of human cutaneous mast cell degranulation by opiates and endogenous opioid peptides : evidence for opiate and nonopiate receptor participation. J. Allergy Clin. Immunol. 73, 775-781.

27. Plotnikoff, N.P., Murgo, A.J., Faith, R.E. (1984). Neuroimmunomodulation with enkephalins : effects on thymus and spleen weight in mice. Clin. Immunol. Immunopathol. 32, 52-56.

28. Lipinski, M., Braham, K., Cailland, J.M., Carlu, C., Tursz, T. (1983). HNK-1 antibody detects an antigen expressed on neuroectodermal cells. J. Exp. Med. 158, 1775-1780.

29. Kruse, J., Mailhammer, R., Wernecke, H., Faissner, A., Sommer, I., Goridis, C., Schachner, M. (1984). Neural cell adhesion molecules and myelin-associated glycoprotein share a common carbohydrate moiety recognized by monoclonal antibodies L2 and HNK-1. Nature. 311, 153-155.

30. Leifer D., Lipton, S.A., Barnstable, C.J., Masland, R.H. (1984). Monoclonal antibody of Thy-1 enhances regeneration of processes by rat ganglional cells in culture. Science. 224, 303-306.

31. Lampson, L., Fisher, C.A. (1984). Weak HLA and β2 microglobulin expression of neuronal cell lines can be modulated by interferon. Proceed. Nat. Acad. Sci. 81, 6476-6480.

32. Bockman,D.E., Kirby, M.L. (1984). Dependence of thymus development on derivates of the neural crest. Science. 223, 498–500.

33. Wybran, J., Schandené, L. : in preparation.

34. Plotnikoff, N.P., Miller, G.C., Nimeh, N.F. : in preparation.

THE INFLUENCE OF ENDOGENOUS OPIOID PEPTIDES

ON VENOUS GRANULOCYTES

Eike G. Fischer and Nora E. Falke

Sekt.Elektronenmikroskopie
Universität Ulm
D-7900 Ulm , Fed.Rep.Germany

POLYMORPHONUCLEAR LEUKOCYTES (PMNs)

History

Ameboid migrating phagocytes represent a phylogenetically ancient defense system. Amebocytes are found throughout the animal kingdom. All functions of the PMNs (aggregation, adherence, polarization, chemokinesis, chemotaxis, phago-cytosis, pinocytosis, endocytosis, exocytosis) are primitive functions, as they occur in most of the protozoa. In mammals they appear in all embryonic cells and in some of the differentiated cells.

In vertebrates the most distinct marker of inflammation is the appearence of granulocytes (PMNs) in tissue. After irritation of the tissue they adhere to the endothelium and after some minutes begin to migrate out of the vessel. This was already observed by Waller(1846) and Cohnheim(1867,1869) in the tongue of the frog. In bacterial inflammations the PMNs and their disintegration products represent the major part of pus. In 1888 Leber interpreted the directed migration towards the source of inflammation as chemotaxis. As a result our present view of PMNs has its origin 100 years ago.

The Cells

In mammals nearly 70 % of the white blood cells are PMNs. In humans PMNs are round-shaped with an average diameter of 8.5 µm . They are specialized in hunting microbes. Granulo-cytes originate from the bone marrow. In the bloodstream they have a short life span of less than 12 hours and a daily turnover rate of about 100.000.000.000. The name polymorphonuclear leukocytes (PMNs) derives from their lobed nucleus. According to their staining reactions granulocytes

are subdivided into neutrophils, basophils and eosinophils.
This division is also based on functional criteria. In the
following only neutrophils, which represent about 95% of all
granulocytes, are taken into account. Neutrophils contain two
different populations of granula (vesicles): i) primary
granules with lysosomal enzymes and ii) secondary (specific)
granules containing lactoferrin (both granula contain of other
mediators and enzymes as well).

Substances modulating PMNs behavior

When one speaks about the brain influence on the immune
system one should not forget that the endogenous opioids
represents only a small voice in a great concert. PMNs respond
with chemotactic migration to numerous inflammatory mediators.
Some endogenous stimulators like the immune-derived factors
(e.g. complement-fragments or the IgG-fragment tuftsin) are
always present in the form of inactive precursors. Other
stimulators derived from irritated tissues can be released by
many cells including PMNs. These factors include denatured
peptides and tissue hormones such as bradykinin, angiotensin,
substance P, neurotensin and the nerve growth factor(NGF) and
are mainly released by peripheral nerve terminal cells. In
physiological concentrations only neurotensin and perhaps NGF
seem to be potent enough to stimulate PMNs (Goldman et.al.´
83, Gee et.al.´83). Microbial degradation products like
N-formylized peptides or oxidized lipids are very potent
stimulators. The most potent N-formylized peptide is N-formyl-
-methionyl-leucyl-phenylalanine (fMLP) and is used as a
reference in our testsystems.

Most stimulators depending on their dose successively
induce all functions. With low concentrations of stimulators
the cells become typically adherent or in suspensions
aggregate. In a concentration gradient they migrate towards
the (presumptive) center of inflammation and are maximal
stimulated to engulf microbes and aberrant autologous cells.
During phagocytosis and with high concentrations of
stimulators the PMNs release lysosomal enzymes and
bacteriocidal oxygen compounds. High concentrations of
stimulators also inhibit a further migration.

Other substances inhibit PMN functions. Migrating is
impaired by epinephrine and some prostaglandins. The
prostaglandin prostacyclin inhibits PMN adherence to
endothelial cells.

One finds a considerable variation in the enzymatic
contents of PMNs in different species. Therefore, we can
expect functional differences and different sensitivities to
various stimulators from one species to another. For example,
PMNs from human beings, rabbits, rats, guinea pigs and sheep
respond well to fMLP, while there is no reaction of PMNs from
horses, cows, pigs or dogs. Everyone who is going to
investigate PMNs has to consider that blood from different
donors can show very different reactions, even if blood from
young healthy students is used.

OPIOIDS

The opiate alkaloids like morphine and their effects on
pain perception and mood are well known for thousands of
years. Since opiate effects can be induced only by active
stereoisomers an opiate receptor in the brain was postulated
and has been described by several groups in 1973. Consequently
an intensive search for an endogenous ligand for this receptor
started. Opioid peptides were first isolated from the brain
and later isolated in the pituitary, the adrenal medulla and
also in the plasma. The opioid peptides include the
enkephalins, ß-endorphin (ßEnd) and the dynorphin-related
peptides.

High concentrations of opiate alkaloids as found in
clinical use and in addicts have inhibitory effects on PMN
functions, particulary on migration (Stanley et.al.´76),
phagocytosis (Zucker-Franklin et.al.´71) and chemoluminescence (Gyires et.al.´85). In 1981/82 several groups
including ourselves started to investigate the effects of
endogenous opioids on immune cells (Fischer and Falke´84).
Let us look at the opioid effects in PMNs which we detected in
our investigations.

WHAT CAN WE SEE ?

Separate the granulocytes from venous blood, suspend them
in Hanks´ buffered salt solution (HBSS). Put a droplet of
such a suspension onto a glass coverslip. Within a few minutes
all granulocytes (more than 95%) will adhere to the glass,
while other cells can be rinsed off with HBSS. Add a droplet
of buffer on the coverslip with the adherent cells and turn it
upside down onto a slide and surround it with paraffin. In
such a preparation most of the PMNs are globular-shaped. Their
surface is slightly ruffeled like an untidy sheet. But some
cells show spontaneous shape changes and random movements.

If ß-End (10^{-8} to $^{-10}$ M) is added and the cells
are observed under a microscope nothing seems to happen within
the first 2 minutes. Only after exact measurement of the cell
diameters on photographs does it become evident that 1/3 of
the cells have an increased diameter of about 20% (Falke and
Fischer´85). The scanning electron microscope shows that many
cells had lost their rounded shape and were flattened on the
substrate, their ruffeled cell membranes were now smoothened,
in short, they appeared like fried eggs. While the pseudopodia
appearing later are clearly visible under the light microscope
the thin layer of hyaloplasma (the ´white of the egg´) could
be observed only under the scanning microscope. With PMNs from
the rat even under the light microscope the ´fried egg´
phenomenon could be observed in 1/3 of the cells. In venous
PMNs from dog, sheep or rabbit this effect did not seem to
appear.

The cell spreading which could be observed with ß-End
could not be induced by opiate alkaloids in equal
concentrations. On the contrary, after addition of levorphanol
or the antagonist diprenorphine the cells increased the
ruffeling of their membrane and also tended to shrink slightly.

Let us compare the opioid effects with the well known early effects of fMLP on PMNs. If we measure human PMNs treated with fMLP (10^{-8} M) an increase in the cell diameter as occurs with ß-End becomes evident. In PMNs of the rat the 'fried egg' phenomenon could not be observed with fMLP. According to reports of Zigmond and Sullivan'79 and Davis'82 PMNs show a cell spreading within two minutes and a simultaneous ruffeling of the surface. Most of the ruffeling dissapears in the following two minutes. As can be seen, there are fundamental differences in the early reaction to opioids and to fMLP. From this it can be concluded that the stimulation by opioids results in a second messenger pattern which differs from that activated by fMLP.

Now we return to our coverslip with PMNs and ß-End. After 3 min from the start of the preparation more and more cells begin to migrate. At 12 minutes nearly all cells are moving. About one third of the cells are now entirely flattened, one third are nearly rounded showing a thin margin of pseudopodia at the front and a short tail-like uropod. The observer's attention is attracted to the remaining one third of the cells which are extremly elongated more than 3 times normal. This comes as no surprise that the cells react in such a variety of ways. Since these cells have a short life span in the blood they undergo a rapid metamorphoses and thus behave differently.

During the whole incubation time control cells incubated in HBSS had a length over width ratio (a/b) between 1.1 and 1.2 on average for each preparation. The same applies to ß-End within the first 2 minutes. Twelve minutes after the addition of ß-End this ratio reached 1.8 for human and ovine PMNs. In PMNs of the rabbit the elongation is less expressed, and in PMNs of the dog and the rat an elongation is not visible. In human PMNs an elongation of 1.8 could also be induced with the alkaloid levorphanol (10^{-8} M) but not with the dextrorotatory isomer dextrorphan. All effects of ß-End could be inhibited by the opiate antagonist diprenorphine in equimolar concentrations. Thus the effects are stereospectific and antagonizable.

To estimate the influence of ß-End on the cell velocity the same cells were photographed every 20 seconds after 15 min of incubation. For human PMNs it could be shown that the cell velocity of nearly all cells was twofold increased as compared to the control. To our surprise the most elongated cells were hardly moving probably because they could not detatch their retraction fibers. The fastest cells were the relativly rounded ones bearing a short uropod.

If we compare the effect of ß-End on cell elongation and cell velocity up to this point there is no difference than with fMLP. To investigate if endogenous opioids are chemotactic stimulators like fMLP we used the Zigmond-chamber (Zigmond'77). A coverslip with adherent PMNs prepared as described above was placed on a special slide similar to a counting chamber. Between two wells of 2 x 4 mm there is a bridge of 1 mm width. The coverslip leaves a space of 0.01 mm above the bridge. Filling one well with HBSS and the other with a stimulatory substance a gradient is established over

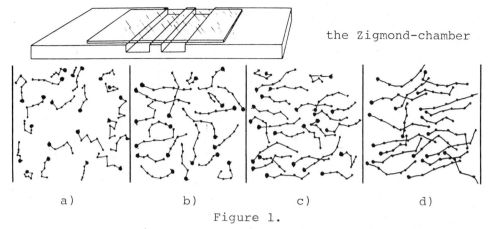

the Zigmond-chamber

a)   b)   c)   d)

Figure 1.

Cells moving in a Zigmond-chamber 20 min after preparation.
Points indicate the centers of the moving cells. The start
of each cell is marked by a fat point. The lines indicate
the distances travelled by single cells within 5 x 20 sec.
a)   control cells in buffer only
b)   in a gradient of ß-End, which is added 10^{-10} M in
      the right well
c)   in a gradient of fMLP, which is added 10^{-8} M
d)   same preparation like c), but with ß-End 10^{-10} M
      homogenously in the medium

the bridge. Filling one well with HBSS and the other with a
stimulatory substance a gradient is established over the
bridge. The cells were monitored by time lapse photography and
the distances travelled and the degree of orientation in the
gradient were measured on a computer tablet.

In a gradient of fMLP nearly all cells were oriented and
migrated directly towards the well with fMLP. This does not
apply for ß-End. One can see the stimulation of the cell
velocity but the cells are moving in all directions. This
means they showed chemokinesis but in contrast to fMLP-treated
PMNs no chemotactic behavior. Their degree of orientation was
the same as in buffer (0.15-0.17 McCutcheon index, McCutcheon´
46) To investigate the effects of a combined administration of
ß-End and fMLP, ß-End was present homogenously while fMLP was
added into only one well. This resulted in an additional
increase in cell velocity. This stimulation was significant at
a ß-End concentrations of 10^{-11} M and higher. Nearly all
cells were stimulated and the maximal effect was achieved with
a concentrations 10^{-9} M. With the addition of ß-End the
cell orientation in the gradient of fMLP remained unchanged
(0.82 - 0.87). The additive effect of ß-End and fMLP was also
observed by Simpkins et.al.´84 in a chemotaxis-under-agarose
assay. Although a different testsystem was used this group
reported equal results and a dose response relationship as was
found in our testsystem. An interesting phenomenon is that the
broadest interassay variance occurred near the optimal dose of
about 10^{-8} M and that with higher doses an inhibitory
effect on cell motility was achieved as confirmed by us. This
suppression acts parallel to the alkaloid effects. They also
showed that the effects of ß-End could be antagonized by
naloxone.

fMLP 10^{-8} M gradient

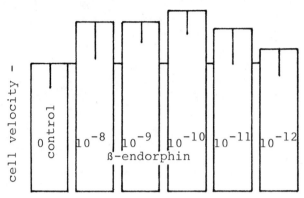

Figure 2.

Zigmond chamber
Additive effect of ß-End on the velocity of cells migrating
orientated in a gradient of fMLP. In each of 7 experiments
50 cells were evaluated. Vertical bars indicate deviation
between individual experiments.

Having observed an invasion of macrophages into the
ventricle after injection of opioid peptides Saland and van
Epps´82 tested the chemotactic effects of these peptides in
the Boyden-chamber (van Epps et.al.´83 and ´84). The Boyden-
-chamber consists of an upper compartment containing the cells
and a lower compartment containing the stimulatory substance
separated by a filter membrane. Using fMLP as a reference this
group described a moderate chemotactic effect of the opioids
on PMNs, and a stronger effect on monocytes. All findings of
this group are consistent with our findings, however, we
disagree with their interpretation. We are sure that opioids
increase the speed of the cells, but they have no influence on
the orientation of a single cell. The Boyden-chamber allows a
rapid evaluation but one can not differentiate between a
biased random locomotion (called klino-kinesis, which is also
found in bacteria) and chemotaxis (the oriented and directed
migration)(Keller et.al.´77).

OTHER FUNCTIONS

The opioid effects on cell shape and motility encouraged
us to test opioid effects on other granulocyte functions. To
investigate if PMNs release the contents of their granula
after stimulation by ß-End human PMNs were incubated with the
addition of 2 ug/ml cytochalasin B (this addition is necessary
for the in vitro test of enzyme release). The release of
lactoferrin and the enzymes ß-glucoronidase and myeloperoxidase were measured. Under these conditions fMLP induced a
dose dependent release from primary (enzymes) and secondary
(lactoferrin) granula, while a release stimulated by ß-End
could not be measured. There were no modulatory effects of
ß-End on the fMLP-induced release. No release was observed
with either ß-End or Met-enkephalin (both at a concentration
of 3 x 10^{-9} M).

To investigate the influence of ß-End (10^{-10} to
10^{-7} M) on phagocytosis PMNs were incubated with

heat-inactivated Candida albicans (yeast cells). The exessive
uptake of candida cells in presence of serum was not inhibited
by ß-End. In incubations without serum there was no
stimulatory effect of ß-End and the fMLP-stimulated
phagocytosis remained unchanged (fMLP 10^{-9} to 10^{-7} M).
There were no effects on oxidization in the NBT-assay (Nitro
blue tetrazolium).

RECEPTORS

There were no morphological effects with dextrorphan, an
inactive stereoisomer of the opiate alkaloid levorphanol. All
effects of ß-End could be inhibited with opiate antagonists.
So the effects were stereospecific and antagonizable. These
findings suggest that the effects are mediated by an opiate
receptor. In contrast to Hazum et.al.´79, who were unable to
find any specific binding of iodinated D-Ala2-ß-End in human
PMNs, Lopker et.al.´80 described stereospecific opiate
binding in human PMNs and monocytes. Our binding studies were
performed on living cells incubated under isotonic conditions.
No specific binding could be found with the enkephalin
analogue DADLE. Specific binding of the opiate antagonists
naloxone and diprenorphine occurred in incubations on ice and
at 37°C. Binding of the natural opioid peptides
Met-enkephalin and dynorphin 1-8 was less at 4°C than at
37°C. These peptides were labeled with tritium at the
N-terminal tyrosine. Their rapid degradation accompanied by a
tyrosine uptake and the minimal effect of various protease
inhibitors made the binding studies rather difficult.
Adsorption chromatography was used to differentiate between
cell-bound intact peptide and tyrosine. At the beginning of
the incubations the major part of the cell bound radioactivity
turned out to be specifically bound intact peptide. In summary
our studies are evidence for opioid receptors in PMNs
(manuscript in preparation).

CONCLUDING REMARKS

Ten years ago it was generally presumed that the various
PMN functions are strictly correlated in their stimulation.
Only the dose of a mediator was thought to be the
discriminating factor. The effects were thought to be mediated
by the same structures of the cytoskeleton and by the same
second messengers like Ca2+ or cyclic nucleotides (Showell
et.al.´76). This view is not unquestioned today (Keller´82)
since numerous mediators are known which stimulate certain
functional patterns. The stimulatory pattern opioids is well
defined among the stimulatory effects of other peptides. To
our knowledge the same functional pattern is achieved only
with the artifical peptide Gly-His-Gly in the high
concentration of 10^{-5} M (Spielberg et.al.´78). In many
animal species nearly all functions can be stimulated by fMLP.
Up to now there was no blood donor in any species whose cells
reacted to opioids but not to fMLP.

In various situations of ´stress´ like sport, sex,
labour, and delivery the plasma level of opioid peptides is
elevated. Assuming that in these situations there is an

increased liability of injury there is a teleological sense in the augmentation of analgesia, wound healing and defense against infections. Other groups working with natural killer cells emphasized an inhibitory effect of stress-induced opioid peptide release (Shavit et.al.´84). According to our investigations there is a short term stimulating effect of opioid peptides between their release and there rapid degradation on the short living PMNs. The results described above indicate that endogenous opioids might play a role in modulating the inital phase of the PMN´s offensive behavior, presumably cell adherence and motility.

The Zigmond-chamber data were partly presented at the Meeting OPIOID PEPTIDES IN PERIPHERY, may 1984, Rome, Italy.

ACKNOWLEDGEMENT

We would like to thank Tony DalleAve for help with the manuscript

REFERENCES

Cohnheim J., 1867, Ueber Entzündung und Eiterung. Virchow´s Arch.path.Anat.40:1-79

Cohnheim J., 1969, Ueber das Verhalten der fixen Bindegewebskörperchen bei der Entzündung. Virchow´s Arch.path.Anat.45.4:333-350

Davis B.H., Walter R.J., Pearson C.B., Becker E.L. and Oliver J.M., 1982, Membrane actitity and topology of f-Met-Leu-Phe-treated polymorphonuclear leukocytes. Am.J.Pathol.108:206-216

Falke N.E. and Fischer E.G., 1985, Cell shape of polymorphonuclear leukocytes is influenced by oipids. Immunobiol.169: in press

Fischer E.G. and Falke N.E., 1984, ß-Endorphin modulates immune functions - A review. Psychother.Psychosom.42:195-204

Gee A.P., Boyle M.D.P., Munger K.L., Lawman M.J.P. and Young M., 1983, Nerve growth factor: Stimulation of polymorphonuclear leukocyte chemotaxis in vitro. Proc.Natl.Acad.Sci.USA 80:7215-7218

Goldman R., Bar-Shavit Z. and Romeo D., 1983, Neurotensin modulates human neutrophil locomotion and phagocytic capability. FEBS Lett.159:63-67

Gyires K., Budavarit I., Fürst S. and Molnar I., 1985, Morphine inhibits the carrageenan-induced oedema and the chemoluminescence of leucocytes stimulated by zymosan. J.Pharm.Pharmacol.37:100-104

Hazum E., Chang K.J. and Cuatrecasas P., 1979, Specific nonopiate receptors for ß-endorphin. Science 205:1033-1035

Keller H.U., Wilkinson P.C., Abercrombie M., Becker E.L.,
Hirsch J.G., Miller M.E., Ramsey W.S. and Zigmond S.H., 1977,
A proposal for the definiton of terms related to locomotion of
leucocytes and other cells. Clin.exp.Immunol.27:377-380

Keller H.U., Hess M.W. and Cottier H., 1982, Leucocyte
activation and the assessment of leucocyte locomotion and
chemotaxis. Adv.Exp.Med.Biol.141:9-17

Leber T., 1888, Ueber die Entstehung der Entzündung und die
Wirkung der entzündungserregenden Schädlichkeiten.
Fortschr.Med.6:460-464

Lopker A., Abood L.G., Hoss W. and Lionetti F.J., 1980,
Stereoselective muscarinic acetylcholine and opiate receptors
in human phagocytic leukocytes. Biochem.Pharmacol.29:1361-1365

McCutcheon M., 1946, Chemotaxis in leukocytes.
Physiol.Rev.26:319-336

Saland L.C., van Epps D.E., Ortiz E. and Samora A., 1983,
Acute injection of opiate peptides into the rat cerebral
ventricle: A macrophage-like cellular response. Brain
Res.Bull.10:523-528

Shavit Y., Lewis J.W., Terman G.W., Gale R.P. and Liebeskind
J.C., 1984, Opioid peptides mediate the suppressive effect of
stress on natural killer cell cytotoxicity. Science
223:188-190

Showell H.J., Freer R.J., Zigmond S.H., Schiffmann E.,
Aswanikumar S., Corcoran B. and Becker E.L., 1976, The
structure-activity relations of synthetic peptides as
chomotactic factors and inducers of lysosomal enzyme secretion
for neutrophils. J.Exp.Med.143:1154-1169

Simpkins C.O., Dickey C.A. and Fink M.P., 1984, Human
neutrophil migration is enhanced by beta-endorphin.
Life-Sci.34:2251-2255

Spielberg I., Mandell B., Mehta J., Sullivan T. and Simchowitz
L., 1978, Dissociation of the neutrophil functions of
exocytosis and chemotaxis. J.Lab.Clin.Med.92:297-302

Stanley T.H., Hill G.E., Portas M.R., Hogan N.A. and Hill
H.R., 1976, Neutrophil chemotaxis during and after general
anesthesia and operation. Anesth.Analg., Cleveland 55:668-673

van Epps D.E., Saland L., Taylor C. and Williams R.C., 1983,
In vitro and in vivo effects of ß-endorphin and Met-enkephalin
on leukocyte locomotion. Prog.Brain Res.59:361-374

van Epps D.E. and Saland L., 1984, ß-Endorphin and
Met-enkephalin stimulate human peripheral blood mononuclear
cell chemotaxis. J.Immunology 132:3046-3053

Waller A., 1846, Microscopic examination of some of the
principal tissues of the animal frame, as observed in the
tongue of the living frog, toad, &c. Philosophical Magazine,
London 29:271-287 and Microscopic observation on the
perforation of the capillaries by the corpuscles of the blood,
and on the origin of mucus and pus-globules. :397-405

Zigmond S.H., 1977, Ability of polymorphonuclear leukocytes to
orient in gradients of chemotactic factors. J.Cell
Biol.75:606-616

Zigmond S.H. and Sullivan S.J., 1979, Sensory adaptation of
leukocytes to chemotactic peptides. J.Cell Biol.82:517-527

Zucker-Franklin D., Elsbach P. and Simon E.J., 1971, The
effect of the morphine analog levorphanol on phagocytosing
leukocytes. Lab.Invest.25:415-421

IMMUNOSUPPRESSIVE EFFECTS OF THE OPIOPEPTINS

Hulon W. McCain,[1,2] Ira B. Lamster[2,3] and Joanne Bilotta[3]

Departments of Pharmacology,[1] Periodontics and Oral Medicine[2] and The Oral Health Research Center,[3] Fairleigh Dickinson University School of Dentistry, Hackensack, New Jersey 07601

INTRODUCTION

The immune system has long been considered an organ system differing significantly from others in the immediacy of its regulation by the central nervous system. Whereas other organs have, to differing degrees, well characterized neural and hormonal afferent as well as efferent regulatory pathways, immune function has traditionally been viewed as an internally regulated effector system essentially devoid of CNS modulation with the possible exception of the CRF-ACTH-corticosteroid link. Such views were reinforced by Jerne's natural antibody selection theory (Jerne, 1955), and the observed ability of immune elements to display significant levels of activity in varied in vitro assay systems (Nowell, 1960). Astute clinicians, however, have for centuries reported antecdotal evidence of increased disease susceptibility associated with diverse physiological and psychological stimuli (Shigami, 1919) including those of stress and emotional distress (Locke, 1982). Patients suffering stressful injury such as burns, and operative or accidental trauma, exhibit decreased immune responsiveness which is often well correlated with post-traumatic susceptibility to bacterial, viral and fungal infections (Constantin et al., 1977; Wolfe et al., 1981; Alexander, 1968; and Goodman et al., 1968). Cancer patients have generally suppressed immunocompetence and, conversely, a large body of experimental data indicates that stress reduces the rate of implanted tumor rejection (Visintaner et al., 1982), and increases tumor growth (Riley, 1981) along with other correlates of invasiveness (Shavit et al., 1983). Recently, intense interest has generated research efforts to elucidate mechanisms by which the central nervous system may modulate normal and stress-induced changes in immune activity, and the physiologic relevance of these putative neuroendocrine-immune system regulatory links. The greatest activity in this regard has been in investigating possible roles of the circulating endorphinergic and enkephalinergic peptides. B-endorphin and several shorter chain products of its enzymatic processing (Akil et al., 1985), as well as numerous high and low molecular weight enkaphalinergic peptides (Evans et al., 1984) are released into peripheral circulation in response to stress, and have as yet undefined biologic relevance. Early studies, however, indicated that cultured human lymphocytes had specific non-opiate binding sites for B-endorphin (Hazum et al., 1979) and that isolated human peripheral blood lymphocytes displayed opiate receptor-like activity with met-enkephalin (Wybran et al., 1979). These cells are key components of immune expression since T-lymphocytes and macrophages are the primary cell types involved in cell-mediated immunity, whereas humoral immunity is characterized by the activity of B-lymphocytes and immunoglobin producing plasma cells. Lymphocytes also play a major role in immunoregulation since when activated they are known to produce regulatory factors influencing the macrophage (i.e., macrophage inhibitory factor), neutrophils (i.e., chemotactic factor), eosinophils (i.e., chemotactic factor), and basophils (i.e., enterleukin-3). They also elaborate compounds controlling activity of other lymphocyte populations (i.e., interleukin-2, suppressing factors and chemotactic factors) (Bellanti and Rocklin, 1985). Ultimate expression of lymphocyte activity may be determined by reciprocal interactions of T-

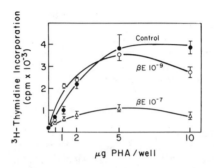

Fig. 1. The effect of B-endorphin on PHA-induced blastogenesis of human T-lymphocytes. Experiments were with lymphocytes freshly isolated from normal healthy volunteers. Lymphocytes were separated from heparinized whole blood by density gradient centrifugation over Lymphoprep. Recovered lymphocytes were washed twice and resuspended in Eagles Minimal Essential Media supplemented with 5% fetal calf serum, glutamine and pen-strep. Cells were cultured in microwells containing 2×10^5 lymphocytes, PHA and/or B-endorphin. Incubations were at $37°C$ for 48 hrs in 95% air/5% CO_2. Each well was pulsed with 1uCi ^{3}H-thymidine and incubations continued for 20 hr. ^{3}H-DNA was collected with a cell harvester and quantitated. Viability of cultured cells was 90% as determined by lactic dehydrogenase assay of culture supernatant. PHA and/or BE were simultaneously. Results are reported as mean ± SEM (N = 4).

cell subsets. T-helper cells may be critical to these interactions producing soluble regulators which stimulate activity of relevant cell types including the T-suppressor population, and T-suppressor cells in turn elaborating soluble modulating factors which suppress activity of both B-cells and T-helper populations. This balance of suppressor and helper activities may provide the necessary precise regulation of this system. Specific immunity therefore results from a multi-faceted, integrated response relying on a complex interplay of regulatory modulators. The internal enhancement, regulation and suppression of this system has been characterized through recent investigation. Neuroendocrine/hormonal immunoregulation has only recently come under intense investigation. Although effects of the corticosteroids on immune function have been defined (Parillo and Fauci, 1978), actions of

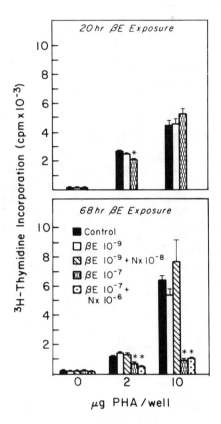

Fig. 2. A. Effect of B-endorphin and naloxone on established blastogenesis of human lymphocytes. BE and/or Nx were added to cultured cells 40 hrs after initiation of mitogenic stimulation. Results are mean ± SEM (N = 4) with significant differences determined by ANOVA. Asterisks indicate P<0.01.

B. Effect of naloxone (Nx) on B-endorphin (BE)-induced suppression of human lymphocyte blastogenesis. Methods were as described in Fig. 1 except when Nx was used, it was added 30 min prior to BE. Results are mean ± SEM (N = 4) with significant differences determined by ANOVA. Asterisks indicate P<0.01.

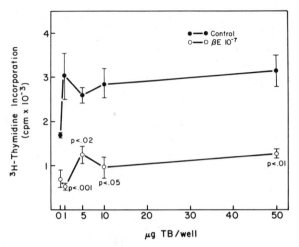

Fig. 3. B-endorphin induced suppression of M. tuberculosis stimulated blastogenesis in sensitized mouse splenocytes. Eight week BALB/c mice were immunized by subcutaneous injection of complete Freund's adjuvant containing M. tuberculosis (TB). Four week later mice were injected with purified protein derivative of tuberculin (PPD). Two weeks after PPD injections, spleens were removed, pressed through a wire mesh, and cells collected, washed and resuspended in RPMI containing fetal calf serum (FCS) and pen-strep. Blastogenesis assay was essentially as described in Fig. 1 except TB was used as antigen. B-endorphin (BE) was added at initiation of cell culture. Results are reported as mean ± SEM (N = 4) with significant differences determined by students T-statistic.

neuroendocrine mediators such as B-endorphin have only recently been studied. This chapter will review our studies of the effects of B-endorphin, its metabolite glycyl-L-glutamine and also isolated adrenal medullary peptides on various aspects of immune functions.

EFFECT OF B-ENDORPHIN AND ITS CARBOXY-TERMINAL DIPEPTIDE ON BLASTOGENESIS OF HUMAN PERIPHERAL BLOOD LYMPHOCYTES AND MOUSE SPLENOCYTES

Our interest in opiopeptin-immunity interactions began following reports by Hazum et al., 1979, of specific non-opiate receptors for B-endorphin on a cultured lymphoid cell line. Our research efforts have since focused on T-helper, T-suppressor and also B-lymphocyte activity assessed by their proliferative and regulatory activities in response to phytohemagglutinin (PHA), concanavalin A (Con-A) Mycobacterium tuberculosis (TB), and partially purified derivative of mycobacterium tuberculosis (PPD). In our human studies we have used normal healthy dental students ranging in age from 20-28 years. Venous blood was collected and used immediately

Table 1.   The Effect of GLG and BE on PHA-induced Blastogenesis of Human PBL[a]
Blastogenesis of Human PBL[a]

GLG(10^{-7}M)	BE(10^{-7}M)	(PHA ug/well)	[b]Response (%Control)
+	–	0.5	50
–	+	0.5	51
+	–	1.0	49
–	+	1.0	33
+	–	2.0	57
–	+	2.0	33
+	–	5.0	55
–	+	5.0	21

a
Glycyl-L-Glutamine (GLG) and B-endorphin (BE) were used in standard
blastogenesis assay with human peripheral blood lymphocyte (PBL) as described
in Fig. 1.
b
Response is reported as % of control (without GLG or BE) and is the mean
of three separate determinations performed in quadruplicate.

for blastogenesis assays utilizing a microculture system.   In our initial studies
(McCain et al., 1982) we reported that B-endorphin produced a dose related inhibition
of PHA-induced blastogenesis (Fig. 1). Low concentrations of B-endorphin (10^{-9}M)
suppressed proliferative responses only with supra-optimal mitogen concentration,
whereas, higher concentrations (10^{-7}M) caused significant suppression at all PHA
doses. With our experimental design, concentrations of B-endorphin less than 10^{-9}M
did not produce reliable suppression of mitogen-induced lymphocyte blast
transformation. In order for the opiopeptin to exert its immunosuppressive effect it
was necessary that it be present at the time of initial mitogenic stimulation (Fig. 2).
When it was added 48 hrs. after culture initiation, minimal effects were observed and
then only at the highest concentration of B-endorphin. A similar temporal association
has been observed when a low molecular weight (< 10,000 daltons) immunosuppressive
plasma peptide was used in studies of PHA-induced blastogenesis of human
lymphocytes (Cooperband, 1976).   This suggests that endorphin may interfere with
events associated with initiation of the PHA "receptor" transduction-amplification
mechanism.   Once the mitogenic signal is expressed, it is apparently difficult to
repress.   The effects of B-endorphin which we observed are not inhibited by the
opiate antagonist naloxone, suggesting interaction of the carboxy-terminal portion of
the peptide with receptors on the lymphoid cells.   A non-opiate receptor for B-
endorphin was originally described on a lymphoid cell line (Hazum, 1979). Although
once seldom reported, similar naloxone insensitive receptors for opiate drugs and
peptides have recently been characterized in rat vas deferens (Wuster el al., 1978),
ileum (Nakatsu et al., 1981), adipocytes (Morley et al., 1980), and brain (Johnson et
al., 1982). B-endorphin also reportedly binds to a nonpeptide, cytolytic membrane-
derived C5b-9(M) complex and also to the serum derived SC5b-9 complex of human
complement (Schweigerer et al., 1982). Also, Gilman et al., 1982, observed that B-
endorphin effects on PHA-induced lymphocyte transformation were not reversed by
treatment with naloxone. It should be noted, however, that there is inconsistency in
reports of the actions of B-endorphins on lymphoid proliferation. Gilman et al.,
(1982) observed that with rat splenocytes 3.2×10^{-8} - 3.3×10^{-9} M B-endorphin
produced enhanced responses to PHA, also Weber and Pert, 1984, reported that with

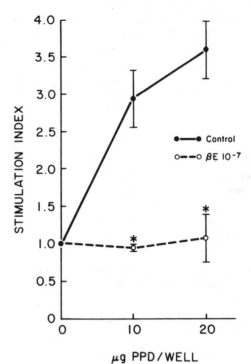

Fig. 4. The effect of B-endorphin on antigen-induced blastogenesis of M. tuberculosis immunized BALB/c mice. Animals were immunized, their splenocytes collected and cultured with or without PPD and/or BE as described in Fig. 3. Results, mean ± SEM (N = 4), are reported as stimulation index (SI).

highly purified, PHA-activated human T-lymphocytes and a mouse derived interleukin-2 dependent T-cell line, B-endorphin enhanced lymphocyte proliferation. Explanation for these discrepancies are at present unclear but may relate to the cellular composition isolated and used in the experiments, since multiple actions (both opiate and non-opiate) for B-endorphin have been demonstrated on various cell types of the immune system (i.e., Wybran, 1979).

Recent studies (Akil et al., 1985) clearly indicate that shorter chained and metabolized forms of B-endorphin may be released from the pituitary differential in chronically stressed rats. Many of these are also devoid of opiate activity and are present in substantial concentrations in the peripheral circulation. Proteolytic cleavage of B-endorphin has also been reported to produce the dipeptide glycyl-L-glutamine within the pituitary (Smyth, 1983). This dipeptide was shown to have widespread inhibitory actions on brainstem neuronal activity which was non-opiate and not related to activation of glycine or glutamate receptive sites. This compound is the carboxy-terminal dipeptide of B-endorphin, and presumably participates in non-opiate interactions of B-endorphin (Schweigerer, 1982). Since the effects of B-endorphin which we observed were non-opiate, we have begun evaluating the effects of this dipeptide on PHA-induced blastogenesis of human lymphocytes (McCain et al., 1985). Glycyl-L-glutamine (GLG) at 10^7 M caused a 50% suppression of lymphocyte proliferation over the test range of mitogen concentrations. This was generally less

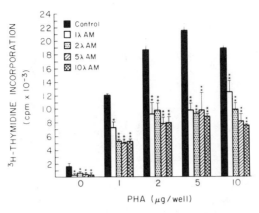

Fig. 5. The effect of adrenal medullary extract on PHA-induced blastogenesis of human peripheral lymphocytes. Adrenals were dissected to provide medallae from which a suspension of chromaffin granules was obtained by differential centrifugation (Smith and Winkler, 1967). Chromaffin granules were lysed, large proteins removed by TCA precipitation and centrifugation, and lipids removed by ether extraction (Stern et al., 1979). Following extensive dialysis and concentration by lyophilization, aliquots were added at initiation of cell culture. Isolation of human lymphocytes and blastogenesis assay were as described in Fig. 1. Results are reported as mean ± SEM (N = 3) with significant differences determined by ANOVA (*$P < .05$, **$P < .01$).

efficacious than B-endorphin in these assays. It appears, therefore, that although stress may be associated with increased intermediate pituitary lobe release of N-acetylated endorphinergic compound devoid of opiate activity, non-opiate interactions may still persist if this dipeptide reaches appreciable concentrations in plasma. It should be noted that numerous small peptides have potent immunoregulatory properties. Common examples are muramyl dipeptide and some tripeptide chemotactic factors (Fraser-Smith et al., 1981; Simpkins et al., 1984).

PHA and other lectins provide a potent nonspecific stimulus for lymphocyte transformation, and assays utilizing this or similar mitogens are popular in vitro indices of in vivo immunologic competence. Mitogen stimulated lymphocyte transformation, however, differs from antigen-stimulated activity in that the latter is both specific and generally less intense. In an effort to more closely approximate the in vivo immunologic response, we have examined the effect of B-endorphin on antigen-stimulated blastogenesis of sensitized mouse splenocytes (Fig. 3). BALB/c mice were appropriately immunized with multiple injections of inactivated Mycobacterium tuberculosis (TB) and a partially purified derivative of Mycobacterium tuberculosis (PPD). TB (1-50 ug/well) was used to induce an antigen-specific lympho-proliferative response and did in fact produce a significant two-fold

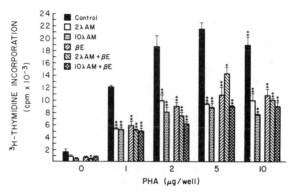

Fig. 6. Interaction of adrenal medullary peptides with B-endorphin in mitogen-induced blastogenesis of human peripheral lymphocytes. Conditions and materials are as described in Fig. 5. Results are reported as means ± SEM (N = 3).

stimulation of ^{3}H-thymidine incorporation with these assays. B-endorphin (10^{-7}M) was added at the initiation of culture, and almost completely prevented the TB dependent blastogenic stimulus. We also used PPD (10-20 ug/well) to induce antigenic stimulation in hopes of eliciting a greater response in the sensitized lymphocytes (Fig. 4). ^{3}H-thymidine incorporation was increased almost four-fold with the higher dose of PPD. B-endorphin (10^{-7}M) completely inhibited antigen-induced proliferation in these assays. While PPD was a more effective antigen than the inactivated bacterial suspension, the immunosuppressive activity of BE was more pronounced for the antigen driven lymphocyte transformation. It should be noted that the degree of stimulation with these antigens was much less than that induced by PHA (stimulation indices of 2-4 as opposed to 10 15 for the lectin). Immunosuppression by B-endorphin was also most prominent with the PPD experiments, confirming our previous observation and also that of others (Gilman et al., 1982) that the effect of this peptide is greater when the stimulus for transformation is mild.

PARTIALLY PURIFIED ADRENAL MEDULLARY PEPTIDES INHIBIT LYMPHOCYTE BLASTOGENESIS

Selye (1956) observed that stress is a complex stimulus resulting in pituitary and adrenal secretions along with other coordinated physiological responses. However, recent studies indicate the truly complex nature of this response and suggest that Selye's original concept may no longer be scientifically acceptable (Terman et al., 1984). Traditional studies have shown stress-associated pituitary release of B-endorphin and ACTH (Rossier et al., 1977) along with concurrent adrenal medullary and cortical secretory activity. The adrenal medulla contains high concentrations of opiate peptides derived from the proenkephalin A and B genes (Udenfriend and Kilpatrick, 1983). Recent reports also suggest that proopiomelanocortin is expressed in human adrenal medulla (Evans et al., 1983). The adrenal enkephalinergic peptides range in size from that of the < 1 kilodalton met- and leu-enkephalins to the > 50

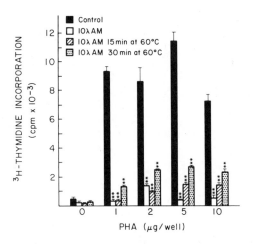

Fig. 7. The effect of heat-treated adrenal medulla extract on PHA-induced blastogenesis of human lymphocytes. Experimental conditions are as described in Fig. 1 except the crude adrenal medulla homogenate was heated at 60°C for 15 or 30 min before isolation of chrommaffin granule proteins.

kilodalton polypeptides (Kilpatrick et al., 1980) and possess widely different opiate receptor binding affinities, as well as biologic activities (Quixion and Weiss, 1983). Although specific proenkephalin converting enzymes have been isolated from adrenal chromaffin granules which produce the free enkephalin pentapeptides, stimulation of the adrenal gland causes release of both high and low molecular weight enkephalinergic peptides (Hanbauer et al., 1982; Chaminade et al., 1983). In the resting condition only the fully processed product of proenkephalin (met-or leu-enkephalin) may be released into peripheral circulation. When more powerful stimuli were utilized, however, greater proportions of higher molecular weight peptides are observed. In recent studies of the pathophysiology of shock, roughly equal quantities of the 31, 8, and 3-5 kilodalton peptides and native enkephalin pentapeptides were found in the plasma of dogs (Evans et al., 1984). Although abundant evidence has been obtained indicating that the enkephalin pentapeptides modify numerous in vitro indices of immune activity (Plotnikoff et al., 1985), no information has been reported regarding possible immunomodulatory activities of the higher molecular weight peptides.

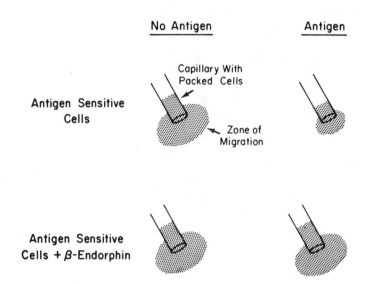

No Antigen   Antigen

Antigen Sensitive Cells

Capillary With Packed Cells

Zone of Migration

Antigen Sensitive Cells + β-Endorphin

$$\text{Migration Index} = \frac{\text{Migration Area With Antigen}}{\text{Migration Area Without Antigen}} \times 100$$

Fig. 8. Cell migration inhibition assay with PPD-sensitive mouse splenocytes. PPD-sensitive mouse (BALB/c) splenocytes were generated and isolated as described in Fig. 3. Cells were packed into capillary tubes by centrifugation and the tubes cut at the cell-fluid interface (David, 1966). The tube was assembled into a Sykes-Moore Culture Chamber filled with RPMI-1640, 15% fetal calf serum, pen-strep with or without PPD (100 ug/ml) and/or B-endorphin. Chambers were incubated for 24 hrs at 37°C and the "migratory fan" enlarged and quantitated by planimetry.

We have recently begun evaluating the actions of adrenal medullary peptides on in vitro assays of human lymphocyte activity. The method of Stern et al., 1979, was used to isolate a fraction containing enkephalinergic peptides from dissected adrenal medullae. Lyophilized adrenal extract was reconstituted (4 ug dry wt/ul) and added to cultures at their initiation. Adrenal medulla extract (AM) produced a prominent suppression of PHA-induced proliferation at all doses of the mitogen tested (Fig. 5). AM in doses of 1-10 ul (4-40 ug) reduced responses by 40-60% in most cases. We also looked for possible interactions of the adrenal-derived peptides and B-endorphin since presumably both may be released into the bloodstream in a coordinated fashion during times of stress (Fig. 6). B-endorphin (10^{-7} M) and/or AM were added to the cultures at their initiation. B-endorphin reduced the proliferation responses by approximately 50% at all mitogen concentrations as did AM. When used in combination, there was no evidence that these peptides possess any interactive characteristics since B-endorphin and/or AM treatment resulted in an approximate 50% suppression of proliferative responses with PHA. We also examined the heat sensitivity of peptides in this crude adrenal extract (Fig. 7). Heating the adrenal medullae homogenate to 60°C for 15 or 30 min prior to isolation of the peptides did not greatly alter their biologic activities in these assays. However, there were clear indications of reduced actions of the extracted compounds with longer heat treatments. The peptides in this extract apparently have significant heat stable characteristics.

Stress, presumably associated with increased levels of adrenal medullary secretion, is clearly associated with diminished immune activity. It is associated with

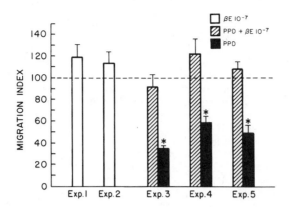

Fig. 9 Effect of B-endorphin on PPD-induced inhibition of cell migration. Experiments 1 & 2 were with normal (not TB immunized) mouse splenocytes. Splenocytes for experiments 3, 4 & 5 were from TB immunized animals. PPD and/or B-endorphin were added at initiation of culture. Results are reported as mean ± SEM (N = 4) with significant differences determined by students T-statistic (* P<0.01).

a markedly reduced lymphoproliferative response to mitogenic stimulation (Shavit et al., 1977; Laudenslager et al., 1983), natural killer cell activities (Shavit et al., 1984) and numerous indices of implanted tumor rejection (Riley, 1981; Sklar and Anisman, 1979). Although the enkephalinergic pentapeptides are generally considered immunopotentiators (Plotnikoff et al., 1985), our studies suggest that adrenal medullary compounds with MW >2000 daltons have significant inhibitory action on human lymphocyte proliferation. In vivo and in vitro models suggest that intense stimuli (stress) may induce release of these high molecular weight peptides from the adrenal medulla. It should be noted, however, that stress-induced immunosuppression has been observed in adrenalectomized rats (Keller et al., 1983). We are continuing to investigate the biologic activities of this group of compounds.

B-ENDORPHIN INHIBITS ANTIGEN SPECIFIC MIGRATION OF MOUSE SPLENOCYTES

Lymphocytes and macrophages participate in a complex interdependent regulatory scheme by which expression of specific activities of each cell type is modulated by the other. Macrophages liberate interleukin-1, which is necessary for full activation and differentiation of T-helper and B-lymphocytes, as well as numerous other monokines (Bellanti, 1985). T-helper cells elaborate interleukin-2 which together with interleukin-1 promote differentiation of the TDTH (T4+) subpopulation of T-lymphocytes. The TDTH (T4+) cells when fully differentiated can, if activated, release a series of lymphokines which direct activity of the macrophage. These lymphokines include macrophage chemotactic factor and also migration inhibition factor (MIF), which inhibits macrophage migration from sites containing activated lymphocytes. In vivo antigenic challenge of sensitized T-cells provides

283

sufficient stimuli to initiate this response. Numerous in vitro tests have been developed for evaluating migratory components of cell-mediated immunity (delayed hypersensitivity), however, one of the oldest and most useful is the cell migration inhibition assay (Likhite and Sehon, 1971). In this assay specific antigen is used to stimulate sensitized lymphocyte production of lymphokines which include MIF (Fig. 8). Antigen-induced in vitro assays of macrophage migration inhibition is in fact an established and sensitive indicator of MIF production by sensitized lymphocytes (Bennett and Bloom, 1968). We have investigated the effects of B-endorphin on cell-mediated immunity using TB sensitized mouse splenocytes in this assay (Fig. 9). Antigen (100 ug/ml PPD) reduced the 24 hr. migration area by 40-60% compared to cultures without antigen. B-endorphin (10^{-7}M) did not significantly alter the migration of nonsensitized splenocytes (Exp 1 & 2). However, when B-endorphin was simultaneously added to cultures of sensitized cells along with PPD, it completely prevented antigen-induced migration inhibition (Exp 3, 4 &5). These results suggest that B-endorphin has no direct effect on nonstimulated migration of mouse splenocytes. The interaction between sensitized (presumably) T-lymphocytes and macrophage may be prevented. Since opiate receptors have been demonstrated on lymphocytes, the initial explanation may be that this opiopeptide inhibits antigen-induced activation of TDTH (T4+) subpopulation which liberates MIF. However, numerous other interactions could produce a similar effect. B-endorphin could interact with macrophage to prevent MIF-induced transduction signal or prevent effective MIF-"receptor" binding. It should be noted that B-endorphin has been reported to act as a neutrophil chemoattractant using the Boyden chamber technique (Van Epps et al., 1983) and to enhance migration of human neutrophils to the chemoattractant peptide N-formyl-methionyl-leucyl-phenylalanine (Simpkins et al., 1984). Regardless of the specific mechanism, it is apparent from our studies that B-endorphin effectively intervenes in this in vitro model of delayed hypersensitivity reaction - a reaction in which subpopulations of T-lymphocytes provide substantial regulatory control.

CONCLUSIONS

It seems clear that the opiopeptins can modulate various components of immune function, however, individual effects as well as physiological relevance of these effects remain uncertain. Our results indicate that B-endorphin and its naturally occurring carboxy terminal dipeptide inhibit mitogen-induced blastogenesis of cultured human peripheral blood lymphocytes. Furthermore, antigen-driven proliferation, and antigen-induced migration inhibition of sensitized mouse splenocytes were potently inhibited by B-endorphin. The immunosuppressive activities of these neuropeptides which we have examined are apparently mediated via non-opiate receptors since the effects were not prevented by naloxone. The adrenal medulla also was shown to contain relatively high molecular weight (> 2000 dalton) compounds which have immunosuppressive action in in vitro blastogenesis assays with human peripheral blood lymphocytes. These compounds were isolated in relatively crude preparations which previously have been shown to contain numerous high molecular weight enkephalinergic peptides.

Stress of varied etiologies induces a myriad of physiological effects including immunosuppression and secretion of "stress hormones" from the pituitary and adrenal glands. The pituitary contains numerous opiatergic peptides including B-endorphin and other products of the proopiomelanocortin gene, many of which contain peptide sequences shared with B-endorphin and the enkephalins. Many of these opiate and non-opiate peptides have been demonstrated in plasma. We have shown that at least two of these compounds, B-endorphin and glycyl-L-glutamine, have potent immunosuppressive activity. However, other products of proopiomelanocortin may be in plasma at higher concentrations than B-endorphin (Akil et al., 1985). Also, numerous non-opiate products of B-endorphin (i.e., N-acetyl-B-endorphin) are released into plasma. None of these acetylated compounds, shorter chained products of B-endorphin metabolism, or larger products of proopiomelanocortin has been evaluated for immuno-modulating activity. Since immunomodulation by these endorphinergic and enkephalinergic neuropeptides apparently occurs via opiate as well as non-opiate interactions with numerous cell types, physiologic effects may well depend upon preferential synthesis and/or release from the pituitary. Recent evidence has suggested that such capacities do exist in pituitary neurosecretory activity (Akil et al., 1985).

The enkephalins are generally reported to potentiate immune activity, and it has been suggested that physiological release of these compounds from the adrenal may serve to counteract immunosuppressive action of the adrenocorticosteroids (Plotnikoff et al., 1985). The adrenal also contains as yet uncharacterized relatively high molecular weight peptides capable of depressing blastogenesis of lymphocytes. Although the fully processed product of proenkephalin (met- or leu-enkephalin) can be released with physiological stimuli, ample evidence has been presented that high molecular weight enkephalinergic compounds may actually predominate in plasma during times of extreme stress such as cardiovascular shock. Also, the adrenal medulla apparently has separate controlling mechanisms for synthesis and processing of its enkephalinergic products (Fleminger et al., 1984). It seems possible therefore that in normal situations the fully processed met- and leu-enkaphalins are released into the peripheral circulation providing positive modulatory influences upon immune expression, perhaps acting in opposition to secreted corticosteroids. However, during particularly stressful situations, secretion of higher molecular weight adrenal peptides may predominate. These compounds may act in unison with the adrenal steroids to induce immunosuppression. Few firm conclusions can be made until systemic investigation determines the contribution of presently uncharacterized adrenal compound(s) to immunologic expression.

Defining the interaction of secretory proopiomelanocortin and proenkephalin derived peptides with the immune system will have a profound impact upon our understanding of immune function and dysfunction. These hormonal regulators may induce multiple immunosuppressive or immunopotentiative effects, as is the situation with the corticosteroids, or more discrete interactions at specific points in the pathways of intrinsic regulatory control. Relatively mild interactions of these putative immunoregulators could induce immunopotentiation or immunodeficiency by shifting the regulatory balance between T-helper and T-suppressor cells. Actions of the endorphins and enkephalins may also summate with ongoing positive and negative regulatory control signals. Nevertheless, the complexity of specific immune expression suggests the need for caution when extrapolating biologic relevance based upon any individual test of immunocompetence.

REFERENCES

Akil, H., Hirohito, S. and Matthews, J., 1985, Induction of the intermediate pituitary by stress: synthesis and release of a nonopioid form of B-endorphin, Sci., 227:424.

Alexander, J.W., 1968, Effect of thermal injury upon the early resistance to infection, J. Surg. Res. 8:128.

Bellanti, J.A., and Rocklin, R.E., 1985, Cell mediated immune reactions, in: "Immunology," J.A. Bellanti, ed., W.B. Saunders, New York.

Bennett, B., and Bloom, B.R., 1968, Reactions in vivo and in vitro produced by a soluble substance associated with delayed-type hypersensitivity, Proc. Natl. Acad. Sci. (USA), 59:756.

Chaminade, M., Foutz, A.S., and Rossier, J., 1983, Co-release of enkephalins and precursors of catecholamines by the perfused rat adrenal in situ, Life Sci., 33:21.

Constantian, M.B., Manzoian, J.O., Nimberg, R.B., Schmid, K., and Mannick, J.A., 1977, Association of a circulating immunosuppressive polypeptide with operative and accidental trauma, J. Surg., 185:73.

Cooperband, S.R., Badger, A.M., and Mannick, J.A., 1976, Non-hormonal serum suppressive factors, in: "Mitogens in Immunobiology," J. Oppeheim and D.L. Rosenstreich, Eds., Acad. Press, New York.

David, J.R., 1966, Delayed hypersensitivity in vitro: its mediation by cell free substances formed by lymphoid cell-antigen interaction, Proc. Natl. Acad. Sci. (USA) 56:72.

Evans, C.J., Erdelyi, E., Weber, E. and Barchas, J.D., 1983, Identification of proopiomelanocortin-derived peptides in the human adrenal medulla, Sci., 221:957.

Evans, S.F., Medbak, S., Hinds, C.J., Tomlin, S.J., Varley, J.F. and Rees, L.H., 1984, Plasma levels and biochemical characterization of circulating met-enkephalin in canine endotoxin shock, Life Sci., 34:1481.

Fleminger, G., Howells, R.D., Kilpatrick, D.L., and Udenfriend, S., 1984, Intact proenkephalin is the major enkephalin-containing peptide produced in rat adrenal glands after denervation, Proc. Natl. Acad. Sci. (USA), 81:7985.

Fraser-Smith, E., and Matthews, T.R., 1981, Protective Effect of muramyl dipeptide analogs against infection of pseudomanas aeruginosa or candida albicans in mice, Infection and Immunity, 34:676.

Gilman, S.C., Schwartz, J.M., Milner, R.J., Bloom, F.E., and Feldman, J.D., 1982, B-endorphin enhances lymphocyte proliferative responses, Proc. Natl. Acad. Sci. (USA), 79:4226.

Goodman, J.S., Schaffner, W., Collins, H.A., Battersby, E.J., and Koenig, M.G., 1968, Infection after cardiovascular surgery: clinical study including examination of antimicrobial prophylaxis, N. Engl. J.Med., 278:117.

Hanbauer, I., Kelly, G.D., Saiani, L., and Yang, H.Y.T., 1982, (Met)-enkephalin-like peptides of the adrenal medulla: release by nerve stimulation and functional implications, Peptides, 3: 469.

Hazum, E., Chang, K., and Cuatrecasas, P., 1979, Specific non-opiate receptors for B-endorphin, Sci., 205:1033.

Ishigami, T., 1919, The influence of psychic acts on the progres of pulmonary tuberculosis, Am. Rev. Tuberculosis, 2:470.

Jerne, N.K., 1955, The national selection theory of antibody formation, Proc. Natl. Acad. Sci. (USA), 41:849.

Johnson, N., Houghten, R., and Pasternack, G., 1982, Binding of ^{3}H-B-endorphin in rat brain, Life Sci., 31:1381.

Keller, S.E., Weiss, J.M., Schleifer, S.J., Miller, N.E., and Stein, M., 1983, Stress-induced suppression of immunity in adrenalectomized rats, Sci., 221:1301.

Kilpatrick, D.L., Lewis, R.V., Stein, S., and Udenfriend, S., 1980, Release of enkephalins and enkephalin-containing peptides from perfused adrenal gland, Proc. Natl. Acad. Sci. (USA), 77:7473.

Laudenslager, M.L., Ryan, S.M., Drugan, R.C., Hyson, R.L., and Mailer, S.F., 1983, Coping and immunosuppression: inescapable but not escapable shock suppresses lymphocyte proliferation, Sci., 221:568.

Likhite, V., and Sehon, A., 1971, Migration inhibition and cell-mediated immunity: a review, Rev. Can. Biol., 30:135.

Lock, S.E., 1982, Stress, adaptation and immunity: studies in humans, Gen. Hospital Psychiatry, 4:49.

McCain, H.W., Bilotta, J.M., and Lamster, I.B., 1985, Life Sci. (submitted for publication).

McCain, H.W., Lamster, I.B., Bozzone, J.M., and Grbic, J.T., 1982, B-endorphin modulates human immune activity via non-opiate receptor mechanisms, Life Sci., 31:1619.

Morely, J., and Levine, A., 1980, Stress-induced eating is mediated through endogenous opiates, Sci., 209:1259.

Nakatsu, K., Goldenburg, E., Penning, D., and Jhamandas, K., 1981, Enkephalin-induced inhibition of the rat ileum is not blocked by naloxone, Can. J. Physiol. Pharmacol., 59:901.

Johnson, N., Houghten, R., and Pasternack, G.W., 1982, Binding of ^{3}H-B-endorphin in rat brain, Life Sci., 31:1381.

Nowell, P.C., 1960, Phytohemagglutinin: indication of mitosis in cutures of normal human leukocytes, Cancer Res., 20:462.

Parillo, J.E. and Fauci, A.S., 1978, Comparison of the effector cells in human spontaneous cellular cytotoxicity and antibody dependent cytotoxicity: Differential sensitivity of effector cells to in vivo and in vitro corticosteroids, Scand. J. Immunol., 8:99.

Plotnickoff, N.P., Murgo, A.J., Miller, G.C., Corder, C.N., and Faith, R.C., 1985, Enkephalins: immunomodulators, Federation Proc., 44:118.

Quirion, R., and Weiss, A., 1983, Peptide E and other proenkephalin-derived peptides are potent kappa opiate receptor agonists, Peptides, 4:445.

Riley, V., 1981, Psychoneuroendocrine influences on immunocompetence and neoplasia, Sci., 212:1100.

Rossier, J., French, E., Rivier, C., Ling, N., Guillemin, R., and Bloom, F.E., 1977, Foot-shock induced stress increases beta-endorphin levels in blood but not brain, Nature, 270:618.

Schweigerer, L., Bhakdi, S., and Teschemacher, H., 1982, Specific non-opiate binding sites for human beta-endorphin on the terminal complex of human complement, Nature, 296:572.

Selye, H., 1956, " The stress of life," McGraw-Hill, New York.

Shavit, Y. Lewis, J.W., Terman, G.W., Gale, R.P., and Liebeskind, J.C., 1984, Opioid peptides mediate the suppressive effect of stress on natural killer cell cytotoxicity, Sci., 223:188.

Shavit, Y., Lewis, J.W., Terman, G.W., Gale, R.P., Liebeskind, J.C., 1983, Endogenous opiates may mediate the effects of stress on tumor growth and immune function, Proc. West. Pharmacol. Soc., 26:53.

Simpkins, C.O., Dickey, C.A., and Fink, M.P., 1984, Human neutrophil migration is enhanced by B-endorphin, Life Sci., 34:2251.

Sklar, L., and Anisman, H., 1979, Stress and coping factors influence tumor growth, Sci. 205:513.

Smith, A.D., and Winkler, H., 1967, A simple method for the isolation of adrenal chromaffin granules on a large scale, Biochem. J., 103:480.

Smyth, D.G., Parish, D.C., Normanton, J.R., and Wolstencroft, J.H., 1983, The C-terminal dipeptide of beta-endorphin: a neuropeptide with inhibitory activity, Life Sci., 33:575.

Stern, A.S., Lewis, R.V., Kimura, S., Rossier, J., Gerber, L.D., Brink, L., Stern, S., and Udenfriend, S., 1979, Isolation of the opioid hepta-peptide met-enkephalin-arg-6, Phe-7 from bovine adrenal medullary granules and striatum, Proc. Natl. Acad. Sci. (USA), 76:6680.

Terman, G.W., Shavit, Y., Lewis, J.W., Cannon, J.T., and Liebeskind, J.C. 1984, Intrinsic mechanims of pain inhibition: activation by stress, Sci., 226:1270.

Udenfriend, S., and Kilpatrick, D.L., 1983, Biochemistry of the enkephalins andenkephalin-containing peptides, Arch. Biochem. Biophys., 221:309.

Van Epps, D., Saland, L., Taylor, C., and Williams, R., 1983, In vitro and in vivo effects of beta-endorphin and met-enkephalin on leukocyte locomation, Prog. Brain Res.. 59:361.

Visintaner, M.A., Volpicelli, T.R., and Seligman, M.E.P., 1982, Tumor rejection in rats after inescapable or escapable shock, Sci., 216:437.

Weber, R.J., and Pert, C.B., 1984, Opiatergic Modulation of the Immune System, in: "Central and peripheral endorphins: Basic and clinical aspects," E.E. Muller and A.R. Genazzani, eds., Ravin Press, New York.

Wolfe, J.H.N., Saporoschetz, I., Young, A.E., O'Connor, N.E., and Mannick, J.A., 1981, Suppressive serum, suppressor lymphocytes, and death from burns, Ann. Sug., 193:513.

Wuster, M., Schulz, R., Herz, A., 1979, Specificity of opioids towards the mu-, delta- and epsilon-opiate receptors. Neurosci. Lett., 15:193.

Wybran, J., Appelboom, T. Famaey, J., and Gavaerts, A.M. 1979, Suggestive evidence for receptors for morphine and methionine-enkephalin on normal human blood T-lymphocytes, J. Immunol., 123(3):1068.

T-Cell E-RECEPTOR MODULATION BY OPIATES, OPIOIDS AND OTHER BEHAVIORALLY

ACTIVE SUBSTANCES

Robert Donahoe, John Madden, Felicia Hollingsworth,
David Shafer, and Arthur Falek

Department of Psychiatry, Emory University
and Georgia Mental Health Institute
1256 Briarcliff Road
Atlanta, Georgia 30306

INTRODUCTION

Homeostasis has been defined as a state of metastable equilibrium wherein the constancy of the internal milieu is forever being challenged [1,2] Using this definition, any antihomestatic stimulus may be regarded as a stressor [2]. As reviewed eleswhere [3,4], the neural and immune systems share many basic physiologic processes in response to environmental stressors. The ultimate purpose of the neuroimmune system is maintenance of homeostasis. Neurons and lymphocytes are pluripotent sensory cells [5] capable of eliciting and responding to various hormone and hormonelike peptides that have systemic and local effects characteristic of endocrine, exocrine, and paracrine functions. The primary physiologic basis for the adaptability of the neuroimmue system resides in a complex network of receptor-response systems. This review focuses on the means by which opiates and other behaviorally active substances, as examples of environmental stressors of known behavioral modifying capacity, can modulate receptor activity on T-cell lymphocytes. This capacity for receptor modulation appears to be a primary means by which opiates and like factors evoke both neurobiological and immunobiological changes in host physiology and responsive behavior.

FIRST EVIDENCE OF T-CELL E-RECEPTOR MODULATION BY OPIATES

About 5 years ago, Wybran et al. [6] reported that in vitro treatment of T-cells with morphine depressed their ability to form active and total E-rosettes with sheep erythrocytes (E). Similar treatment with methionine enkephalin enhanced active E-rosette formation. They demonstrated that these effects were reversible by the opiate receptor antagonist, naloxone, which confirmed their probable mediation through opiate receptors. Contemporary with these observations, McDonough et al. [7] from our laboratory demonstrated that T-cells of heroin addicts were similarly depressed in regard to total T-cell E-rosette formation and that this effect was reversible in vitro with naloxone. Table 1 shows recent data which indicates that active T-cell E-rosettes are also depressed in heroin addicts. In addition, Miller et al. [8] have shown that treatment of peripheral blood lymphocytes from cancer patients with methionine-enkephalin significantly enhanced active E-rosette formation. These observations have established that opiates and their endogenous congeners alter T-cell function by affecting expression of the E-receptor. We have since explored these phenomena through kinetic analyses of E-rosette formation.

Table 1. Effect of heroin addiction on active
T-cell E-rosette formation[a].

Experimental group	% Active E-rosettes
Addicts n = 21	18.6 ($\pm$ 10.2) ($p\leq$ 0.05)
Controls n = 11	30.1 ($\pm$ 10.4)

[a] Active E-rosettes were formed in accordance with procedures of Wybran and Fudenberg[11] with the following modifications: 25/1 E/T-ratio; centrifugation at 600 x g for 3 min; assessment of rosettes 2 min after centrifugation.

DESIGN OF KINETIC ANALYSES OF E-ROSETTE FORMATION

Various investigators[9,10] have reported methods for kinetic analyses of E-rosetting based on variations of the active E-rosette protocol of Wybran and Fudenburg[11]. However, these kinetic assessments did not account for events occurring in the earliest stages of binding of E to T-cells. Consequently, we developed assays to assess early interactions of E with T-cells. Our first approach to this end involved mixing of E with T-cells in a 25:1 E/T ratio along with 50% fetal bovine serum (heat inactivated and pre-adsorbed with E); incubating the mixture

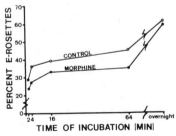

Fig. 1. Effect of in vitro treatment of leukocytes with 10^{-9}M morphine on the rate of E-rosette formation. The kinetic active E-rosette assay was used as described in the text.

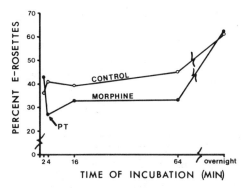

Fig. 2. Effect of in vitro treatment of leukocytes with $10^{-9}M$
morphine on the rate of E-rosette formation. The kinetic
active assay, adapted by first incubating cells on wet ice
for 10 min, was used.

for 5 minutes at 37°C; and then centrifuging at 2,000 x g for 20
seconds. By centrifuging rapidly for brief duration, assessment of the
kinetics of E-rosette formation was possible soon after E and T-cells made
initial contact. A typical result with this kinetic active assay, when
used to determine the effects of in vitro treatment of leukocytes with
morphine ($10^{-9}M$, 1 hr, 23°C before mixing with E), is shown in
Fig. 1. Morphine inhibited the extent and rate of active E-rosette
formation; but, unlike Wybran et al.[6], not the formation of total T-cells.

We then examined the effects of varying assay temperatures on
rosetting kinetics in the presence and absence of morphine. Using the
kinetic active assay as defined above, altered so that the reaction
mixture of E and T-cells was chilled on wet ice for 10 minutes before
initiating the 37°C incubation, we found that morphine actually enhanced
E-rosette number relative to the control (Fig. 2) at the 2-minute
assessment time in the kinetic procedure. However, this E-rosette
enhancement shifted to depression by 4 minutes which continued thereafter
throughout the portion of the kinetic curve representative of active types
of E-rosettes (up to 64 minutes). Again, no effect of morphine on total
T-cell E-rosettes was seen.

To understand how morphine could cause phase transition kinetics of
E-rosette formation by simply shifting pre-test incubation conditions as
in the preceding experiment (Fig. 2), we examined effects of thermal
changes on E-rosetting kinetics. In the kinetic active assay, the time
before the 37°C incubation step was regarded as the pre-incubation
stage. During this stage, cells are normally kept at room temperature
(~23°C). We changed these thermal conditions by holding cells on wet
ice until the start of centrifugation while eliminating incubations at
both 37°C and 23°C before centrifugation. For this procedure,
centrifugation was conducted at 4°C and at 600 x g for 3 minutes. In

291

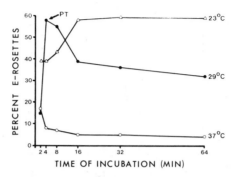

Fig. 3. Kinetic rates of E-rosetting measured with a 0-29°C kinetic
assay as described in the text. The different temperatures
represent the varied incubation conditions used during the
kinetic assessment phase.

this way, the cells were kept chilled throughout the assay up to the point
when kinetic assessments were begun. Then E-rosetting kinetics were
examined for purposes of determining the effects of variation in
incubation temperatures during the kinetic assessment stage, at either
23°C, 29°C, or 37°C. As shown in Fig. 3, kinetics of E-rosetting at
23°C were biphasic and devoid of phase transitions. At 29°C, kinetics
of E-rosette formation were multiphasic with obvious phase transitions
cycling between increases and decreases in E-rosette percentages. At
37°C, biphasic kinetics of the loss of E-rosettes through capping events
was apparent.

    This experiment defined conditions for a new type of kinetic assay
(the 0-29°C kinetic assay) that accentuates phase transition kinetics.
When this assay was employed along with variation in conditions of
centrifugation of E with T-cells, it was found that the magnitude
(amplitude) and duration (frequency) of phase transitions differed with
respect to the intensity of contact between E and T-cells. These
observations indicated that E modulate expression of their own T-cell
receptor as a function of thermal and physical conditions that affect the
ability of E and T-cells to initiate and maintain contact with each other.
This is a notable observation because self modulation of receptor activity
is a common feature in cell surface receptor-ligand systems[12]. Thus, we
found that centrifugation at 600 x g for 1 1/2 minutes in the 0-29°C
kinetic assay accentuated phase transitional kinetics of E-rosette
formation and that, under these conditions, morphine (10^{-9}M) caused
extension of the transitional phases of E-rosette formation and ultimate
depression of active E-rosetting (Fig. 4). This slowing or extension of
the phase transition effect identified with the way morphine affected
E-rosette formation when cells were first chilled on wet ice before the
kinetic active assay as in Fig. 2.

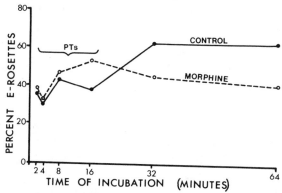

Fig. 4. Effect of in vitro treatment of leukocytes with 10^{-9}M on the rate of E-rosette formation with the 0-29°C kinetic assay adapted by centrifuging for 90 sec at 600 x g (see text).

AN EXPLANATION FOR THE PHASE TRANSITION PHENOMENON

As shown above, observation of phase transitions in the kinetics of E-rosette formation was owing primarily to judicious application of assay thermal and centrifugation conditions. Phase transitions in kinetics of E-rosette formation with untreated lymphocytes were only seen when active-assay thermal and centrifugation conditions were adjusted to accentuate this effect as in Figs. 3 and 4. However, in the presence of morphine, phase transitions were even more easily demonstrated if initial thermal conditions were cold, as in Figs. 2 and 4. Because of these thermal restrictions on expression of phase transitions, it was concluded that the portion of phase transitory kinetic curves wherein the percentage of E-rosettes was in decline was related to capping as described by Yu[9].

Capping involves the lateral mobilization of patched receptor-ligand complexes (E bound to the T-cell E-receptor) through the cell membrane into a cap at the polar end of the cell[9,13,14]. Patching and capping are both temperature dependent requiring physiologically warm conditions for their efficient expression, but only capping is energy dependent[14]. Following capping, E-rosettes are typically stripped from the cell as receptor-ligand complexes undergo endocytosis. T-cell E-rosettes are particularly susceptible to the processes of patching, capping and endocytolytic stripping because of their innate ability to serve as a receptor crosslinker.

Because of this probable involvement of capping in the phase transition phenomenon, we examined the kinetics of E-rosette capping. Yu[9] has described similar studies but did not document the very early events of this phenomenon. We studied kinetics related to 2-fold geometrically progressive increases in E-rosette assessment times beginning at 0.5 minutes. Total T-cell E-rosettes were generated by standard procedures[7] and placed in a water bath at 37°C. Then E-rosettes were evaluated at the appropriate intervals thereafter.

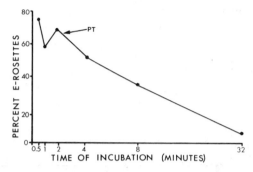

Fig. 5. Derosetting response generated by incubating total T-cell E-rosettes at 37°C before pellet disruption and E-rosette ascertainment.

Surprisingly, even during derosetting, phase transition kinetics were observed (Fig. 5).

Together, the preceding findings appeared somewhat dichotomous. When E-rosettes formed in the 0-29°C kinetic assay, there was a steady increase of E-rosettes with periods of intermittent losses of E-rosettes. On the other hand, when total T-cell E-rosettes were derosetted at 37°C, there was a steady decline in E-rosettes with intermittent periods where gain in E-rosette number occurred.

Explanation for these findings has been constructed in a model (Fig. 6) based on the assumption that E-receptor expression by T-cells is controlled by cytological processes of E-receptor microdisplacement (as originally defined by Bernard et al.[15], see later discussion) together with patching, capping and endocytolytic stripping of E-receptor-ligand complexes. It is assumed that a normal sample of peripheral blood lymphocytes is comprised of a variety of T-cells in various states of differentiation related in part to the level of expression of E-receptors[16,17], both in terms of affinity[18] and density[16]. Thus, lymphocytes initially exist in a receptor-level gradient. Within this gradient, some T-cells have a high density of high-affinity E-receptors. Others have lesser numbers of E-receptors on their surface and/or E-receptors of lower affinity. Under satisfactory thermal conditions, when E and T-cells make adequate contact for receptor-ligand binding, receptor microdisplacement processes that change the E-binding capacity of T-cells are activated so that more avid binding occurs across the T-cell gradient. T-cells lower on the E-receptor gradient would need time to reach optimal expression of ligand receptivity so that stable E-rosettes could form. This stability, however, would be dictated by thermal conditions. At temperatures of 23°C or lower (to 0°C) capping of E-rosettes would essentially cease and efficient microdisplacement of dormant E-receptors would result in accumulation of E-rosettes over time

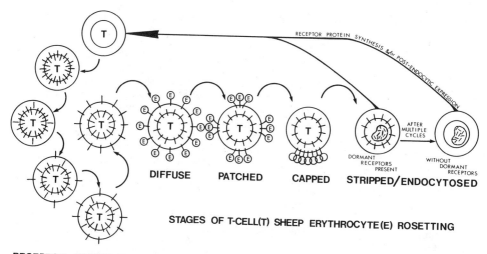

STAGES OF T-CELL(T) SHEEP ERYTHROCYTE(E) ROSETTING

RECEPTOR MICRODISPLACEMENT

Fig. 6. Gradient of T-cell receptor expression. Lines attached to the inner circles of T-cells represent E-receptors that are lying dormant within the cell membrane probably attached to a transducer-effector complex. Those protruding from the cell represent ligand-receptive receptors capable of binding E. Others are floating within the lipid bilayer in the process of being microdisplaced. This gradient correlates with phase transition kinetics in that T-cells accumulate rosettes after sufficient expression of E-receptors through microdisplacement (the gain portion of phase transitions); then the loss portion of the phase transitions will occur when thermal conditions are conducive to capping and endocytolytic stripping of E-rosettes. As long as these stripped T-cells have dormant E-receptors available for microdisplacement, the processes described for gaining and losing E-rosettes will occur cyclically. When dormant E-receptors are expended as the result of these processes new receptors will have to be synthesized and/or re-expressed from endocytic vesicles before new E-rosettes can be formed, and the gradient and receptor cycling re-activated.

(see Fig. 1-3). At 37°C, capping of E-rosettes would be so efficient that microdisplacement of E-receptors would occur too rapidly for detection, as in Fig. 3 where assessment of active types of E-rosettes was involved, or only be barely perceptible if total T-cell E-rosettes were examined through kinetic analysis of derosetting (Fig. 5). However, at temperatures intermediate between 23°C and 37°C (in our studies 29°C), the rates of E-receptor microdisplacement and E-rosette capping would be nearly equal allowing both processes to be observable in kinetic analyses of E-rosette formation as cyclical phase transition kinetics (Figs. 2-4). Thus, gain portions of the phase transition kinetics occur when dormant E-receptors are recruited into the rosetting process via microdisplacement processes. Losses occur when sufficient ligand-receptive receptors are constituitively expressed or have become expressed via microdisplacement of dormant receptors so that when these receptors bind E they will initiate patching, capping and endocytolytic stripping if thermal conditions are warm enough for the successful activation and maintenance of these post-binding processes.

As mentioned previously, capping of E-rosettes is a well documented phenomenon[9,13,14]. However, microdisplacement of E-receptors has not been studied intensively since originally described by Bernard et al.[15]. By using monoclonal antibodies that bind the 9.6 and D66 E-receptor epitopes, they[15] showed that E-receptors lying dormant within the sugar layer of the cell membrane assume a new molecular conformation after capping of E-receptors which makes them highly E-ligand receptive. They[15] also showed that microdisplacement and capping events can be cyclical, as we have seen by observations of phase transition kinetics of E-rosette formation and loss. Our kinetic E-rosetting data further show that the interdependency of microdisplacement and capping processes is related to the metabolic and physiologic state of the T-cell. Contrary to the need for active metabolic conditions requiring energy sources to drive capping events[14], we have seen that microdisplacement of E-receptors occurs efficiently at all temperatures between 4°C and 37°C; and, thus, that receptor microdisplacement appears not to be strictly reliant on capping. In fact, microdisplacement occurs most efficiently at cooler temperatures, as does E-rosetting. This circumstance probably relates to increases in membrane fluidity because of relaxation of metabolic constraints upon the lipid bilayer. Indeed, the division of T-cell biotypes into early (active, high affinity) E-rosette formers and late formers[6,18,19] is most likely a reflection of variable metabolic and physiologic constraints on E-receptor expression on one T-cell type versus another. These considerations also help explain why total T-cells, as determined by E-rosetting, require relatively long durations of incubation of E with T-cells and are best expressed when assayed at relatively cool temperatures (4°C usually, and up to 23°C). That is, given sufficient time and relaxation of metabolic and physiological constraints on E-receptor expression, enough E-receptors will become microdisplaced on all T-cells to allow for total T-cell E-rosette formation.

INTERPRETATION OF THE EFFECTS OF OPIATES ON E-ROSETTE FORMATION

In accordance with the E-receptor gradient model in Fig. 6, both the initial state of T-cells within this receptor gradient and their state during and after assay, as regards E-receptor expression, would be a reflection of the influence of various factors that affect homeostasis. Such factors as listed below would interdependently modulate the metabolic and physiologic set-points of receptor expression: 1. assay thermal conditions; 2. the intensity of the E-ligand and T-cell E-receptor interaction as dictated by the relative concentrations of each reactant and the centrifugal forces used to bring them into contact; 3. metabolites, ions and other nutrients in the assay medium; 4. presence of, or previous exposure of T-cells to drugs and the like which influence membrane functions either nonspecifically or through specific receptor-ligand interaction; 5. genetic restriction of receptor expression on the T-cell surface.

Opiates represent a type of factor as listed above in the fourth category. By examining the data in Figs. 1-5, it can be surmised that opiates affect E-rosette formation by altering the configurational expression of E-receptors through interference with their microdisplacement. This explanation accounts for the ability of opiates to both slow phase transition kinetics (Figs. 2 & 4) and the rate of E-rosetting (Figs. 1, 2, 4); and, also, for their ability to reduce the absolute number of active E-rosettes.

There are several observations about the physiological and metabolic changes that accompany binding of morphine to its receptor that support the possibility that morphine inhibits E-receptor microdisplacement.

Morphine receptors couple with adenylate cyclase through a guanine nucleotide-sensitive regulatory protein[20]. Much evidence supports the notion that coupling of membrane receptors and transducer-effector molecules of a variety of receptor systems occurs in a shared manner[21,22], which indicates that activation of coupling processes by morphine may result in coordinate coupling of both morphine receptors and E-receptors within the cell membrane. This coupling event could inhibit the ability of the E-receptor to undergo microdisplacement. An essential element in efficient coupling of receptors to their transducer-effector systems, at least with opiate receptors and others like them that are inhibitory for adenylate cyclase, is that Na^+ and GTP are required as cofactors[20]. This leads to the possibility that Na^+ fluxes are critical in determining the outcome of E-rosetting, especially under the influence of morphine. In fact, E-rosettes are poorly formed when the assay medium is deficient in Na^+ (unpublished data). The potential role of sodium is further suggested by the fact that receptor affinity for agonists is influenced by Na^+ concentrations[23]. Such effects could be mediated through receptor microdisplacement. Also, Na^+ has been reported to alter the reactivity of sulfhydryl groups at or near the binding site for opiates[24]. This finding, along with the fact that crosslinking of receptor-ligand complexes occurs through joining of sulfhydryl bonds[25], indicates that Na^+ may also be a controlling element in the E-receptor patching phenomenon, as also suggested by Yu[19]; and that such effects are relevant to the phase transition process. The notion of coupling of E-receptors and the potential role of Na^+ are represented schematically in Fig. 7.

AN EXPLANATION FOR THE NATURE OF ACTIVE E-ROSETTING ASSAYS

The nature of the active E-rosetting process is better understood because of the preceding considerations. For generation of the data for Fig. 1, thermal conditions of assay were identical to those used in 'classical' active E-rosetting assays, while, for the data in Fig. 2, cells were first chilled on wet ice (not held at room temperature, as was done for the data in Fig. 1) before active assay conditions were pursued (i.e., incubation at 37°C for 5 minutes before centrifugation). These thermal differences account for the ability of morphine to cause phase transitions in kinetics of E-rosette formation in the second experiment, but not in the first. Thus, it appears that the cooler conditions of the second experiment combined with an ability of morphine to slow E-receptor microdisplacement processes led to sufficient slowing of the phase transition processes to make them observable by kinetic assessment of E-rosette formation. This implies that in active assays, in situ (during centrifugation of E with T-cells), E-receptors normally cycle between dormancy, full expression consequent to microdisplacement, and endocytolytic stripping after formation, patching and capping of E-rosettes. However, this cycling is dependent on the initial warm thermal conditions promoted by incubating the cells at 37°C immediately before centrifugation. In this way, the cycling will stop during a late stage of centrifugation because the thermal conditions of centrifugation at that time will have reached ambient temperature of approximately 23°C which results in the essential discontinuation of capping processes. The consistency of results in active assays, therefore, appears to be dependent on the relative efficiency of the E-receptor cycling processes. Indeed, the findings of West et al.[18] that active assays are more reproducible if pelleted E and T-cells are incubated after centrifugation for 1 hour at 29°C (their high-affinity E-rosette assay procedure) are probably a consequence of the fact that these procedures promote stability of the E-receptor cycling processes under discussion here. Because of these interpretations, one can view active assays as a measure of the metabolic and physiologic equilibrium between microdisplacement and

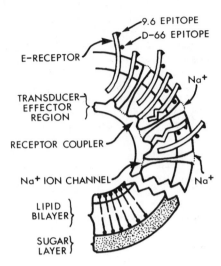

Fig. 7. Illustration of hypothetical receptor conformations in the T-cell membrane based on the observations of Bernard et al.[15]. This illustration is a magnified projection of what happens to E-receptors during their microdisplacement. Some E-receptors are linked to a transducer-effector complex, some are floating freely in various states of expression, and some are fully expressed. As shown by Bernard et al.[15], partial expression indicates that only the 9.6 E-receptor epitope is exposed at the cell surface while full expression requires that both the 9.6 and D66 epitopes be expressed. The latter fully expressed receptors bind E with high affinity. It is possible (see text) that binding of ligands such as E itself or morphine (not shown) to their respective T-cell receptors would activate physiological changes via opening of Na^+ channels, thereby modulating E-receptor coupling to a transducer-effector complex within the cell membrane and thus influencing the ability of the receptor to undergo microdisplacement.

capping processes. In this way, factors, like morphine, that inhibit active E-rosetting[6] can be envisioned as inducing metabolic and physiologic changes that inhibit microdisplacement while those, like enkephalins, which enhance active E-rosetting[6] enhance this receptor modulating process.

FURTHER EVIDENCE FOR RECEPTOR MODULATION BY BEHAVIORALLY ACTIVE DRUGS

In a recent study we showed that alcohol use by pregnant women and treatment of normal leukocytes in vitro with alcohol associate with enhancement in the rate of E-rosette formation[26]. We have also found that heroin use by addicts associates with enhanced expression of T4 markers on T-helper lymphocytes[27]; and that, if addicts also use cocaine regularly, depression in E-rosetting rate that is otherwise apparent can be reversed[28]. In conjunction with the information presented in this report, these observations suggest that modulation of receptors on the surface of T-cells is a characteristic property of behaviorally active drugs to which they are sensitive. Such conclusions identify well with the fact that enkephalins modulate E-receptor expression[6],[8] while endogenous opioids and other neurotransmitters and neurohormones are known to serve as modulators of neuronal receptors[3],[4],[29]. Likewise, these conclusions are compatible with the fact that alcohol modulates both E-receptor[26] and neuronal receptor expression[30],[31] through an apparent enhancement of the fluidity of cell membranes[30],[31]. Indeed, many receptor-ligand systems are autoregulatory[12],[21], as are E-receptors in response to E; and many are regulated by secondary receptor interaction[21],[22], as are E-receptors in conjunction with opiate receptors. These observations suggest that receptor modulation is a fundamental property of behaviorally active substances regardless of their tissue tropisms. These conceptualizations fit well with the notion that lymphocytes like neurons may be regarded as receptor-responsive sensory cells[5].

CONCLUSIONS

The foregoing discussion has indicated how study of the kinetics of T-cell E-rosette formation and loss can lead to better understanding of the cytological processes involved in receptor modulation. A new phenomenon of phase transition kinetics has been described which shows that E-receptors are regulated both independently and co-jointly with other receptors by processes of receptor microdisplacement along with patching, capping and endocytolytic stripping of receptor ligand complexes. It is possible that such findings identify microdisplacement processes with the concept of interconversion of receptor specificity and affinity as proposed to occur with mu and delta opiate receptors[32]. Notably, fibroblast receptors for insulin and epidermal growth factor have also been shown to undergo up-down regulation through capping processes[33] which further attests to the probability that our findings about E-receptor regulation can be generalized for most, if not all, cell surface receptor systems. Indeed, the link between up-down regulation of receptors and capping and endocytosis of receptor ligand complexes has been well established [22],[34]. This information indicates that homeostatic maintenance relates in large measure to the ability of an organism to alter its receptor expression in response to changes in its environment and consequently that the ability of stressors to cause aberrant changes in receptor expression might lead to homeostatic dysfunction and disease. In as much as the findings reported here show that modulation of receptor expression is often tantamount to modulation of the differentiation status of cellular elements of a given organism, the concepts presented in this report seem as relevant to the study of cell differentiation as they are for investigation of immunomodulation and behavioral expression.

Because the endogenous opioid system is activated during stressful situations along with adrenocorticotropin and cortisol production[35], the present findings are of particular relevance to understanding how stress events might precipitate immunological dysfunction. That is, one might suspect that chronically stress-induced opioids might alter T-cell functioning in much the same way as chronic heroin abuse has been shown to alter the differential expression of E-receptors[7] and T4 antigenic markers[27] with the possible effect of making heroin addicts more susceptible to opportunistic infections and cancers [27],[36].

E-receptors are physiological regulators of T-cell function which emphasizes their relevance in homeostatic regulation of immune response systems. They serve as negative feedback receptors for T-cell division[37] and are associated with the differential expression of thymocytes, and of T-suppressor/cytotoxic and T-helper/inducer lymphocytes[16,38]. E-receptors are also functionally linked to expression of the T-cell antigen receptor[39], Fc receptors[18,40], Ia antigens[40], gamma-interferon receptors[41] and interleukin-2 receptors[41,42]. Consequently, one can envision numerous ways by which E-receptor modulation might influence the normal functioning of T-cells as well as immune dysfunction. However, the complexities of T-cell function extend well beyond the inter-receptor linkages outlined here. T-cells have receptors for a variety of neurotransmitters and neuroendocrine hormones[3,4,6,43] as well as foreign antigens and numerous immunohormones and immunotransmitters. Therefore, it is likely that all these receptor-response systems interact to maintain homeostatic balance within the neuroimmune system and that the cytological mechanisms described in this report are broadly relevant in moderating these inter-receptor processes.

Recently Nadi et al.[44] showed that the familial association of affective disorder was genetically linked with enhanced expression of acetylcholine receptors. Such information leads to an appreciation of the potential importance of genetic restriction of receptor expression as a variable in determining the means by which individuals mount receptor-mediated responses to changes in their environment. This information in conjunction with the data and other conclusions in the present report indicate that future investigation into the mechanisms of homeostatic maintenance can profit considerably by detailed examination of the processes involved in receptor and inter-receptor function within the neuroimmune system.

REFERENCES

1. W. B. Cannon, Organization for physiological homeostasis, Physiol. Rev. 9:399 (1929).
2. T. L. Sourkes, Neurotransmitters and central regulation of adrenal functions, Biol. Psychiatry 20:182 (1985).
3. R. Ader, "Psychoneuroimmunology," Academic Press, N.Y. (1981).
4. R. Guillemin, M. Cohn, and T. Melnechuk, "Neural modulation of immunity," Raven Press, N. Y. (1984).
5. J. E. Blalock, The immune system as a sensory organ, J. Immunol. 132:1067 (1985).
6. J. Wybran, T. Appelboom, J.-P. Famaey, and A. Govaerts, Suggestive evidence for receptors for morphine and methionine-enkephalin on normal human T-lymphocytes, J. Immunol. 123:1068 (1980).
7. R. J. McDonough, J. J. Madden, A. Falek, D. A. Shafer, M. Pline, D. Gordon, P. Bokos, J. C. Kuehnle, and J. Mendelson, Alteration of T and null lymphocyte frequencies in the peripheral blood of human opiate addicts: In vivo evidence for opiate receptor sites on T lymphocytes, J. Immunol. 125:2539 (1980).
8. G. C. Miller, A. J. Murgo, and N. P. Plotnikoff, Enkephalin-enhancement of active T-cell rosettes from lymphoma patients, Clin. Immunol. Immunopathol. 26:446 (1983).
9. D. T. Y. Yu, Human lymphocyte receptor movement induced by sheep erythrocyte binding: Effect of temperature and neuraminidase treatment, Cell Immunol. 14:313 (1974).
10. D. T. Y. Yu, J. B. Peter, H. E. Paulus, and K. M. Nies, Human lymphocyte subpopulations. Study of T and B cells and density distribution, Clin. Immunol. Immunopathol. 2:333 (1974).
11. J. Wybran and H. H. Fudenberg, Thymus-derived rosette-forming cells in various human disease states: Cancer, lymphoma, bacterial and viral infections, and other diseases, J. Clin. Investig. 52:1026 (1972).

12. E. Loumaye and K. J. Catt, Homologous regulation of gonadotropin-releasing hormone receptors in cultured pituitary cells, Science 215:983 (1982).

13. E. R. Unanue, W. D. Perkins, and M. J. Karnovsky, Ligand-induced movement of lymphocyte membrane macromolecules. I. Analysis by immunofluorescence and ultrastructural radioautography, J. Exp. Med. 136:885 (1972).

14. G. B. Ryan, E. R. Unanue, and M. J. Karnovsky, Inhibition of surface capping of macromolecules by local anaesthetics and tranquilizers, Nature (London) 250:56 (1974).

15. A. Bernard, C. Gelin, B. Raynal, D. Pham, C. Gosse, and L. Boumsell, Phenomenon of human T-cell rosetting with sheep erythrocytes analyzed with monoclonal antibodies. "Modulation" of a partially hidden epitope determining the conditions of interaction between T-cells and erythrocytes, J. Exp. Med. 155:1317 (1982).

16. F. D. Howard, J. A. Ledbetter, J. Wong, C. P. Bieber, E. B. Stinson, and L. A. Herzenberg, A human T-lymphocyte differentiation marker defined by monoclonal antibodies that block E-rosette formation, J. Immunol. 126:2117 (1981).

17. R. B. Ashman, M. F. L. LaVia, S. Sawanabori, and A. J. Nahmias, Studies on the mechanism of E-rosette formation and inhibition, Clin. Immunol. Immunopathol. 16:39 (1980).

18. W. H. West, S. M. Payne, J. L. Weese, and R. B. Herberman, Human T-lymphocyte subpopulations: Correlation between E-rosette-forming affinity and expression of the Fc receptor, J. Immunol. 119:548 (1977).

19. D. T. Y. Yu, Human lymphocyte subpopulation: Early and late rosettes, J. Immunol. 115:91 (1975).

20. G. Koshki, R. Streaty, and W. A. Klee, Modulation of sodium-sensitive GTPase by partial opiate agonists. An explanation for the dual requirement for Na^+ and GTP in inhibitory regulation of adenylate cyclase, J. Biol. Chem. 257:14035 (1982).

21. C. R. Kahn, Membrane receptors for hormones and neurotransmitters, J. Cell Biol. 70:261 (1976).

22. M. Bornens, E. Karsenti, and S. Avrameas, Receptor mobility and its cooperative restriction by ligands, in: "Immunology of Receptors," B. Cinader, ed., Immunol. Series 6:41 (1977).

23. C. B. Pert, G. Pasternak, and S. H. Snyder, Opiate agonists and antagonists discriminated by receptor binding in brain, Science 182:1359 (1973).

24. E. J. Simon and J. Groth, Kinetics of opiate receptor inactivation by sulfhydryl reagents: Evidence for conformational change in presence of sodium ions, Proc. Natl. Acad. Sci. USA 72:2402 (1975).

25. E. Hazum, K.-J. Chang and P. Cuatrecasas, Role of disulphide and sulfhydryl groups in clustering of enkephalin receptors in neuroblastoma cells. Nature (London) 282:626 (1975).

26. J. J. Madden, R. M. Donahoe, I. E. Smith, D. E. Martinson, S. Moss-Wells, L. Klein, and A. Falek, Increased rate of E-rosette formation by T-lymphocytes of pregnant women who drink alcohol, Clin. Immunol. Immunopathol. 33:67 (1984).

27. R. M. Donahoe, J. K. A. Nicholson, J. J. Madden, F. Hollingsworth, A. Falek, D. A. Shafer, D. Gordon, and P. Bokos, Drug abuse, leukocyte antigenic markers, and AIDS, (submitted 1985).

28. R. M. Donahoe, J. J. Madden, F. Hollingsworth, D. A. Shafer, A. Falek, J. K. A. Nicholson, and P. Bokos, Immunomodulation by behaviorally active drugs provides a paradigm for connecting AIDS-like processes and psychoneuroimmunology, Proc. 1st Int. Workshop Neuroimmunol. (in press 1985).

29. W. Shain and D. O. Carpenter, Mechanisms of synaptic modulation, Int. Rev. Neurobiol. 22:205 (1981).

30. J. M. Hiller, L. M. Angel, and E. J. Simon, Multiple opiate receptors: Alcohol selectively inhibits binding to delta receptors, <u>Science</u> 214:468 (1981).

31. M. E. Charness, A. S. Gordon, and I. Diamond, Ethanol modulation of opiate receptors in cultured neural cells, <u>Science</u> 222:1246 (1983).

32. W. D. Bowen, S. Gentleman, M. Herkenham, and C. B. Pert, Interconverting μ and δ forms of the opiate receptor in rat striatal patches, <u>Proc. Natl. Acad. Sci. USA</u> 78:4818 (1981).

33. J. Schlessinger, Y. Shechter, M. C. Willingham, and I. Pastan, Direct visualization of binding, aggregation and internalization of insulin and epidermal growth factor on living fibroblast cells. <u>Proc. Natl. Acad. Sci. USA</u> 75:2659 (1978).

34. G. M. Edelman, Surface modulation in cell recognition and cell growth, <u>Science</u> 192:218 (1976).

35. R. Guillemin, T. Vargo, J. Rossier, S. Minnick, N. Ling, C. Rivier, C. Vale, and F. Bloom, β-Endorphin and adrenocorticotropin are secreted concomitantly by the pituitary gland, <u>Science</u> 197:1367 (1977).

36. J. D. Sapira, J. C. Ball, and H. Penn, Causes of death among institutionalized narcotic addicts, <u>J. Chron. Dis.</u> 22:733 (1970).

37. R. Palacios and O. Martinez-Maza, Is the E-receptor on human T-lymphocytes a "negative signal receptor"?, <u>J. Immunol.</u> 129:2479 (1982).

38. R. Mandle, R. E. Birch, S. H. Polmar, G. M. Kammer, and S. A. Rudolph, Abnormal adenosine-induced immunosuppression and cAMP metabolism in T-lymphocytes of patients with systemic lupus erythematosus, <u>J. Immunol.</u> 79:7542 (1982).

39. S. C. Meuer, R. E. Hussey, M. Fabbi, M. Fox, D. Acuto, O. Fitzgerald, K. A. Hodgdon, J. C. Protentis, S. F. Schlossman, and E. L. Reinherz, An alternate pathway of T-cell activation: A functional role for the 50 KD T11 sheep erythrocyte receptor protein, <u>Cell</u> 36:897 (1984).

40. G. Semenzota, G. Basso, V. Fagiolo, A. Pezzutto, C. Agostini, M. G. Cocito, and G. Gasparotto, Active and later rosette-forming cells: Immunological and cytochemical characterization, <u>Cell. Immunol.</u> 64:227 (1981).

41. M. Wilkinson and A. Morris, The E-receptor regulates interferon-gamma production: Four receptor model for human lymphocyte activation, <u>Eur. J. Immunol.</u> 14:708 (1984).

42. G. H. Reem and N. H. Yeh, Interleukin 2 regulates expression of its receptor and synthesis of gamma interferon by human T-lymphocytes, <u>Science</u> 225:429 (1984).

43. D. G. Payan, J. D. Levine, and E. J. Goetzl, Modulation of immunity and hypersensitivity by sensory neuropeptides, <u>J. Immunol.</u> 132:1601 (1984).

44. N. S. Nadi, J. I. Nurnberger, Jr., and E. S. Gershon, Muscarinic cholinergic receptors on skin fibroblasts in familial affective disorder, <u>New Engl. J. Med.</u> 311:225 (1984).

SIGNIFICANT ROLE OF RECEPTOR COUPLING IN THE

NEUROPEPTIDE-INDUCED ALTERATIONS OF MACROPHAGE CYTOTOXICITY

Gabriella Foris*, George A. Medgyesi**, and
Jozsef I. Szekely***

First Department of Medicine, University Medical School
Debrecen*, Institute of Heaematology and Blood Transfusion
Budapest** and Institute for Drug Research, Budapest***
Hungary

INTRODUCTION

Although in 1975 (Hughes et al., 1975) the year of discovery of the endogenous opiates, great expectations accompanied the research of these peptides, our knowledge regarding the central and peripheric effects of these compounds remain incomplete and superficial. Presumably the un-expected difficulties are due partly to the fact that the "secret" of the complex function of the opiate receptors has not been revealed, and on the other hand, some smaller peptide hormones derived from the large precursor molecules and displaying various biological effects could always confuse the interpretation of the essential processes.

In spite of the great amount of data regarding the function of the peptidergic system and published during the recent years, the exact role opioid peptides in the endocrine regulation cannot be defined unequivocally.

Obviously, nobody could predict 10 years ago that just the discovery of the opioid peptides would lead to the recognition of the fact that the peptidergic regulation of the neuroendocrine and the immune systems are closely related to each other. The serial discoveries of the recent years clarifying the immunomodulator functions of the opioid peptides on one hand, and the evidence showing that stimulated lymphocytes produce neuropeptides or neuropeptide-like factors on the other hand, may further stimulate both the endocrinological and immunological research activities.

This chapter will report on the results obtained when studying the effects of Met-enkephalin and its analogue D-Met^2-Pro^5 enkephalinamide on the peritoneal macrophages of rats. This type of study was also performed by using 2 other neuropeptides, angiotensin II and somatostatin, and the conclusion was reached that all these peptides affect the macrophages in a strongly similar way, and this effect resembles partly also that of the chemotactic peptides. The most important reason for such a similarity of their effect is probably the fact that all these peptides act through re-ceptors being negatively coupled to the adenylate-cyclase system, and this coupling determines unequivocally their effects on the phagocytic cells.

Obviously, it was possible to reach a correct interpretation of the similar effects of neuropeptides and chemotactic peptides only when considering the results of the recent years, which clarify the intracellular regulatory mechanisms of phagocytes.

INTRACELLULAR REGULATING MECHANISM OF PHAGOCYTIC CELLS (PC)

The two major types of PC dependent effector functions are the extracellular and intracellular degradation of antigen (target) following its adherence through specific receptors. The first step of this process is the binding of target (either directly or by the mediation of antibody and/or complement) to one or more specific receptors of PCs. In the next step, signals induced by receptors upon target binding trigger processes leading to the destruction of target. Depending on the cell type, the size and physicochemical nature of target, two different kinds of reaction -cascade may follow: 1. The incorporation of target gets started involving concerted changes in microfilaments (MF) and microtubules (MT) or, 2. The attached target remains fixed on the other surface of PC. In the former process membrane ruffling is followed by invagination and phagosome formation, whereas in the later case the lysosomes cumulate at the inner site of PC membrane. The participation of cytoskeletal elements in these early steps of effector functions are well documented. Cytochalasin B (CB) known to disrupt MF inhibits markedly all kinds of incorporation, rosette formation, however, is diminished only slightly by relatively high concentration of this drug. On the other hand, CB stimulates the extracellular cytotoxicit indicating that lysosome-migration is not MF-dependent process. Colchicin and Vinblastin which inhibit MT assembly are able to augment rosette formation even in low concentration with a subsequent inhibition of incorporation, whereas the ADCC (antibody dependent cellular cytotoxicity) of PCs are only slightly affected by these drugs (Oliver, 1978; Foris et al., 1981; Medgyesi et al., 1980, 1984). The accumulation of lysosomes in the proximity of phagosome seems also to be independent on cytoskeleton, therefore the later steps of effector functions are not affected by drugs which damage cytoskeleton (Lowrie et al., 1980).

What kinds of regulation operate in PCs, which affect surface receptors through the directed assembly/disassembly of cytoskeletal elements? During yeast cell phagocytosis in PCs an early enhancement of intracellular cAMP level was recorded (Stolz, 1981; Fülöp et al., 1984) and furthermore all drugs which stimulate adenylate cyclase as well as the lipophilic cAMP analogues are able to stimulate the rosette formation and the early phase of incorporation (Vogel et al., 1981; Oliver and Zurier, 1976; Ogmundsdottir and Weir, 1980; Hartwig et al., 1980). On the other hand, lysosomal enzyme release during the extracellular cytotoxicity and the fusion of lysosomes with the phagosomes during the phagocytosis are associated with a significant elevation of intracellular cGMP (Fülöp et al., 1984; Ogmundsdottir and Weir, 1980). Drugs, which stimulate guanylate cyclase and lipophilic cGMP analogues augment both extracellular cytotoxicity and the intracellular killing activity of PCs (Lowrie et al., 1980; Oliver and Zurier, 1976)

It should be pointed out that enhancement of effector function by stimuli elevating cGMP level is only partly accounted for the mechanism described above. Important messenger functions of cyclic nucleotides are directed to the oxidative processes, in so far as cGMP stimulates and cAMP inhibits the activation of NADPH oxidase (McPhah et al., 1983), an initial step in the respiratory burst. However, during activation of Fcγ receptors by immune complexes, Ca^{2+} influx into the cells ensues, although the phagocytosis does not depend on the extracellular Ca^{2+} content of medium, as the intracellular level of free Ca^{2+} may also be increased using intracellular pools (Onazaki et al., 1983).

Summarizing the data available on the intracellular regulating mechanism of PCs, specific receptors mediating effector functions appear to be coupled to adenylate cyclase resulting in a transient stimulation, which is followed by a switch of receptors to the inositol triphosphate -diacylglycerol system (Berridge, 1984). Therefore, agents recognized by specific receptors on the surface of PCs and consequently trigger intracellular messenger production, are able to modulate the effector functions of PCs.

ALTERATIONS OF PC FUNCTIONS BY NATURAL CHEMOTACTIC PEPTIDES (CP)

A wide variety of natural and synthetic peptides affect PCs through specific receptors in a similar way: they stimulate the phagocytosis through Fc and C3 receptors (Najjar and Nishioka, 1970; Foris et al., 1984a), induce respiratory burst, aggregation and spreading inhibition (Holian and Daniele, 1979; Fehr and Huber, 1984; Keller et al., 1976), positive chemotaxis and lysosomal enzyme release. Binding to their specific receptors these peptides cause Na^+ influx, K^+ and Ca^{2+} efflux from cells, and an elevation in intracellular free Ca^{2+} level by mobilization from the intracellular Ca^{2+} pools (Holian and Daniele, 1982; Gennaro et al., 1984). All these specific receptors are coupled positively to inositol triphosphate-diacylglycerol system resulting in increase of intracellular cGMP level (Berridge, 1984; Gilman, 1984). These CPs are of various origin, they may be cleaved from large molecules during the immue response such as C5a from complement component C5 (Damerau, 1978) tuftskin and other fragments from immunoglobulins (Najjar and Nishioka, 1970; Kolb et al., 1982) and CP s from lymphokine components (Honda and Havashi, 1982; Coleman et al., 1984; Foris et al., 1983c, 1983b). Lymphokine derived oligopeptides (isolated from rat lymphokine by purification on Sephadex G 150 column) in higher than 10 µg/ml concentrations stimulated phagocytosis by elicited macrophages through Fcγ and C3b receptors, whereas in lower than 10 µg/ml concentrations they inhibited the Fcγ receptor mediated engulfment of [51] Cr-labeled sheep erthrocytes (Foris et al., 1983c).

In the last decade, a large number of formyl and muramyl di and tri-peptides were isolated from bacterial cell walls (Wahl et al., 1979; Wilkinson, 1979) and in addition, their synthetic analogues were also prepared. For experimental studies the synthetic f-Met-Leu-He (FMLP) is applied the most frequently, since it has a pronounced influence on phagocytic cells under in vitro circumstances (Keller et al., 1981). FMLP exerts its effect on PCs through specific receptors with "high" and "low" affinity for the ligand, however, the former type of receptors are in strong and even morphologically recognizable association with the cytoskeletal structure of cells (Jesaits et al., 1984). The FMLP-triggered processes in PCs are similar or even identical with those which are induced by the natural CPs mentioned above.

The question arose about the physiological role of natural CPs released during the immune response either in circulation or in tissues? It is evident, that in consequence of their chemotactic effect they are able to accumulate PCs at the site of inflammation. Furthermore, their stimulating effect on the activity of both Fc and C3b receptors, as well as on the respiratory burst of PCs attach a great importance to these immune mediators. These peptides released from lymphokines, complement components and from immunoglobulins represent a significant amplifying mechanism that may be involved in the fine regulation of the effector cell functions during the immune response. It is reasonable to assume that they exert their effect more intensively at the site of their formation and that they are inactivated immediately or shortly after their generation by peptidases. Consequently, some of the most effective amino acid sequences might not have been determined so far.

As suggested by the earlier reviews of David and Remold (1976) it is possible that both "activating" and "inhibiting" peptides are released from lymphokines at the same time and site during the macrophage-lymphokine interaction. The same authors found the sensitivity of guinea pig macrophages to be increased in the presence of protease inhibitors such as soybean trypsin inhibitor, which acts only extracellularly. The assumption that peptides which are split from larger lymphokine components by macrophage proteases exert inhibitory effect on lymphokine induced activation, seems plausible.

Information on the role of these natural CPs beyond the immune system is scarce. As it is well documented, fragments released during complement activation (C3a, C5a, earlier called "anaphylatoxins"), may exert vasoconstriction at the periphery (Hugli et al., 1981). Furthermore, CPs are able to stimulate NA^+ leak-influx and consequently, the ATPase dependent Na^+ pumping mechanism (Korchak and Weissmann, 1980). Indeed, Na, K-ATPase stimulating factor or factors were demonstrated in sera of patients suffering from essential hypertension with low renin activity (Horky et al., 1984) and factor(s) was detected in supernatant of Concanavalin A-stimulated blood lymphocytes of the patients (unpublished data). Therefore, CPs or pepetides released together with CPs can also play some role in the development of essential hypertension. On the other hand, not only gamma interferon (Blalock and Smith, 1981) but also tuftsin and muramyl peptides exert morphin-like effects after intracerebral administration in mice (Herman et al., 1981; Krueger et al., 1984).

Summarizing the available knowledge about natural CPs, they are significant amplifying components of the immune response, but they may also have some undefined hormone-like effects outside the immune system.

GENERAL ASPECTS OF IMMUNOMODULATION BY OPIOID PEPTIDES (OP)

The immunodeficiency of morphine addicts has been known for a long time. However, because of the living conditions of these subjects, this observation could not be considered as an evidence of the immunosuppressive effect of morphine (Sheagran and Tuazon, 1977). On the other hand, both the immunosuppression caused in animals with large doses of morphine (Hung et al., 1973) and the existence of specific morphine receptors in leukocytes (Merishi and Mills, 1983) represents the most important proofs for a direct immunosuppressive effect of morphine. Moreover, morphine administration decreased the mean survival time of tumor bearing mice. Therefore, one may conclude that the immune system is suppressed unambigously by morphine (Fischer and Falke, 1985). In addition, OPs administered to animals and elevation of the OP level induced by stress, caused immunosuppression and an increase of tumor growth in most of the cases (Lewis et al., 1984). On the other hand, the survival time of mice treated with low doses of heroin increased after transplantation of neuroblastoma cells. It should be noted, however, that neuroblastoma cells possess also morphine receptors, therefore a direct effect of morphine on tumor growth may not be excluded (Zagon and McLaughlin, 1981). A significant increase in number of survivors was observed by Plotnikoff and Miller (1983), if BDF_1 mice inoculated with L 1210 cells were treated with enkephalins. It has been found that the subcutaneous injection of either methionine-enkephalin or leucine-enkephalin in healthy BDF_1 mice resulted in a significant increase in thymus weight and a significant decrease in spleen weight (Plotnikoff et al., 1984). According to the in situ model experiment of Moore (1984) carried out in sheep popliteal lymph node, the output of lympocytes increased under the effect of acute infusion of serotonin, substance P, bombesin, metenkephalin, isoprenaline and phenylephrine: all these compounds elevate cGMP level both in monocytes and the nervous tissue. Casale et al. (1984) demonstrated that the immediate skin response of healthy volunteers to endogenous OPs-occured as a consequence of mast cell degranulation. Similarly, in a number of in vitro experiments, it was found that opioid peptides stimulate leukocytes: lymphocyte proliferation (Gilman et al., 1982) and the number of active T cell rosettes obtained from healthy volunteers and lymphoma patients (Miller et al., 1984, 1983) were enhanced. In addition, OPs appeared to augment the natural killer activity of human lymphocytes in vitro (Faith et al., 1984; Mathews et al., 1983). Fischer and Falke (1985), have found a stimulated random migration of human granulocytes in the presence of beta endorphin, whereas Epps and Saland (1984), reported on the chemotactic effect of this peptide. Recently, Foris et al. (1984b), reported that Met-enkephalin stimulated the macrophage cytotoxicity by a calmodulin dependent process. Experiments with the opioid receptor antagonist naloxone suggest that both opioid and non-opioid receptors may be involved in this effect. Some of the multiple effects of OPs may be abolished by their antag-onist naloxone, however, specific opioid and also non-opioid receptors for beta endorphin were detected on human phagocytic leukocytes (Lopkor et al., 1980).

Despite the above contradictory findings, it can definitely be stated that OPs possess a significant immunomodulating effect (Weber and Pert, 1984; Faith et al., 1985). However, the immunomodulation may manifest itself either as a stimulation or a suppression, possibly dependent on the applied concentrations.

The main starting point of our study was that the OPs and also some other NPs have specific leukocyte receptors with positive coupling to inositol triphosphate-diacylglycerol system and possess a common mechanism of action. In lower concentration-range they have a stimulating effect on the immune system like the CPs, whereas the suppressive effect of the higher concentrations of OPs may represent a special kind of down regulation of their receptors.

COMPARATIVE STUDIES WITH THREE NEUROPEPTIDES (NP) ON THE EFFECTOR
FUNCTIONS OF ELICITED RAT PERITONEAL MACROPHAGES (PM)

The starting point of our work was an earlier finding in our laboratory, namely that oligopeptides obtained from a rat lymphokine (Foris et al., 1984c) had an effect on the Fcγ receptor mediated processes of rat PMs like angiotensin II (At II) (Dezsö and Foris, 1981; Foris et al., 1983a). In addition, both peptides have chemotactic activity (Honda and Hayashi, 1982; Goetzl et al., 1980). Experiments were carried out applying two further peptides which bind to specific receptor on the surface of leukocytes (Thomas and Hoffman, 1984; Bhathena et al., 1981) and which are well known immunomodulators (Weinstock and Kassab, 1984; Payan et al., 1984; Foris et al., 1985). Like At II, somatostatin (SS) and Met-enkaphalin (ME) exert their effect on target tissues through specific receptors which are coupled to the adenylate cyclase system in an inhibiting way, since all of the applied NPs affect their targets elevating the intracellular level of cGMP (Gilbert and Richelson, 1983; Wodcock and Johnston, 1982; Spada et al., 1984).

The IgG mediated phagocytosis and antibody dependent cellular cyto-toxicity (ADCC) of PMs are their most significant function in the defense against pathogens and tumor cells and they are regulated intracellularly by secondary messengers with help of cytoskeleton. We assumed that NPs like CPs may influence these effector functions altering cation transport and/ or triggering enzyme activities in phagocytic cells. In Fig. 1. the concentra-tion dependent effect of At II, SS and ME is demonstrated on the Fcγ receptor mediated phagocytosis and ADCC activity of rat PMs elicited by thioglycolate administration. Firstly, it should be noted that all of the applied NPs affected PMs in a similar way: in the 10^{-9}-10^{-7}M range of concentrations they stimulated the extracellular lysis of IgG2a coated ^{51}Cr-sheep erythrocytes, whereas their incorporation was diminished in the

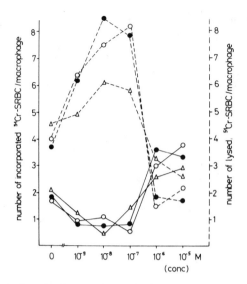

Fig. 1. The NP-induced alterations in Fcγ receptor mediated phagocytosis and ADDC of PMs after 60 min preinculbation. Experiments were carried out on PM monolayers applying IgG2a coated ^{51}Cr-sheep red blood cells (SRBC) as earlier described (Foris et al., 1983c). The target: effector ratio was 16:1. Each point represents the mean of six experiments. At II Δ, SS ● and ME ○.

same range of concentrations. By contrast, the ADCC activity of PMs was significantly decreased by higher concentrations of NPs (10^{-6}-10^{-5}M), and the incorporation of SRBC was augmented.

Furthermore, the intracellular killing capability of PMs was also found altered upon a 60 min pretreatment with NPs (Fig. 2.). Namely, At II, SS and ME in higher, phagocytosis stimulating concentrations (10^{-6}-10^{-5}M) markedly diminished the killing of [51]chromium labeled Candida albicians, whereas they had no effect on killing capability of PMs when applied in lower concentrations. The ability of oligopeptides to stimulate phagocytosis accompanied by a decreased intracellular degradation, may play an important role in the prolonged survival of pathogens during chronic infections as well as in the pathomechanism of different storage disorders. In Fig. 3. the total number of incorporated +lysed + adhered erythrocytes is demonstrated as a function of the hormone concentration applied. Data show that all of the applied NPs were able to increase the number of "affected" SRBCs only in the lower (10^{-9}-10^{-7}M) concentration-range, whereas when the higher concentrations were applied the number of these target cells was similar to the control levels or even slightly lower. The question arose therefore whether NPs induce an increase in the Fcγ receptor expression. As the capacity of PM monolayers to bind ^{125}I-IgG2a was not changed after treatment with the peptides (Table 1), NPs do not appear to affect the rosette formation, phagocytosis or ADCC by enhancing the number and/or affinity of Fcγ receptors, but by modulating the functional activity of these receptors possibly through the cytoskeleton. Although the ADCC activity enhancing effect of NPs applied in the 10^{-9}-10^{-7}M concentration range could have been explained by a functionally enhanced Fcγ receptor activity one should take into account that beyond receptor activity, ADCC depends on the production of biologically active oxygen species (BAOS) which play an essential role in both the intracellular and extracellular degradation of targets (Babior, 1984). In addition, various types of natural and synthetic CPs are known stimulants of BAOS production (Tanabe et al., 1983). Therefore, a study

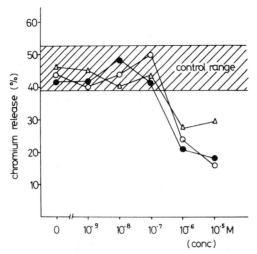

Fig. 2. The alteration of intracellular killing activity of PMs after 60
min preincubation with NPs. Experiments were carried out according
to the method of Yamamura et al. (1976) in the presence of 5% fresh
rat serum. ^{51}Cr release from Candida albicans was calculated as
percentage of total releasable radioactivity. At II Δ, SS ● and
ME o. Each value represents the mean of five experiments.

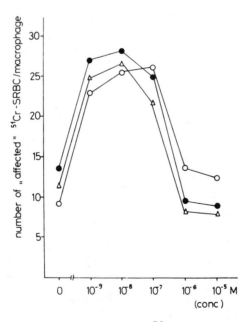

Fig. 3. The elevated number of "affected" ^{51}Cr-erythrocytes through Fcγ
receptors under the effect of NPs. The number of adhered + lysed +
engulfed erythrocytes was calculated as "affected" cells. Each point
represents the mean of five experiment. At II o, SS ● and ME Δ.
Experimental conditions see on Fig. 2.

Table I. The effect of NPs in different concentrations on the
^{125}I-labeled IgG2 a binding capacity of PM monolayers

^{125}I-labeled rat IgG2a^x bound (% of control)

conc M	At II	SS	ME
none	100.0	100.0	100.0
10^{-9}	96.3	108.6	89.6
10^{-8}	109.0	102.7	104.3
10^{-7}	100.5	95.3	96.5
10^{-6}	91.2	101.1	111.2
10^{-5}	98.8	93.8	94.8

^{x}IgG2 a was separated from rat immune sera according to the
method of Medgyesi et al. (1983). Each value represents the
mean of four experiments.

Summarizing the available data on the modulating effect of NPs on
phagocyte function, NPs stimulate macrophage ADCC in the 10^{-9}–10^{-7}M range
of concentration. Both an enhancement of Fcγ receptor activity and stimulation of respiratory burst may underlie this effect. In higher concentrations both ADCC and intracellular killing activity were inhibited by these
hormones in parallel with a suppression of superoxide anion production.

of the effect of NPs on superoxide generation looked warrented (Fig. 4.).
The effect of NPS was assessed on the phorbol myristate acetate (PMA)-
stimulated superoxide anion production of PMs, since the low level of the
spontaneously generated superoxide anion was not sufficient to study an
inhibiting effect. Indeed, all of the applied NPs enhanced markedly the
superoxide generation, i.e. the NADPH oxidase activity in rat PMs, but only
in the concentration range in which an ADCC stimulating effect was observed,
whereas the amount of superoxide anion produced was inhibited by higher
concentrations. These data are not easy to interpret as the most well
characterized CPs such as C5a and FMLP did not suppress BAOS production in
the same concentration range. On the other hand, some synthetic substrates
for peptidases such as N-benzoyl-L-tyrosine ethyl ester and L-1-tosylamide
-2-phenylethyl chloromethyl ketone exert a respiratory burst suppressing
effect on PCs, as a consequence of an increase in the H$^+$ concentration in
the extracellular space upon the cleavage of these substrates (Dri et al.,
1981; Kitagawa et al., 1979). The lowered pH at the outer site of membrane
inhibits the H$^+$ excretion from cells resulting in an enhancement of intracellular H$^+$ concentration (Lynn and Mohapatra, 1980). The activity of
glutathione peroxidase (GSH·Px) which is involved in the elimination of
the most significant BAOS, i.e. H_2O_2 (Baker and Cohen, 1983) was slightly
diminished by the higher (inhibiting ADCC and intracellular killing) concentrations of NPs. The present experimental data do not allow an answer
to the question, whether intracellular elevation of H$^+$ concentration exerts
its effect through inhibition of GSH·Px activity or affects NADPH oxidase
by a direct way. Baker and Cohen (1983) reviewed the problem of a feed
back mechanism between GSH·Px and NADPH oxidase as it was demonstrated in
granulocytes of rats fed by a selenium deficient diet.

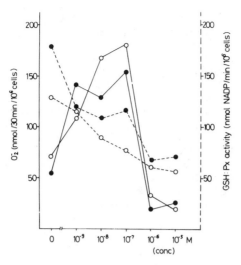

Fig. 4. The SS($\bullet$) and ME (o) induced changes in PM suspension O_2^- generation (——) and glutathione peroxidase (GSH·Px) activity (– –). The
GSH·Px activity was measured in the 30th min of incubation according
to the method of Holmes et al. (1970).

MECHANISMS WHICH ARE INVOLVED IN THE DUAL EFFECT OF OPs

Finding a correct explanation for the effects of the higher ME concentrations is a real challenge. On one hand, ME may be subject of enkephalinase present in the membrane of PMs and a decrease of BAOS production is
induced either by inhibition of H^+ excretion from cells or by releasing
biologically active break down products of ME. On the other hand, it was
reported by Gilbert and Richelson (1983) that delta opiate receptors which
are coupled inhibiting to adenylate cyclase in cultured murine neuroblastoma
clones and their glioma hybrids, after incubation with the high concentrations of ME may form clusters with a positive coupling to the adenylate
cyclase system. This change in the receptor coupling serves as a form of
down regulation at the post-receptor level without any reduction in the
number of affinity of delta receptors. As it was observed by the same
authors, cluster formation depends on the membrane fluidity of cells.
Prompted by these data, we determined the cyclic nucleotide level in PMs
during incubation with low (10^{-8}M) and high (10^{-6}M) concentrations of ME
(Fig.5.). The intracellular cAMP level was increased only in the presence
of 10^{-6}M) of ME with a peak in the 30th min of incubation. The cGMP level
rose progressively during the 120 min incubation period in the presence of
10^{-8}M of ME. This finding is in good agreement with the observations of
the above mentioned authors, that ME is able to stimulate adenylate cyclase
in higher concentrations through the guanylate cyclase stimulating delta
opiate receptors. (In Fig. 6.) the intracellular cAMP levels are presented
after 30 min incubation with different concentrations of ME and it was
evident that ME in 10^{-6}-10^{-5}M concentrations increased the adenylate
cyclase activity of PMs. In our system the altered receptor coupling was
abolished with the acetylated form of low density lipoprotein (LDL)
isolated from sera of healthy human volunteers. acLDL after binding to

scavenger receptors is endocytosed and degraded intracellularly with a subsequent increase of membrane cholesterol, i.e. membrane rigidity (Zechner et al., 1984). Cytochalasin B (CB) which disrupts the contractile elements of cytoskeleton and blocked in many cells all forms of receptor movement in the plane of membrane lipid bilayer also abolished the cAMP elevation induced by the higher concentrations of ME. To elucidate the role of enkephalinase in the ME-triggered adenylate cyclase activation, the effect of the known enkephalinase inhibitor puromycin (Hersch, 1982) was also investigated. Puromycin was found to abolish the cAMP increasing effect of ME in 10^{-6}M concentration. In addition, a potent ME analogue (D-Met^2, Pro^5) enkephalinamide (MP-EA) with high resistence against proteolysis (Bajusz et al., 1977) did not induce adenylate cyclase activation even in higher concentrations. Therefore, the change in the receptor coupling does not depend only on the membrane fluidity but also on ME processing by enkephalinase. Undoubtedly, ME appears to affect PMs through two different ways depending on the concentration applied, however, at this point of our experiments the mechanism of action induced by the higher concentrations, i.e. this special form of down regulation remains a puzzle.

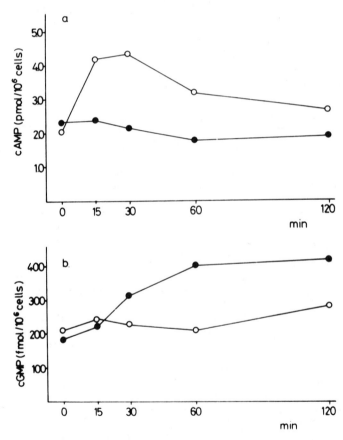

Fig. 5. The alteration of cAMP (a) and cGMP (b) level in PMs under the effect of 10^{-8}M (-•-) and 10^{-6}M (-o-) of ME. Each point represents the mean of four experiments. Experiments were carried out according to the method of Stabinsky et al. (1980).

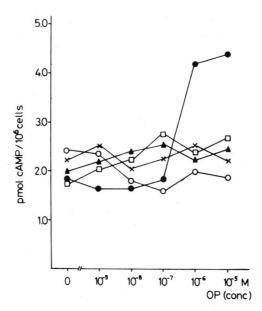

Fig. 6. The inhibition of ME induced cAMP elevation in PMs measured in the 30th min of incubation. ME alone ● , (D-Met^2, Pro^5) EA alone ▢ , ME 50 µg/ml acLDL x , ME + 5 µg/ml CB ▲ , ME + 10^{-5}M puromycin o . Each value represents the mean of four experiments.

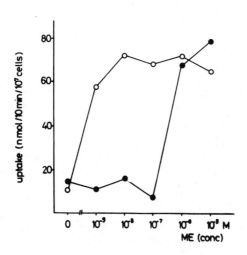

Fig. 7. The ^{22}Na$^+$ (o) and ^{45}Ca^{2+} (●) uptake by PM monolayers from the medium containing 140 Na$^+$, 5 K$^+$, 1.4 Ca^{2+}, and 1.2 Mg^{2+} Each value represents the mean of four experiments.

313

Examining the early cation uptake, ME was found to enhance the ^{22}Na$^+$ influx into cells when applied in low concentrations (found to activate guanylate cyclase). No. Ca^{2+} influx was found at the same ME concentrations (Fig.7.). However, a pronounced ^{45}Ca^{2+} influx was measured upon exposure of PMs to $10^{-6}-10^{-5}$M ME. One can conclude therefore, that opioid receptor clustering triggered by the higher concentrations of ME may induce Ca channel opening. Alternatively, binding a large amount of extracellular Ca^{2+} by the Ca^{2+} dependent enkephalinase in the presence of high ME concentrations can be assumed (Pant et al., 1982). To clarify the role of enkephalinase and of membrane fluidity dependent receptor clustering in the cAMP level elevating effect of the higher concentrations of ME, the enkephalinase activity of living PMs was measured applying fluorogenic substrate L-alanine-beta naphthylamide (ABNA). Enzyme which cleaves ABNA is the common peptidase for both ME and At II and in the presence of its natural substrates the cleavage of the synthetic substrate is markedly diminished (Fig. 8.). Thus, enhancing the concentration of ME in the system the enkephalinase activity of living PMs by the inhibition of cleaved beta naphtylamide may be determined. ME was able to inhibit the cleavage of ABNA only in the higher ($10^{-9}-10^{-5}$M) concentrations and this inhibition was not merely augmented by the addition of enkephalinase-inhibitor puromycin or EGTA (Hersch, 1982). The cleavage of ABNA was not inhibited by MP-EA, corroborating the earlier observed resistence of this analogue against peptidases (Bajusz et al., 1977). However, At II in 10^{-5}M concentration resulted a similar inhibition of ABNA-cleavage, the inhibition induced by ME and At II was not additive. It should be noted, that ABNA specific peptidase which was not inhibited by ME, At II or by puromycin was located in the lysosome fraction of PMs and it was inhibited by epsilon amino caproic acid (unpublished data). We assume that the crucial point of our observations is the abolition of Me induced inhibition of ABNA cleavage by both LDL and CB. In other words, both the normal condition of membrane fluidity and an intact cytoskeletal structure are required not only for cAMP elevation, but for the sufficient ME processing by enkephalinase. Based upon earlier results (Fig. 6.) that in the presence of $10^{-6}-10^{-5}$M of ME the increase in cAMP level was abolished by puromycin as well as our further observations about the role of membrane fluidity in the ME processing by enkephalinase indicate that both delta opioid receptor clustering and enkephalinase activity are involved in the modified signallization triggered by high concentrations of ME.

It has been pointed out, that enkephalinase of living PMs is able to cleave ME if its natural ligand is processed by clustered receptors. Consequently, if no receptor clustering has occurred, enkephalinase is not able to split ME. Ca^{2+} uptake resulted either by cluster formation of by enkephalinase activation may serve as trigger for adenylate cyclase stimulation. This hypothesis is corroborated by data of Fig. 9. in so far as the ME induced enhancement of ADCC was abolished by the opiate antagonist naloxone applied in 10^{-5}M concentration, whereas the inhibition of ADCC resulting from the higher concentrations of ME was not abolished by this drug. On the other hand puromycin, CB and acLDL inhibited markedly the concentration dependent decrease of ADCC activity, however, the nalaxone sensitive stimulation of ADCC remained unaltered by these agents. In addition, the enkephalinase resistent analogue MP-EA increased the ADCC even if it was added to the PMs in higher than 10^{-7}M concentration. Lastly, the calmodulin inhibitor trifluoperazine (Smith et al., 1981) abolished both suppressing and inhibiting effects of ME indicating the role of calmodulin in the ME-triggered alterations of effector functions.

Concluding our considerations, the unique form of receptor down regulation with change of receptor coupling appear by a good explanation for the dual effect of ME on phagocyte function which is observed both in vivo and in vitro.

314

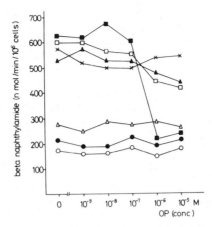

Fig. 8. The effect of various drugs on the enkephalinase activity of living
PM suspension measured by cleavage of fluorogenic substrate L-ala-
nine–beta naphthylamide (ABNA in the presence of different concentrations of ME.   The assay was performed in Hitachi–NK spectro-
fluorimeter at 480 nm ME alone ■, ME + 10^{-6}M At II Δ ME + 10^{-5}M
Puromycin ●, ME+5 mM EGTA o, ME+5µg/ml CB ▲, ME+50 µg/ml
acLDL x (D–Met,Pro/EA alone □.   Each value represents the mean
of four experiments.

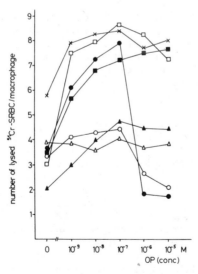

Fig. 9. The effect of various agents on the ME–induced alterations of ADCC
activity of PM–monolayers.   Each value represents the mean of five
experiments.   The monolayers were preincubated with different agents
for 30 min before the 60 min incubation with different concentration
of ME.
ME alone ●, 10^{-5}M naloxone+ ME o, 10^{-6}M trifluoperazine+ ME Δ,
50 µg/ml acLDL + ME ▲, 10^{-5} µ puromycin + ME □, 5 µg/ml CB + ME
x, (D–Met^2, Pro^5) EA alone ■.

315

Our investigations on human neutrophil granulocytes obtained from aged, arteriosclerotic and diabetic patients as well as from patients suffering from Alzheimer disease corroborated our assumption that one of the most vulnerable points in the regulation of phagocytic function is the post-receptor signallization (unpublished data). We suggest that this is also the case with opioid receptors. It must be kept in mind, that the final effect brought about by OPs is not only determined by their actual dose, but also individual changes of cellular sensitivity defined by the membrane fluidity and/or by the effective peptidase activity.

CONCLUSION

The in vitro effect of three neuropeptides (At II, SS and ME) was investigated on rat PMs elicited by thioglycolate provocation. All of the applied peptides equally affected PMs. In lower concentrations (10^{-9}-10^{-7}M) they markedly inhibited the phagocytosis through Fc γ receptors whereas the ADCC activity of PMs was stimulated by both the increased Fc γ receptor activity and the enhancement of oxidative processes. On the other hand, these NPs in higher concentrations (10^{-6}-10^{-5}M) inhibited both ADCC and intracellular killing capability of PMs possibly as a consequence of diminished respiratory burst of PMs.

In the case of ME the mechanism of this dual effect appear to be based on the presence of naloxone sensitive opioid receptors on PMs with negative coupling to adenylate cyclase. These receptors are able to form clusters and positive coupling to the adenylate cyclase in the presence of high concentrations of ligand. The incubation with higher concentrations (10^{-6}-10^{-5}M) of ME caused an elevation of the intracellular cAMP level which was abolished by acLDL, CB as well as by the enkephalinase inhibitor puromycin. Therefore we concluded that the adenylate cyclase stimulating (and consequently ADCC suppressing) effects of ME are caused by changes in the post-receptorial coupling. It should be noted that this type of coupling is strongly dependent on the actual state of the cell membrane fluidity and membrane-cyto-skeleton interaction. In addition, the enkephalinase activity of PMs may play a significant role in this special form of down regulation, because (D-Met, Pro) EA (an ME analogue with high resistence to enkephalinase) exerts only stimulating effect on PM cytotoxicity. Furthermore, puromycin as a potent inhibitor of enkephalinase, abolished the cAMP elevation and ADCC suppression induced by the higher concentrations of ME.

REFERENCES

Babior, B.M., 1984, The respiratory burst of phagocytes, J. Clin. Invest., 73:599.
Bajusz, S., Ronai, A.Z., Szekely, J.I., Graf, L., Dunai-Kovacs, Z., and Berzetei, I., 1977, A superactive antinociceptive pentapeptide, (D-Met^2, Pro^5) enkephalinamide, Febs Letters, 76:91.
Baker, S.S.,and Cohen, H.J., 1983, Altered metabolism in selenium deficient rat granulocytes, J. Immunol., 130:2856.
Berridge, MJ., 1984, Inositol triphosphate and diaclyglycerol as second messengers, Biochem. J., 220:345.
Bhathena, S.J., Loule, J., Scheitter, G.P., Redman, R.S., Wahl, I., and Recant, L., 1981, Identification of human mononuclear leukocytes bearing receptors for somatostatin, and glucagon, Diabetes, 30:127.
Blalock, J.E., and Smith, E.M., 1981, Human leukocyte interferon: potent endorphin-like opioid activity, Bioch. Biophys. Res. Commun., 101:472.
Casale, T.B. Bowman, S., and Kaliner, M., 1984, Induction of human cutaneous mast cell degranulation by opiates and endogenous opioid peptides: evidence for opiate and non opiate receptor participation, J.Allergy Clin. Immunol., 73:775.

Coleman, D.L., Culver, K.E., and Ryan, J.L., 1984, Enhancement of macrophage immune and non immune receptor mediated phagocytosis by a low molecular weight soluble factor from resident thymocytes, J. Immunol., 133:3121.

Damerau, B., Grünefeld, E., and Vogt, W., 1978, Chemotactic effect of complement-derived peptides C3ai, C5a (classical anaphylatoxin) in rabbit and guinea pig polymorphonuclear leukocytes, Naunyn-Schemeideberg's Pharm., 305:181.

David, J.R., and Remold, H.G., 1976, Macrophage activation by lymphocyte mediators and studies on the interaction of macrophage inhibitory factor (MIF) with its target cells, In: "Immunobiology of the Macrophage," D.S. Nelson, ed., Academic Press, New York, San Francisco.

Dezso, B., and Foris, G., 1981, Effect of angiotensin II on the Fc receptor activity of rat macrophages, Immunology, 42:277.

Dri, P., Berton, G., and Patriarca, P., 1981, A twofold effect of L-tosylamide-2-phenylethyl chloromethyl ketone on the oxidative metabolism of guinea pig phagocytes, Inflammation, 5:223.

Epps, D.E., and Saland, L., 1984, β endorphin and Met-enkephalin stimulate human peripheral blood mononuclear cell chemotaxis, J. Immunol., 132:3046.

Faith, R.E., Liang, H.J., Murgo, A.J., and Plotnikoff, N.P., 1984, Neuroimmunomodulation with enkephalins: enhancement of human natural killer (NK) cell activity in vitro, Clin. Immunol. Immunopathol., 31:412.

Faith, R.E., Plotnikoff, N.P., and Murgo, A.J., 1985, Effects of opiates and enkephalins-endorphins on immune functions, In: "NIDA Technical Meeting on Mechanisms of Tolerance and Dependence"(In Press).

Fischer, E.G., and Falke, N.E., 1985, β endorphin modulates immune functions In:"Psychotherapy and Psychosomatics, II," World Congress of the International College of Psychosomatic Medicine, (In Press).

Foris, G., Dezso, B., Medgyesi, G.A., and Bazin, H., 1981, Role of cytoskeleton in the Fc receptor activity of rat peritoneal macrophages, Int. Archs. Allergy appl. Immun., 65:138.

Foris, G., Dezso, B., Medgyesi, G.A., and Füst, G., 1982a, Effect of angiotensin II on macrophage functions, Immunology, 48:529.

Foris, G., Füst, G., and Medgyesi, G.A., 1983b, The effect of oligopeptides on the C3b receptor-mediated functions of rat macrophages, Immunol. Letters, 6:7

Foris, G., Hauck, M., Dezso, B., Medgyesi, G.A., and Füst, G., 1983c, Effect of low-molecular weight lymphokine components on the Fc and C3b receptor mediated macrophage functions, Cell. Immunol., 78:276.

Foris, G., Medgyesi, G.A., and Fust, G., 1984a, Regulating role of natural peptides in the Fc and C3b receptor mediated functions of resident and provoked macrophages, In: "Tissue Culture and RES," P. Rohlich and E. Baczy, eds., Publishing House of the Hung. Acad. Sci.

Foris, G., Medgyesi, G.A., Gyimesi, E., and Hauck, M., 1984b, Met-enkephalin induced alterations of macrophage functions, Mol. Immunol., 21:747.

Foris, G., Gyimesi, E., and Komaromi, I., 1985, The mechanism of antibody dependent cellular cytotoxicity stimulation by somatostatin in rat peritoneal macrophages, Cell. Immunol., 90:217.

Fülöp, T., Foris, G., and Leövey, A., 1984, Age related changes in cAMP and cGMP levels during phagocytosis in human polymorphonuclear leukocytes, Mech. Ageing Develop., 27:233.

Gennaro, R., Pozzan, T., and Romeo, D., 1984, Monitoring of cytosolic free Ca^{2+} in C5a-stimulated neutrophils: Loss of receptor modulated Ca^{2+} uptake in granule-free cytoplasts, Proc. Natl. Acad. Sci. USA, 81:1416.

Gilbert, J.A., and Richelson, E., 1983, Function of delta opioid receptors in cultured cells, Mol. Cell. Biochem., 55:83.

Gilman, S.C., Schwartz, J.M., Milner, R.J., Bloom, F.E., and Feldman, J.D., 1982, endorphin enhanced lymphocyte proliferative responses, Proc. Natl. Acad. Sci. USA, 79:4226.

Gilman, A.G., 1984, Guanine nucleotide binding regulatory proteins and dual control of adenylate cyclase, J. Clin. Invest., 73:1.

Goetzl, E.J., Klickstein, L.B., Watt, K.W.K., and Wintroub, B.U., 1980, The preferential human mononuclear chemotactic activity of the substituen tetrapeptides of angiotensin II. Bioch. Biophys. Res. Commun., 97:1097.

Hartwig, J.H., Yin, L., and Stossel, T.P., 1980, Contractile proteins and mechanism of phagocytosis in macrophages, In: "Mononuclear Phago-cytes," R. van Furth, ed., Martinus Nijhoff, The Hague, Boston, London.

Herman, Z.S., Stachure, Z., Opielka, L., Siemion, I.Z., and Nawrocka, E., 1981, Tuftsin and D-Arg^3-tuftsin possess analgesic action, Experientia, 37:76.

Hersch, L.B., 1982, Degradation of enkephalins: the search for an enkepha-linase, Mol. Cell. Biochem., 47:35.

Holian, A., and Daniele, R.P., 1979, Stimulation of oxygen consumption and superoxide anion production in pulmonary macrophages by N-formyl methionyl peptides, Febs Letters, 108:47.

Holian, A., and Daniele, R.P., 1982, Formyl peptide stimulation of super-oxide anion release from lung macrophages: sodium and potassium involvement, J. Cell. Physiol., 113:413.

Holmes, B., Prk, D.H., Malavista, S.E., Qui, P.G., Nelson, D.L., and Good, R.A., 1970, Chronic granulomatous disease in females. A deficiency of glutathione peroxidase, N. Engl. J. Med., 283:217.

Honda, M., and Hayashi, H., 1982, Characterization of three macrophage chemotactic factors from PPD-induced delayed hypersensitivity reaction sites in guinea pigs, with special reference to a chemo-tactic lymphokine, Am. J. Pathol., 108:171.

Horky, K., Schreiber, V., and Pribyl, T., 1984, Radioactive [86]Rubidium influx into red blood cells in essential hypertension in relation to the plasma renin activity, Horm. Metab. Res., 16:41.

Hughes, J., Smith, T.W., Kosterlitz, H.W., Fothergill, L.A., Morgan, B.A., and Morris, H.R., 1975, Identification of two related pentapeptides from the brain with potent opiate agonist activity, Nature, 258:577.

Hugli, T.E., Gerard, C., Kawahara, M., Scheetz, M.E., Barton, R., Briggs, S., Koppel, G., and Russel, S., 1981, Isolation of three separate anaphylatoxins from complement activated human serum, Moll. Cell. Biochem., 41:59.

Hung, C.Y., Lefkowitz, S.S., and Geber, W.F., 1973, Interferon inhibition by narcotic analgestics, Proc. Soc. Exp. Biol. Med., 142:106.

Jesaits, A.J., Naemura, J.R., Sklar, L.A., Cohrane, C.G., and Painter, R.G., 1984, Rapid modulation of N-formyl chemotactic peptide receptors on the surface of human granulocytes: formation of high-affinity ligand-receptor complexes in transient association with cytoskeleton, J. Cell. Biol., 98:1378.

Keller, H.U., Gerber, H., Hess, M.W., and Cottier, H., 1976, Studies on the regulation of neuthrophil chemotactic response using a rapid and releable method for measuring random migration and chemotaxis of neutorphil granulocytes, Agents and Actions, 6:326.

Keller, H.U., Wissler, J.H., and Damarau, B., 1981, Diverging effects of chemotactic serum peptides and synthetic f-Met-Leu-Phe on neutrophil locomotion and adhesion, Immunology, 42:379.

Kitagawa, S., Takaku, F., and Sakamoto, S., 1979, Possible involvement of proteases in superoxide production by human polymorphonuclear leuko-cytes, Febs Letters, 99:275.

Kolb, G., Köppler, H., Gramse, M., and Haveman, I., 1982, Cleavage of IgG by elastase-like protease (ELP) of human polymorphonuclear leuko-cytes (PMNL): isolation and characterization of Fab and Fc fragments and low molecular weight peptides stimulation of granulocyte function by ELP-derived Fab and Fc fragments, Immunobiol., 161:507.

Korchak, H.M., and Weissmann, G., 1980, Stimulus response coupling in the human neutrophil. Transmembrane potential and the role of extra-cellular Na⁺, Biochem. Biophys. Acta, 601:180.

Krueger, J.M., Walter, J., Karnovsky, M.L., Chediak, L., Choay, J.P., Lefrancier, P., and Lederer, E., 1984, Muramyl peptides. Vatiation of somnogenic activity with structur, J. Exp. Med., 159:68.

Lewis, J.W. Shavit, Y., Terman, G.W., and Gale, R.P., 1984, Stress and morphine affect survival of rats challenged with a mamary ascites tumor (MAT 31762B), Nat. Immun. Cell. Growth Regul., 3:43.

Lopkor, A., Abood, L.G., Hass, W., and Lionetti, F.J., 1980, Stereo-selective muscarinic acethylcholine and opiate receptors on human phagocytic leukocytes, Biochem.Pharmacol., 29:1361

Lowrie, D.B., Jackett, P.S., Aber, V.K., and Carol, M.E.W., 1980, Cyclic nucleotides and phagosome-lysosome fusion in mouse peritoneal macrophages, In: "Mononuclear Phagocytes," R. van Furth, ed., Martinus Nijhoff, The Hague, Boston, London.

Lynn, W.S., and Mohapatra, N., 1980, Control of leukocyte functions. Role of internal H⁺ concentration and a membrane-bound esterase, In-flammation, 4:329.

Mathews, P.M., Froelich, C.J., Sibbit, W.L., and Bankhurst, A.D., 1983, Enhancement of natural cytotoxicity by β endorphin, J. Immunol., 130:1658.

McPah, L.C., and Snyderman, R., 1983, Activation of the respiratory burst enzyme in human polymorphonuclear leukocytes by chemoattractants and other soluble stimuli, J. Clin. Invest., 72:192.

Medgyesi, G.A., Foris, G., Dezso, B., Gergely, J., and Bazin, H., 1980, Fc receptors of rat peritoneal macrophages: immunoglobulin class specificity and sensitivity to drugs affecting the microfilament and microtubule system, Immunology, 40:317.

Medgyesi, G.A., Miklos, K., Kulich, J., Fust, G., Gergely, J., and Bazin, H., 1981, Classes and subclasses of rat antibodies: reaction with the antigen and interaction of the complex with the complement system, Immunology, 43:171.

Medgyesi, G.A., Foris, G., Fust, G., and Bazin, H., 1984, Regulation of Fc receptor mediated functions of resident and provoked peritoneal macrophages, Immunobiol., 167:293.

Merishi, J.N., and Mills, I.H., 1983, Opiate receptors on lymphocytes and platelets in man, Clin. Immunol. Immunopathol., 27:240.

Miller, G.C., Murgo, A.J., and Plotnikoff, N.P., 1983, Enkephalins - enhancement of active T-cell rosettes from lymphoma patients, Clin. Immunol. Immunophathol., 26:446.

Miller, G.C., Murgo, A.J., and Plotnikoff, N.P., 1984, Enkephalins - enhancement of active T-cell rosettes from normal volunteers, Clin. Immunol. Immunopathol. 31:132.

Moore, T.C., 1984, Modification of lymphocyte traffic by vasoactive neuro-transmitter substances, Immunology, 52:511.

Najjar, V.A., and Nishioka, K., 1970, A natural phagocytosis stimulating peptide, Nature, 228:672.

Oliver, J.M., 1978, Cell biology of leukocyte abnormalities-membrane and cytoskeletal function in normal and defective cells, Am. J. Pathol., 93:221.

Oliver, J.M., and Zurier, R.B., 1976, Correction of characteristic abnor-malities of microtubule function and granule morphology in Chediak-Higashi syndrome with cholinerg agonist, J. Clin. Invest., 57:1239.

Onazaki, K., Takenawa, T., Homma, Y., and Hashimoto, T., 1983, The mechanism of macrophage activation induced by Ca^{2+} ionophore, Cell Immunol., 72:242.

Ogmundsdottir, H.M., and Weir, D.M., 1980, Mechanism of macrophage activa-tion, Clin. Exp. Immunol., 40:223.

Pant, H.C., Gallant, P.E., Gould, R., and Gainer, H., 1982, Distribution of calcium-activated protease activity and endogenous substrates in the squid nervous system, J. Neurosci., 2:1587.

Payan, D.G., Hes, C.A., and Goetzl, E.J., 1984, Inhibition by somatostain of the proliferation of T-lymphocytes and Molt-r lymphoblasts, Cell. Immunol., 84:433.

Plotnikoff, N.P., and Miller, G.C., 1983, Enkephalins as immunomodulators, Int. J. Immunopharmac., 5:437.

Plotnikoff, N.P., Murgo, A.J., and Faith, R.E., 1984, Neuroimmunomoduation with enkephalins: effects on thymus and spleen weights in mice, Clin. Immunol. Immunopathol., 32:52.

Sheagran, J.N., and Tuazon, C.U., 1977, Immunological aspects, In: "Drug Abuse. Clinical and Basic Aspects," S.N. Pradhan and S.N. Dutta, eds., C.V. Mosby Co., St. Louis.

Smith, R.J., Bowman, B.J., and Iden, S.S., 1981, Effects of trifluoperazine on human neutrophil function, Immunology, 44:677.

Spada, A., Vallar, L., and Giannatasio, G., 1984, Presence of an adenylate cyclase dually regulated by somatostain and human pancreatic growth hormone GH-releasing factor in GH-secreting cells, Endocrinology, 115:1203.

Stabinsky, Y., Bar-Shavit, Z., Fridkin, M., and Goldman, R., 1980, On the mechanism of action of the phagocytosis-stimulating peptide, tuftsin, Mol. Cell. Biochem., 30:71.

Stolz, V., 1981, Stimulatory effect of latex and zymosan particles on cAMP content in human granulocytes, Mol. Immunol., 18:773.

Tanabe, A., Kobayashi, Y., and Usui, T., 1983, Enhancement of human neutrophil oxygen consumption by chemotactic factors, Experientia, 39:604.

Thomas, D.W., and Hoffman, M.D., 1984, Identification of macrophage receptors for angiotensin: a potential role in antigen uptake for T-lymphocyte responses, J. Immunol., 132:2807.

Vogel, S.N., Weedon, L.L., Oppenheim, J.J., and Rosenstreich, D.Z., 1981, Defecive Fc-mediated phagocytosis in C3HeJ macrophages II. Correction by cAMP agonists, J. Immunol., 126:441.

Wahl, S.M., Wahl, L.M., McCarthy, J.B., Chedid, L., and Mergehagen, S.E., 1979, Macrophage activation by mycobacterial water soluble compounds and synthetic muramyl dipeptides, J. Immunol., 122:2226.

Weber, R.J., and Pert, C.B., 1984, Opiaterg modulation of the immune system, In: "Central and peripheral endorphins: basic and clinical aspects," E.E. Müller and A.R. Genezzani, eds., Raven Press, New York.

Weinstock, J.V., and Kassab, J. T., 1984, Angiotensin II stimulation of granuloma macrophage phagocytosis and actin polymerization in murine Schistosomiasis mansoni, Cell Immunol., 89:46.

Wilkinson, P.C., 1979, Synthetic peptide chemotactic factors for neutrophils: the range of active peptides, their efficacy, inhibitory and susceptibility of the cellular response to enzymes and bacterial toxins, Immunology, 36:579.

Woodcock, E.A., and Johnston, C.I., 1982, Inhibition of adenylate cyclase by angiotensin II in rat renal cortex, Endocrinology, 111:1687.

Yamamura, M., Boler, J., and Valdimarsson, H., 1976, A [51] chromium release assay for phagocytic killing of Candida albicans, J. Immunol. Meths., 13:227.

Zagon, I.S., and Mc Laughlin, P.J., 1981, Heroin prolongs survival time and retards tumor growth in mice with neuroblastoma, Brain Res. Bull., 7:25.

Zechner, R., Dieplinger, H., Roscher, A., and Kostner, G.M., 1984, The low density lipoprote in pathway of native and chemically modified low density lipoprotein isolated from plasma incubated in vitro, Biochem. J., 224:569.

HORMONAL MODULATION OF THE HUMAN AUTOLOGOUS MIXED LYMPHOCYTE REACTION

Georges J.M. Maestroni

Laboratory of Cellular Pathology
Istituto cantonale di patologia
6604 Locarno, Switzerland

INTRODUCTION

"Mens sana in corpore sano". This roman proverb expresses beautifully the ancient recognition of the organism unity and it implies awareness of mutual influences between mind and body. As a consequence, it should not be surprising to find, in our analytical era, specific connections between the major homestatic device of the mind - the neuroendocrine system- and the major homestatic device of the body - the immune system. In fact, several years details of these connections are increasingly piled to give a complicated and still confusing picture. A rather exhaustive review of our knowledge of the field may be found in the recently published book "Psychoneuroimmunology" (R. Ader, ed., 1981). Most recently however, the field of neuroimmunomodulation has become fashionable and the list of neurohormones known to have important immunomodulatory properties has increased (Johnson et al., 1982; Mathews et al., 1983; Plotnikoff and Miller, 1983; Miller et al., 1984; Faith et al and Murgo et al., 1984). On the other hand, the already proposed view of lymphocytes producing messengers for the neuroendocrine system (Pierpaoli and Maestroni, 1977; Maestroni and Pierpaoli, 1981) has been further confirmed and detailed (Smith and Blalock, 1981; Smith et al., 1983). The mechanisms by which both the neuroendocrine and the immune system synergizes in order to preserve the organism from environment challenges are thus becoming slowly clearer. The so called psychosomatic integrity appears as a finely tuned balance of neuroendocrine and immune interactions. It becomes also more conceivable that a deranged or exaggerated psychoneuroendocrine response to environmental stimuli or a continuous exposure to stress events may lead to pathological alterations of the immune system.

Concrete examples of such situations might be those autoimmune diseases whose etiology clearly involves hormonal factors such as rheumatoid arthritis (RA) and systemic lupus erythematosis (SLE). As a matter of fact, most connective tissue autoimmune diseases are far more frequent in females than in males (Theophilopoulos and Dixon, 1982). For example, the incidence of SLE in sexually mature women is nine times that in men (Dubois, 1974).

The reasons for such differences are not clear but experimental and clinical evidence incriminate, at least in part, female hormones (Yocum et al., 1975; Lahita et al., 1970; Steinberg et al., 1979). Pregnancy and oral contraceptives are known to affect onset and development of autoim-

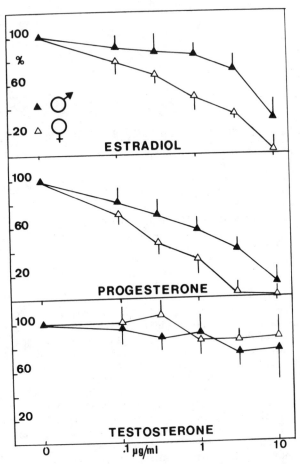

Fig. 1.   Sex steroid effect on the human AMLR- Human blood cells were
obtained from buffy coats of normal, healthy male and female
blood donors. Mononuclear cells were separated by Ficoll centrifugation and subsequently layered on discontinuous Percoll
gradients for the separation of T cells from non-T cells according to the method of Gutierrez et al. (1979). Two separate
fractions of T cells are obtained by this method. The cultures
were set up by mixing the non-T cell fraction with the second
T cell fraction.

One hundred μl of medium containing 10^5 non-T cells were added
to the same volume and to the same number of T lymphocytes in
round bottomed microplates. In order to be closer to a possible
in vivo situation, non-T cells were not irradiated. On the other
hand, irradiation was found not to affect the AMLR as reported
also by Katz and Fauci (1979). Culture medium was RPMI 1640
supplemented with 10% pooled serum from untransfused healthy
men, 2mM L-glutamine and 50 μl/ml gentamycin. Each culture was
set up in quintuplicate. The cells were incubated for 6 days at
37 C in a 5% CO_2 atmosphere before pulsing with 1 μCi/well.
Twenty hours later the cells were harvested and the activity
measured by liquid scintillation. The steroid hormones were
dissolved in 100% ethanol and then diluted in culture medium.
The volume added was 20 μl/well for any final concentration
tested. At the concentrations used, ethanol alone did not
affect the AMLR. The values represent the mean ± standard

mune diseases. For instance, RA is often ameliorated by pregnancy and oral contraceptives seem to lower significantly its incidence (Persellin, 1977; Vandenbroucke, 1982). Moreover, inability to cope with stressful stimuli has been listed amongst personality features of RA patients (Solomon, 1981). A sex specific difference in the neuroendocrine response to stress has also been shown (Frankenhauser et al., 1978).

On the other hand, amongst the various immunological abnormalities found in patients suffering from autoimmune diseases, a most interesting alteration of the in vitro T cell reaction in response to autologous antigens has been found to correlate with active phases of the disease. This in vitro T lymphocyte reaction is called autologous mixed lymphocyte reaction (AMLR) and has been found decreased in most autoimmune diseases as well as in other pathological situations including cancer (Weksler et al., 1981; Smith and deHoratius, 1982). The AMLR is the in vitro proliferation of T lymphocytes in response to autologous B lymphocytes and monocytes. It has been found in both experimental animals and man. The stimulation is mediated by HLA-DR or Ia glycoproteins and the response displays memory and specificity (Opelz et al., 1975; Weksler et al., 1981). Helper, suppressor and cytotoxic functions may be generated during the AMLR (Opelz et al., 1975; Miller and Kaplan, 1978; Smith and Knowlton, 1979; Weksler et al., 1981; Kotani et al., 1984). Thus the AMLR may represent basic immunoregulatory circuits taking place also in vivo. Helper and suppressor mechanisms may regulate humoral responses while cytotoxicity may serve a surveillance mechanism.

In this context we investigated the effect of steroid, pituitary and hypothalamic hormones on the human AMLR.

EFFECT OF SEX STEROID HORMONES

All the autologous cultures (AMLR) used for the experiments described in this chapter were set up by mixing peripheral blood T lymphocytes with autologous non-T cells isolated from buffy-coats of normal healthy female and male blood donors (see legend to fig. 1).

Here, different concentrations of progesterone, beta-estradiol and testosterone (Sigma Co., St. Louis, USA) were added to the cultures. The results are shown in fig. 1. Pharmacological concentrations of female sex steroid hormones (> 1 µg/ml) produced a significant ($P<0.01$) depression of the AMLR of both male and female cells. Similar effects have been already described in a variety of immunological in vitro models (Mendelsohn et al., 1977; Wyle and Kent, 1977; Herr, 1982). However, here it has to be noted that both progesterone and beta-estradiol depressed significantly ($p < 0.1$ and $p < 0.02$) more the AMLR of female than that of male cells. The inhibition produced by testosterone was weaker and no significant sex difference was apparent.

deviation of 3 experiments and are expressed as percentage of the ^{3}H-thymidine incorporation given by the relative controls. The depression of female AMLRs was significantly different from that of male cultures for estradiol ($p < 0.02$) and for progesterone ($p < 0.01$).

The human polypeptide hormones used in this study were a generous gift from the National Institute of Arthritis, Diabetes and Digestive and Kidney Diseases (NIADDK), Bethesda, Ma, U.S.A., except vasopressin (VP), oxytocin (OT) and somatostatin that were purchased from Sigma, Co., St. Louis, MO. USA. The human pituitary hormones growth hormone (GH), prolactin (PRL), follicle stimulating hormone (FSH), luteinizing hormone (LH), thyroid stimulating hormone (TSH), adrenocorticotropic hormone (ACTH), beta-lipotropin (β -LPH), alpha-endorphin (α -EN), VP, OT, estrogen stimulated neurophysin (ESN), nicotine stimulated neurophysin (NSN) and the hypothalamic tetradecapeptide somatostatin were tested at different concentrations for their effect on the human AMLR.

Table 1 illustrates the results of three experiments. The majority of the hormones tested did not affect the human AMLR, only ESN and NSN showed a decided inhibition. However, in contrast with the other hormones human neurophysins were sent by NIADDK already dissolved and containing 1 % NaN_3 as preservative. Therefore, in order to establish whether the observed inhibition was due to NaN_3 we performed experiments where similar dilutions of a NaN_3 solution were added to the AMLR as controls. NaN_3 is known to be an energy poison and therefore its profound inhibition of the human AMLR was not surprising. On the contrary, the surprising thing was that at certain dilutions the NaN_3-mediated inhibition was counteracted by the presence of ESN but not of NSN (table 2). These puzzling findings suggested continued studies in two directions. The investigation of a possible effect of NaN_3-free ESN was the first one. In order to get rid of NaN_3, ESN was exhaustively dialyzed against sterile phosphate buffer at 4 C and the dialyzate tested in the AMLR. The second approach was to go more deeply investigate the interesting NaN_3-ESN competition. The next paragraphs illustrates the results of these studies.

Human neurophysins: a brief description

Neurophysins are specific proteins of about 100 aminoacids synthetized in association with the well known neurohypophyseal nonapeptides arginine-vasopressin (VP) and oxytocin (OT). These hormone- bound proteins are packed with the hormones in neurosecretory granules and transported along axonal pathways to the site of secretion. Neurophysins are released into the blood stream and it is postulated that their secretion always accompanies hormone secretion. Two human neurophysins have been identified, nicotine-stimulated-neurophysin (NSN) and estrogen - stimulated-neurophysin (ESN). NSN secretion is associated to VP release while ESN is postulated to appear in plasma at times when would expect OT release (Robinson, 1978 a, b). Stress seems to inhibit ESN and stimulates NSN secretion (Robinson, 1978 a,b). The concentration of plasma ESN increases as response to pharmacological doses of estrogen and to physiological changes in estrogen. In fact, ESN is elevated in plasma of women on oral contraceptives (Robinson, 1974) and during pregnancy (Robinson et al., 1973). In spite of these interesting relationships of ESN with estrogen and of NSN with stressfull stimuli, no physiological function of circulating neurophysins is known.

Table 1. Effect of human polypeptide hormones on the AMLR

CONCENTRATION ng/ml

(% of ^{3}H-thymidine incorporation of controls $\pm$ SD)

HORMONES	10^{-3}	5×10^{-3}	10^{-2}	10^{-1}	0.5	1	5	10	50	10^2	5×10^2	10^3
GH				103$\pm$6	-	90$\pm$16	112$\pm$7	115$\pm$12	95$\pm$8			
PRL						106$\pm$19	-	101$\pm$9	100$\pm$4	93$\pm$6	120$\pm$7	
LH						98$\pm$11	-	110$\pm$9	87$\pm$9	89$\pm$11	104$\pm$16	
FSH								95$\pm$12	106$\pm$8	74$\pm$20	107$\pm$6	83$\pm$4
TSH								73$\pm$27	118$\pm$12	95$\pm$8	95$\pm$7	114$\pm$8
ACTH						68$\pm$32	-	78$\pm$25	90$\pm$36	89$\pm$30	78$\pm$12	
β-LPH						76$\pm$7	-	125$\pm$12	81$\pm$11	68$\pm$20	74$\pm$22	
δ-EN						94$\pm$33	-	76$\pm$33	108$\pm$12	73$\pm$25	89$\pm$31	
VP	112$\pm$20	92$\pm$8	89$\pm$16	123$\pm$30	98$\pm$10							
OT	78$\pm$18	102$\pm$9	91$\pm$4	107$\pm$8	102$\pm$11							
ESN				96$\pm$12	82$\pm$20	39$\pm$10	8$\pm$5	4$\pm$5				
NSN				35$\pm$7	19$\pm$3	5$\pm$6	6$\pm$2	5$\pm$3				
ST						79$\pm$20	102$\pm$13	97$\pm$23	87$\pm$20	85$\pm$29		

Cultures were set up with cells obtained from healthy blood donors. Hormone concentrations were chosen in order to include and exceed physiological plasma levels. The data represent the mean $\pm$ standard deviation (SD) of three experiments and are expressed as percentage of the values of ^{3}H-thymidine incorporation given after 6 days of incubation (see legend of fig. 1) by control cultures in which no hormone was added.

Table 2. Human, estrogen stimulated neurophysin prevents the NaN_3-mediated inhibition of the AMLR

Hormone concentration ng/ml	ESN + NaN_3 % of controls	NSN + NaN_3 % of controls	NaN_3 % of controls	NaN_3 concentration μg/ml
1	116+4	8+2	8+3	100
0.1	118+18	20+9	11+4	10
0.05	174+87	30+13	27+16	5
0.01	103+13	107+6	75+51	1
0.005	94+10	85+17	106+23	0.5

The hormones and NaN_3 were diluted in supplemented medium and the volume added was 20 μl/well for any final concentration tested. The values represent the mean $\pm$ standard deviation of three experiments and are expressed as percentage of ^{3}H-thymidine incorporation given by controls.

Concentrations of NaN_3-free ESN higher than that shown in table 2 were tested in the human AMLR. In the series of experiments performed with the first two neurophysins batches sent by the NIADDK we obtained encouraging results showing that ESN alone may affect the AMLR as reported in fig. 2. Physiological concentrations of human ESN significantly ($p < 0.005$) increased T cell proliferation during the AMLR.

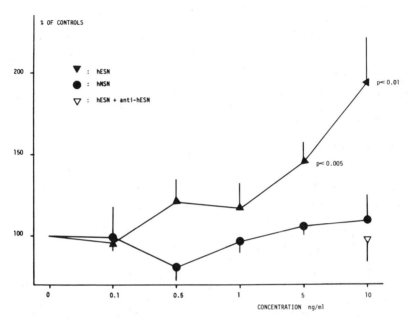

Fig. 2. Effect of ESN and NSN on the human AMLR - The values represent the mean ± standard deviation of 5 experiments and are expressed as percentage of the incorporation of ^{3}H-thymidine given by the relative controls. Cultures were set up with cells obtained from healthy donors. The AMLR was evaluated as described. The final dilution of the anti-ESN antiserum was 1:10,000.

IS THE MEMBRANE ENZYME ATPase (E.C.3.6.1.3) THE TARGET OF HUMAN ESN ?

At concentrations in the range of 10^{-1}-10^{-4}M, NaN_3 has been reported to interfere with a variety of membrane associated phenomena including inhibition of ATPase activity (Kobayashi, 1977) antigenic modulation (Schlesinger and Chaovat, 1972) and capping of surface immunoglobulins (Stackpole et al., 1978). ATPase activity is associated with energy utilization and ion transport. In particular the ATPase moiety showing sensitivity to the glycoside ouabain is known as Na^+, K^+ pump. The activity of this enzyme appears therefore fundamental for most cellular events. From the immunological point of view it seems that membrane receptors and ion transport mechanisms have important roles in lymphocyte activation leading to T-lymphocyte proliferation (DeCoursey et al., 1984). Increased production of interleukin 2 (IL 2) by stimulated normal human lymphocytes has been reported to occur in presence of 0.01 % NaN_3 (Feldman et al., 1983). Ouabain has been reported to inhibit mitogen or alloantigen activated T cells, production and utilization of IL 2 and binding of cytotoxic T cells to their target (Stoek et al., 1983).

By these considerations, the observed ESN-azide competition appears extremely interesting. In order to confirm the phenomenon, normal human peripheral blood mononuclear cells (PBMC) have been stimulated by suitable concentrations of pokeweed mitogen (PwM) in presence of various concentrations of NaN_3 or NaN_3+ESN and at three different concentrations of fetal calf serum (FCS). The results of this experiment are reported in table 3 and show that ESN is capable of reversing the NaN_3-mediated inhibition of B cell polyclonal stimulation. We have no explanation for the apparent correlation between FCS concentration and degree of the NaN_3-mediated inhibition (table 3). This result confirms that human ESN competes with azide at concentrations of the poison known to inhibits ATPase activity, therefore the enzyme ATPase might be, if not the cellular target of ESN, at least closely connected with it. This possibility was investigated by measuring the ouabain-sensitive and insensitive ATPase activity of normal human PBMC after addition of ESN and/or an equal amount of phosphate saline as control. Table 4 illustrates the results of these experiments and shows that ESN seems to interfere with the ouabain-mediated inhibition of the (Na,K) ATPase activity. Alternatively one might infer that ESN selectively stimulates the ouabain insensitive (Mg)ATPase activity while keeping the level of total ATPase constant.

ARE HORMONE-ASSOCIATED HUMAN NEUROPHYSINS THE ACTIVE AGENTS IN NIADDK PREPARATIONS ?

The experiments described above were performed using the first two batches of human neurophysins sent by NIADDK. The investigation was obviously continued in order to establish the modalities of the observed ESN effects on the AMLR. But with our great disappointment, the successive batches of NIADDK human neurophysins were found completely inactive. ESN apparently lost any activity in the AMLR and as azide inhibitor. At this point we reasoned that the activity previously observed might be due to contaminants contained in variable amounts in human neurophysins preparations. In fact, NIADDK human neurophysins are extracted from human neurohypophysis. Furthermore, neurophysins are synthetized in association with VP or OT. Hence, nobody may exclude that small and variable amounts of OT and/or VP "contaminate " some neurophysins preparations and that the activity observed was indeed due to these hormone-associated forms of ESN rather than to ESN alone. Both neurophysins bind OT and VP in vitro (Breslow, 1984). Therefore, different concentrations of OT and/or VP were mixed with a rather high concentration of ESN and NSN because of the low binding affinity at 37 C and physiological pH (Breslow, 1984). The mixtures were added to the AMLRs. The results are shown in fig. 3 and indicate that ESN-OT had the most significant although contrasting effects. OT-associated -ESN showed the ability of modulating human AMLRs. In fact, out of 10 AMLRs, 3 cultures were enhanced, 4 depressed and 3 unaffected by the presence of ESN-OT. Also, 2 cultures were enhanced and 2 depressed by ESN-VP. The ESN-OT dependent positive and negative alterations of the AMLRs were significant with a $p < 0.05$ (100 mg neurophysins / ml) if confronted with the values given by the other hormone combinations (fig. 3).
OT and ESN alone had no effect while anti-ESN antiserum completely abolished the ESN-OT action as shown in fig. 4. Also OT associated NSN never showed significant effects as well as the specific anti-NSN antiserum (Fig. 4). Therefore it seems that the immunomodulatory properties of OT-ESN mainly depended on the neurophysin, or perhaps on the precursor molecule of both OT and ESN. We cannot possibly know whether the stimulation given by the first batches of ESN depended on the presence of this precursor protein.

Table 3. ESN reverses the NaN$_3$-mediated inhibition of PwM-induced proliferation of peripheral blood mononuclear cells.

Hormone concent. ng/ml	FCS 1%		FCS 5%		FCS 10%		NaN$_3$ concent. µg/ml
	ESN+NaN$_3$ CPM±SD (% of control)	NaN$_3$ CPM±SD (% of control)	ESN+NaN$_3$ CPM±SD (% of control)	NaN$_3$ CPM±SD (% of control)	ESN+NaN$_3$ CPM±SD (% of control)	NaN$_3$ CPM±SD (% of control)	
0.5	73476±10522 (83%)	65056±2329 (72%)	57561±4073 (58%)	47061±6097 (47%)	49498±5559 (49%)	45449±4754 (45%)	50
0.1	99576±11141 (110%)	59106±3235 (65%)	69444±10610 (69%)	48303±5535 (48%)	64189±6218 (64%)	36293±2653 (36%)	10
0.05	100495±10085 (111%)	63216±5280 (70%)	89050±5328 (89%)	49266±4449 (49%)	89987±6525 (89%)	41724±7148 (41%)	5
0 (control)	90281±4758		9952±11591		100729±8804		0 (control)

The experiment shown is one of three experiments yielding similar results. FCS: fetal calf serum, CPM: counts per minute, SD: standard deviation.

Table 4. Human, estrogen-stimulated-neurophysin prevents the ouabain-mediated inhibition of the (Na,K) ATPase activity of peripheral blood mononuclear cells

	(Na,K,Mg) ATPase total ATPase	(Mg) ATPase ouabain-insensitive	(Na,K) ATPase ouabain-sensitive
	(nmole / hr / 10^6 cells)		
PBMC + 10 ng/ml ESN	77.79 $+$ 7.1	76.47 $+$ 8.9	1.33 $+$ 1.8
PBMC	72.41 $+$ 8.6	41.80 $+$ 1.9	30.71 $+$ 7.6

(Na,K,Mg) adenosine-triphosphatase (EC.3.6.1.3) and (Mg) adenosine triphosphatase were assayed according to the method described by Losa et al. (1982). The difference between the total and the ouabain-insensitive ATPase activity was considered as the activity of the ouabain-dependent (Na,K)ATPase. A preincubation was performed in duplicate at 37 C for 10 min in a total volume of 0.5 ml. $2x10^6$ human PBMC suspended in 0.2 ml of 0.9% NaCl were added to a mixture containing 1mM EDTA, 25 mM Tris-HCl buffer at pH 7.4 and 0.02% of Na-deoxycholate at this concentration allowed the maximal activity to be reached. A further incubation at 37 C for 30 min was performed after adding to the preincubation mixture 0.5 ml of an aqueous solution containing 10 mM $MgCl_2$, 6mM ATP-Tris, 100 mM NaCl, 40 mM KCl, 2 mM EDTA and 100 mM Tris, adjusted to pH 7.5. The reaction was stopped with 1 ml of ice-cold TCA 10%. After centrifugation, the inorganic phosphate was determined in an aliquot of supernatant by the method of Chen et al. (1956). Enzyme activity was expressed as nanomole of substrate liberated per hour and per 10^6 peripheral blood mononuclear cells (PBMC). The values represent the mean $+$ SD of three experiments. The hormone diluted in phosphate buffer pH 7.4 was added to cell suspensions 1 hr before initiating the assay. The same volume of phosphate buffer (10 μl) was added to the controls.

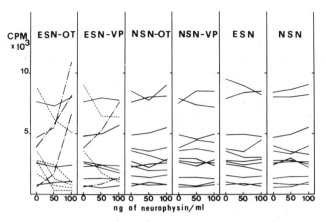

Fig. 3. Oxytocin-associated ESN modulates the human AMLR - Each curve
represent the data from one single AMLR performed in presence of
different concentrations of neurophysins and of OT and/or VP at a
given final concentration of 100 pg/ml. The values are expressed
in counts per minute (CPM) relative to the ^{3}H-thymidine incorporation after 6 days of culture. ——————— : no change,·————·———— :
significant (p < 0.05, 100 ng of neurophysin / ml) increase,
- - - - - - - -: significant (p < 0.02, 100 ng of neurophysin / ml)
decrease.

As a matter of fact, those previous preparations never inhibited AMLRs,
but this might depend on the relative small number of experiments performed. Anyhow, OT-associated ESN seems to possess powerful immunomodulatory
properties whose sense changes according to unknown individual variables. In
the attempt to investigate the nature of these variables, experiments were
devised in which human AMLRs were performed with a monocyte depleted non-T
cell fraction. Monocytes are known to have various influence on the AMLR.
The presence of monocytes has been reported to lower T cell proliferation
in the AMLR (Smolen et al., 1981) but, on the other hand, the Ia+ monocytes
subpopulation is known to stimulate the AMLR (Weksler et al., 1981). We
reasoned that the ESN-OT action might be mediated by monocytes, implying
that monocytes would have been the cellular targets of ESN-OT. However,
the results of such experiments were negative (data not shown). The presence or absence of monocytes did not change the sense and the extent of
the ESN-OT effect on the AMLR.
A recent paper by Kotani et al. (1984) reports that T lymphocytes that had
been activated for three days in AMLR helped PwM stimulated immunoglobulin
synthesis by autologous B cells. However, cells activated for 6 days preferentially exerted strong suppressor activity. It is thus conceivable that
intrinsic individual differences in functions activated in the AMLR may
account for the different sense of the ESN-OT mediated modulation. Inhibition of suppressor cell activation and stimulation of helper cell formation would have contrasting effect on proliferation (and thus on ^{3}H-
thymidine incorporation as measured in the AMLR) but an identical final

immunoregulatory effect. Experiments to investigate this important point are in progress. The first and simplest attempt consisted in adding the hormone-associated neurophysins to Concanavalin A stimulated PBMC. No effect was apparent in this model (data not shown). However, mitogen stimulated PBMC might be sensitive to higher concentrations of hormone-associated neurophysins. A similar situation is already known: physiological concentrations of corticosteroids almost abolish the AMLR while effect on alloantigen or mitogen stimulated lymphocytes (Ilfeld et al., 1977).

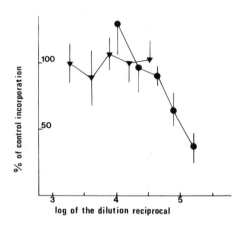

Fig. 4. Anti-ESN antiserum abolish the ESN-OT mediated effect on the AMLR
The curves represent the results of one AMLR in which different dilutions of anti-NSN and anti-ESN specific antisera were added to a given concentration of NSN+OT (100 ng/ml + 100 pg/ml) and of ESN+OT (100 ng/ml + 100 pg/ml). The values are expressed as percentage of the control cultures without antiserum and are the mean of the quintuplicate of each dilution tested ± standard deviation. Similar experiments gave identical results. The antisera were a gift from the NIADDK, Bethesda, Ma, U.S.A.
▲: (NSN+OT) + anti-NSN, ●: (ESN+OT) + anti-ESN.

CONCLUSIONS

Effect of steroid hormones

The most interesting observation is the sex difference in the steroid-mediated depression of the AMLR. Although the effect was apparent at rather high concentrations this sex difference seems to reflect a different cellular sensitivity to female steroid hormones. Estrogen receptors have been recently found on human lymphocytes (Danel et al., 1983), however it seems unlikely that hormone receptors are involved in our case because of the high level of the effective steroid concentrations. The major depression of the AMLR might thus express an intrinsic and receptor independent major weakness of female cells toward sex steroid hormones. It has been reported that human monocytes-macrophages produce a factor that protects lymphocytes from the direct toxic effect of corticoid hormones (Blomgren, 1974). As the composition of male and female AMLRs was very similar with respect to the concentration of monocytes, it follows that female monocytes might be less able to produce this factor. A deficient production of this factor would render lymphocytes much more sensitive to the effect of sex steroid hormones. The possibility that such a mechanism might play a role in autoimmunity deserves attention.

In general, depression of the AMLR might mean impaired regulation of immune responses and thus major susceptibility to disturbances such as autoimmunity. As a matter of fact it has been recently reported that 6 days long AMLRs as those performed in this study, preferentially express suppressor functions (Kotani et al., 1984). Depression of suppressor functions means enhanced immune responses and possibly autoimmunity. In this respect, the weaker depression of the AMLR given by testosterone may assume a particular relevance.

Effect of polypeptide hormones

Although interesting, the results of this section appears rather puzzling. First of all, human pituitary hormones previously reported to affect in vitro and in vivo immune responses as for example, GH, ACTH and endorphins (Ahlqvist, 1981; Solomon and Amkraut, 1981; Johnson et al., 1982; Mathews et al., 1983) had no effect on human AMLR. Then, the variable effects of ESN and of ESN-OT bring several questions to the fore.

We do not know whether the active batches of ESN contained OT or were "contaminated" by other substances or forms of precursor hormone that actually would be the covalent association of ESN with OT. However, ESN maintains a weak in vitro affinity for OT (Breslow, 1984). It is so conceivable that ESN and OT might act on their targets in the associated form.

Anyhow, the ESN or ESN-OT mediated activity seems important for a series of reasons:

a) Plasma concentration of ESN is elevated ($>$ 10 ng/ml) in situations such as pregnancy and use of oral contraceptives that are associated with changes in onset and development of autoimmune diseases (Persellin, 1977; Vandenbroucke et al., 1982).

b) Secretion of ESN and/or OT is inhibited by stress. Stress factors are clearly implicated in the etiopathogenesis of autoimmune diseases (Solomon, 1981; Solomon and Amkraut, 1981).

c) A poorly explained sex difference in normal immune responses is well recognized. Generally human and animal females respond significantly better than males to a given antigen.

COMMENTS

The individual variability of the effects shown by ESN-OT might reflect two situations: a basic inconsistency of the model used or real immunomodulatory properties. Further in vitro and in vivo investigations are clearly needed to answer this question. The ESN-OT affected immune functions, the cellular targets and the suggested ESN-ATPase connection have to be better defined and confirmed.

The confirmation of ESN dependent biological effects might mean more than a mere addition of a polypeptide to the list of neurohormones affecting in some way the immune system. The modulation of a putative immunoregulatory reaction (AMLR) by estrogen stimulated polypeptides might represent a neuroendocrine buffer against variations of the immune performance induced by other factors just as it may happen during the female hormonal cycle.

Chronic disturbance of this buffer system such as those that, for example, stress events may induce, might lead to basic alterations of the immune reactivity including autoimmunity.

ACKNOWLEDGEMENTS

I am grateful to Mrs. E. Hertens for her skillful technical assistance and to Miss T. Bacciarini for typing the manuscript. I thank Dr. A. Conti for the ATPase determination and Dr. D. Castelli with the technical staff of the Centro Trasfusione Sangue della Croce Rossa Svizzera for providing the buffy coats used in this study.

REFERENCES

Ahlqvist, J., 1981, Hormonal influences on immunologic and related pheno-
    mena, in: "Psychoneuroimmunology," R. Ader, ed., Academic Press,
    New York.
Blomgren, H., 1974, Steroid sensitivity of the response of human lympho-
    cytes to phytohemagglutinin and pokeweed mitogen: role of phagocytic
    cells, Scand. J. Immunol., 3:655.
Breslow, E., 1984, Neurophysin: biology and chemistry of its interactions,
    in: "Cell biology of the secretory process," M. Cantin, ed., S.
    Karger, Basel.
Chen, P. S., Toribara, T. Y., and Warner, H., 1956, Microdetermination of
    phosphorus, Anal. Chem., 28:1756.
Danel, L., Souweine, G., Monier, J.C., and Saez, S., 1983, Specific estro-
    gen binding sites in human lymphoid cells and thymic cells, J.
    Steroid Biochem., 18:559.
DeCoursey, T. E., Chandy, K. G., Gupta, S., and Cahalan, M. D., 1984,
    Voltagegated K$^+$ channels in human T lymphocytes: a role in mitoge-
    nesis ?, Nature, 307:465.
Dubois, E. L., 1974, The clinical picture of systemic lupus erythematosus,
    in: "Lupus erythematosus," 2nd edition, E. L. Dubois, ed., Univer-
    sity of Southern California Press, Los Angeles.
Feldman, S. P., Mertelsman, R., Venuta, S., Andreed, M., Welte, K., and
    Moore, A. S. M., 1983, Sodium azide enhancement of interleukin-2
    production, Blood, 61:815.
Frankenhauser, M., Rauste-von Wright, M., Collins, A., von Wright, J.,
    Sedvall, G., and Swahn, C. G., 1978, Sex differences in psychoneu-
    roendocrine reactions to examination stress, Psychosom. Med.,
    40:334.
Gutierrez, C., Bernabe, R. R., Vega, J., and Kreisler, M., 1979, Purifica-
    tion of human T and B cells by a discontinuous density gradient of
    percoll, J. Immunol. Meth., 29:57.
Herr, H. W., 1982, Effect of estrogen on the mixed lymphocyte reaction in
    normal individuals and prostatic cancer patients, The Prostate,
    3:17.
Ilfeld, D. N., Krakauer, R. S., and Blaese, M. R., 1977, Suppression of
    the human autologous mixed lymphocyte reaction by physiologic con-
    centrations of hydrocortisone, J. Immunol., 119:428.
Johnson, H. M., Smith, E. M., Torres, B. A., and Blalock, J. E., 1982,
    Regulation of the in vitro antibody response by neuroendocrine
    hormones, Proc. Natl. Acad. Sci. U.S.A., 79:4171.
Katz, P., and Fauci, A. S., 1979, Autologous and allogeneic intercellular
    interactions: modulation by adherent cells, irradiation, and in
    vitro and in vivo corticosteroids, J. Immunol., 123:2270.

Kobayashi, H., Maeda, M., and Anraku, Y., 1977, Membrane-bound adenosine triphosphatase of Echerichia Coli. IV effect of sodium azide on the enzyme functions, J. Biochem., 81:1071.

Kotani, H., Takada, S., Ueda, Y., Murakawa, Y., Suzuki, N., and Sakane, T., 1984, Activation of immunoregulatory circuits among OKT4+ cells by autologous mixed lymphocyte reactions, Clin. Exp. Immunol., 56:390.

Lahita, R. G., Bradlow, H. L., Kunkel, H. G., and Fishman, J., 1979, Alterations of estrogen metabolism in systemic lupus erythematosus, Arthritis Rheum., 22:1195.

Losa, G., Morell, A., Barandun, S., 1982, Correlations between enzymatic and immunologic properties of human peripheral blood mononuclear cells, Am. J. Pathol., 107:191.

Maestroni, G. J. M., and Pierpaoli, W., 1981, Pharmacological control of the hormonally mediated immune response, in: "Psychoneuroimmunology," Ader, ed., Academic Press, New York.

Mathews, P. M., Froelich, G. J., Sibbit, W. L., and Bankhurst, D., 1983, Enhancement of natural cytotoxicity by β-endorphin, J. Immunol., 130:1658.

Mendelsohn, J., Multer, M. M., and Bernheim, J. L., 1977, Inhibition of human lymphocyte stimulation by steroid hormones: cytokinetic mechanisms, Clin. Exp. Immunol., 27:127.

Miller, R. A., and Kaplan, H. S., 1978, Generation of cytotoxic lymphocytes in the autologous mixed lymphocyte culture, J. Immunol., 121:2165.

Miller, G. C., Murgo, A. J., and Plotnikoff, N. P., 1984, Enkephalins-Enhancement of active T-cells rosettes from normal volunteers, Clin. Immunol. Immunopath., 31:132.

Opelz, G., Kiuchi, M., Takasugi, M., and Terasaki, P. I., 1975, Autologous stimulation of human lymphocytes subpopulations, J. Exp. Med., 142:1327.

Persellin, R. H., 1977, The effect of pregnancy on rheumatoid arthritis, Bull. Rheum. Dis., 27:922.

Pierpaoli, W., and Maestroni, G. J. M., 1977, Pharmacological control of the immune response by blockade of the early hormonal changes follo-wing antigen injection, Cell. Immunol., 31:355.

Plotnikoff, N. P., and Miller, G. C., 1983, Enkephalins as immunomodulators, Int. J. Immunopharmac., 5:437.

"Psychoneuroimmunology," 1981, R. Ader, ed., Academic Press, New York.

Robinson, A. G., Archer, D. F., and Tolstoi, L. F., 1973, Neurophysin in women during oxytocin-related events, J. Clin. Endocrinol. Met., 37:645.

Robinson, A. G., 1974, Elevation of plasma neurophysin in women on oral contraceptives, J. Clin. Invest., 54:209.

Robinson, A. G., 1978a, Neurophysins, an aid to understanding the structure and function of the neurohypophysis, in: "Frontiers in Neuroendo-crinology," Vol. 5, W. F. Ganong and L. Martini, eds., Raven Press, New York.

Robinson, A. G., 1978b, Neurophysins, in: "Clinical Neuroendocrinology," L. Martini, and G. M. Besser, eds., Academic Press, New York.

Schlesinger, M., and Chaovat, M., 1972, Modulation of the H-2 antigenicity on the surface of murine peritoneal cells, Tissue Antigens, 2:427.

Smith, J. B., and Knowlton, R. P., 1979, Activation of suppressor T cells in human autologous mixed-lymphocyte culture, J. Immunol., 123:419.

Smith, E. M., and Blalock, J. E., 1981, Human Lymphocyte production of ACTH and endorphin-like substances: association with leukocytes interferon, Proc. Natl. Acad. Sci. U.S.A., 78:7530.

Smith, J. B., and DeHoratius, R. J., 1982, Deficient autologous mixed lymphocyte reactions correlate with disease activity in systemic lupus erythematosus and rheumatoid arthritis, Clin. Exp. Immunol., 48:155.

Smith, E. M., Phan, M., Coppenhaver, D., Kruger, T. E., and Blalock, J. E., 1983, Human lymphocyte production of immunoreactive thyrotropin, Proc. Natl. Acad. Sci. U.S.A., 80:6010.

Smolen, J. S., Sharrow, S. O., Roeves, J. P., Boegel, W. A., and Steinberg, A. D., 1981, The human autologous mixed lymphocyte reaction I suppression by macrophages and T cells, J. Immunol., 127:1987.

Solomon, G. F., 1981, Emotional and personality factors in the onset and course of autoimmune disease, particularly rheumatoid arthritis, in: "Psychoneuroimmunology," R. Ader, ed., Academic Press, New York.

Solomon, G. F., and Amkraut, A. A., 1981, Psychoneuroimmunological effects on the immune response, Ann. Rev. Microbiol., 35:155.

Stackpole, C. W., Jacobson, J. B., and Smith, M. P., 1978, Two distinct types of capping of surface receptors on mouse lymphoid cells, Nature, 248:232.

Steinberg, A. D., Melez, K. A., Raveche, E. S., Reeves, J. P., Boegel, W. A., Smathers, P. A., Taurog, J. D., Weinlein, L., and Duvic, M., 1979, Approach to the study of the role of sex hormones in autoimmunity, Arthritis Rheum., 22:1170.

Stoeck, M., Northoff, H., and Resh, K., 1983, Inhibition of mitogen-induced lymphocyte proliferation by ouabain interference with interleukin-2 production and interleukin-2 action, J. Immunol., 131:1433.

Theophilopoulos, A. N., and Dixon, F. J., 1982, Autoimmune diseases. Immunopathology and etiopathogenesis, Am. J. Pathol., 108:321.

Vandenbroucke, J. P., Valkenburg, H. A., Boersma, J. W., Cats, A., Festen, J. J. M., Huber-Bruning, O., and Rasker, J. J., 1982, Oral contraceptives and rheumatoid arthritis; further evidence for a preventive effect, The Lancet, ii:839.

Weksler, M. E., Moody, Jr. C. E., and Kozak, R. W., 1981, The autologous mixed-lymphocyte reaction, Adv. Immunol., 31:271.

Wyle, F. A., and Kent, J. R., 1977. Immunosuppression by sex steroid hormones I the effect upon PHA- and PPD-stimulated lymphocytes, Clin. Exp. Immunol., 27:407.

Yocum, M.W., Grossman, J., Waterhouse, C., Abraham, G. N., May, A. G., and Condemi, J. J., 1975, Monozygotic twins discordant for systemic lupus erythematosus, Arthritis Rheum., 18:193.

IMPLICATIONS INVOLVING AUTOIMMUNE MECHANISMS TO THE PCP RECEPTOR IN

SCHIZOPHRENIA

H.D. Whitten, K.Y. Tsang, P. Arnaud, N.K. Khansari, and
H.H. Fudenberg
Department of Basic and Clinical Immunology, Medical
University of South Carolina, 171 Ashley Avenue
Charleston, S.C.

INTRODUCTION

Substantial evidence indicates that autoimmune mechanisms may
either accompany or even precipitate some forms of psychoses. Such
findings include: 1. Up to 50% of systemic lupus erythematosus (SLE)
patients demonstrate some kind of neuropsychiatric disease; the most
commom symptom (psychotic alteration in behavior or thinking) is not due
to any known pre-existing psychiatric illness.[1] 2. The deposition of
immune complexes in the choroid plexus is common in such cases and often
has been shown to culminate ultimately in both DNA-anti-DNA antibody
complexes in the cerebrospinal fluid (CSF)[2] and lymphocytic perivascular
cuffing of small blood vessels in the frontal cortex and hippocampus.[1]
Interestingly, although CNS involvement usually develops late in the
course of SLE, it often occurs early and can appear as a sporadic
disturbance of mental function.[3] Thus, evidence exists supporting the
concept of altered blood-brain barrier permeability accompanying immune
complex disease.[1,4] In fact, Rudin has suggested that every SLE
patient would develop psychosis if other lethal complications were
avoided.[5] 3. Anti-brain antibodies are commonly detected in SLE and
schizophrenia. Bluestein[6] reported that 78% of SLE sera contain IgM
antineuronal antibody and 17% had IgG antineuronal antibody. Antibrain
antibodies have been detected in the sera and sometimes the CSF of 48%
of schizophrenics by Pandey and co-workers.[7] Others have found 17%,
25%, 21%, 29%, 86%, and 63%[8-14] depending on the sensitivity of the test
utilized for antibody detection. One of the most interesting studies
came from Luria and Domashneva[15] in which sera (1:32 dilution) of
schizophrenics demonstrated a 100% positive immunofluorescence toward
mouse thymocytes in contrast to no reactivity from healthy donors. This
finding was later confirmed and extended by Goldstein et al.[16]

Thus, it is apparent that the CNS choroid plexus blood-brain
barrier can at times be transgressed. Whether it be an emphatic assault
with overt lesion as in SLE or of a more subtle nature as in schizophrenia, the "target" antigen to which the immune response is directed may
be of paramount importance. The most obvious candidates for immune
attack in the psychoses would appear to involve one or more of the
neurotransmitter receptors. In this chapter, we chose to emphasize the
PCP(phencyclidine,"angel dust")receptor that may be akin or synonymous with
the sigma(σ) receptor for several reasons. First, it has been proposed

that PCP and adenosine may compete for a subpopulation of receptor sites in that adenosine receptor agonists have been shown capable of blocking the discriminative properties of PCP.[17] Interestingly, adenosine receptors are apparently localized to the axon terminals of the only excitatory type neuron in the cerebellum – the granule cell. The remaining four neuronal types are inhibitory in nature.[18] Second, the PCP receptor itself is a pharmacologically excitatory receptor (vide infra). Third, PCP reportedly induces diverse effects on several neurotransmitter systems.[19] And finally, a small but certain percent of PCP abusers are ultimately diagnosed as chronic schizophrenics. These individuals, although a very circumscribed patient group, may well comprise a unique model system in that symptomology follows the interaction of PCP with specific receptors on cells. This cell membrane sigma receptor site has been well characterized by binding, saturation, and inhibition studies[20-22] and is purportedly the prototype excitatory ligand among the five major pharamacological classes of opiate receptor.[23] The sigma receptor may well be a class of entities instead of a single receptor site at which chemically diverse psychoactive drugs can produce various effects; these include some benzomorphans as well as PCP and some of its analogs. Conceptual support for this resides in the fact that PCP-binding materials include; 1) cell membrane sigma σ receptor sites on brain slices and various neurotumor cell lines, 2) the alpha and delta subunits of the acetylcholine receptor, 3) a ninety-five thousand dalton synaptosome protein involved in potassium channeling, 4) a forty-three thousand dalton protein in the synaptosome of uncertain function and 5) low and high affinity binding sites within the synaptosome complex.[24,25] PCP-binding to any of these receptors might well result in an anti-receptor process, especially in genetically predisposed individuals. Interesting, the development of anti-nuclear antibodies in psychiatric patients chronically treated with chlorpromazine was strikingly increased in the HLA-BW44 type compared to non-BW44 controls.[26] A similar genetic susceptibility to PCP-induced psychoses is an intriguing possibility.

Most contemporary hypotheses concerning neurotransmission dysfunction in schizophrenia emphasize dopaminergic hyperactivity.[27,28] Schizophrenics who respond to anti-psychotic drugs have recently been speculated to possess "autoantibodies" which interact with and stimulate dopamine receptors.[29] However, dopamine receptors appear to be heterogeneous and the increased dopamine (D-2) receptors observed in the schizophrenic brain may be due to neuroleptic drug treatment. This has been experimentally confirmed in rats.[28] Yet, it is probable that these receptors are somehow linked anatomically or physiologically to the cell membrane sigma receptor since chronic PCP administration in vivo leads to a down regulation or diminution of dopamine and acetylcholine as well as PCP receptors.[30]

We have postulated also that some subsets of schizophrenia have an immune basis[31] in that multiple forms of schizophrenia may have deficiencies in receptor number and/or function in common. Human diabetes is the relevant analogy; one type is associated with high levels of antibody against insulin receptors; a second (insulin dependent diabetes) is associated with antibodies to the pancreatic islet cells producing insulin that arises in a genetically predisposed group after cell damage by cytomegalovirus infection; a third, adult-onset noninsulin-dependent diabetes, appears due to deficiency in numbers and/or affinity of insulin receptors. The second type is associated with pancreatic islet cell damage following coxsackievirus infection suggesting that both genetic prediposition (high incidence of the gentically determined histocompatability antigen, HLA-B8), and an environmental triggering agent (the virus) are prerequisites for development of diabetes.

In PCP-induced chronic schizophrenia, PCP might block a receptor which is normally present, so that a naturally occurring PCP-like "orphin" cannot bind to the PCP receptor. Candidates for such an endogenous ligand have been detected in preliminary experiments and tentatively termed "angeldustin".[20,31] Additional forms of chronic schizophrenia may result from other mechanisms including viruses whose "epitopes" (antigenic determinants) are partially similar to the receptor, analogous to the situation in which a selective affinity of rabies virus exists for the acetylcholine receptor.[32]

Other schizophrenia subsets might be analogous to autoantibodies to the receptor in myasthenia gravis (in which patients have antibodies to acetylcholine receptors), and some forms of "autoimmune" thyroiditis, in which patients have antibodies to the receptors for the thyroid stimulating hormone. Thus, we postulate that immunological parameters can be productively applied also to an analysis of the schizophrenic syndrome.

Antigenically distinct immunocytes regulate the immune response by simultaneously helping and suppressing and some share antigens with neural cells but no other body cells. In autoimmune disease a number or functional decrease of suppressor T cells is often accompanied by increased autoantibodies and immune complexes, i.e., agents interfering with suppressor cell physiology. Removal or inactivation of suppressor cells may induce the hypergammaglobulinemia observed in systemic lupus erythematosus (SLE). Suppression can be exerted by T cell and/or monocyte subsets; for instance, suppressor T cells are defective in human SLE[33-36] and certain monocyte subsets appear to suppress B cell function.[37] The decrease in suppressor T cell subsets and/or suppressor monocytes may culminate in increased autoantibodies.

The murine theta antigen is present on both T lymphocytes and brain cells (indeed on synaptosomes); also a monoclonal antibody against human suppressor T cells also binds specifically to oligodendrocytes[38] indicating the sharing of some brain cell surface structures with those of lymphocytes. Receptors for morphine and met-enkephalin have also been detected recently on a human T lymphocyte subset.[39] Also, the neurotransmitter "Substance P"[40] and beta-endorphin[41] have been shown to bind and stimulate proliferation of T lymphocytes and to greatly enhance natural killer cell activity, respectively. The specificity of binding of these ligands to these receptors was implied by the reversibility of binding in the presence of suitable concentrations of naloxone, an antagonist of the ligand drugs. These competition studies suggest that at least some of the drug binding sites on human lymphocytes are specific, identical or cross-reactive with opiate receptors and lend credence to the hypothesis that opioid receptors on lymphoid cells are likely to be similar in their physicochemistry to the brain receptors. Resolution of the enigmas of immunogenetic subgroups in some subsets of schizophrenia, of sigma and/or PCP receptor structure, and of susceptibility of some genetically defined groups to mental disorders may well be clarified upon scrutiny of the impact that these opioids have on particular immunocyte subpopulations.

Pharmacological studies have incriminated PCP as an indirect dopamine agonist in that PCP has been shown to release a pool of intracellular dopamine. Thus, PCP-induced chronic psychoses in humans and stereotypy in animals have been stated to respond to administration of dopamine receptor blockers.[27,29] Therefore, an alteration in the PCP receptor through direct stimulation or blocking effects by antibody binding might lead to symptoms similar or identical to that seen in schizophrenia. In addition, since PCP has been shown to bind and block the K^+ channels of synaptosomes, it may be that autoantibodies to this receptor might also prevent the naturally occurring endogenous ligand from binding to these sites. The knowledge gained from a scrutiny of the human PCP-induced schizophrenia model might be applied to an examination of endogenous ligand-induced autoimmune receptor alteration. Indeed, several investigators have emphasized that of those currently available the PCP-model most closely approximates human schizophrenia.[42,43]

In the transfer of information between nerve cells in schizophrenia, aberrations may well result from the selective blockage of certain potassium (K^+) channels in the brain cells or in the synaptosomes.[24,25] Recent startling and provocative studies indicate that PCP binds to such channels and can be used to photoaffinity label them. This binding of PCP to particular brain ion channels appears to increase the nerve impulse duration, leading to elevated amounts of released neurotransmitter. It is obvious that autoantibodies directed against such PCP-binding ligands could cause topographical rearrangements resulting in clustering and an imbalance in the local molecular environment leading to neurotransmitter release dysfunction.

Plotz[44] recently suggested that autoantibodies are in reality anti-idiotypic antibodies to antiviral antibodies. He suggested that a cell membrane receptor (designed for some particular cell function) is recruited by a virus for its own use and that to the extent that the viral structure is different from the host, it is a potential immunogen. The antiviral antibodies elicited will resemble in structure the host element with which the viral immunogen interacts. If these antiviral antibodies elicit anti-idiotypic antibodies (via heightened helper T cell or defunct suppressor T cell activity) some may be able to interact with the initial host receptor. It is a simple extension to envision that in addition to interacting with the neuronal sigma receptor and/or synaptosome K^+ channels, PCP could possibly have a similar effect on immunocyte populations if they possessed sigma-like receptors. It is interesting in this regard to note that purified B lymphocytes were the lymphocyte subpopulation most heavily labelled with [^{3}H]PCP (Table 2).

To determine if PCP (sigma) receptors were present on human peripheral blood lymphocytes (PBL), the NCB-20 mouse neuroblastoma-chinese hamster brain clonal hybrid cell line known to have sigma receptors was used as a prototype control sigma receptor positive cell line. The saturability of the receptor and the reversibility of binding (cold inhibition) were measured both in the NCB-20 cell line and in peripheral blood lymphocytes. The results of these experiments are shown in Figures 1 and 2. Interestingly, partial inhibition of PCP binding to lymphocytes was accomplished by lymphocyte preincubation with dopamine; this may indicate either the proximity of the dopamine-sigma receptor, partial identity, or an allosteric effect. Saturability and reversibility of PCP binding to the NCB-20 cell sigma receptor is similar to that of peripheral blood lymphocytes, indicating that sigma-like receptors are present on both cells. Therefore, it can be contended that human PBL possess sigma receptors approximating those on NCB-20 cells. Thus, the major difficulty of tissue availability in conducting research within the neuropsychiatric field can be circumvented by looking for opiate receptors on lymphoid tissues. In addition, adenosine receptors have been detected on human peripheral blood T cell and perhaps null cell subpopulations[45]. The activities of these receptors (PCP, dopamine and adenosine) are easily quantifiable with immunological parameters.

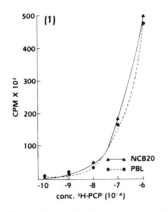 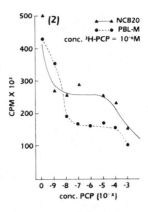

Fig. 1. Binding curve of radiolabelled PCP to peripheral blood lymphocytes and NCB20 neurotumor cells.

Fig. 2. Inhibition of binding of radiolabelled PCP by various concentrations of unlabelled PCP.

In other experiments, preliminary indications hint the existence of PCP-binding materials in both NCB-20 supernatants and normal human serum. When concentrated (100X) and incubated with [^{3}H] PCP, the following percentages (Table 1) of radioactive counts were found to be trichloroacetic acid (TCA) precipitable:

Table 1

Source (100X)	Incubation time (hrs)	Temperature (°C)	% counts ppt.
NCB-20 supernate	6	4	23
NCB-20 supernate	18	37	56
Human serum	6	4	35
Human serum	18	37	40
RPMI-1640 Media Control	6 and 18	4 and 37	0.2%

These above findings indicate that the sigma receptor positive NCB-20 cell line may be releasing their membrane PCP-receptors into the super- natant and can be compared with the results of Bailey and Zettner[46] using equilibrium dialysis; these investigators found that PCP can bind to some undefined component in normal human serum (more than 50% bound at 4°C). This binding apparently was not to α-globulins, γ-globulins (or albumin?) at the physiological concentrations of these proteins. These PCP-binding entities may have been circulating PCP receptors per se and the fact that γ-globulin containing immunoglobulin showed no binding does not negate the possibility that anti-PCP antibodies would be detected had the human serum been obtained from drug abusers and/or those with chronic PCP-induced psychosis. Further investigations in this area are underway in our laboratory.

Of further interest is our preliminary findings indicating that [^{3}H] PCP binds selectively to certain subpopulations of human T lympho- cytes (non-autologous rosette forming cells, non-ARFC) and to a greater extent to B cells (Table 2). The binding profiles of these "autologous" rosette forming T and B cells suggest that PCP can indeed interact with unknown consequences with certain immunocompetent cell subpopulations.

Table 2

[³H] PCP Binding* to Human Lymphocytes

Cells	CPM
ARFC-T	5,040 cpm
non-ARFC-T	34,731 cpm
B cells	88,671 cpm

*250 X 10³ cpm total added

[See Khansari, N., Whitten, H.D. and Fudenberg, H.H.: Phency-clidine (PCP)-induced immunodepression. Science 225: 76-78, 1984].

The small, but significant binding of ARFC-T is particularly interesting in that this T cell subpopulation appears to exert suppressor activity.[49] Although comprising a small percentage of peripheral blood lymphocytes, their numbers are greatly increased by Concanavalin A (ConA) activation. Hence the ARFC have been regarded as the ConA-inducible suppressor cell.[47,48] PCP-induced anomalies in their immuno-regulatory capacities could lead to autoantibody formation. Possible consequences of PCP-immunocyte interactions are shown in Figure 3.

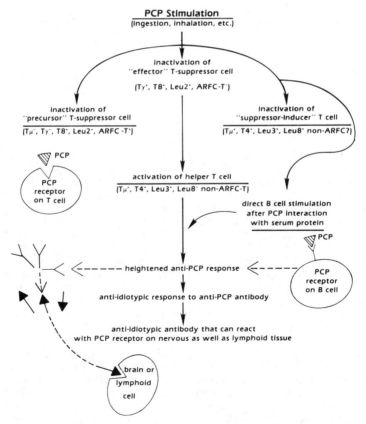

Fig. 3. PCP-immunocyte hypothetical interactions and sequalae.

Also an accelerated $^{86}Rb^+$ (K^+) release has been noted to be the
first physiologic event associated with the lethal hit on target cells
delivered by cytotoxic T lymphocytes.[50] If PCP should block lymphocyte
K^+ channels in an analogous fashion to that of synaptosome K^+ channels
(with resultant increased neurotransmitter production), then helper T
lymphocytes may well be induced by PCP to form excessive helper factors.
This too is a potential mechanism of autoantibody production. Currently
studies are underway to clarify these interactions and to investigate
the mitogenic activity of PCP on different lymphocyte subpopulations.

REFERENCES

1. D.A.S. Compston, "Neurological Disease", in: Immunology in Medicine
   Medicine, E.J. Holborow and W. Reeves, ed., Grune & Stratton,
   New York, N.Y. (1983).

2. R.J. Harbeck, A.A. Hoffman, S.A. Hoffman and D.W. Shucarel, CSF and
   and the choroid plexus during acute immune complex disease,
   Clin. Immunol. Immunopathol. 13:413 (1979).

3. R.T. Johnson and E.P. Richardson, The neurological manifestations
   of SLE, Medicine 47:337 (1968).

4. L.D. Petz, G.C. Sharp, N.R. Cooper and W.S. Irwin, Serum and CSF
   complement and serum autoantibodies in SLE, Medicine 50:259
   (1971).

5. D.O. Rudin, The choroid plexus and system disease in mental illness.
   II. Systemic lupus erythematosus: a combined transport dysfunction model for schizophrenia, Biol. Psychiat. 16:373 (1981).

6. H.G. Bluestein, Neurocytotoxic antibodies in serum of patients with
   with systemic lupus erythematosus, Proc. Natl. Acad. Sci. (USA)
   75:3965 (1978).

7. R.S. Pandey, A.K. Gupta and U.C. Chaturvedi, Autoimmune model of
   schizophrenia with special reference to antibrain antibodies,
   Biol. Psychiat. 16:1123 (1981).

8. R.T. Rubin, Investigation of precipitins to human brain in sera of
   psychotic patients, Brit. J. Psychiat. 110:84 (1965).

9. N.I. Kuznetoza and S.F. Semenov, Detection of antibrain antibodies
   in the sera of patients with neuropsychiatric disorders,
   Zh. Neuropatol. Psikhiatr. 61:869 (1961).

10. M. Yokoyama, E.G. Trams and R.O. Brady, Sphingolipid antibodies in
    animals and patients with central nervous system lesions, Proc.
    Soc. Exptl. Med. 111:350 (1962).

11. R.G. Heath and I.M. Krupp, Schizophrenia as an immunologic disorder.
    I. Demonstration of antibrain globulins by fluorescent antibody
    techniques, Arch. Gen. Psychiat. 16:1 (1967).

12. M. Stern, R. Anavi and J.P. Witz, Tissue-binding factor in schizo-
    phrenic sera: A clinical and genetic study. Biol. Psychiat.
    12:199 (1977).

13. R.F. Willikens, R.R. Whitaker, R.V. Anderson and D. Berven,
    Significance of antinuclear factors in older persons. Ann.
    Rheumatic Diseases 26:306 (1967).

14. N.I. Kuznetzova, "Some data concerning the immunological properties of brain mitochondria", in: "Biological Research in Schizophrenia", M. Vartanian, ed., Ordina Lennia, Moscow (1967).

15. E.A. Luria and I.V. Domashneva, Antibodies to thymocytes in sera of patients with schizophrenia. Proc. Natl. Acad. Sci. (USA) 71:235 (1974).

16. A.L. Goldstein, J. Rossio, G.I. Kolyeskina, L.E. Emory, J.E., Overall, G.B. Thurman and J. Hatcha, "Immunological components in schizophrenia", in: "Perspectives in Schizophrenia Research, C. Baxter and T. Melnechuk, eds., Raven Press, N.Y. (1980).

17. R.G. Browne and W.M. Welch, Stereoselective antagonism of phencyclidine's discriminative properties by adenosine receptor agonists, Science 217:1157 (1982).

18. R.R. Goodman, M.J. Kuhar, L. Hester and S.H. Synder, Adenosine receptors: autoradiographic evidence for their location on axon terminals of excitatory neurons, 220:967 (1983).

19. L.L. Hsu, R.C. Smith, C. Rolstein and D.E. Leelavathei, Effects of acute and chronic PCP on neurotransmitter enzyme in rat brain, Biochem. Pharmacol. 29:2524 (1980).

20. J.P. Vincent, J. Vignon, B. Kartalouski and C.B. Pert, "Receptor sites for phencyclidine in mammalian brain and peripheral organs", in: "PCP: Historical and Current Perspectives", E.F. Domino, ed., Ann Arbor, Michigan (1981).

21. R. Quirion, R.P. Hammer, M. Horkenham and C.B. Pert, Phencyclidine (angel dust/sigma "opiate" receptor): Visualization by tritium-sensitive film, Proc. Natl. Acad. Sci. U.S.A. 78:5881 (1981).

22. R.S. Zukin and S.R. Zukin, Multiple opiate receptors: Emerging concepts, Life Sciences 29:2681 (1981).

23. A.R Gintzler, R.S. Zukin and S.R. Zukin, Effects of phencyclidine and its derviatives on enteric neurons, Brit. J. Pharmacol. 75:261 (1982).

24. R. Oswald and J.P. Changeux, Ultraviolet light-induced labeling by noncompetitive blocking of the acetylcholine receptor from Torpedo marmorata, Proc. Natl. Acad. Sci. U.S.A. 78:3925 (1981).

25. E.X. Albuquerque, L.G. Aguayo, J.E. Wannick et al., The behavioral effects of phencyclidines may be due to their blockade of potassium channels, Proc. Natl. Acad. Sci. U.S.A. 78:7792 (1981).

26. R.T. Canoso, M.E. Lewis and E.J. Yunis, Association of HLA-Bw44 with chlorpromazine-induced autoantibodies, Clin. Immunol. Immunopathol. 25:278 (1982).

27. T.J. Crow, Molecular pathology of schizophrenia: More than one disease process? Brit. Med. J. 280:66 (1980).

28. R. Rodnight, Schizophrenia: Some current neurochemical approaches, J. Neurochem. 41:12 (1983).

29. J.G. Knight, Dopamine-receptor-stimulating autoantibodies: A possible cause of schizophrenia, The Lancet ii:1073 (1982).

30. R. Quirion, M.A. Bayorh, R.L. Zorlie and C.B. Pert, Chronic phen-
    cyclidine treatment decreases phencyclidine and dopamine
    receptors in rat brain, Pharmacol. Biochem. Behav. 17:699
    (1982).

31. H.H. Fudenberg, H.D. Whitten, E. Merler and O. Farmati, Is
    schizophrenia an anti-receptor disorder? Medical Hypothesis
    12:85 (1983).

32. T.L. Lentz, T.E. Burrage, A.L. Smith, J. Crick and G.H. Tignor,
    Is the acetylcholine receptor a rabies-virus receptor?
    Science 215:182 (1982).

33. M.F. Hamilton and J.B. Winfield, T gamma cells in systemic lupus
    erythematosus, Arth. Rheumatol. 22:1 (1979).

34. C. Morimoto, Loss of suppressor T-lymphocyte function in patients
    with systemic lupus erythematosus, Clin. Exp. Immunol. 32:125
    (1978).

35. A.S. Fauci, A.D. Steinberg, B.F. Haynes and G. Whalen, Immunoregula-
    tory aberrations in systemic lupus erythematosus, J. Immunol.
    121:1473 (1978).

36. A. Sagawa and N.T. Abdou, Suppressor-cell dysfunction in systemic
    lupus erythematosus, J. Clin. Invest. 62:789 (1978).

37. F. Gmelig-Meyling, and T.A. Waldman, Human B cell activation in
    vitro: Augmentation and suppression by monocytes of the immuno-
    globulin production induced by various B cell stimulants, J.
    Immunol. 126:529 (1981).

38. J. Oger, J. Szudhet, J. Antel, B.G.W. Arnason, A monoclonal antibody
    against human T suppressor lymphocytes binds specifically to the
    surface of cultured oligoendrocytes, Nature 295:66 (1982).

39. J. Wybran, T. Appelboom, J.P. Famasy and A. Govaerts, Suggestive
    evidence for receptors for morphine or methionine-enkephalin in
    normal human blood lymphocytes, J. Immunol. 123:1068 (1983).

40. D.G. Payan, D.R. Brewster and E.F. Goetzl, Specific stimulation of
    human T lymphocytes by Substance P, J. Immunol. 131:1613 (1983).

41. P.M. Matthews, C.J. Froehlick, W.L. Sibbitt and A.D. Edmonds,
    Enhancement of natural cytotoxicity by beta-endorphin, J.
    Immunol. 131:1658 (1983).

42. E.D. Luby, Phencyclidine revisited: PCP research and functional
    psychoses, Psychopharmacol. Bull. 16:85 (1980).

43. S.H. Synder, Phencyclidine, Nature 285:355 (1980).

44. P.H. Plotz, Autoantibodies are anti-idiotype antibodies to antiviral
    antibodies, Lancet 290:824 (1983).

45. C. Moroz, H. Bessler, M. Djaldetti and R.H. Stevens, Human adenosine
    receptor bearing lymphocytes: enumeration, characterization and
    distribution in peripheral blood lymphocytes, Clin. Immunol.
    Immunopathol. 18:47 (1981).

46. D.N. Bailey and A. Zettner, PCP binding in human serum, Res. Commun. Subst. Abuse 3:237 (1982).

47. R. Palacios, Role of autologous rosette-forming T cells in the concanavalin A-induced supppressor cell functions, Cell. Immunol. 61:273 (1981).

48. T. Sakane, M. Honda, Y. Taniguchi and H. Kotani, Separation of concanavalin A-induced human suppressor and helper T cells by the autologous erythrocyte rosette technique, J. Clin. Invest. 68:447 (1981).

49. N. Khansari, M. Petrini, F. Ambrogi et al., Role of autorosette forming cells in antibody synthesis in vitro: suppressive activity of ARFC in humoral immune response, Immunobiology 166:1 (1984).

50. J.H. Russell and C.B. Dobos, Accelerated ^{86}Rb$^+$ (K$^+$) release from the cytotoxic T lymphocyte is a physiologic event associated with delivery of the lethal hit, J. Immunol. 131:1138 (1983).

EFFECTS OF MORPHINE OPIATES ON IMMUNE FUNCTION

Hikmet Koyuncuoğlu and Mehmet Güngör

Department of Pharmacology and Clinical Pharmacology
Istanbul Medical Faculty
Çapa, Istanbul

The general anesthesia and surgery on the morphine opiate addicts, in which total blood volume and blood cell mass had been found to be less than normal, were more problematic and complicated than on the patients and prisoners in similar health conditions (Williams and Oberst, 1946; Isbell, 1947; Eiseman et al., 1964). There is substantial evidence that opiate addicts suffer from a mortality rate considerably higher that what would be expected in relation to their age. The follow-up studies of opiate addicted persons discharged from the treatment institutions reveal that a marked proportion died shortly after discharge although they were mostly young adults. Among the causes of death found in postmortem examinations the major medical complications of opiate addiction mostly related to the use and administration routes such as abscesses, cellulitis, endocarditis, hepatitis, pneumonia, septic pulmonary embolism, tetanus, thrombophlebitis etc. were called up (Tolentino et al., 1961; Cherubin, 1967; Louria et al., 1967; Cherubin et al., 1968; Espiritu and Medina, 1980; Tarr, 1980; Sequeira et al., 1982) ignoring the fact that opiate addicts are highly prone to infectious diseases and death (Cherubin, 1967).

It has long been known (Clouet and Ratner, 1967; 1968) that either a single dose of morphine or its long-term administration decrease the rate of removal of the labeled leucine from the free amino acid pool of brain and the rate of incorporation of labeled leucine into protein. In HeLa cells, morphine congeners, levorphanol and levallorphan, also inhibit protein synthesis (Noteboom and Müller, 1966 a; b). The mechanism underlying this inhibition was then reported to be the inhibitory effects of morphine and its surrogates on uridine and thymidine incorporating abilities, on RNA polymerase activity and on aminoacyl-tRNA synthethase (Datta and Antopol, 1972; 1973).

Postpartum studies of the hamster offspring that were exposed to morphine opiates in utero indicate deficiencies in growth rates and possible increased susceptibility to infections (Geber and Schramm, 1974). Additionally morphine and related opiates, administered to the pregnant hamster during the critical period of organogenesis, have been reported to be capable of altering the embryonic developmental pathways to such an extent as to produce a variety of important anatomical malformations especially in the central nervous system. When they were given to the weanling hamster

347

offspring they have been demonstrated to be powerful inhibitors of the ability of the tissue cells to rise the serum titer of interferon, an integral component of the host-defense mechanism (Geber and Schramm, 1975). Morphine opiates exert the effects similar to those of immunosuppressive agents not only during the gestation (Harpel and Gautieri, 1968; Dawis and Lin, 1972; Buchenauer, 1974) but before mating as well. Treatment of male or female rats with morphine opiates prior to mating reduces neonatal viability and increases the number of stillborns (Friedler and Cochin, 1972; Smith and Joffe, 1975). The antagonism by opiate antagonists of growth retardation brought about by morphine opiates (Smith et al., 1977) and the interesting experimental findings of Zagon and McLaughlin, who have previously showed the inhibitory effect of morphine on growth rate and the increasing effect of morphine on the percentage of stillborns and infant mortality (Zagon and McLaughlin, 1977 a; b) regarding the increase in brain size and brain cellular content in infant rats treated with naltrexone, an opiate antagonist (Zagon and McLaughlin, 1983) can be considered as experimental results supporting the idea that the administration and/or free intake of morphine opiates, and the normal or excessive release of their endogenous ligands may play a substantially important role in the development of immunity and immune system, and in the acquisition of immune response.

In spite of the suggestive experimental findings and clinical observations some of which have been mentioned above, very few experimental and clinical studies concerning the effects of morphine opiates on the immune system have been reported. In one of them (Güngör et al., 1980) chronic morphine administration has been demonstrated to inhibit the primary immune response in mice, and an impaired cellular immunity, a markedly decreased ratio of T helper/inducer cells to T suppressor/cytotoxic cells and associated viral infections in drug abusers have been reported in the other (Small et al., 1983). It has also been shown that morphine markedly inhibits the in vitro mitogenic response of human lymphocytes unstimulated as well as stimulated by phytohaemagglutinin (Brown et al., 1974; Zagon and McLaughlin, 1977).

Furthermore, opiate addicts were found to have a considerable reduction in the total number of T-lymphocytes as investigated by the ability of the lymphocytes to form rosettes with sheep erythrocytes (McDonough et al., 1980). The results of the experiments showing that in vitro treatment of peripheral blood lymphocytes obtained from normal human subjects with morphine decreases the ability of the lymphocytes to form rosettes with sheep erythrocytes probably through the presence of opioid receptors on lymphocytes (Wybran et al., 1979), the inhibition of natural killer cytotoxicity (Shavit et al., 1984) and the decrease of antibody dependent cellular cytotoxicity (Morgan et al., 1984) provide additional support for the idea that opiates alter immune system.

Even though none of the productive parts of the mammalian immune system are located in the central nervous system the immune system and immune response are greatly regulated by the central nervous system via the secretion of different hormones and/or the release of the neurotransmitters from the autonomic nervous system innervating the organs and tissues which provide the essential humoral and cellular elements of the immunity against microorganisms and degenerated cells giving access to tumor development. Thus, morphine opiates which cause many changes in the functions and hormonal status of the brain cannot be thought ineffective on the immune system and the preparation of immune response. Because of the very limited number of the experimental works concerning the direct or indirect effects of morphine opiates on the immune system we only have to overview the nearly well-established central actions of morphine opiates which can influence the immune system and response to give informations about the possible actions of morphine opiates on the immune system and immune response. Nevertheless, some direct effects of morphine opiates, unrelated to the functioning of the cent. ner. sys. which may be regarded to be rather peripheral, will be added to others. On the other hand, the actions of the chronic administration or intake of morphine opiates will be emphasized even though their single dose also can, rather for a very short time, alter the immune system and immune response through the effect on the release of acetylcholine, dopamine, noradrenaline, adrenaline, 5-hydroxytryptamine and the secretion of some hormones (Vogt, 1954; Beleslin and Polak, 1965; Akera and Brody, 1968; Inturrisi and Fujimoto, 1968; Jhamandas et al., 1971; Fennessy and Lee, 1972; Fukui and Takagi, 1972). The small percentage of morphine opiates used as a single dose especially for medical purposes in the huge amount of opiates consumed largely for non-medical aims is the other reason to take this decision.

The brain regulation and modulation of the immune system and immune response are possibly mediated by direct secretion of brain peptides into the general circulation and/or by the release of the neurotransmitters of the autonomic nervous system. Not only the relationship between the secretion of the peptides and the peripheral release of the neurotransmitters has to be taken into consideration but the modulation of the secretion of the peptides by the neurotransmitters within the central nervous system and viceversa has to be emphatically pointed out. Among the neurotransmitters and peptides by which the brain might modulate immune functions and processes acetylcholine, dopamine, noradrenaline, adrenaline, 5-hydroxytrytamine growth hormone, vasopressin, corticotropin, thyrotropin stimulating hormone, follicule stimulating hormone and luteinizing hormone have mostly been subject to the studies of the effects of morphine opiates.

In addition to the decreasing effect of single dose morphine opiates on the release of acetylcholine from brain neurons (Beleslin and Polak, 1965; Jhamandas et al., 1971) Maynert (1967) observed an increase in brain levels of acetylcholine, presumably due to the inhibition of acetylcholine release, in chronically morphinized rats. It has similarly been found that striatal acetylcholine and acetylcholinesterase were increased after chronic administration of morphine (Merali et al., 1974). On the basis of these central effects of morphine opiates and their effects on gastrointestinal tract it has almost generally been accepted that morphine opiates decrease the release of acetylcholine from the cholinergic nerve endings. The decrease of acetylcholine release may influence immune system as acetylcholine stimulates cyclic guanosine monophosphate which in turn has been demonstrated to activate B-cell as well as T-cell responses (Bourne et al., 1974; Goldberg et al., 1974). Furthermore, several investigators have reported the existence of acetylcholine receptors in thymus tissue (Eremina and Devoino, 1973; Lindstrom et al., 1976). Singh (1979) showed that thymocytes also contain cholinergic receptors and cholinergic stimulation can increase the cell yield from thymus tissue (Sing, 1979). Additionally it has been revealed that bone marrow stem cells bear cholinergic receptors which might be involved in the activation of these precursor cells (Byron, 1975; 1976) and cholinergic innervation might influence the production and/or release of thymic hormones via the stimulation of cholinergic receptors on epithelial cells in the thymus which produce thymic hormones as a consequence of the increase cyclic guanosine monophosphate content (Oosterom et al., 1979; Oosterom and Kater, 1980; Kater et al., 1980).

From the reported changes that occur in the immune system and immune response in the patients with neurologic disorders involving the dopaminergic pathways and dopamine metabolism, as well as experimental manipulation and determination of dopamine in animals it has been concluded that the central dopaminergic system has an evident stimulatory effect on various components of the immune system. The total number of T-lymphocytes as well as their ability to respond to mitogenic stimulation and in T-dependent skin tests were shown to be reduced in the patients with Parkinson's disease in which neuropathology is associated with dopaminergic neurons in the Substantia nigra (Hoffman et al., 1980). The production of immunoglobulins in response to the antigen of Salmonella-Nashua strain, which never causes an infection in human, was found to be much slower and lower level in the chronic and defective schizophrenic patients than in the controls, and in the psychotic patients treated with antipsychotics the level of immunoglobulins reached the control level after a letancy period (Özek et al., 1971). Moreover the administration of the antigens to animals which causes an increase in dopamine-stimulated adenyl cyclase activity in Nucleus caudatus was considered as an experimental finding supporting the fact that the decrease in brain dopaminergic activity increases the mortality in the mice bearing mammary tumors (Cotzias and Tang, 1977). As morphine opiates inhibits dopamine release, augments brain dopamine content and brain dopamine turnover, and blocks dopamine receptors (Clouet and Ratner, 1970; Kuschinsky and Hornykiewicz, 1972; Perez-Cruet et al., 1972; Puri and Lal, 1973; Lal, 1975; Lal and Numan, 1976; Koyuncuoğlu et al., 1977; Puri et al., 1978) their single or multiple doses is expected to exert an inhibitory action on immune system and immune response.

Noradrenaline and adrenaline have long been regarded as the neurotransmitters modulating immune system and immune response rather periferically. Adrenergic fibers innervating the interlobular septa of the rat thymus have been demonstrated (Fujiwara et al., 1966). The surfaces of T-cells, B-cells and macrophages contain a considerable amount of beta-adrenergic receptors (Bourne et al., 1974). Kasahara et al. (1977) and Hall et al. (1979) reported that chemical sympatectomy by 6-hydroxydopamine resulted in a significant depression of antibody production lasting till the return to normal of splenic noradrenaline content. On the other hand, Anderson and Slotkin (1975) found that the administration of morphine to rats produces a biphasic change in catecholamine content of adrenal medulla; in acute phase there is a reflex stimulation-induced depletion and during chronic administration the depletion is followed by an increase in the catecholamine content indicating an inhibition of catecholamine release (Anderson and Slotkin, 1975). Recently, it has been shown that endogenous opiates diminish the release of catecholamines from sympathetic nerve endings and the adrenal medulla by acting on the opiate receptors present in the membranes of the nerves and adrenal chromaffin cells (Weiner, 1979; Kumakura et al., 1980). On the basis of these experimental results the inhibition of immune system and immune response would be occurred during chronic administration or intake of morphine opiates by their blocking effect on catecholamine release from sympathetic nerve endings and adrenal medulla, in addition to others.

The experimental findings, resulted from the inverse relationship between antibody production and brain 5-hydroxytryptamine contents, suggest that 5-hydroxytryptamine exerts a clear inhibitory influence over immunogenesis. After administration of 5-hydroxytryptamine and its immediate precursor 5-hydroxytryptophan an increase in the latent period of antibody formation and a decrease in the intensity of both the primary and secondary response have been observed (Devoino et al., 1970; Idova and Devoino, 1972). In contrast to the inhibition by increased brain 5-hydroxytryptamine contents of the immunogenesis the reduction of brain 5-hydroxytryptamine levels appeared to have a stimulatory action on immune system. The destruction of the nucleus of the midbrain raphe, which has 5-hydroxytryptamine rich neurons, stimulates antibody production to bovine serum albumin (Eremina and Devoino, 1973). The extirpation of pineal gland which contains very high levels of 5-hydroxytryptamine is able to enhance the growth of certain tumors (Rodin, 1963; Lapin 1974; 1976). Although the ability of 5-hydroxytryptamine to alter immune system and immune response has saticfactorily been shown no conclusive conciliation has come out yet from the experimental results to say whether single dose or long-term use of morphine opiates can cause increases or decreases in the brain level of 5-hydroxytryptamine or its metabolism (Cochin and Axelrod, 1959; Maynert and Klingman, 1962; Gunne, 1963; Sloan et al., 1963; Algeri and Costa, 1971; Koyuncuoğlu et al., 1977). Therefore it is not possible, at the moment, to say in which direction, stimulation or inhibition, chronic use of morphine opiates may influence immune system and/or immune response by means of the changes in central 5-hydroxytryptamine metabolism.

Experimental findings have revealed that the intensity of immunologic responses such as antibody production, anaphylactic shock, skin reaction of the delayed type etc., are dependent on the action of neurohumoral factors. It has been shown that the intensity of the process of immunogenesis is affected by the actions of the hypothalamus, limbic system, pituitary body, adrenal glands, thymus and thyroid gland (Kanda, 1959; Luparello et al., 1964; Tsypin and Maltzev, 1967; Stein et al., 1969; Spector et al., 1975; Stein et al., 1976; Filipp, 1973; Amkraut and Solomon, 1974). Hormonal alterations generally follow antigenic challenge and they provide basic conditions for the pharmacologic control of the immunogenesis. Indeed, it appears logical to assume that a drug-mediated interference with neuroendocrinological events related to the central nervous system presumably promoting the hormonal variations observed would affect the immunogenesis and immune response to the antigen that triggers this very complex chain of reactions. Morphine opiates as the agents influencing directly the hypothalamus as well as the limbic system, to a lesser extent, indirectly the peripheral hormonal systems may play an important role in the orientation of the immune response. Without going in details of the interactions of the hormonal systems with the chemical neurotransmitters which take part in their release and/or metabolism, and the relationships between the neurotransmitters and hormonal systems and viceversa, the probable actions of morphine opiates on immune system and immune response via their effects on hormonal systems will shortly be reviewed.

It has been reported that growth hormone increases the weight of the thymus after hypophysectomy in neonatal Snell pituitary dwarf mice (Okouchi, 1976) Growth hormone has been found to stimulate rat thymocyte mitosis in vitro (Ahlqvist, 1976). Gisler (1974) showed that growth hormone reverses the immunosuppressive effects of corticosteroids in the plaque-forming cell assay. Moreover, growth hormone enhances graft rejection (Comsa et al., 1975). In spite of these experimental findings favouring the stimulatory effect of growth hormone on immune system there have been other contradictory reports (Dougherty, 1952; Ahlqvist, 1976; 1981). Growth hormone has long been regarded as a prophylogistic hormone enhancing a large number of different experimental vasculitic, arthritic, carditic and other inflammatory reactions, prevented tuberculosis in cortisone-treated rats, and turning monilial foci into proper granulomas (Ahlqvist, 1981). Growth hormone increases the fibrinogen level and erythrocyte sedimentation rate and it induces a neutrophilic reaction in dogs and it stimulates hepatic fibrinogen synthesis in rats (Ahlqvist, 1976). Even though it cannot surely be said that growth hormone inhibits the immune system, on the basis of the information mentioned above, it may be concluded that the direct evidence seems to be in favour of an inhibition. Therefore, the long-term administration of morphine opiates may be considered to have an inhibitory effect or at least contributory effect to the other inhibitory factors on immune system through the increased growth hormone secretion since the release of growth hormone is stimulated by exogenous as well as endogenous opioids and since opiate antagonists abolish the stimulatory effects of opioids on growth hormone release (Brown and Vale, 1975; Bruni et al., 1977; Koenig et al., 1980; Okajima et al., 1980; Sarne et al., 1981).

Antidiuresis, which follows the administration of morphine opiates, has been attributed to the direct action of these opiates on the hypothalamoneurohypophyseal axis, causing the release of vasopressin (DeBodo, 1944; Inturrisi and Fujimoto, 1968; Meites et al., 1979). Recently it has been shown that morphine, D-aspartic acid and PLG (prolyl-leucyl-glycinamide), all of which are the inhibitors of the brain L-asparaginase activity (Koyuncuoğlu et al., in press), elevate the urine osmolality (Koyuncuoğlu et al., 1984 c) and cause the release of vasopressin also in homozygous Brattleboro rats suffering from severe diabetes insipidus due to the lack of vasopressin. It has been concluded that the mechanism underlying the release of vasopressin is the inhibition of the brain L-asparaginase activity which was claimed to be the mechanism of physical dependence on morphine (Koyuncuoğlu, 1983; Koyuncuoğlu et al., 1984 b) . Vasopressin has not only antidiuretic effect at the level of kidneys but it has many other effects and functions inside and/or outside of the central nervous system. Vasopressin is one of the main factors causing the release of corticotropin from the anterior part of the pituitary gland (Hahmeier et al., 1980; Lutz-Bucher et al., 1980; Knepel et al., 1982).. It also can alter the turnover of the catecholamines in various brain regions (Meisenberg and Simmons, 1983). Vasopressin stimulates Na^+,K^+-ATPase and adenylate cyclase activity (Roy, 1979; Radominska-Pyrek et al., 1982; Courtney and Raskind, 1983) and it induces the increase of cAMP level. Moreover, vasopressin affects directly and/or indirectly carbohydrate, protein and lipid metabolism (Caisova et al., 1980 a, b; Edwards et al., 1981; Wood, 1981; Kneer and Lardy, 1983; Knudtzon,1983; Rofe and Williamson, 1983). So, from the information given above it is possible to reach the conclusion that morphine opiates may negatively affect immune system also via the release of vasopressin which increases the release of corticotropin and exerts direct metabolic effects.

As well known, hypothalamic lesions have a protective effect on anaphylaxis presumably related to changes in endocrine activity. It has been reported that the administration of thyroxine partially restores the sensitivity to anaphylaxis of actively immunized guinea pigs with lesions in the tuberal area of the hypothalamus (Filipp and Mess, 1969). When thyroxine in combination with metopirone, an inhibitor of adrenocorticol hormone synthesis, is administered to the sensitized guinea pigs with lesions in the tuberal region the protective action of the lesions from anaphylactic state is completely abolished, suggesting that the antianaphylactic effect of hypothalamic damage is connected with the combined effect of decreased thyroid function and increased adrenocortical activity (Filipp and Mess, 1969). It has also been demonstrated that thyroid enhances immune processes in the rat, mouse, and guinea pig. The resistance to anaphylaxis is increased in thyroidectomized rats, mice and guinea pigs. Inhibition of thyroid activity suppresses local and systemic anaphylaxis, abolishes circulating precipitins, and decreases the susceptibility of the animals to histamine administration (Leger and Masson, 1947; Nilzen, 1955; Csaba et al., 1977; Denckla, 1978). Thyroxine and triiodothyronine increase the phagocytic activity (Luri, 1960). Even though the direct effects of thyrotropin on tissues, other than the thyroid gland, such as the stimulation lipolysis in fat, and the inflammation in orbital muscle and connective tissue have been demonstrated, the effects of thyrotropin on the immunogenesis, a part from the effects mediated by thyroid hormones, have not been shown yet (Maclean and Reichlin, 1980). Administration of morphine opiates results in decreased thyrotropin secretion (Kim and Michael, 1975; Krulich et al., 1977; Tache et al., 1977). The activation by morphine of an inhibitory hypothalamic system under basal conditions has been claimed to be the mechanism of the inhibitory effect of morphine on thyroid functions (Lomax and George, 1966). While morphine prevents the cold stimulated rise in TSH it significantly increases thyrotropin releasing hormone content of the medial-basal hypothalamus reflecting morphine suppression of TRH release (Krulich et al., 1977). These findings are most consistent with a hypothalamic site for morphine action on thyrotropin secretion is mediated through decreased portal thyrotropin releasin hormone. No tolerance develops to the inhibitory effect of morphine on thyrotropin release (Morley et al., 1979). Chronic administration of morphine inhibits ^{131}I uptake and release of ^{131}I-labeled hormone by the thyroid (George and Lomax, 1965). Morphine addiction decreases thyroxine levels measured by radioimmunoassay (Morley et al., 1979).

The acute involution of the rodent thymus following stressful events is generally attributed to the increase in glucocorticoid levels (Dieckhoff et al., 1965). Rat thymus size is inversely correlated with plasma levels of unbound corticosterone, the main glucocorticoid in rodents (Westphal, 1971). Elevations of plasma corticosterone levels cause thymus involution, lymphocytopenia, alterations in amino acid metabolism and may produce various effects upon tumor growth, latent period and incidence (Spackman and Riley, 1974; Spackman et al., 1974; Fauci, 1975; Monjan and Collector, 1977). One of the most important effects of corticosteroids is their influence on amino acid metabolism and on protein synthesis. Elevated blood levels of these hormones significantly alter the levels of amino acids in physiological fluids and tissues, and result in an increased excretion of urinary nitrogen and a negative nitrogen balance presumably due to both an inhibition of protein synthesis and increased protein catabolism causing the elevated concentrations of plasma amino acids, as well as increased gluconeogenesis (White et al., 1968; Turner and Hagnara, 1971). These alterations in protein and amino acid metabolism have potential influences upon disease processes, via their adverse effects on the synthesis of enzymes and cellular proteins needed for normal immune surveillance. In may experiments it has been shown that the basic cellular elements forming the immunological system, involving macrophages, T cells and B cells, are all subject to modification, impairment and/or destruction by glucocorticoids (Santisteban and Dougherty, 1954; Gisler and Schenkel-Hullinger, 1971; Monjan and Collector, 1977). The lymphocytopenia resulting from elevated plasma glucocorticoids undoubtedly indicates destruction of T cells and probably also B cells (Monjan and Collector, 1977; Solomon and Amkraut, 1979). On the other hand, adrenalectomy increases the size of thymus (Dougherty, 1952), and seems to stimulate the mitotic index in both epithelial cells and thymocytes after X-ray-induced involution (Gregoire and Duchateau, 1956). Adrenalectomy may also enhance antibody formation and susceptibility to anaphylaxis and Arthus reaction (Ahlqvist, 1976). When glucocorticoids are administered before antigen challenge they suppress antibody formation (Ahlqvist, 1976). Although there have been reports claiming that exogenous and endogenous opioids have an inhibitory effect on the pituitary-adrenal axis (Blankstein et al., 1980; Grossman and Besser, 1982) it has generally been ascribed that acute administration of morphine stimulates corticosterone release (Lotti et al., 1969; George, 1971; George and Kokka, 1976). The corticotropin releasing action of morphine is mainly mediated via the hypothalamus; lesions of the median eminence blocks the adrenal cortical response to morphine (George and Way, 1959; Kokka and George, 1974). Recently morphine has been demonstrated to potentiate the adrenal steroidogenic response to corticotropin (Heybach and Vernikos, 1981). However, the release by morphine opiates of vasopressin may also play an important role in the secretion of corticotropin (DeBodo, 1944; George and Way, 1959; Inturrisi and Fujimoto, 1968; Meites et al., 1979; Koyuncuoğlu et al., 1984 b). Even though tolerance to the corticosterone releasing effect of morphine opiates develops and higher doses are required to elevate corticosterone levels (Kokka and George, 1974) the parallel increase in compulsory intake by addicts because of the development of tolerance may not cause any significant change in the elevations of plasma glucocorticoid levels.

Although gonadectomy in experimental animals of both sexes has been reported to increase the size of the thymus and to counteract the thymic

involution induced by stress and fasting (Dougherty, 1952; Ahlqvist, 1976)
quite a large number of experimental findings is in favour of the enhancing
effects of sex hormones especially androgens on antibody formation. The "anti-infective" action of 4-chloro testosterone in experimental infections was
first demonstrated by Ghione (1958). The androgen prolonged the survival tim
of the experimentally infected animals and it provided a more rapid healing
of infectious lesions. Using metyrapone, an 11-beta-hydroxylase blocker,
which decreases the synthesis of cortisol and increases the synthesis of
adrenal androgens, it has been shown that androgens stimulate the antibody
formation (Tolentino et al., 1961). Then the confirming data obtained from
the experiments performed on experimental animals as well as on human beings
utilizing different antigens and different anabolic agents helped to reach
the almost generally accepted conclusion that sex hormones stimulate immune
system especially by means of their anabolic action (Sawyer et al., 1955;
Coraggio et al., 1962; Heboyan and Messeri, 1962; Jannuzzi and Bassi, 1962;
1964; Terragna and Januzzi, 1963; Dieckhoff et al., 1965; Januzzi and Gemme,
1965; Wakabayashi, 1966). On the other hand morphine and opioid peptides
consistently produce naloxone reversible suppression of luteinizing hormone
and to a lesser extent of follicle stimulating hormone (Cicero et al., 1975;
Zimmerman and Pang, 1976; Bruni et al., 1977). Chronic morphine administration causes regressive changes in Leydig cells with minimal alterations in
testicular weight (Hohlweg et al., 1961; Cicero et al., 1975). Morphine and
methadone both suppress the growth of sex organs (Cicero et al., 1975; 1976)
No tolerance to the inhibitory effects of morphine on luteinizing hormone,
follicle stimulating hormone and testosterone levels was demonstrated 14
days after the continuous morphine administration (Cicero and Badger, 1977;
 Morley et al., 1979).

   Malnourished animals and humans appear to be more susceptible to all
forms of infection and recovery is often delayed. Infections occur more often and may be more severe in chronically undernourished populations. Based
on this often observed coincidence it has been suggested that undernutrition
predisposes to infections and malnutrition has generally been accepted as
one of the main factors causing secondary immunodeficiency. As most studies
have been on malnourished children they have been found particularly prone
to septicaemia with Gram negative organisms or disseminated herpes simplex
infections (Harmon et al., 1963; Scrimshaw et al., 1968; McFarlane, 1976;
Hayward, 1977; Suskind, 1977; Murray and Murray, 1979; Gross and Newberne,
1980; Chandra, 1983). Furthermore it has been shown that caloric restriction
can increase tumour incidence and growth rates (Vissher et al., 1942; Rusch,
1944; Tannenbaum and Silverstone, 1953). In spite of many studies the nature
of increased infection, and of the high tumour incidence and growth rate in
malnutrition is not quite clear. Whereas the majority of malnourished individuals have been reported to have normal concentrations of the serum immuno
globulins (Smythe et al., 1971) the deprivation of certain amino acids in
the diet has been shown to cause an impaired synthesis of antibodies (Jose
and Good, 1973). In addition various alterations of host defense in anorecti
patients such as blood polymorphonuclear granulocyte glucose oxidation, adherence and bactericidal capacity (Gotch et al., 1975; Kjösen et al., 1975;
Palmblad et al., 1977) and depression of factors Cl, C2, C3, Cls inactivator
B and total hemolytic complement (Kim and Michael, 1975) have been described
and the decrease in numbers of lymphoid cells in spleen and thymus of rats
with malnutrition has been suggested as an impaired cell-mediated immune
response (McFarlane and Hamid, 1973). Malnutrition is almost always accompanied by deficiencies of vitamins some of which have an important function
in immune response. Deficiencies of the B group vitamins have long been associated with reduction in antibody production to antigenic stimuli. Vitamin
B6 (pyridoxine) deficiency causes a much more complete inhibition of the
immune response (Axelrod and Trakatellis, 1964). The effects of Vitamin B6
deficiency on tumour suppression have also been shown (Mihich, 1962; Mihich
and Nichol, 1965). Vitamin B12 also has been reported as affecting the immun

response (Ludovici and Axelrod, 1951). Recently some more experimental findings regarding the stimulation by Vitamin C supplements of the immune system
have been added to previous ones (Feigen et al., 1982; Kennes et al., 1983).

Long term use of morphine opiates by subjects, physically dependent
or not, is usually detrimental to the users for many important reasons also
in terms of nutrition. Although the malnutrition seems to be related, to
some extent, with financial, social and familial problems the most prevalent
factor is the effect of morphine opiates on appetite. Even though it has
been hypothesized that opioid systems take part in the regulation of behaviour in association with acquisition of nutrients and in the conservation
and expenditure of energy (Margules, 1979) and morphine like agents have,
in favour of the hypothesis, been reported to increase food and fluid intake
(Grandison and Guidotti, 1977; Maickel et al., 1977; Belluzzi and Stein,
1978) several other studies have generally found a decrease (Kumar et al.,
1971; Chance and Rosecrans, 1977; Mark-Kaufman and Kanarek, 1980; Koyuncuoğlu et al., 1984 a). This is why the users of morphine opiates generally
lose appetite, and the majority of them are thin even cachectic, and malnourished.

As known, interferon is a small protein which takes part in the general
cellular defense mechanisms against chemically induced carcinogenesis, solid
tumour growth, both cancer and noncancer-inducing virus invasion in animals.
It can be effective in the therapy of respiratory and other virus infections
in humans. Animal experimental work showed that a single administration of
morphine is capable of depressing or inhibiting the circulating serum interferon level for 3-9 days which can render the body more susceptible to
virus-induced pathology (Hung et al., 1973; Geber et al., 1976 a,b).

As most actions, including vasopressin release, of the acute and
chronic administration of morphine opiates have been attributed to the inhibitory effect of these substances on the activity of L-asparaginase
(Koyuncuoğlu et al., 1979; 1982 a,b; 1984 b; Koyuncuoğlu 1983; Koyuncuoğlu
et al., in press) which has long been used in the treatment of lymphomas
because of the catalytic effect on the deamidation of asparagine and, to a
lesser extent, glutamine resulting in the depletion of these amino acids
required for peptides and proteins synthesis, it seems to be logical to
think that the inhibitory effect of morphine opiates on L-asparaginase activity can be one of the main factors in their modulating action on immune
function. The promising experimental studies regarding the discovery of the
physical dependence development on morphine opiates via their effects on
L-asparaginase can be taken into consideration as the basis of the additional innovative experimentations in connection with immunity in all senses
of the word, and the resistance to experimental pyelonephritis of homozygous
Brattleboro rats suffering from a genetic severe hypothalamic diabetes insipidus (Güngör et al., in press) and having a higher L-asparaginase activity than normal rats (Koyuncuoğlu et al., 1984 b) can be regarded as one
of the primary experimental findings in favour of this suggestion.

REFERENCES

Ahlqvist, J., 1976, Endocrine influences on lymphatic organs, immune respon-
      ses, inflammation and autoimmunity, Acta Endocrinol. (Copenhagen),
      Suppl., 206.
Ahlqvist, J., 1981, Hormonal Influences on Immunologic and Related Phenomena,
      in: "Psychoneuroimmunology", R. Ader and R.A. Good, Eds., Academic
      Press, New York.
Akera, T., and Brody, T.M., 1968, The addiction cycle to narcotics in the rat
      and its relation to catecholamines, Biochem. Pharmacol., 17:675.
Algeri, S., and Costa, E., 1971, Physical dependence on morphine fails to

increase serotonin turnover in rat brain, Biochem.Pharmacol., 20:877.

Amkraut, A., and Solomon, G.F., 1974, From the symbolic stimulus to the pathophysiologic response: Immune mechanisms, Int.J.Psychiatry Med., 5:542.

Anderson, T.R., and Slotkin, T.A., 1975, Maturation of the adrenal medulla -IV. Effects of morphine, Biochem.Pharmac. 24:1469.

Axelrod, A.E., and Trakatellis, A.C., 1964, Relationship of pyrodoxine to immunological phenomena, Vitamins Hormones 22:591.

Beleslin, D., and Polak, R.L., 1965, Depression by morphine and chloralose of acetylcholine release from the cat's brain, J.Physiol.(Lond.), 177:411.

Belluzzi, J.D., and Stein, L., 1978, Do enkephalin systems mediate drive reduction? Soc.Neurosci.Abstr., 8:405.

Blankstein, J., Reyes, F.I., Winter, J.S.D., and Faiman, C., 1980, Effects of naloxone upon prolactin and cortisol in normal women, Proc. Soc.Exp.Biol.Med., 164:363.

Bourne, H.R., Lichtenstein, L.M., Melmon, K.L., Henney, C.S., Weinstein, Y., and Shearer, G.M., 1974, Modulation of inflammation and immunity by cyclic AMP, Science, 184:19.

Brown, M., and Vale, W., 1975, Growth hormone release in the rat: Effects of somatostatin and thyrotropin-releasing factor, Endocrinology, 96: 1333.

Brown, S.M., Stimmel, B., Taub, R.N., Kochwa, S., and Rosenfield, R.E., 1974, Immunologic dysfunction in heroin addicts, Arch.Intern.Med., 134:1001.

Bruni, J.F., Van Vugt, D., Marshall, S., and Meites, J. 1977, Effects of naloxone, morphine and methionine enkephalin on serum prolactin, luteinizing hormone, follicle stimulating hormone, thyroid stimulating hormone and growth hormone, Life Sci., 21:461.

Buchenauer, D., Turnbow, M., and Peters, M.A., 1974, Effects of chronic methadone administration of pregnant rats and their offspring, J.Pharmac.Exp.Ther., 189:66.

Byron, J.W., 1975, Manipulation of the cell cycle of the hamopcietic stem cell, Exp.Hematol., 3:44.

Byron, J.W., 1976, Cyclic nucleotides and the cell cycle of the hematopoietic stem cell. in: "Cyclic Nucleotides and the Regulation of Cell Growth", M.Abou-Sade, ed., Dowden, Hutchinson and Ross, Pennsylvania.

Caisova, D., Stajner, A., and Suva, J., 1980 a, Modification of fat and carbohydrate metabolism by neurohypophyseal hormones: I.Effects of lysine-vasopressin on non-esterified fatty acid, glucose, triglyceride and cholesterol levels in the serum of female rats, Endokrinologie, 76:315.

Caisova, D., Suva, J. and Stajner, A., 1980 b, Modification of fat and carbohydrate metabolism by neurohypophyseal hormones: II. Effect of lysine-vasopressin on non-esterified fatty acid, glucose triglyceride and cholesterol levels in the serum of male rats, Endokrinologie, 76:326.

Chance, W.T., and Rosecrans, J.A., 1977, Inhibition of drinking by intrahypothalamic administration of morphine, Nature, 270:167

Chandra, R.K., 1983, Nutrition and immune responses, Can.J.Physiol.Pharmacol. 61:290.

Cherubin, C.E., Baden, M., Kavaler, F., Lerner, S., and Cline, W., 1968, Infective endocarditis in narcotic addicts, Ann.Int.Med. 69:1091.

Cherubin, C.E., 1967, The medical sequelae of narcotic addiction, Ann.Int. Med., 67:23.

Cicero, T.J., and Badger, T.M., 1977, A comparative analysis of the effects of narcotics, alcohol and the barbiturates on the hypothalamic-pituitary-gonadalaxis, Adv.Exp.Med.Biol., 85:95.

Cicero, T.J., Meyer, E.R., and Bell, R.D., 1976, Effects of morphine on serum testosterone and luteinizing hormone levels and on secondary sex organs of the male rat, Endocrinology, 98:367.

Cicero, T.J., Meyer, E.R., and Wiest, W.A., 1975, Effects of chronic morphine administration on the reproductive system of the male rat, J.Pharmacol.Exp.Ther., 192:542.

Clouet, D.H., and Ratner, M., 1967, The effect of the administration of morphine on the incorporation of ^{14}C-leucine into the proteins of rat brain in vivo, Brain Res., 4:33.

Clouet, D.H., and Ratner, M., 1968, The effect of morphine administration on the incorporation of ^{14}C leucine into protein in cell-free system from rat liver and brain, J.Neurochem., 15:17.

Clouet, D.H., and Ratner, M., 1970, Catecholamine biosynthesis in brains of rats treated with morphine, Science, 168:854.

Cochin, J., and Axelrod, J., 1959, Biochemical and pharmacological changes in the rat following chronic administration of morphine, nalorphine and normorphine, J.Pharmacol.Exp.Ther., 125:105.

Comsa, J., Leonhardt, H., and Schwarz, J.A., 1975, Influence of the thymus -corticotropin-growth hormone interaction on the rejection of skin allografts in the rat, Ann.N.Y.Acad.Sci., 249:387.

Coraggio, F., Coto, V., Oriente, P., De'Longis, G., and Galeota, C.A., 1962, Influenza del 19-norandrostenolone sulla produzione di anticorpi antimorbillosi nel coniglio, Boll.Soc.Ital.Biol.Sper., 38:1316.

Cotzias, G.C., and Tang, L.C., 1977, An adenylate cyclase of brain reflects propensity for breast cancer in mice, Science, 197:1094.

Courtney, N., and Raskind, M., 1983, Vasopressin affects adenylate cyclase activity in rat brain: A possible neuromodulator, Life Sci., 32: 591.

Csaba, G., Sudar, F., and Dobozy, O., 1977, Triiodothyronine receptors in lymphocytes of newborn and adult rats, Horm.Metab.Res. 9:499.

Datta, R.K., and Antopol, W., 1972, Inhibitory effect of chronic administration of morphine on uridine and thymidine incorporating abilities of mouse liver and brain subcellular fractions, Toxicol.appl.Pharmacol., 23:75.

Datta, R.K., and Antopol, W., 1973, Effect of chronic administration of morphine on mouse brain aminoacyl-tRNA synthetase and tRNA-amino acid binding, Brain Res., 53:373.

Dawis, W.M., and Lin, C.H., 1972, Prenatal morphine effects of survival and behaviour of rat offspring, Res.Commun.Chem.Pathol.Pharmacol., 3:205.

DeBodo, R.C., 1944, The antidiuretic action of morphine, and its mechanism, J.Pharmacol.Exp.Ther., 82:74.

Denckla, W.D., 1978, Interactions between age and neuroendocrine and immune systems, Fed.Proc.Fed.Am.Soc.Exp.Biol., 37:1263.

Devoino, L.V., Eremina, O.F.N., and Ilyutchenok, R.Yu., 1970., The role of the hypothalamopituitary system in the mechanism of action of reserpine and 5-hydroxytryptophan on antibody production, Neuropharmacology, 9:67.

Dieckhoff, J., Schneeweiss, B., Schicke, R., and Hübschmann, K., 1965, Tierexperimentelle Untersuchungen über die Antikörperbildung unter gleichzeitiger, Anabol.Applikation,Mschr.Kinderheilk., 113:468.

Dougherty, T.F., 1952, Effects of hormones on lymphatic tissue, Physiol. Rev., 32:379.

Edwards, M.W., Brooks, S.L., Gove, C.D., Hems, D.A., and Cawthorne, M.A., 1981, Effects of vasopressin on lipogenesis in obese mice, FEBS Letters, 127:25.

Eiseman, B., Lam, R.C., and Bush, B., 1964, Surgery on the narcotic addict, Ann.Surg., 159:748.

Engel, W.K., Trotter, J.L., McFarlin, D.E., and McIntosh, C.L., 1977, Thymic epithelial cell contains acetylcholine receptor, Lancet, 1:1310.

Eremina, O.F., and Devoino, L.V., 1973, Production of humoral antibodies in rabbits with destruction of the nucleus of the midbrain raphe, Bull.Exp.Biol.Med.(Engl Transl.), 75:149.

Espiritu, M.B., and Medina, J.E., 1980, Complications of heroin injections of the neck, Laryngoscope, 90:1111.

Fauci, A.S., 1975, Mechanisms of corticosteroid action on lymphocyte subpopulations. I.Redistribution of circulating T and B lymphocytes to the bone marrow, Immunology, 28:669.

Feigen, G.A., Smith, B.H., Dix, C.E., Flynn, C.J., Peterson, N.S., Rosenberg, L.T., Pavlovic, S., and Leibovitz, B., 1982, Enhancement of antibody production against systemic anaphylaxis by large doses of vitamin C, Res.Comm.Chem.Path.Pharmac., 38:313.

Fennessy, M.R., and Lee, J.R. 1972, Comparison of the dose-response effects of morphine on brain amines, analgesia and activity in mice, Brit.J.Pharmacol., 45:240.

Filipp, G., 1973, Mechanism of suppressing anaphylaxis thorough electrolytic lesion of the tuberal region of the hypothalamus, Ann.Allergy, 31: 272.

Filipp, G., and Mess, B., 1969, Role of the adrenocortical system in suppressing anaphylaxis after hypothalamic lesion, Ann.Allergy, 27:607.

Friedler, C., and Cochin, J., 1972, Growth retardation of offspring of female rats treated with morphine prior to conception, Science, 175:654.

Fujiwara, M., Muryobayashi, T., and Shimamoto, K., 1966, Histochemical demonstration of monoamines in the thymus of rats, Jpn.J.Pharmacol., 16:493.

Fukui, K., and Takagi, H., 1972, Effect of morphine on the cerebral contents of metabolites of dopamine in normal and tolerans mice: its possible relation to analgesic action, Brit.J.Pharmacol., 44:45.

Geber, W.F., Lefkowitz, S.S., and Hung, C.Y., 1976 a, Action of naloxone on the interferone lowering activity of morphine in the mouse, Pharmacology, 14:322.

Geber, W.F., Lefkowitz, S.S., and Hung, C.Y., 1976 b, Role of spleen in the interferon-lowering action of morphine, Gen.Pharmac., 7:255.

Geber, W.F., and Schramm, L.C., 1974, Postpartum weight alteration in hamster offspring from females injected during pregnancy with either heroin, methadone, a composite drug mixture, or mescaline, Am.J. Obstet.Gynecol., 120:1105.

Geber, W.F., and Schramm, L.C., 1975, Congenital malformation of the central nervous system produced by narcotic analgesics in the hamster, Am.J. Obstet.Gynecol. 123:705.

George, R., 1971, Hypothalamus: Anterior Pituitary Gland. in: "Narcotic Drugs, Biochemical Pharmacology", D.M.Clouet, ed., Plenum Press, NewYork.

George, R., and Lomax, P., 1965, The effects of morphine, chlorpromazine and reserpine on pituitary-thyroid activity in rats, J.Pharmacol. Exp.Ther., 150:129.

George, R., and Way, E.L., 1959, The role of the hypothalamus in pituitary -adrenal activation and antidiuresis by morphine, J.Pharmacol.Exp. Ther., 125:111.

Ghione, M., 1958, Anti-infective action of an anabolic steroid, Proc.Soc. Exp.Biol.Med., 97:773.

Gisler, R.H., 1974, Stress and the hormonal regulation of the immune response in mice, Psychother.Psychosom., 23:197.

Gisler, R.H., and Schenkel-Hullinger, L., 1971, Hormonal regulation of the immune response. II.Influence of pituitary and adrenal activity on immune responsiveness in vitro, Cell. Immunol., 2:646.

Goldberg, N.D., Haddox, M.K., Estensen, R., White, J.G., Lopez, C., and Hadden, J.W., 1974, Evidence of a dualism between cyclic GMP and cyclic AMP in the regulation of cell proliferation and other cellular processes, in: "Cyclic AMP, Cell Growth, and the Immune Response", W.Braun, L.M.Lichtenstein and C.W.Parker, eds., Springer -Verlag, NewYork.

George, R., and Kokka, N., 1976, The Effects of Narcotics on Growth Hormone,

ACTH and TSH Secretion, in: "Tissue Responses to Addictive Drugs", D.M.Ford ·and D.H.Clouet, eds., Spectrum Publications, NewYork.

Gotch, F.M., Spry, C.J.F., Mowat, A.G., Beeson, P.M., and MacLennan, I.C.M., 1975, Reversible granulocyte killing defect in anorexia nervosa, Clin.Exp.Immunol., 21:244.

Grandison, S., and Guidotti, A., 1977, Stimulation of food intake by muscimol and beta-endorphin, Neuropharmacology, 16:533.

Gregoire, C., and Duchateau, G., 1956, Study on lympho-epithelial symbosis in thymus. Reactions of the lymphatic tissue to extracts and to implants of epithelial components of thymus, Arch.Biol. 67:269.

Gross, R.L., and Newberne, P.M., 1980, Role of nutrition in immunologic function, Physiol.Rev., 1:188.

Grossman, A., and Besser, G.M., 1982, Opiates control ACTH through a noradrenergic mechanism, Clin.Endocrinology, 17:287.

Gunne, L.-M., 1963, Catecholamines and 5-hydroxytryptamine in morphine tolerance and withdrawal, Acta physiol.scand. 58:Suppl., 204.

Güngör, M., Genç, E., Sagduyu, H., Eroglu, L. and Koyuncuoğlu, H., 1980, Effect of chronic administration of morphine on primary immune response in mice, Experentia, 36:1309.

Güngör, M., Ang, Ö., Uysal, V., Sagduyu, H., Inanç, D., Anğ, M., and Koyuncuoglu, H., Comparison of experimental pyelonephritis in homozygous Brattleboro diabetes insipidus, heterozygous control and normal Wistar rats, Infection (in press).

Hahmeier, W., Fenske, M., Pitzel, L., Holtz, W., and König, A., 1980, Corticosteroids and testosterone in adult male pig, Acta Endocrinologica, 95:518.

Hall, N.R., McClure, J.E., Hu, S.-K., Tick, N.T., Seales, C.M., and Goldstein, A.L., 1979, Effects of chemical sympathectomy upon thymus dependent immune responses, Soc.Neurosci.Abstr., 26.4.

Harmon, B.G., Miller, E.R., Hoeffer, J.A., Ullrey, D.E., and Luecke, R.W., 1963, Relationship of specific nutrient deficiencies to antibody production in swine. I.Vitamin A, J.Nutr., 79:263.

Harpel, H.S., and Gautieri, R.F., 1968, Morphine-induced malformations, J. Pharm.Sci., 57:1590.

Hayward, A.R., 1977, "Immunodeficiency", Edward Arnold Ltd, London.

Heboyan, M., and Messeri, E., 1962, Variazioni immunitarie in ratti tenuti a dicta normale e a dicta di Handler, vaccinati con Salmonella typhi e trattati con 4-idrossi-19-nortestosterone-17-ciclopentilpropionato, Rass.Ital.Gastroenter., 11:590.

Heybach, J.P., and Vernikos, J., 1981, Naloxone inhibits and morphine potentiates the adrenal steroidogenic response to ACTH, Eur.J.Pharmacol., 75:1.

Hoffman, P.M., Robbins, D.S., Nolte, M.T., Gibbs, jr, C.S., and Gajdusek, D.C., 1980, Immunity and immunogenetics in Guamanians with amyotrophic lateral aclerosis (ALS) and Parkinsonism-dementia, J. Supramol.Struct., 8:Suppl. 2.

Hohlweg, W., Knappe, G., and Domer, G., 1961, Tierexperimentelle Untersuchungen ueber den Einfluss von Morphine auf die gonadotrope und thyrectrope Hypophysenfunktion, Endokrinologie 40:152.

Hung,C.Y., Lefkowitz, S.S. and Geber, W.F., 1973, Interferon inhibition by tion of morphine in the rat, Eur.J.Pharmacol. 2:301.

Idova, C.V., and Devoino, L.V., 1972, Dynamics of formation of M- and ₲-antibodies in mice after administration of serotonin and its precursor 5-hydroxtryptophan, Bull.Exp.Biol.Med.(Engl.Transl.), 73:294.

Inturrisi, C.E., and Fujimoto, J.M., 1968, Studies on the antidiuretic acnarcotic analgesics, Proc.Soc.Exp.Biol.Med., 142:106.

Isbell, H., 1947, The effect of morphine addiction on blood plasma and extracellular fluid volumes in man, Public Health Reports, 62:1499.

Jannuzzi, C., and Bassi, A., 1962, Ormoni steroidei ed anticorpopoiesi. Nota III. Potenziamento della vaccinazione antidifterica nel bambino da parte di ormoni anabolizzanti, Boll.Ist.Sieroter.Mil., 41:221.

Jannuzzi, C., and Bassi, A., 1964, Vaccinazione antitetanica e ormoni ana-
bolizanti, G.Mal.Inf., 16:748.
Jannuzzi, C., and Gemme, G., 1965, Tentativi di immunizzazione attiva del
neonato verso i ceppi enteritogeni di E.coli, G.Mal.Inf., 17:74.
Jhamandas, K., Phillis, J.W., and Pinsky, C., 1971, Effects of narcotic
analgesics and antagonists on the in vivo release of acetylcholine from the cerebral cortex of the cat, Brit.J.Pharmacol.,
43:53.
Jose, D.G. and Good, R.A., 1973, Quantitive effects of nutritionally essential amino acid deficiencies upon immune responses to tumors in mice,
J.Exp.Med., 137:1.
Kanda, R., 1959, Studies of the regulation centre on promotion of antibody
II. On the migration and relation of normal precipitin antibody and
leucocyte in the peripheral blood by electric stimuli in the hypothalamus of rabbit, Jpn.J.Bacteriol., 14:542.
Kater, L., Oosterom, R., McClure, J., and Goldstein, A.L., 1980, Presence
of thymosin-like factors in human thymic epithelial conditioned me-
dium, Int.J.Immunopharmacol. 1:273.
Kasahara, K., Tanaka, S., Ito, T., and Hamashima, Y., 1977, Suppression of
the primary immune response by chemical sympathectomy, Res.Commun.
Chem.Pathol.Pharmacol. 16:687.
Kennos, B., Dumont, I., Brohee, D., Hubert, C., and Neve, P., 1983, Effect
of Vitamin C supplements on cell-mediated immunity in old people,
Gerontology 29:305.
Kim, Y., and Michael, A.E., 1975, Hypocomplementemia in anorexia nervosa,
J.Pediatr., 87:582.
Kjösen, B., Bassoe, H.H., and Myking, O., 1975, The glucose oxidation in
isolated leukocytes from female patients suffering from overweight
or anorexia nervosa, Scand.J.Clin.Lab.Invest., 35:447.
Kneer, N.M., and Lardy, H.A., 1983, Regulation of gluconeogenesis by nor-
epinephrine, vasopressin, and angiotensin II: A $_2$ comparative study
in the absence and presence of extracellular Ca^{2+}, Arch.Biochem.
Biophys. 225:187.
Knepel, W., Benner, K., and Hertling, C., 1982, Role of vasopressin in the
ACTH response to isoprenaline, Eur.J.Pharmacol., 81:645.
Knudtzon, J., 1983, Acute effects of oxytocin and vasopressin on plasma levels of glucogon, insulin and glucose in rabbits, Horm.metabol.
Res., 15:103
Krulich, L., Giachetti, A., Marchlewska-Koj., Hefco, E., and Jameson, H.E.
1977, On the role on the central noradrenergic and dopaminergic
systems in the regulation of THS secretion in the rat, Endocrinology, 100:496.
Koenig, J., Mayfield, M.A., Coppings, R.J., McCann, S.M., and Krulich, L.,
1980, Role of central nervous system neurotransmitters in mediating
the effects of morphine on growth hormone-and prolactin-secretion
in the rat, Brain Res., 197:453.
Kokka, N. and George, R., 1974, Effects of Narcotic Analgesics, Anesthetic
and Hypothalamic Lesions on Growth Hormone and Adrenocorticotrophic
Secretion in Rats, in:"Narcotics and the Hypothalamus", E.Zimmerman
and R.George, eds., Raven Press, NewYork.
Koyuncuoğlu, H., 1983, The treatment with L-aspartic acid on persons addicted to opiates, Bull.Narcotics (United Nation Publication), 35:
11.
Koyuncuoğlu, H., Berkman, K., Wildmann, J., and Matthaei, H., Antagonistic
effect of L-aspartic acid on decrease in body weight, food and
fluid intake, and naloxone reversible rectal temperature caused
by D-aspartic acid, Pol.J.Pharmacol.Pharm., 34:333.
Koyuncuoğlu, H., Berkman, K., and Sabuncu, H., 1984 a, Feeding, drinking,
urine osmolality in DI Brattleboro rats: Changes by morphine,
naloxone, D-amino acids, prolyl-leucyl-glycinamide (PLG),

Pharmacol.Biochem.Behav., 20:29.

Koyuncuoğlu, H., Berkman, K., Hatipoğlu, I., and Sabuncu, H., 1984 b, Vasopressin release by D-aspartic acid, morphine and prolyl-leucyl-glycinamide (PLG) in DI Brattleboro rats, Pharmacol.Biochem.Behav., 20:519.

Koyuncuoğlu, H., Berkman, K., and Matthaei, H., Effects of morphine, D-aspartic acid, d phenylalanine, D-leucine and PLG on L-asparaginase activity in rats, Med.Bull.Ist.Med.Fac. (in press).

Koyuncuoğlu, H., Berkman, K., and Sabuncu, H., 1984 c, Feeding, drinking, urine osmolality in DI Brattleboro rats: Changes by morphine, naloxone, D-amino acids, prolyl-leucyl-glycinamide (PLG), Pharmacol.Biochem.Behav., 20:29.

Koyuncuoglu, H., Genç, E., Güngör, M., Eroglu, L., and Sağduyu, H., 1977, The antagonizing effect of aspartic acid on the brain levels of monoamines and free amino acids during the development of tolerance to and physical dependence on morphine, Psychopharmacology, 54:187.

Koyuncuoğlu, H., Keyer-Uysal, M., Berkman, K., Güngör, M., and Genç, E., 1979, The relationship between morphine, aspartic acid and L-asparaginase, Eur.J.Pharmacol., 60:369.

Koyuncuoğlu, H., Wildmann, J., Berkman, K., and Matthaei, H., 1982 b, The effects of D- and/or L-aspartic acid on the total weight of body and the weights of certain organs, and their protein, triglyceride and glycogen contents, Drug Res., 32:738.

Kumakura, K., Karoum, F., Guidotti, A., and Costa, E., 1980, Modulation of nicotinic reseptors by opiate receptor agonists in cultured adrenal chromaffin cells, Nature, 283:489.

Kumar, R., Mitchell, E., and Stolerman, I.P., 1971, Disturbed patterns of behavior in morphine tolerant and abstinent rats, Br.J.Pharmacol. 42:473.

Kuschinsky, K., and Hornykiewicz, O., 1972, Morphine catalepsy in the rat: Relation to striatal dopamine metabolism, Eur.J.Pharmacol. 19: 119.

Lal, H., 1975, Narcotic dependence, narcotic action and dopamine receptors, Life Sci. 17:483.

Lal, H., and Numan, R., 1976, Blockade of morphine-withdrawal body shakes by haloperidol, Life Sci., 18:163.

Lapin, V., 1974, Influence of simultaneous pinealectomy and thymectomy on the growth and formation of metastases of the Yoshida sarcoma in rats, Exp.Pathol., 9:108.

Lapin, V., 1976, Pineal gland and malignancy, Österr.Z.Onkol., 3:51.

Leger, J., and Masson, G., 1947, Factors influencing an anaphylactoid reaction in the rat, Fed.Proc.Fed.Am.Soc.Exp.Biol., 6:150.

Lindstrom, J.M., Lennon, V.A., Seybold, M.E., and Whittingham, S., 1976, Experimental autoimmune myasthenia gravis and myasthenia gravis: Biochemical and immunochemical aspects, Ann.N.Y.Acad.Sci., 274: 254.

Lomax, P., and George, R., 1966, Thyroid activity following administration of morphine in rats with hypothalamic lesions, Brain Res., 2:361.

Lotti, V.J., Kokka, N., and George, R., 1969, Pituitary-adrenal activation following intrahypothalamic microinjection of morphine, Neuroendocrinology, 4:326.

Louria, D.B., Hensle, T., and Rose, J., 1967, The major medical complications of heroin addiction, Ann.Int.Med., 67:1.

Ludovici, P.P., and Axelrod, A.E., 1951, Circulating antibodies in vitamin-deficiency states: Pteroylglutamic acid, niacin-tryptophan, vitamin B12 and D deficiencies, Proc.Soc.Exp.Biol.Med., 77:526.

Luparello, T.J., Stein, M., and Park, C.D., 1964, Effect of hypothalamic lesions on rat anaphylaxis, Am.J.Physiol., 207:911.

Luri, M.B., 1960, The reticuloendothelial system, cortisone, and thyroid function: Their relation to native resistance to infection, Ann.N. Y.Acad.Sci., 88:83.

Lutz-Bucher, B., Koch, B., Mialhe, C., and Briaud, B., 1980, Involvement of vasopressin in corticotropin-releasing effect of hypothalamic median eminence extract, Neuroendocrinology, 30:178.

Maclean, D., and Reichlin, S., 1980, Neuroendocrinology and the Immune process, in: "Psychoneuroimmunology" R.Ader and R.A.Good, eds., Academic Press, NewYork.

Maickel, R.P., Braude, M.C., and Zabit, J.E., 1977, The effects of various narcotic agonists and antagonists on deprivation-induced fluid consumption, Neuropharmacology, 16:863.

Maravelias, C.P., and Coutselinis, A.S., 1984, Suppressive effects of morphine on human blood lymphocytes: an in vitro study, IRCS Med. Sci., 12:106.

Margules, D.L., 1979, Beta-endorphin and endoloxone. Hormones of the autonomic nervous system for the conservation or expenditure of bodily resources and energy in anticipation of famine or feast, Neurosci. Biobehav.Rev., 3:155.

Mark-Kaufman, R., and Kanarek, R.B., 1980, Morphine selectively influences macronutrient intake in the rat, Pharmacol.Biochem.Behav., 12:427.

Maynert, E.W., 1967, Effect of morphine on acetylcholine and certain other neurotransmitters, Arch.Biol.Med.exp.(Santiago), 4:36.

Maynert, E.W., and Klingman, G.I., 1962, Tolerance to morphine. I.Effects on catecholamines in the brain and adrenal glands, J.Pharmacol.Exp. Ther., 135:285.

McFarlane, H., 1976, Malnutrition and impaired response to infection, Proc. Nutr.Soc., 35:263.

McFarlane, H., and Hamid, J., 1973, Cell-mediated immune response in malnutrition, Clin.Exp.Immunol. 13:153.

McFarlane, H., Reddy, S., Adcock, K.J., Adeshina, H., Cocke, A.E., and Akene, J., 1970, Immunity, transferrin and survival in kwashiorkor, Brit.Med.J., 4:268.

McDonough, R.J., Madden, J.J., Falek, A., Shafer, D.A., Pline, M., Gordon, D., Bokos, P., Kuehnle, J.C., and Mendelson, J., 1980, Alteration of T and null lymphocyte frequencies in the peripheral blood of human opiate addicts: In vivo evidence for opiate receptor sites on T lymphocytes, J.Immunol., 125:2539.

Meisenberg, G., and Simmons, W.H., 1983, Centrally mediated effects of neurohypophyseal hormones, Neurosci.Biobehav.Rev., 7:263.

Meites, J., Bruni, J.F., VanVugt, D.A., 1979, Relation of endogenous opioid peptides and morphine to neuroendocrine functions, Life Sci., 24: 1325.

Merali, Z., Chosh, P.K., Hrdina, P.D., Singhal, R.L., and Ling, G.M., 1974, Alterations in striatal acetylcholine esterase, and dopamine after methadone replacement in morphine-dependent rats, Eur.J.Pharmacol., 26:375.

Mihich, E., 1962, Host defense mechanisms in the regression of sarcoma 180 in pyridoxine deficient mice, Cancer Res., 22:218.

Mihich, E., and Nichol, C.A., 1965, Differences in the selective antitumor effects of 4-deoxypyridoxine and dietary pyridoxine deficiency, Cancer Res. 25:153.

Monjan, A.A., and Collector, M.I., 1977, Stress-induced modulation of the immune response, Science, 196:307.

Morgan, D.R., DuPont, H.L., Wood, L.V., and Kohl, S., 1984, Cytotoxicity of leucocytes from normal and Shigella-susceptible (opium-treated) Guinea pigs against Shigella sonnei, Infect.Immun., 46:22.

Morley, J.E., 1981, The endocrinology of the opiates and opioid peptides, Metabolism, 30:195.

Morley, J.E., Yamada, T., and Shulkes, A., 1979, Effects of morphine addiction and withdrawal on thyrotropin releasing hormone (TRH), somatostatin (SLI) and vasoactive intestinal peptide (VIP), Clin.Res., 27:75A.

Murray, M.J., and Murray, A.B., 1979, Anorexia of infection as a mechanism of host defense, Am.J.Clin.Nutr. 32:593.

Needham, W.P., Shuster, L., Kanel, C.C., and Thompson, M.L., 1981, Liver damage from narcotics in mice, Toxicol.Appl.Pharmacol. 58:157.

Nilzen, A., 1955, The influence of the thyroid gland on hypersensitivity reactions in animals, Acta Allergol., 7:231.

Noteboom, W.D., and Müller, G.C., 1966 a, Effect of levallorphan on RNA and protein in Hela cells, Fed.Proc., 25:646.

Noteboom, W.D., and Müller, G.C., 1966 b, Inhibition of protein and RNA synthesis in Hela cells by levallorphan and levorphanol, Molec.Pharmacol., 2:534.

Okajima, T., Motomatsu, T., Kato, K., and Ibayashi, H., 1980, Naloxone inhibits prolactin and growth hormone release induced by intracellular glucopenia in the rats, Life Sci., 27:755.

Okouchi, E., 1976, Thymus, peripheral tissue and immunological responsiveness of the pituitary dwarf mice, J.Physiol.Soc.Jpn., 38:325.

Oosterom, R., and Kater, L., 1980, Target cell subpopulations for human thymus, Clin.Immunol.Immunopathol., 17:183.

Oosterom, R., Kater, L., and Oosterom, J., 1979, Effects of human thymic epithelial conditioned medium on mitogen responsiveness of human and mouse lymphocytes, Clin.Immunol.Immunopathol., 12:460.

Özek, M., Töreci, K., Akkök, I., and Güvener, Z., 1971, Die Wirkung der Neuroleptica-Behandlung auf die Antikörperbildung, Psychopharmacologia (Berl.), 21:401.

Palmblad, J., Fohlin, L., and Lundström, M., 1977, Anorexia nervosa and polymorphonuclear (PMN) granulocyte reactions, Scand.J.Haematol., 19:334.

PerezCruet, J., Chiara, G.D., and Gessa, G.L., 1972, Accelerated synthesis of dopamine in the rat brain after methadone, Experientia, 28:926.

Puri, S.K., and Lal,H., 1973, Effect of dopaminergic stimulation or blockade on morphine-withdrawal aggression, Psychopharmacologia, 32:113.

Puri, S.K., Spaulding, T.C., and Mantione, C.R., 1978, Dopamine antagonist binding: A significant decrease with morphine dependence in the rat striatum, Life Sci., 23:637.

Radominska-Pyrek, A., Kraus-Friedmann, N., Lester, R., Little, J., and Denkins, Y., 1982, Rapid stimulation of Na^+,K^+-ATPase by glucagon, epinephrine, vasopressin and cAMP in perfused rat liver, FEBS Letters 141:56.

Rodin, A.E., 1963, The growth and spread of Walker 256 carcinoma in pinealectomized rats, Cancer Res., 23:1545.

Rofe, A.M., and Williamson, D.H., 1983, Metabolic effects of vasopressin infusion in the starved rat: Reversal of ketonaemia, Biochem.J., 212:231.

Roy, C., 1979, Vasopressin-sensitive adenylate cyclase: Reversibility of hormonal activation, Biochim.Biophys.Acta, 587:433.

Rusch, H.P., 1944, Extrinsic factors that influence carcinogenesis, Physiol.Rev., 24:177.

Santisteban, G.A., and Dougherty, T.F., 1954, Comparison of the influences of adrenocortical hormones on the growth and involution of lymphatic organs, Endocrinology, 54:130.

Sarne, Y., Gilt-Ad, I., and Laron, Z., 1981, Regulation of hypophysial secretion by endogenous opiates: Humoral endorphin stimulates the release of growth hormone, Life Sci., 28:681.

Sawyer, C.H., Critchlow, B.V., and Barrclough, C.A., 1955, Mechanism of blockage of pituitary activation in the rat by morphine, atropine and barbiturates, Endocrinology, 57:345.

Scrimshaw, N.S., Taylor, C.E., and Gordon, J.E., 1968, "Interactions of nutrition and infection", World Health Organization, Geneva.

Sequeira, W., Jones, E., Siegel, M.E., Lorenz, M., and Kallick, C., 1982,

Pyogenic infections of the pubis symphysis, Ann.Int.Med., 96:604.

Sing, U., 1979, Effect of catecholamines on lymphopoiesis in fetal mouse thymic explants, J.Anat., 129:279.

Shavit, Y., Lewis, J.W., Terman, G.W., Gale, R.P., and Liebeskind, J.C., 1984, Opioid peptides mediate with suppressive effects of stress on natural killer cell cytotoxicity, Science, 223:188.

Sloan, J.W., Brooks, J.W., Eisenman, A.J., and Martin, W.R., 1963, The effect of addiction to and abstinence from morphine on rat tissue catecholamine and serotonin levels, Psychopharmacologia(Berl.), 4:261.

Small, C.B., Klein, R.S., Friendland, G.H., Moll, B., Emerson, E.E., and Spigland, I., 1983, Community-acquired opportunistic infectious and defective cellular immunity in heterosexual drug abusers and homosexual men, Am.J.Med., 74:433.

Smith, A.A., Hui, F.W., and Crofford, M.J., 1977, Inhibition of growth in young mice treated with d,l-methadone, Eur.J.Pharmacol., 43:307.

Smith, D.J., and Joffe, J.M., 1975, Increased neonatal mortality of offspring of male rats treated with methadone or morphine before mating, Nature, 253:202.

Smythe, P.M., Shonland, M., Brereton-Stiles, G.G., Coovadia, H.M., Grace, H.J., Loening, W.E.K., Mafoyame, A., and Pavent, M.A., 1971, Thymolymphatic deficiency and depression of cell-mediated immunity in protein-calorie malnutrition, Lancet, II:939.

Spackman, D.H., and Riley, V., 1974, Increased corticosterone, a factor in LDH-virus induced alterations of immunological responses in mice, Proc.Am.Assoc.Cancer Res., 15:143.

Spackman, D.H., Riley, V., Santisbetan, G.A., Kirk, W., and Bredburg, L., 1974, The role of stress in producing elevated corticosterone levels and thymus involution in mice, Abstr.Int.Cancer.Congr., 11th, 3:382.

Spector, N.H., Cannon, L.T., Diggs, C.L., Morrison, J.E., and Koob, G.F., 1975, Hypothalamic lesions: Effects on immunological responses, Physiologist, 18:401.

Solomon, G.F., and Amkraut, A.A., 1979, Neuroendocrine aspects of the immune response and their implications for stress effects on tumor immunity, Cancer Detect.Prev., 2:197.

Stein, M., Schiavi, R.C., and Camerino, M.S., 1976, Influencer of brain and behavior on the immune system, Science, 191:435.

Stein, M., Schiavi, R.C., and Luparello, T.J., 1969, The hypothalamus and immune process, Ann.N.Y.Acad.Sci., 164:465.

Suskind, R., 1977, in: "Malnutrition and the Immune Response", RavenPress, NewYork.

Tache, Y., Lis, M., and Collu, R., 1977, Effects of thyrotropin-releasing on behavioral and hormonal changes induced by β-endorphin, Life Sci., 21:841.

Tannenbaum, A., and Silverstone, H., 1953, Nutrition in relation to cancer, Adv.Cancer Res., 1:451.

Tarr, K.H., 1980, Candida endophthalmitis and drug abuse, Aust.J.Ophthalmol. 8:303.

Terragna, A., and Jannuzzi, C., 1963, Ormoni steroidei e anticorpopoiesi. Nota II. Valutazione comparativa di vari ormoni anabolizzanti, G.Mal.Inf., 15:360.

Tolentino, P., Terragna, A., and Jannuzzi, C., 1961, Ormoni steroidei e anticorpopoiesi. Nota I. Blocco enzimatico della 1. idrossilasi surrenalica. Effetto della somministrazione di androgeni, G.Mal. Inf., 13:561.

Tsypin, A.B., and Maltzev, V.N., 1967, The effects of irritation of the hypothalamus on the concentration of normal antibodies in blood, Patol.Fiziol., 11:83.

Turner, C.D., and Hagnara, J.T., 1971, in: "General Endocrinology" 5th ed., Saunders, Philadelphia.

Visscher, B., Ball, Z., Barnes, R.H., and Silvertsen, I., 1942, The influence of caloric restriction upon the incidence of spontaneous
mammary carcinoma in mice, Surgery, 11:48.

Vogt, M., 1954, The concentration of sympathin in different parts of the
central nervous system under normal conditions and after the administration of drugs, J.Physiol.(Lond.), 123:451.

Wakabayashi, M., 1966, On the effect of hormones on antibody production, J.
Jap.Obstet.Gynaec.Soc., 13:209.

Weiner, N., 1979, Multiple factors regulating the release of norepinephrine
consequent to nerve stimulation, Fed.Proc., 38:2193.

Westphal, U., 1971, in: "Steroid-Protein Interactions", Springer-Verlag,
NewYork.

White, A., Handler, P., and Smith, E.L., 1968, in: "Principles of Biochemistry" 4th ed. McGraw-Hill, NewYork.

Williams, E.G., and Oberst, F.W., 1946, A cycle of morphine addictions, I:
Biological investigations, Public Health Reports, 61:1.

Wood, C.L., Babcock, C.J., and Blum, J.J., 1981, Effects of vasopressin on
fructose and glycogen metabolism in hepatocytes from fed and fasted
rats, Arch.Biochem.Biophys., 212:43.

Wybran, J., Appleboom, T., Famaey, J.P., and Govaerts, A., 1979, Suggestive
evidence for receptors for morphine and methionine-enkephalin on
normal blood T lymphocytes, J.Immunol., 123:1068.

Zagon, I.S., and McLaughlin, P.J., 1977, Morphine and brain growth retardation in the rat, Pharmacology 15:276.

Zagon, I.S., and McLaughlin, P.C., 1977 b, Effects of chronic morphine administration on pregnant rats and their offspring, Pharmacology, 15:
302.

Zagon, I.S., and McLaughlin, 1983, Increased brain size and cellular content
in infant rats treated with an opiate antagonist, Science, 221:1179.

Zimmerman, E., and Pang, C.N., 1976, Acute Effects of Opiate Administration
on Pituitary Gonadotrophin and Prolactin Release, in: "Tissue
Response to Addictive Drugs", D.M.Ford and D.H.Clouvet, eds.,
Spectrum Publications, NewYork.

OPIOID PEPTIDE EFFECTS ON LEUKOCYTE MIGRATION

S. Lori Brown*, Sei Tokuda,** Linda C. Saland,*** and
Dennis E. Van Epps*

*Departments of Pathology and Medicine
**Department of Microbiology
***Department of Anatomy

The University of New Mexico School of Medicine
Albuquerque, New Mexico 87131

INTRODUCTION

The recognition that morphine bound stereospecifically to receptors
in the brain to exert its effects led to a concerted search for an
endogenous ligand for the opiate receptor (Terenius and Wahlstrom,
1975). In 1975, peptides which bound to the opiate receptor were
isolated from porcine brain extracts and characterized (Hughes et al.,
1975; Hughes et al., 1976). The first opioid peptides characterized were
the pentapeptides methionine-and-leucine enkephalin (met- and
leu-enkephalin). Simultaneously, a larger (31 amino acid), more active
peptide containing the amino acid sequence of met-enkephalin as its first
5 N-terminal amino acids was isolated from porcine and camel pituitary
and was named beta-endorphin (a contraction for "endogenous morphine")
(Teschemacher et al., 1975; Li and Chung, 1976). Beta-endorphin and
alpha-endorphin (amino acids 1-16 of beta-endorphin), gamma-endorphin
(amino acids 1-17 of beta-endorphin), (Ling et al., 1976), as well as
other neuropeptides, may arise from a 31 Kd glycoprotein, the
proopiomelanocortin molecule (reviewed by Frederickson and Geary, 1982).
The discovery that beta-endorphin is released from the pituitary along
with the steroidogenic hormone, adrenocorticotropin (ACTH) in response to
acute stress suggests that in addition to its numerous actions in the
central nervous system, beta-endorphin, like ACTH, also has peripheral
hormonal effects (Guillemin et al., 1977; Rossier et al., 1977). The
release of both ACTH and beta endorphin may be under the control of the
hypothalamic peptide, corticotropin releasing factor (CRF) in some
species (Hook et al, 1982 and Knepel et al, 1984).

Endogenous ligands for the opiate receptor are traditionally defined
as ligands which compete for binding at the opiate receptor with the
agonist morphine or with naloxone, the opiate receptor antagonist.
Leukocytes have both classical receptors as defined by morphine and
naloxone binding (Lopker et al., 1980; Mehrishi and Mills, 1983) and a
specific non-opiate receptor for beta-endorphin (Hazum et al., 1979). In
addition, leu-enkephalin binds to Jurkat cells, a human lymphoid line,

and binding is not prevented by morphine or naloxone suggesting the existence of other lymphocyte receptors which are specific for opioid peptides but unreceptive to exogenous ligands (Ausiello and Roda, 1984).

That leukocytes possess receptors for opiates and opioid peptides suggests that these cells may be targets for peripheral hormonal effects of opioid peptides. A multitude of recent studies have suggested that plasma beta-endorphin levels rise in response to stressful stimuli in both humans and experimental animals (Genazzani et al., 1981; Puolakka et al., 1982; Wilkes et al., 1980; Cosontos et al., 1979; Goland et al., 1981; Mueller, 1981; Wardlaw et al., 1981; Nakao et al., 1981; Fraioli et al., 1980; Colt et al., 1981; Dubois et al., 1981). In humans, the "stressed" level of circulating beta-endorphin has been reported to be as high as 10^{-10} M. Like beta-endorphin, met-enkephalin is also found in the plasma (Clement-Jones et al., 1980; Shanks et al., 1981). Though its relationship to stress is not known, met-enkephalin has recently been detected in bovine adrenal glands (Kilpatrick et al.,1980; Livett et al., 1982; Pelto-Huikko et al., 1982). Because the adrenal glands are activated in response to stressful stimuli, one may cautiously posit that the adrenal glands may be a source of stress-provoked circulating met-enkephalin. Leu-enkephalin is also found circulating in plasma, and its concentration increases in response to stress (Ryder and Eng, 1981).

Another possible source of circulating opioids are leukocytes themselves. Smith and Blalock (1981) have discovered that in response to viral infection human peripheral blood lymphocytes produce a protein which is immunologically indistinguishable from gamma endorphin. Utilizing immunofluorescence and radioimmunoassay, Lolait et al (1984) have shown that mice spleen cells produced a beta endorphin like peptide.

Evidence for a Role for Opioid Peptides in Immunomodulation

Since the discovery of the opioid peptides in 1975, numerous studies have been devoted to determining the location of endogenous opioids and to understanding their role in the central nervous system (reviewed by Smith and Simon, 1981; Hughes et al., 1980; Frederickson and Geary, 1982; Olson et al., 1984). In addition to their analgesic properties centrally administered endogenous opioids mediate numerous behavioral effects (Barchas et al., 1978). Because beta-endorphin and enkephalin have been shown to be released into the peripheral circulation, this suggests that in addition to their numerous roles in the central nervous system, these opioid peptides also act as peripheral hormones (Amir et al., 1980). In the past few years, accumulating evidence indicates that endogenous opioids modulate numerous measurable immune functions (reviewed by Fischer and Falke, 1984; Weber and Pert, 1984). To date, receptors for opiates or opioid peptides have been found on both mononuclear and polymorphonuclear leukocytes (Ausiello and Roda, 1984; Hazum et al., 1979; Lopker et al., 1980; Mehrishi and Mills, 1983). Likewise, opiates and opioid peptides have been found to exert effects on each of these cell types. A summary of in vitro studies is presented in Table 1 and briefly in the following text.

The earliest report that an opioid peptide could bind to and modulate leukocyte function was by Wybran et al (1979). They demonstrated that both the exogenous opiate morphine and the endogenous opioid, met-enkephalin, affected the formation of active T-cell rosettes with sheep red blood cells. Though these drugs had opposing effects on active rosette formation, the effects of either were prevented by naloxone, the opiate receptor antagonist. Miller et al (1984) have confirmed the finding that met-enkephalin enhances active T-cell rosette

TABLE 1: OPIOID PEPTIDES AND OPIATE EFFECTS ON LEUKOCYTES IN VITRO

IMMUNE PARAMETER	β	α	γ	M	L	MO	N	REF
Active T-Rosette Formation				↑*	↓	↓*		Wybran et al, 1979
Active T-Rosette Formation				↑	↑		↑	Miller et al, 1984
Total T-Rosette Formation				↑		↓*		Wybran et al, 1979
Human Peripheral Blood Lymphocyte Proliferation	↓						↑	McCain et al, 1982
Human Peripheral Blood Lymphocyte Proliferation	↑					↑	↑	Bocchini et al, 1983
Rat Spleen Lymphocyte Proliferation	↑	↑		↑			↓±	Gilman et al, 1982
Mouse Spleen Lymphocyte Proliferation	↑			↑	↑			Plotnikoff & Miller, 1983
Mouse Spleen-Specific Antibody Production	↓	↓*	↑	↓	↓		↓±	Johnson et al, 1982
Human Antibody-Dependent Cellular Cytotoxicity	↑						↑	Froelich & Bankhurst, 1984
Human Natural Killer-Mediated Cytotoxicity	↑*	↑		↑*	↑	↑	↑	Mathews et al, 1983
Human Natural Killer-Mediated Cytotoxicity	↑*			↑	↑			Faith et al, 1984
Human Natural Killer-Mediated Cytotoxicity	↑*	↑	↑*	↑	↑		↑	Kay et al, 1984
Rat Mast Cell Serotonin Release	↑*			↑*		↑*	↓	Yamasaki et al, 1982
Human Leukocyte Chemotaxis								
Mononuclear Cells	↑*			↑*			↑	Van Epps & Saland, 1984
Neutrophils	↑			↑				Van Epps et al, 1983
Response to Chemotactic Factor After Preincubation in Opioid:								
Mononuclear Cells	↓							Van Epps & Saland, 1984
Neutrophils	↑							Van Epps & Saland, 1984
Neutrophils	↑*						↑±	Simpkins et al, 1984
Production of Lymphocyte Chemotactic Factor	↓	↑		↓			↓	Brown & Van Epps, 1985
Leukocyte Adherence	↑			↑				Van Epps (unpublished)

Key:

α = Alpha-Endorphin	M = Met-Enkephalin
β = Beta-Endorphin	L = Leu-Enkephalin
γ = Gamma-Endorphin	MO = Morphine
	N = Naloxone

↑ Enhanced
↓ Inhibited
→ No Effect
± Insignificant Effect

*Effect prevented by naloxone

369

formation and have shown that leu-enkephalin has similar effects in this assay. Met- and leu-enkephalin not only increase the percentage of T-lymphocytes forming active rosettes from normal human donors but have similar effects on T cells from lymphoma patients (Miller et al., 1983).

Opioid peptides and opiates also have effects on in vitro T-lymphocyte proliferation in response to the mitogenic lectins, phytohemmaglutinin (PHA) and concanavalin A (Con A). McCain et al (1982) have shown that 10^{-7}M beta-endorphin suppressed the human peripheral blood lymphocyte (PBL) blastogenic response to PHA. The suppressive effects of beta-endorphin were not prevented by 10^{-6}M naloxone which, alone, had no effect on PHA mitogenesis. Bocchini et al (1983) have shown that naloxone and morphine both enhance the proliferative response of human PBL to PHA. Phencyclidine, a drug which may bind to opiate receptors (Vincent et al, 1978), has suppressive effects on mitogen-induced proliferation of human lymphocytes (Khansari et al., 1984). Though human PBL proliferation was suppressed by some concentrations of beta-endorphin, rat spleen lymphocyte (RSL) proliferation appears to be enhanced (Gilman et al., 1982). In these experiments, naloxone, which slightly suppressed RSL proliferation itself, did not prevent the effects of beta-endorphin. Mouse spleen lymphocyte proliferation has also been shown to be enhanced by leu- and met-enkephalin (Plotnikoff and Miller, 1983).

The response to the B-cell mitogen, lipopolysaccharide/dextran sulfate, by RSL was not affected by beta-endorphin (Gilman et al., 1982). However, production of antibody by B cells in response to a T-cell-dependent antigen was depressed by alpha-endorphin, met- and leu-enkephalin and to a lesser degree by beta- and gamma-endorphin (Johnson et al., 1982). Naloxone prevented the suppressive effect of alpha-endorphin on antibody production by B cells in this system.

Beta-endorphin has been shown to have no effect on antibody-dependent cellular cytotoxicity (Froelich and Bankhurst, 1984), but beta-endorphin, met-enkephalin, leu-enkephalin and gamma-endorphin enhance human natural killer (NK) activity against the NK-sensitive K562 cell line (Mathews et al., 1983; Faith et al., 1984; Kay et al., 1984). The enhancing effects of beta-endorphin, met-enkephalin and gamma-endorphin were prevented by naloxone. Others, however, have reported that opioid peptides depress human NK activity as well as killing by cytotoxic T-lymphocytes (Prete and Levin, 1985).

In addition to the effects of opioids on lymphocytes, opioids may also bind to mast cells and cause degranulation. Yamasaki et al (1982) have shown that beta-endorphin, met-enkephalin, and morphine reverse or prevent the PGE_1-mediated inhibition of serotonin release from rat mast cells. Others have shown that opiates and opioid peptides induce wheal and flare reactions in skin testing and enhance histamine-induced itch and flare (Casale et al., 1984; Fjellner and Hagermark, 1982).

All of these findings indicate that leukocytes have functional opiate receptors or receptors for opioid peptides which when bound by ligand may modulate the function of these cells. Furthermore, taken together, these studies indicate that opioid peptides may potentially affect both the afferent and efferent limbs of the immune response. One aspect of the expression of immunity which may be influenced by the opioid peptides is leukocyte chemotaxis. The directional locomotion of cells in response to a gradient of chemotactic factor is a functional characteristic of polymorphonuclear leukocytes (PMN), monocytes and lymphocytes and will be the subject of the remainder of this review.

LEUKOCYTE CHEMOTAXIS AND OPIOID PEPTIDES

Chemotaxis is the directional movement of cells in response to a chemical gradient. The ability of leukocytes to sense and respond to chemotactic factors may, in part determine the outcome of immune or inflammatory responses. In vivo, this mobilization of leukocytes to a source of chemotactic factor is believed to be the major mechanism of accumulating PMN, monocytes or lymphocytes at an inflammatory focus or site of antigenic challenge. The chemotactic factors may be generated as a result of complement activation and the consequent generation of C5a, activation of arachidonic acid metabolism to produce leukotrienes, or by antigen or mitogen triggering of lymphocytes to release chemotactic factors for neutrophils, monocytes or lymphocytes.

The elaboration of chemotactic lymphokines by inflammatory or immune cells may be important in stimulating the migration of immunocytes to sites of inflammation or of antigen deposition. The type of cell accumulating at the inflammatory site is probably dictated by a number of factors, one of which is the cell specificity of the chemotactic factor generated at that site. For example, antigen-antibody complex deposition and the release of C5a derived from the activation of the complement system stimulates predominantly a neutrophil influx. A monocyte-specific chemotactic factor can also be derived from antigen- or mitogen-challenged lymphocytes and may be responsible for the influx of monocytes and macrophages of cellular immune reactions. More recently, the release of a T-cell-specific chemotactic factor from antigen- or mitogen-challenged lymphocytes has been described which may account for the concentration of T cells at sites involving cellular immune reactions, such as delayed cutaneous hypersensitivity reactions, allograft rejections, or tumor rejections. It is apparent that any agents that may alter the migration of leukocytes to an inflammatory site may potentially result in a compromised or, alternatively, an enhanced expression of immunity in the host.

Several recent studies have shown that opioid peptides can directly stimulate leukocyte chemotaxis. In addition, more recent studies from this laboratory indicate that opioids can also modulate the production of a T-lymphocyte chemotactic factor by human mononuclear cells.

Beta-endorphin and Met-enkephalin Stimulate Leukocyte Locomotion In Vivo

Acute injection of the opioid peptides beta endorphin and met enkephalin into the cerebral ventricle of cannulated rats, results in the rapid influx of macrophage-like cells (Saland et al, 1983 and Van Epps et al, 1983). Within an hour following infusion of these opioid peptides into the ventricle, scanning and transmission electron microscopy revealed numerous cells exhibiting a typical macrophage morphology (high cytoplasmic to nuclear ratio, multiple granules and vacuoles, pseudopod-like projections, and ruffled membrane) atop the ependyma. In these previous studies, beta endorphin was much more effective than met enkephalin at stimulating migration of these cells into the ventricle. Alpha endorphin infused animals were indistinguishible from saline infused controls who displayed only a minimal cellular infiltration. The origin of these macrophage-like cells is not known but they could conceivably arise from peripheral blood monocytes (Baldwin, 1980) or from a pool of macrophage-like microglial cells residing in close proximity to the ventricle (Bleier and Marsh, 1978).

More recent studies (Saland et al, 1984) demonstrate that chronic infusion of beta endorphin into the rat cerebral ventricle, using osmotic pumps over 24- or 48-hours, induces an inflammatory-like cellular

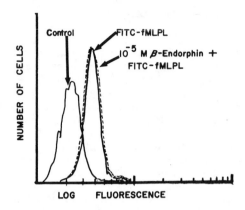

Figure 1. Beta-endorphin does not bind to the f-MLP receptor on
neutrophils. Control neutrophils were incubated in media alone
and represent autofluorescence of neutrophils. Neutrophils
treated with FITC-fMLPL bind the fluorescent probe (solid
line). Those neutrophils pretreated for 15 minutes with
beta-endorphin (broken line) bind the f-MLPL equally well
indicating that the endorphin is not binding at the f-MLP
receptor.

response, including the appearance of neutrophils, lymphocyte-like cells,
and macrophages. Infusion of other related compounds (naloxone, alpha
endorphin, met enkephalin) or saline produced little or no cellular
response.

That these opioids stimulated a cell infiltration indicated that
they could be chemotactic for leukocytes and suggested that macrophages
have a mechanism for recognizing and responding to opioid peptides.
Although it is difficult to visualize how a gradient of opioid peptide
may form spontaneously in vivo, the effects of opioid peptides on
leukocytes may be particularly relevent to the recent clinical use of
endogenous opiates. Several reports have described the use of opioid
peptides as an analgesic by infusion into cerebral spinal fluid (CSF)
during labor and delivery (Oyama et al, 1980) or into individuals with
chronic pain (Hosobuchi and Li, 1978). The potential also exists for
interaction of opiate drugs, such as morphine or its derivatives, with
cells of the immune system within the CSF during administration to
patients via a lumbar puncture route (Stoelting, 1980 and Hughes et al,
1984).

Opioid Peptides Stimulate Chemotaxis of Human Leukocyte In Vitro

Numerous methods for studying chemotaxis in vitro are currently used
(Gee, 1984). The response of human peripheral blood leukocytes can be
measured in vitro using a modification of the Boyden assay (Boyden,
1962). In this assay, factors being assessed for their ability to

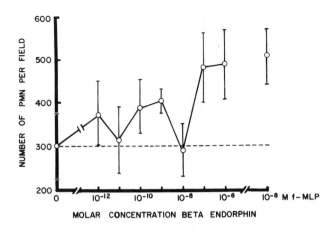

Figure 2. Beta-endorphin enhances neutrophil adherance. Data are expressed as the number of neutrophils adhering per high power field. The adherence of neutrophils in response to 10^{-8}M f-MLP is shown for comparison. Each point represents the Mean±SD of 3-experiments.

stimulate locomotion are placed in the lower chamber of a blind well chemotaxis chamber. A membrane of known pore size is laid over the test solution, and separates leukocytes, in the upper compartment, from the test solution. The distance that leukocytes migrate into the nitrocellulose membrane in response to the test solution can be assessed by using a microscope with micrometer. These techniques have been applied to evaluate the response of human neutrophils, lymphocytes and monocytes to opioid peptides _in vitro,_ and results of these studies are summarized below.

Previous studies from this laboratory have shown that both beta endorphin and met enkephalin stimulated migration of human peripheral blood mononuclear cells _in vitro_ (Van Epps et al, 1983C and Van Epps and Saland, 1984). It was determined that the effect of these opioid peptides on cell locomotion was due to an enhanced directional locomotion (chemotaxis) and not due to enhanced random migration (chemokinesis). This response was dose-dependent and attributable to the glass adherent population in the mononuclear cell preparation. When beta endorphin or met enkephalin were tested in concentrations ranging from 10^{-14} to 10^{-7}M an interesting phenomenon was observed. Both opioids stimulated bimodal peaks of mononuclear cell locomotion. The significance of a bimodal peak is not clear but could be due to, 1.) multiple opiate receptor types on mononuclear cells, 2.) differential binding of opioid peptides by mononuclear cell subsets, or 3.) a combination of 1 and 2. The observed migration of freshly isolated mononuclear cells to 10^{-8}M beta endorphin in these studies was approximately 80% of that seen in response to 10^{-8}M formyl-methionyl-leucyl-phenylalanine (f-MLP). F-MLP is a synthetic peptide which is a relatively potent chemotactic factor for monocytes (Cianciolo and Snyderman, 1980) and for neutrophils (Showell et al, 1976). Although neutrophils have been shown to have more receptors for dihydromorphine than monocytes (Lopker et al, 1980), similar measurements of neutrophil migration in responses to beta endorphin showed variable response averaging only 30% of that observed utilizing f-MLP as a chemotactic stimulus. This may reflect the differences in PMN and monocyte responsiveness to f-MLP since monocytes do not migrate as far in response to fMLP as neutrophils. In the same study, monocytes also showed enhanced migration in response to met-enkephalin, but the magnitude of the response was less than that seen in response to a gradient of beta endorphin. These studies imply that monocytes recognize and respond more effectively to opioid peptides than neutrophils. It is feasible that the lower responsiveness of neutrophils may be due to their demonstrated ability to oxidize met-enkephalin to its sulfoxide derivative (Turkall et al, 1982) and render it inactive. This may also hold true for beta-endorphin which also contains methionine.

In our previous studies experiments were performed to determine whether the migration of mononuclear cells to beta-endorphin and met-enkephalin was opiate receptor mediated. Monocytes were preincubated in naloxone and then placed in the upper compartment of chemotaxis chambers containing beta endorphin or met enkephalin in the lower compartment. Naloxone prevented the migration of mononuclear cells to both of the opioid peptides. Naloxone also showed some slight inhibition of the mononuclear cell response to f-MLP, although not approaching that seen with the opioid peptide-mediated chemotaxis.

Because of the presence of some similar amino acids in met-enkephalin (Tyr-gly-gly-phe-met), beta-endorphin, and f-met-leu-phe, we wished to determine whether opioids were binding at the f-MLP receptor. Studies were performed to determine if either met enkephalin or beta endorphin could block the binding of the f-MLP analog, FITC-f-met-leu-phe-lysine (Van Epps and Saland, 1984). By flow cytometry, 30% of the mononuclear cells bound the fluoresceinated conjugate of f-MLPL which binds to the f-MLP receptor. This binding is attributable to monocytes of which approximately 70-80% bind f-MLP. Neither beta endorphin nor met enkephalin blocked the binding of FITC-f-MLPL indicating that these opioid peptides were not interacting with the f-MLP receptor on monocytes. Similar studies were conducted using human neutrophils. Isolated neutrophils were preincubated for 15 minutes in media alone or with 10^{-5}M beta-endorphin. FITC-fMLPL was then added to the neutrophils for 15 minutes at 25°C, washed and fixed with paraformaldehyde, and binding of the fluorescent fMLP analog to neutrophils was analyzed by flow cytometry. As can be seen in Figure 1, the f-MLPL binding to neutrophils was not blocked by beta-endorphin, indicating that endorphin was not binding to f-MLP receptors on neutrophils. Similar experiments performed with 10^{-5}M met-enkephalin indicated that it did not reduce the binding of f-MLPL to its receptor.

In vivo, one can imagine that leukocytes may be exposed to circulating opioids prior to their migrating from the blood to an inflammatory focus. This type of pre-exposure was simulated in an in vitro model in which leukocytes were preincubated in 10^{-8}M beta endorphin for 15 minutes and their chemotactic response to a second stimulus, such as f-MLP or the chemotactic factor casein, is tested (Van Epps et al, 1983c). When mononuclear cells or isolated lymphocytes were tested in this fashion, there was an inhibition of the migration in response to f-MLP or casein. This phenomenon of decreased responsiveness to a second chemotactic stimuli after exposure to a first chemotactic stimuli is known as down regulation or desensitization and has been previously reported (Nelson et al, 1978). In the modified Boyden assay, beta-endorphin did not down regulate the response of neutrophils to a second chemotactic stimulus (Van Epps et al, 1983c). However, others have reported an enhanced response to f-MLP by neutrophils preincubated in beta endorphin when chemotaxis was measured by the chemotaxis under agarose technique (Simpkins et al, 1984). In their studies the migration response of neutrophils to 10^{-7} M f-MLP was significantly enhanced when PMN were preincubated in beta endorphin. It is interesting that although naloxone alone tended to enhance the chemotactic response of neutrophils, it antagonized the effects of beta endorphin on neutrophils. Is it possible that naloxone alone exerts some agonistic effects but in the presence of an agonist for the opiate receptor, such as beta endorphin, it acts as an antagonist? An alternative explanation for these seemingly incongruent effects of naloxone may be that additive effects of the two factors result in a suppression of the response. Similar mixed effects of naloxone have been observed in other systems. In studies by Johnson et al (1982), naloxone mildly inhibited specific antibody production, while it prevented the inhibitory effects of alpha endorphin in this same system. Likewise, naloxone, like the opiate agonist morphine, enhanced the proliferative response of human lymphocytes (Bocchini et al, 1983). It may be that naloxone is not a pure antagonist for the opiate receptor.

One critical requirement for leukocyte chemotaxis is the necessity for adherence. It is well known that chemotactic factors enhance neutrophil adherence (O'Flaherty et al., 1978; Hoover et al., 1980) and that variation in the adherence of neutrophils to a substratum will influence their ability to migrate (Wilkinson et al., 1982). In view of the fact that our previous studies of PMN and monocyte responses to opioid peptides and those of Simpkins et al, (1984) indicate that the chemotactic response of these cells may be influenced by opioid peptides, experiments were designed to determine the effects of both beta-endorphin and met-enkephalin on human neutrophil adherence. In these studies, 1.5 X 10^5 isolated human PMN were placed in 1 X 2 cm compartments on 5% fetal calf serum-coated tissue culture slides and incubated for 20 minutes at 37°C with or without opioid peptide. Slides were then washed gently, fixed with paraformaldehyde, and the number of cells per 100X field quantified. As shown in Figure 2, when 10^{-12} to 10^{-6} M beta-endorphin is added to neutrophils, a marked increase in the number of cells adhering to glass slides following a 20-minute incubation was observed. This response was dose dependent, and the titration curve was suggestive of a bimodal response like that seen previously in the chemotaxis assays. The adherence of neutrophils in the presence of 10^{-8} M f-MLP is shown for comparison. Met-enkephalin, too, enhanced the adherence of neutrophils to the coated slides. The observed enhancing effects of opioid peptides on neutrophil adherence may account in part for some of the effect on PMN locomotion observed by Simpkins et al where enhancement of neutrophil migration to f-MLP was observed.

The demonstration that opioid peptides directly influence leukocyte migration and that these effects are naloxone reversible is additional evidence for the existence of functional opioid receptors on leukocytes. It can be imagined that in vivo exposure of leukocytes to circulating beta endorphin or met enkephalin may result in an altered response to chemotactic factors which might affect the host's immune status.

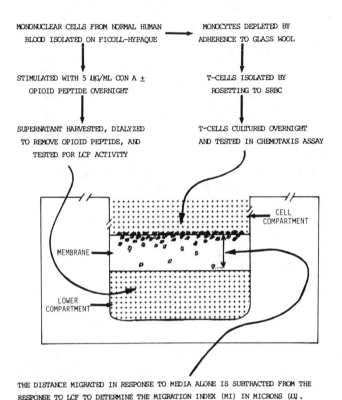

MONONUCLEAR CELLS FROM NORMAL HUMAN BLOOD ISOLATED ON FICOLL-HYPAQUE → MONOCYTES DEPLETED BY ADHERENCE TO GLASS WOOL

STIMULATED WITH 5 µG/ML CON A ± OPIOID PEPTIDE OVERNIGHT

T-CELLS ISOLATED BY ROSETTING TO SRBC

SUPERNATANT HARVESTED, DIALYZED TO REMOVE OPIOID PEPTIDE, AND TESTED FOR LCF ACTIVITY

T-CELLS CULTURED OVERNIGHT AND TESTED IN CHEMOTAXIS ASSAY

CELL COMPARTMENT

MEMBRANE

LOWER COMPARTMENT

THE DISTANCE MIGRATED IN RESPONSE TO MEDIA ALONE IS SUBTRACTED FROM THE RESPONSE TO LCF TO DETERMINE THE MIGRATION INDEX (MI) IN MICRONS (µ).

Figure 3   The production and measurement of T-lymphocyte chemotactic factor (LCF).

EFFECTS OF OPIOID PEPTIDES ON T-LYMPHOCYTE CHEMOTACTIC FACTOR PRODUCTION

In recent years, the central role of lymphokines in regulating the immune response has become apparent. The T-lymphocyte chemotactic factor (LCF) is a lymphokine produced by Con A or antigen stimulated mononuclear cells (Van Epps, 1982, Van Epps et al, 1983A, Van Epps et al, 1983B, Center and Cruikshank, 1982, Cruikshank and Center, 1982) This lymphokine is produced by lymphocytes and is chemotactic for T-lymphocytes. Because only a small number of the lymphocytes that are attracted to a site of antigen deposition are antigen specific (McCluskey et al, 1963), it may be hypothesized that this chemotactic lymphokine is important in recruiting unsensitized lymphocytes to a site of antigenic challenge. The fact that this or a similar lymphokine is produced in the human mixed lymphocyte reaction (El-Naggar et al, 1982) suggests that recruiting lymphocytes to the site of an allograft may be a critical step in allograft rejection.

Our recent studies show that the production or secretion of this lymphokine is inhibited by both beta endorphin and met enkephalin (Brown and Van Epps, 1985). LCF is produced by Con A-stimulated human mononuclear cells and can be measured utilizing the leading front T-cell chemotaxis assay (Van Epps et al, 1983a). Figure 3 outlines the procedure for generating LCF containing supernatants and measuring its activity in the T-cell chemotaxis assay. Both beta endorphin and met enkephalin suppressed the generation of this lymphokine by mononuclear cells. On the contrary, alpha-endorphin did not significantly alter the production of this lymphokine. The effect of high concentrations

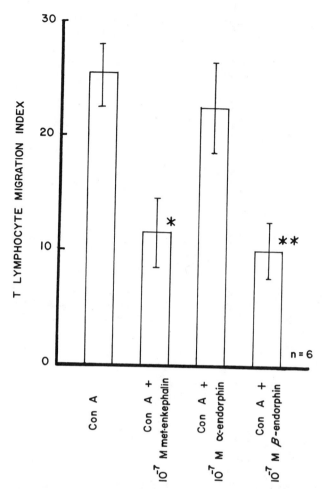

Figure 4. LCF production in the presence and absence of opioid peptides. The production of LCF by opioid containing cultures is compared to the control (Con A) supernatant. *p $\leq$ .05, **p $\leq$ .001. Supernatants generated with alpha-endorphin do not differ significantly from the control.

(10^{-7}M) of beta endorphin, met enkephalin, and alpha endorphin on LCF production are shown in Figure 4. These data are expressed as the migration index: the difference in the distance in microns (u) migrated by T lymphocytes in response to LCF containing supernatants and to media alone. As can be seen, the distance that T cells migrated in response to supernatants generated with 10^{-7}M beta-endorphin or met-enkephalin present is significantly decreased, reflecting a decrease in the generation of LCF in these supernatants. Alpha-endorphin, however, had no significant effect on the production of LCF (Brown and Van Epps, 1985). As can be seen in Figure 5, a titration of beta endorphin resulted in bimodal peaks of inhibition of LCF production. In the two representative experiments shown, it should be noted that peak inhibition varied slightly, but the bimodal curve was a consistent finding and the peaks of inhibition were between 10^{-6} - 10^{-8}M and 10^{-10} to 10^{-12}M. This variability probably represents differences in the sensitivity of mononuclear cells from different donors to opioid peptides as well as differences in responding T-cell preparations. The same effect was seen with met enkephalin. Again, the phenomenon of a bimodal

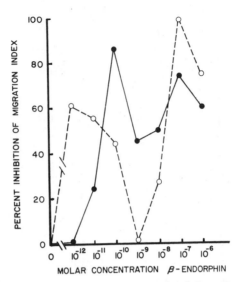

Figure 5. Inhibition of LCF production is bimodal. Experiment 1 and experiment 2 demonstrate that although the peak inhibition may vary from donor to donor, it is a consistent finding.

peak may be due to multiple types of receptors for opioids on these cells or to different receptors on mononuclear cell subpopulations which in turn may influence LCF production.

Experiments to determine whether the effect of these peptides on LCF production were mediated by the opiate receptor showed that naloxone, like the opioid peptides, inhibited the production of LCF. However, unlike the opioid peptides, mononuclear cells titrated with naloxone exhibited only a single peak of inhibition at 10^{-9}M. It was surprising then, that although naloxone exhibited some agonistic qualities, it was a partial antagonist with respect to the effects of both beta endorphin and met enkephalin as is shown in Figure 6. For instance, the migration index in response to the control LCF supernatant (Con A alone) was 35 ± 6u. When 10^{-8}M naloxone was tested, the migration index was decreased to 13 ± 7u. LCF supernatants generated in the presence of 10^{-8}M beta-endorphin stimulated a response of 17 ± 6u. However, when both 10^{-8}M naloxone and 10^{-8}M beta-endorphin were included in culture, mononuclear cells produced slightly more LCF activity than was seen in response to beta-endorphin alone, but not as much as was seen in control supernatants. This finding was consistent with several concentrations of naloxone and opioid peptide suggesting that it was not an artifact. Again, this speaks strongly for a re-evaluation of naloxone's status as a pure antagonist of the opiate receptor. Indeed it has been suggested that naloxone may exert effects independent of the opiate receptor (Badawy et al, 1983) or in some circumstances act as an agonist (Ferreira and Nakamura, 1979).

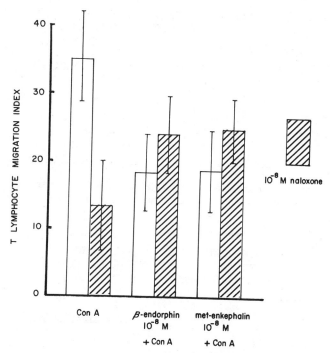

Figure 6. Naloxone alone inhibits the production of LCF but in the presence of opioid peptide acts as a partial antagonist. These data are the mean ± S.E. of 3 experiments.

When glass adherant monocytes are depleted from mononuclear cells resulting in a monocyte-depleted lymphocyte preparation (MDL), there was a pronounced loss of the inhibitory effects of both beta endorphin and met enkephalin on LCF production. When the production of LCF by MDL is compared to that by mononuclear cells (MNC) in the presence of opioid peptide ranging in concentration from 10^{-12} to 10^{-6} M, the suppression of LCF production is diminished. For instance, it was shown that with 10^{-7} M beta endorphin, MNC production of LCF was inhibited by 57±13% (n=6). In response to LCF generated by MDL preparations from the same donors, the migration index of T-cells was only inhibited by 2±1%. The efficacy of met enkephalin, too, was diminished when monocytes were depleted from mononuclear cell preparations. These data suggested that the inhibitory effects of opioids on LCF production were mediated by monocytes.

Like monocyte depletion, inclusion of the cyclooxygenase inhibitor, indomethacin, also prevented the inhibitory effects of opioids on LCF production. As is shown in Table 2, indomethacin prevented the effects of both beta endorphin and met enkephalin in a dose dependent manner when used in concentrations between 10^{-6} M and $5X10^{-6}$ M. A major product of monocyte cyclooxygenase activity is PGE_2 (Bonney et al 1979 and Kurland et al , 1978). PGE_2, but not other prostaglandins (PGA, PGF_2) inhibit the production of LCF (Van Epps et al, 1985).

The PGE_2 mediated suppression of LCF production is dose dependent between 10^{-9} - 10^{-6} M with lower doses of PGE_2 being less effective. In the presence of inodomethacin and either beta-endorphin or met-enkepahlin subinhibitory concentrations of PGE_2 were inhibitory as is shown in Table 3. These data suggested an opioid peptide mediated enhancement of mononuclear cell sensitivity to the suppressive effects of

TABLE 2: INDOMETHACIN PREVENTS OPIOID PEPTIDE
SUPPRESSION OF LCF PRODUCTION*

INDOMETHACIN CONCENTRATION	BETA-ENDORPHIN		MET-ENKEPHALIN	
	0	10^{-7} M	0	10^{-7} M
0	22±3	11±4	25±5	13±5
1×10^{-6}M	23±4	19±4	31±4	20±4
5×10^{-6}M	23±4	20±8	28±5	26±4

*Expressed as the migration index (u). Beta endorphin data represent the
Mean±SE of 5 experiments and the met enkephalin data of 3 experiments.

TABLE 3: SUBINHIBITORY DOSES OF PGE_2 RECONSTITUTE THE
SUPPRESSIVE EFFECT OF OPIOID PEPTIDES
IN THE PRESENCE OF INDOMETHACIN*

OPIOID PEPTIDE	PGE_2 CONCENTRATION[#]		
	0	10^{-12}M	10^{-10}M
Control	0±0%	15±3%	19±8%
10^{-8}M Beta Endorphin	11±4%	53±8%	49±8%
10^{-8}M Met Enkephalin	15±6%	42±13%	40±8%

* All LCF supernatants were generated in the presence of
5×10^{-6}M indomethacin.
The data is expressed as the percent inhibition of the migration
index.
** Each point represents the Mean ± SE from 6-experiments.

PGE_2 on LCF production. It was not determined whether this was a
direct effect of PGE_2 on LCF producing cells or an indirect effect
mediated by another cell type. Enhanced sensitivity to PGE_2 mediated
effects on mononuclear cells has been reported by others to occur in a
stressed and an aged population (Goodwin et al, 1981 and Goodwin and
Messner, 1979).

CONCLUSIONS

These studies indicate that opioid peptides may modulate the immune
response under some circumstances. Opioid peptides are found circulating
in normal individuals and at higher concentrations in stressed
individuals. Their binding to leukocytes may modulate the expression of
immunity in these individuals.

The continued study of these interactions will enhance our
understanding of the effects of neuroendocrine hormones on the immune
system in stressed as well as in healthy individuals and will define the
link between the neuroendocrine and immune systems.

ACKNOWLEDGEMENTS

We gratefully acknowledge Jeff Potter and Susan Griewe for their expert technical assistance. We thank Patricia Eckhardt for her skill and patience in preparing this manuscript.

REFERENCES

Amir, S., Brown, Z. W., and Amit, Z., 1980, The role of endorphins in stress: Evidence and speculations, Neurosci. Biobehav. Rev., 4:77.

Ausiello, C. M., and Roda, L. G., 1984, Leu-enkephalin binding to cultured human T lymphocytes, Cell Biol. Intern. Rep., 8:97.

Badawy, A. A., Evans, M., Punjani, N. F., and Morgan, C. J., 1983, Does naloxone always act as an opiate antagonist? Life Sci., 33 (suppl.):739.

Baldwin, F., The reticuloendothelial system. A comprehensive treatise, in: Vol. 1 "Morphology, Microglia and Brain Macrophages," I. Carr and W. T. Daems, eds., Plenum Press, New York (1980).

Barchas, J. D., Akil, H., Elliottt, G. R., Holman, R. B., and Watson, S. J., 1978, Behavioral neurochemistry: Neuroregulators and behavioral states, Science, 200:964.

Bleier, R., and Albrecht, R., 1980, Supraependymal macrophages of third ventricle of hamster: Morphological, functional and histochemical characterization in situ and in culture, J. Comp. Neurol., 192:489.

Bocchini, G., Bonanno, G., and Canevari, A., 1983, Influence of morphine and naloxone on human peripheral blood T lymphocytes, Drug and Alchol. Depend., 11:233.

Bonney, R. J., Naruns, P., Davies, P., and Humes, J. L., 1979, Antigen-antibody complexes stimulate the synthesis and release of prostaglandins by mouse peritoneal macrophages, Prostaglandins, 18:605.

Boyden, S. V., 1962, The chemotactic effect of mixtures of antibody and antigen on polymorphonuclear leukocytes., J. Exp. Med., 115:453.

Brown, S. L., and Van Epps, D. E., 1985, Suppression of T-lymphocyte chemotactic factor production by the opioid peptides beta endorphin and met enkephalin, J. Immunol., 134:3384.

Casale, T. B., Bowman, S., and Kaliner, M., 1984, Induction of human cutaneous mast cell degranulation by opiates and endogenous opioid peptides: Evidence for opiate and non-opiate receptor participation, J. Allergy Clin. Immunol., 73:775.

Center, D. M., and Cruikshank, W., 1982, Modulation of lymphocyte migration by human lymphokines. Identification and characterization of chemoattractant activity for lymphocytes from mitogen-stimulated mononuclear cells, J. Immunol., 128:2563.

Cianciolo, G. J., and Snyderman, R., 1981, Monocyte responsiveness to chemotactic stimuli is a property of a subpopulation of cells that can respond to multiple attractants, J. Clin. Invest., 67:60.

Clement-Jones, V., Lowry, P. J., Rees, L. H., and Besser, G. M., 1980, Met enkephalin circulates in human plasma, Nature, 283:295.

Cohen, M., Pickard, D., Dubois, M., Roth, Y. F., Naber, D., and Bunney, W. E. Jr., 1981, Surgical stress and endorphins, Lancet, 1:213.

Colt, E. W., Wardlaw, S. L., and Frantz, A. G., 1981, The effects of running on plasma beta endorphin, Life Sci., 28:1637.

Cosontos, K., Rust, M., Hollt, V., Mahr, W., Kromer, W., and Teschemacher, H.J., 1979, Elevated plasma beta endorphin levels in pregnant women and their neonates, Life Sci., 25:835.

Cruikshank, W., and Center, D. M., 1982, Modulation of lymphocyte migration by human lymphokines. II. Purification of a lymphotactic factor, J. Immunol., 128:2569.

Dubois, M., Pickar, D., Cohen, M. R., Roth, Y. F., Macnamara, T., and Bunney, W. E. Jr., 1981, Surgical stress in humans is accompanied by an increase in plasma beta endorphin immunoreactivity, Life Sci., 29:1249.

El-Naggar, A., Van Epps, D. E., and Williams, R. C. Jr., 1982, A human lymphocyte chemotactic factor produced by the mixed lymphocyte reaction, J. Lab. Clin. Med., 100:4.

Faith, R. E., Liang, H. J., Murgo, A. J., and Plotnikoff, N. P., 1984, Neuroimmunomodulation with enkephalins: Enhancement of human natural killer (NK) cell activity in vitro, Clin. Immunol. and Immunopath., 31:412.

Ferreira, S. H., and Nakamura, M., 1979, Prostaglandin hyperalgesia: The peripheral analgesic activity of morphine, enkephalins, and opioid antagonists, Prostagland., 18:191.

Fischer, E. G., and Falke, N. E., 1984, Beta-endorphin modulates immune function, Psychother. Psychosom., 42:195.

Fjellner, B., and Hagermark, O., 1982, Potentiation of histamine-induced itch and flare responses in human skin by the enkephalin analogue FK 33-824, beta-endorphin, and morphine, Arch. Derm. Res., 274:29.

Fraioli, F., Moretti, C., Paolucci, D., Alicicco, E., Crescenzi, F., and Fortunio, G., 1980, Physical exercise stimulates marked concomitant release of beta endorphin and adrenocorticotropic hormone (ACTH) in peripheral blood in man, Experientia, 36:987.

Frederickson, R. C. A., and Geary, L. E., 1982, Endogenous opioid peptides: Review of physiological, pharmacological and clinical aspects, Progress in Neurobiol., 19:19.

Froelich, C. J., and Bankhurst, A. D., 1984, The effect of beta endorphin on natural cytotoxicity and antibody dependent cellular cytotoxicity, Life Sci., 35:261.

Gee, A. P., 1984, Advantages and limitations of methods for measuring cellular chemotaxis and chemokinesis, Mol. Cell. Biochem., 62:5.

Genazzani, A. R., Facchinetti, F., and Parrini, D., 1981, beta-lipotrophin and beta endorphin plasma levels during pregnancy, Clin. Endocrin., 14:409.

Giagnoni, G., Santagostino, A., Senini, R., Fumagalli, P., and Gori, E., 1983, Cold stress in the rat induces parallel changes in plasma and pituitary levels of endorphin and ACTH, Pharm. Res. Comm., 15:15.

Gilman, S. C., Schwartz, J. M., Millner, R. J., Bloom, F. E., and Feldman, J.D., 1982, Beta endorphin enhances lymphocyte proliferative responses, Proc. Natl. Acad. Sci., 79:4226.

Goland, R. S., Wardlaw, S. L., Stark, R. I., and Frantz, A. G., 1981, Human plasma beta endorphin during pregnancy, labor and delivery, J. Clin. Endocrin. Metab., 52:74.

Goodwin, J. S., Bromberg, J., Staszak, C., Kaszubowski, P., Messner, R. P., and Neal, J. F., 1981, Effect of physical stress on sensitivity of lymphocytes to inhibition of prostaglandin E_2, J. Immunol., 132:246.

Goodwin, J.S., and Messner, R. P., 1979, Sensitivity of lymphocytes to prostaglandin E_2 increases in subjects over age 70, J. Clin. Invest., 64:434.

Guillemin, R., Vargo, T., Rossier, J., Minick, S., Ling, N., Rivier, C., Vale, W., and Bloom, F., 1977, Beta endorphin and adrenocortico-tropin are secreted concomitantly by the pituitary gland, Science, 197:1367.

Hazum, E., Chang, K., and Cuatrecasas, P., 1979, Specific nonopiate receptors for beta endorphin, Science, 205:1033.

Hook, V. Y. H., Heisler, S., Sabol, S. L., and Axelrod, J., 1982, Corticotropin releasing factor stimulates adrenocorticotropin and beta-endorphin release from AtT-20 mouse pituitary tumor cells, Biochem. Biophys. Res. Comm., 106:1364.

Hoover, R. L., Folger, R., Haering, W. A., Ware, B. R., and Karnovsky, M. J., 1980, Adhesion of leukocytes to endothelium: Roles of divalent cations, surface changes, chemotactic agents and substrate, J. Cell. Science, 45:73.

Hosobuchi, Y., and Li, C. H., 1978, The analgesic activity of human Beta-endorphin in man, Communications in Psychopharmacology, 2:33-37.

Hughes, J., Beaumont, A., Fuentes, J. A., Malfroy, B., and Unsworth, C., 1980, Opioid peptides: Aspects of their origin, release and metabolism, J. Exp. Biol., 89:239.

Hughes, J., Smith, T. W., and Kosterlitz, H. W., 1975, Identification of two related pentapeptides from the brain with potent opiate agonist activity, Nature, 258:577.

Hughes, J., Smith, T., Morgan, B., and Fothergill, L., 1975, Purification and properties of enkephalin--the possible endogenous ligand for the morphine receptor, Life Sci., 16:1753.

Hughes, S. C., Rosen, M. A., Shnider, S. M., Abboud, T. K., Stefani, S. J., and Norton, M., 1984, Maternal and neonatal effects of epidural morphine for labor and delivery, Anesthesia and Analgesia, 63:319-324.

Johnson, H. M., Smith, E. M., Torres, B. A., and Blalock, J. E., 1982, Regulation of the in vitro antibody response by neuroendocrine hormones, Proc. Natl. Acad. Sci., 79:4171.

Kay, N., Allen, J., and Morley, J. E., 1984, Endorphins stimulate normal human peripheral blood lymphocyte natural killer activity, Life Sci., 35:53.

Khansari, N., Whitten, H. D., and Fudenberg, H. H., 1984, Phencyclidine-induced immunodepression, Science, 225:76.

Kilpatrick, D.L., Lewis, R.V., Stein, S., and Udenfriend, S., 1980, Release of enkephalins and enkephalin containing polypeptides from perfused beef adrenal glands, Proc. Natl. Acad. Sci., 77:7473.

Knepel, W., Homolka, L., Vlaskovska, M., and Nutto, D., 1984, Stimulation of adrenocorticotropin/beta-endorphin release by synthetic ovine corticotropin-releasing factor in vitro. Enhancement by various vasopressin analogs, Neuroendocrin., 38:344.

Kurland, J. I., and Bockman, R., 1978, Prostaglandin E production by human blood monocytes and mouse peritoneal macrophages, J. Exp. Med., 147:952.

Li, C. H., and Chung, D., 1976, Isolation and structure of an untriakontapeptide with opiate activity from camel pituitary glands, Proc. Natl. Acad. Sci. (USA), 73:1145.

Ling, N., Burgus, R., and Guillemin, R., 1976, Isolation, primary structure, and synthesis of alpha-endorphin and gamma-endorphin, two peptides of hypothalmic-lypophysial origin with morphomimetic activity, Proc. Natl. Acad. Sci., 73:3942.

Livett, B. G., Day, R., Elde, R. P., and Howe, P. R. C., 1982, Co-storage of enkephalins and adrenaline in the bovine adrenal medulla, Neuroscience, 7:1323.

Lolait, S. J., Lim, A. T., Toh, B. H., and Funder, J.W., 1984, Immunoreactive beta-endorphin in a subpopulation of mouse spleen macrophages, J. Clin. Invest., 73:277.

Lopker, A., Abood, L. G., Hoss, W., and Lionetti, F. J., 1980, Stereoselective muscarinic, acetylcholine and opiate receptors in human phagocytic leukocytes, Biochem. Pharmacol., 29:1361.

Mathews, P. M., Froelich, C. J., Sibbitt, W. L., Jr., and Bankhurst, A. D., 1983, Enhancement of natural cytotoxicity by beta endorphin, J. Immunol., 130:1658.

McCain, H. W., Lamster, I. B., Bozzone, J. M., and Grbic, J. T., 1982, Beta endorphin modulates human immune activity via non-opiate receptor mechanisms, Life Sci., 31:1619.

McCluskey, R. T., Benacerraf, B., and McCluskey, J. W., 1963, Studies on the specificity of the cellular infiltrate in delayed hypersensitivity reactions, J. Immunol., 90:466.

Mehrishi, J. N., and Mills, I. H., 1983, Opiate receptors on lymphocytes and platelets in man, Clin. Immunol. and Immunopath., 27:240.

Miller, G.C., Murgo, A. J., and Plotnikoff, N. P., 1983, Enkephalins-- enhancement of active T-cell rosettes from lymphoma patients, Clin. Immunol. Immunopath., 26:446.

Miller, G. C., Murgo, A. J., and Plotnikoff, N. P., 1984, Enkephalins-- enhancement of active T-cell rosettes from normal volunteers, Clin. Immun. and Immunopath., 31:132.

Mueller, G.P., 1981, Beta endorphin immunoreactivity in rat plasma: Variations in response to different physical stimuli, Life Sci., 29:1669.

Nakao, K., Nakai, Y., Jingami, H., Oki, S., Fukata, J., Imura, H., 1979, Substantial rise of plasma beta endorphin levels after insulin induced hypoglycemia in human subjects, J. Clin. Endocrin. Metab., 49:838.

Nelson, R. D., McCormack, R. T., Fiegel, V. D., and Simmons, R. L., 1978, Chemotactic deactivation of human neutrophils: Evidence for non-specific and specific components, Infect. Immun., 22:441.

O'Flaherty, J. T., Showell, H. J., Becker, E. L., and Ward, P. A., 1978, Substances which aggregate neutrophils, Am. J. Pathol., 92:155.

Olson, G. A., Olson, R. D., and Kastin, A. J., 1984, Endogenous opiates: 1983, Peptides, 5:975.

Oyama, T., Matsuki, A., Taneichi, T., Ling, N., and Guillemen, R., 1980, Beta-endorphin in obstetric analgesia, Am. J. Obstet. Gynecol., 137:613-617.

Pelto-Huikko, M., Salminen, T., and Hervonen, A., 1982, Enkephalin-like immunoreactivity is restricted to the adrenaline cells in the hamster adrenal medulla, Histochemistry, 73:493.

Plotnikoff, N. P., and Miller, G. C., 1983, Enkephalins as immunomodulators, Int. J. Immunopharm., 5:437.

Prete, P., and Levin, E., 1985, In vitro effect of neuropeptides on human natural killer and cytotoxic T-cell function and T-cell subsets, Clin. Res., (abstr.) 33:54A.

Puolakka, J., Kauppila, A., Leppaluoto, J., and Vuolteenaho, O., 1982, Elevated beta endorphin immunoreactivity in umbilical cord blood after complicated delivery, Acta Obstet. Gynecol. Scand., 61:513.

Rossier, J., French, E. D., Rivier, C., Ling, N., Guillemin, R., and Bloom, F. E., 1977, Footshock induced stress increases beta endorphin levels in blood but not brain, Nature, 270:618.

Ryder, S. W., and Eng., J., 1981, Radioimmunoassay of leucine enkephalin-like substance in human and canine plasma, J. Clin. Endocrin. Metab., 52:367.

Saland, L. C., Van Epps, D. E., Ortiz, E., and Samora, A., 1983, Acute injections of opiate peptides into the rat cerebral ventricle; a macrophage-like cellular response, Brain Res. Bull., 10:523.

Saland, L. C., Ortiz, E., and Samora, A. 1984. Chronic infusion of opiate peptides to rat cerebrospinal fluid with osmotic pumps, Anat. Rec., 210:115.

Shanks, M.M., Clement-Jones, V., Linsell, C.J., Mullen, P.E., Rees, L.H., and Besser, G.M., 1981, A study of 24 hour profiles of plasma met enkephalin in man, Brain Res., 212:403.

Shavit, Y., Lewis, J. W., Terman, G. W., Gale, R. P., and Liebeskind, J. C., 1984, Opioid peptides mediate the suppressive effect of stress on natural killer cell cytotoxicity, Science, 223:188.

Showell, H. J., Freer, R. J., Zigmond, S. M., Schiffman, E., Aswanikumar, S., Corcoran, B., and Becker, E. L., 1976. The structure activity relationship of synthetic peptides as chemotactic factors and inducers of lysosomal secretion for neutrophils, J. Exp. Med., 143:1154.

Simpkins, C. O., Dickey, C. A., and Fink, M. P., 1984, Human neutrophil migration is enhanced by beta-endorphin, Life Sci., 34:2251.

Smith, E.M., and Blalock, J.E., 1981, Human lymphocyte production of corticotropin and endorphin-like substances: Association with leukocyte interferon, Proc. Natl. Acad. Sci., 78:7530.

Smith, J.R., and Simon, E.J., 1981, Endorphins, opiate receptors, and their evolving biology, Pathobiol. Ann., 11:87.

Stoelting, R. K., 1980, Opiate receptors and endorphins: Their role in anesthesiology, Anesthesia and Analgesia, 59:874-880.

Terenius, L., and Wahlstrom, A., 1975, Search for an endogenous ligand for the opiate receptor, Acta Physiol. Scand., 94:74.

Teschemacher, H., Opheim, K. E., Cox, B. M., and Goldstein, A., 1975, A peptide like substance from the pituitary that acts like morphine, Life Sci., 16:1771.

Tubaro, E., Borelli, G., Croce, C., Cavallo, G., and Santiangelli, C., 1983, Effect of morphine on resistance to infection, J. Infect. Dis., 148:656.

Turkall, R. M., Denison, R. C., and Tsan, M., 1982, Degradation and oxidation of methionine enkephalin by human neutrophils, J. Lab. Clin. Med., 99:418.

Van Epps, D. E., 1982, Mediators and modulators of human lymphocyte chemotaxis, Agents and Actions, 12 (suppl.):217.

Van Epps, D. E., Durant, D. A., and Potter, J. W., 1983a, Migration of human helper/inducer T cells in response to supernatants from Con A-stimulated suppressor/cytotoxic T cells, J. Immunol., 131:697.

Van Epps, D. E., Potter, J., and Brown, S. L., 1985, Production and regulation of human T-lymphocyte Chemotactic factor (LCF), in: "Mediators of Inflammation," G. A. Higgs and T. J. Williams, eds., MacMillan, London (in press).

Van Epps, D. E., Potter, J. W., and Durant, D. A., 1983b, Production of human lymphocyte chemotactic factor by T-cell subpopulations, J. Immunol., 130:2727.

Van Epps, D. E., and Saland, L., 1984, Beta endorphin and met enkephalin stimulate human peripheral blood mononuclear cell chemotaxis, J. Immunol., 132:3046.

Van Epps, D. E., Saland, L., Taylor, C., and Williams, R. C. Jr., 1983c, In vitro and in vivo effects of beta endorphin and met enkephalin on leukocyte locomotion, Prog. Brain Res., 59:361.

Vincent, J. P., Cavey, D., Kamenka, J. M., Geneste, P., and Lazdunski, M., 1978, Interaction of phencyclidines with the muscarinic and opiate receptors in the central nervous system, Brain Res., 152:176.

Wardlaw, S. L., Stark, R. I., Daniel, S., Frantz, A. G., 1981, Effects of hypoxia on beta endorphin and beta lipotropin release in fetal, newborn and maternal sheep, Endocrin., 108:1710.

Weber, R. J., and Pert, C. B., Opiatergic modulation of immune system, in: "Central and Peripheral Endorphins: Basic and Clinical Aspects," E. E. Muller and A. R. Genazzini, eds., Raven Press, (New York) (1984).

Wilkes, M. M., Stewart, R. D., Bruni, J. F., Quigley, M. E., Yen, S. S. C., Ling, N., and Chretien, M., 1980, A specific homologous radioimmunoassay for human beta endorphin: Diect measurement in biological fluids, J. Clin. Endocrin. Metab., 50:309.

Wilkinson, P. C., Haston, W. S., and Shields, J. M., 1982. Some determinants of the locomotor behavior of phagocytes and lymphocytes in vitro, Clin. Exp. Immuno., 50:461.

Wybran, J., Appelboom, T., Famaey, J. P., and Govaerts, A., 1979, Suggestive evidence for receptors for morphine and met enkephalin on normal human blood T lymphocytes, J. Immunol., 123:1068.

Yamasaki, Y., Shimamura, O., Kizu, A., Nakagawa, M., and Ijichi, H., 1982, IgE-mediated ^{14}C-serotonin release from rat mast cells modulated by morphine and endorphins, Life Sci., 31:471.

NEUROPEPTIDES ARE CHEMOATTRACTANTS FOR HUMAN MONOCYTES AND TUMOR CELLS:

A BASIS FOR MIND-BODY COMMUNICATION

Michael R. Ruff and Candace B. Pert

Cellular Immunology Section, Laboratory of Microbiology and
Immunology, National Institute of Dental Research, NIH and
Section on Brain Biochemistry, Clinical Neuroscience
Branch, NIMH, Bethesda, Maryland 20892

INTRODUCTION

Monocytes, or their non-circulating counterparts, macrophages, are a
heterogeneous population of cells which regulate many aspects of immune
functioning including antigen processing, T cell activation, lymphokine
and antibody production, as well as defense against neoplastic cells[1].
Recently, several other cell types, histologically and morphologically
different from classical macrophages, have come to be included into this
family of cells. They include the several minor cell populations present
in skin (called Langerhans cells), brain (microglia), and dendritic cells
sparsely distributed throughout basal epithelial layers of numerous
organs and endocrine tissues[2], as well as osteoclasts in joints. The
functions of these macrophages are less clear although a role of the
Langerhans cell in local immune reactions has been inferred.

All of these cells derive from bone marrow stem cell precursors and
a particularly interesting aspect of their physiology is their ability to
egress from bone marrow into the circulation and migrate to various body
sites where they undergo final differentiation. These cells can also be
actively recruited to specific locations during pathological states by
chemotactic signals where, in a programmed sequence, they combat infection and participate in the repair of damaged tissue during wound
healing[3]. Many stimuli have been shown to induce migration of macrophages including bacterial products, peptides generated during clotting
and complement activation, proteolytic fragments of structural matrix
proteins such as collagen, elastin, and fibronectin, as well as lymphocyte and fibroblast products[1]. The signals which regulate the normal
trafficking and ultimate localization of these related but discrete
macrophage populations is, however, largely unknown. Recently, we have
begun to document the receptor-mediated abilities of human monocytes to
migrate toward very low concentrations of several neuropeptides including
the opiates[4,5], bombesin[6], substance P[7], and the benzodiazepines[8] (whose
endogenous ligand is a neuropeptide only recently sequenced). These
agents are not currently considered to be products of inflammatory
reactions (with the possible exception of substance P)[9], and thus it
seems that although neuropeptides may have roles in the inflammatory,
wound healing aspects of macrophage function they likely also have
broader function in the day-to-day maintenance of health and homeostasis[10] throughout the organism by virtue of their action on the

387

disseminated members of the macrophage population. Because neuropeptides have been postulated to be the biochemical mediators of behavior and emotion[11] it seems plausible that these same mediators of various mood states in brain also communicate to macrophages and other cells involved in healing and thus offer a potential mechanism for the effect of emotional states[11] on the course and outcome of illness.

METHODS

Mononuclear cells, obtained from heparinized blood from healthy human volunteers, were isolated by sedimentation over Ficoll-Paque (Pharmacia). This population of cells was comprised of approximately 30% monocytes and 70% lymphocytes as determined by specific antibody and esterase staining. Lymphocytes do not migrate in this assay. Migration was studied using blind-well chemotaxis chambers (Neuro Probe, Bethesda, MD) in which the upper and lower compartments were separated by a 5 μM pore size nucleopore polycarbonate membrane[7]. Mononuclear cells (5.5×10^4) in Geys balanced salt solution (GBSS) (pH 7.4) containing 2% bovine serum albumin were placed in the upper wells and test attractants in the lower wells of the chambers. All drugs were diluted into GBSS containing 2% BSA and were prepared from a 10^{-4} stock solution stored in 0.02 M acetic acid at $-20°C$ and diluted just prior to assay. Monocyte migration was assessed after a 90 min incubation at 37°C by fixing and staining the distal membrane-adherent cells. These migrating cells were enumerated by counting three fields in triplicate utilizing an optical image analyzer (Optomax Inc., Hollis, NH). Data are expressed as the migration index, which is the ratio between migration toward test attractants and buffer alone. The number of migrating cells in the buffer alone controls generally ranged from 20-60 cells/field. The values shown represent the mean and S.E.M. of the migration indices of multiple individual experiments, as indicated. Some experiments report results as actual number of migrating cells. All experiments have been repeated three to twelve times with similar results.

RESULTS

Opiate Receptor. Utilizing the modified Boyden chamber method it was possible to demonstrate that opiate peptides and drugs are chemoattractants for human monocytes (Fig. 1). Results show that the naturally occurring opiate peptides β-endorphin and dynorphin were most potent in this assay with EC_{50} (concentration of half-maximal response) values of 5×10^{-13}M. The peptide met-enkephalin was only slightly less active, EC_{50} of 10^{-12}M, although this comparison may reflect the greater lability of the enkephalins relative to endorphins. Stereospecificity of opiate chemotaxis is demonstrated by the results which show that levallorphan (a synthetic opiate) is greater than 10,000 times more active than its enantiomer dextrallorphan, which was largely inactive in this assay. Bremazocine, another synthetic opiate, showed intermediate activity, EC_{50} of 5×10^{-11}M. Interestingly, morphine, the oldest and perhaps best known opiate was largely inactive in promoting chemotaxis. This apparent selectivity in opiate pharmacologic response (e.g., endorphins vs. morphine) has been used to operationally define subtypes of receptor specificity[11] although the relationship of these varied functional responses to the actual receptor structure is as yet unknown. The responses to β-endorphin, dynoprhin [1-13], and D-ala^2-D-1eu^5-enkephalin (DADL) are stereospecifically reversed by the opiate antagonist naloxone (Fig. 2) thereby indicating that the responses measured are mediated through an opiate receptor. The inactive enantiomer of naloxone did not reverse opiate monocyte chemotaxis.

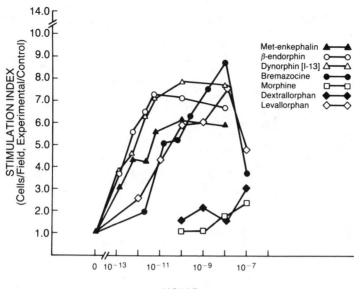

Fig. 1.   Chemotactic response of human monocytes to opiates and
           opiate peptides[5]. Chemotaxis was performed as
           described. Data is expressed as a stimulation index.
           The maximal response for all analogs occurred at 10^{-8}M,
           although the peptides β-endorphin, D-Ala-D-Leu enke-
           phalin, and dynorphin [1-13] were similarly active at
           10^{-10}M. The EC_{50} for these agents was 5×10^{-12}M.
           Stereospecificity is demonstrated in this figure by
           levallorphan, which shows intermediate activity com-
           pared to opiate peptides, while its enantiomer,
           dextrallorphan, is inert. The stimulation index for
           the chemotactic peptide f-Met-Leu-Phe, 10^{-7}M, was 14.2.

Substance P Receptor.   Substance P, an undecapeptide ligand first
sequenced by Leeman and colleagues[13] and recently proposed to stimulate
hypersensitivity and inflammation[9] is also active in promoting monocyte
chemotaxis. This result, therefore, supports a role for substance P in
the development of experimental arthritis and provides an additional
mechanism to explain the monocyte inflammatory infiltrate of arthritic
lesions. In order to establish the receptor mediated nature of substance
P responses a series of closely related analogs was evaluated for their
effect on chemotaxis (Fig. 3). Substance P showed a biphasic response,
also observed with N-formyl peptides[1] as well as other neuropeptide-
induced chemotaxis[4-8], with maximal activity occurring in the range
between 5×10^{-11}M and 10^{-12}M. As was shown for opiate peptides[4,5], chemotaxis is an extremely sensitive bioassay and substance P showed a
significant enhancement of chemotactic activity even at 5×10^{-14}M,
the lowest concentration tested. Lack of effect at high concentrations
has been attributed to receptor desensitization or gradient breakdown[1].
Thus, substance P at concentrations higher than 10^{-10}M elicited reduced
chemotactic responsiveness. Other analogs (e.g., SP[3-11]) showed
similar or reduced potency in this assay; peak responses are shown for
all compounds and no increase in activity over the range $[10^{-14}-10^{-6}$M]
of tested concentrations was observed (data not shown) for any of the
indicated analogs. Intact substance P had greatest potency in this assay
and the results suggest that the C-terminal amino acid residues are
required for maximal biological activity. Thus, increasingly N-terminus

deleted analogs showed increasing loss of activity; e.g., SP[3-11] > SP[9-11], and C-terminal-deleted peptides were largely inactive, e.g., SP[1-9] or SP, free acid. Interestingly, the ability of these analogs to induce monocyte chemotaxis is consistent with previous studies demonstrating specificity of binding to other tissues or cells. Thus, the rank potency orders of substance P analogs in chemotaxis induction were comparable to their potencies in displacing substance P binding to brain membranes[14], and slices[15]; SP > SP[3-11] > SP[8-11] ≅ SP[9-11] >> SP[1-9], SP, free acid. Although these exact analogs were not used, a recent report on substance P binding to a human T lymphocyte line also yielded comparable results[16]; SP > SP[4-11] >> SP[1-4] for rank potency orders in binding displacement.

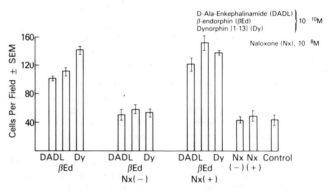

Fig. 2. Stereospecific reversibility of opiate chemotaxis by naloxone. Peptides (10^{-10}M) were co-incubated with active (-) or inactive (+) enantiomers of the antagonist naloxone (10^{-8}M). Controls contained diluent or naloxone only.

Benzodiazepine chemotaxis. Our observations of opiate and substance P mediated chemotaxis suggested the possibility that other behavior and mood modifying drugs which work through neuropeptide receptors might also have effects on macrophage and immune function. The benzodiazepines are a group of drugs widely used for their anxiolytic, hypnotic, and anticonvulsant properties – effects which are mediated through high affinity receptors present in the central nervous system[17]. Recently, an 18 amino acid endogenous peptide ligand has been proposed for the benzodiazepine receptor[18]. We tested a number of benzodiazepines for their effects on monocyte chemotaxis (Fig. 4) and we were able to show responses for this family of drugs as well[8]. Thus, the benzodiazepine receptor ligands diazepam (valium) and Ro5-4864 had potent activity, while clonazepam was largely inert. These results suggested that the monocyte benzodiazepine receptor was of the "peripheral" type (operationally the peripheral benzodiazepine receptor is defined as having selectivity for Ro5-4864 compared to clonazepam). A suitable antagonist exists for the peripheral receptor, the compound PK-11195, and it was possible to show antagonism of both Ro5-4864 and diazepam chemotaxis by this drug. Thus, (Fig. 5) equimolar mixtures of the antagonist with either Ro5-4864 or diazepam resulted in complete inhibition of chemotaxis. This inhibition is specific for benzodiazepine ligands since PK-11195 did not inhibit chemotaxis to the N-formyl peptide receptor. In this case we have been able to directly demonstrate high affinity benzodiazepine receptors on human monocytes utilizing receptor binding methods (Fig. 4 inset)[8]. The

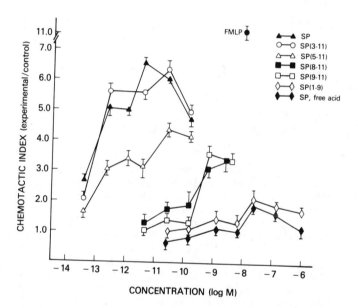

Fig. 3. Human monocyte chemotaxis to substance P and its analogs. Indicated test attractants were evaluated for their ability to stimulate monocyte migration over a broad concentration range. Data are expressed as a stimulation index, which is the ratio of the number of cells/field in experimental compared to control wells, ± S.E.M. Determinations were made as described. Data for substance P (SP) was averaged from three replicate experiments, SP[3-11], SP[5-11], SP[8-11] and SP[9-11] were averaged from two replicate experiments, while data for SP[1-9] and SP, free acid were from a single experiment which was repeated with similar results. The background cell migration, in the absence of specific attractants, ranged from 20-40 cells/field for these experiments. f-Met-Leu-Phe (FMLP) was also tested at 10^{-7}M.

potencies in binding were in agreement with chemotactic activity shown here. Thus the binding activity of Ro5-4864 > diazepam >> clonazepam confirm that chemotaxis is mediated through a peripheral type benzodiazepine receptor.

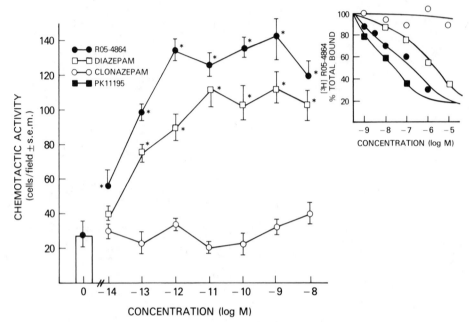

Fig. 4. The effects of various benzodiazepines on the chemotaxis of human peripheral blood mononuclear cells. The data represent the mean ± S.E.M. of the cell migration of an individual experiment that was replicated with similar results. The responses with Ro5-4864 and diazepam were significantly different from control (*) (p<0.01, t test). (Inset). Displacement of specific ^{3}H-labeled Ro5-4864 bound to purified monocytes by various drugs. Displacement potencies of Ro5-4864, PK-11195, diazepam, and clonazepam were determined by incubating 4×10^6 monocytes in 0.05M tris and 0.15M NaCl, pH 7.4 (final volume, 0.5 ml) with ^{3}H-labeled Ro5-4864 (4 nM; specific activity, 82.7 Ci/mmol) and various concentrations of unlabeled drug as described. After a 45 minute incubation at 0°C, the reactions were terminated by rapid vacuum filtration of the solution over GF/B glass fiber filters (Whatman) and then by washing the filters twice with 5.0 ml of ice-cold buffer. Specific binding, defined as the total binding minus that observed in the presence of 10^{-5}M unlabeled Ro5-4864 (nonspecific binding), was approximately 75% at a ligand concentration of 4 nM. Displacement curves for each drug were computed as a percentage of the maximal specific ^{3}H-labeled Ro5-4864 binding in the presence of each drug over the indicated concentration ranges. IC_{50} values were estimated from displacement curves such as those shown here. Values are from a typical experiment repeated three times with similar results.

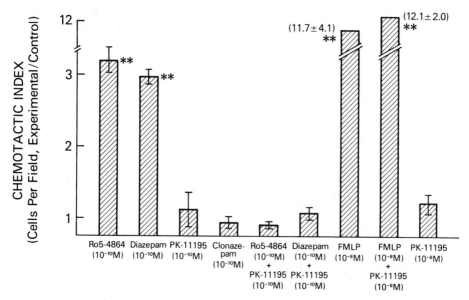

Fig. 5. Benzodiazepine receptor-mediated chemotaxis of human
monocytes. Chemotaxis assays were performed by using
modified Boyden chambers as described. Data are
expressed as a migration index. The number of migrating cells in the buffer alone controls was 40 cells/
field (200X). Values shown represent the mean and
S.E.M. of four experiments. Ro5-4864, (4-chloro-
diazepam), and diazepam yielded statistically significant responses compared to control (**, p<0.001).
Clonazepam, a benzodiazepine analog with low activity
on non-neural cells, was not active in this assay.
These receptor-mediated events were blocked by the
appropriate antagonist, PK-11195, when co-mixed with
the agonist Ro5-4864 or diazepam. The response of the
tripeptide, f-Met-Leu-Phe (FMLP) was not inhibited when
co-mixed with equimolar (10^{-8}M) PK-11195.

Tumor cell chemotaxis. In an attempt to gain some insight into the
factors which may affect metastatic neoplastic diseases we have also
examined the role of neuropeptides as chemoattractants for human tumor
cells[6]. In these experiments a modification of the monocyte chemotactic
methodology was employed[6]. Chemotaxis time was extended to four hours
and filters were coated with collagen IV to promote cell adherence.
Small cell lung cancer (SCLC) cells were used in this study. SCLC
accounts for almost 25% of all human lung cancers and is a rapidly pro-
gressing disease with widespread and early metastases observed. These
cells and tumors have been proposed to be derived from macrophage
precursors[19]. Results (Fig. 6) revealed that SCLC cells express chemotactic receptors for several neuropeptides. Among the active peptides
were bombesin[6], β-endorphin, substance P, and arg-vasopressin. Not all
peptides were active in this assay. For example, oxytocin, which is
closely related to vasopressin, did not appear to be active. Other
peptides such as neurotensin and melanocyte stimulating hormone were not
active (data not shown) further indicating the specificity of the
responses and supporting the concept that unique neuropeptide receptors

are responsible for these results. Interestingly, these tumor cells also seem to express chemotactic receptors for N-formyl peptides since f-Met-Leu-Phe was active.

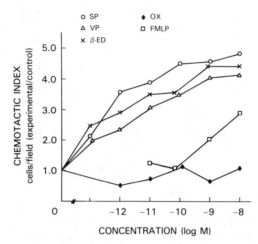

Fig. 6.   Chemotaxis of small cell lung cancer (SCLC) cells to various neuropeptides. Results are expressed as a stimulation index, the ratio of experimental to control migration. SP; substance P, VP; arg-vasopressin, β-ED; β-endorphin, OX; oxytocin, FMLP; f-Met-Leu-Phe. Background migration in this experiment was 6±2 cells/field. Chemotaxis was performed for four hrs on collagen IV coated filters[6].

DISCUSSION

We have previously emphasized that careful structure-activity analysis of the correlation between binding and physiological activity is a useful strategy for demonstrating receptor mediated events[20]. Thus, it has been previously shown that N-formyl peptides, which are potent chemoattractants, bind specifically to rabbit neutrophils with a structure-activity correlation between binding and chemotaxis of p<.001[21]. In this present review we have utilized this principle to infer the receptor-mediated effects of several neuropeptides or drugs on chemotaxis of human monocytes. In at least one case (benzodiazepines) it has been possible to directly demonstrate binding sites on monocytes, the pharmacology of which is in agreement with the functional chemotactic effects[8]. By these arguments and methods we have been able to show that human monocytes express receptors for multiple and distinct neuropeptides. Some tumor cells, such as SCLC, also express functional neuropeptide receptors. The existence of discrete neuropeptide receptors on monocytes is further suggested by observations of blockade by selective antagonists for a given neuropeptide. Rather than speculate on the role of the individual ligands on monocyte function, which at this time is largely unknown, we will focus this discussion on what we perceive to be the major conceptual themes of this work.

Neuropeptides, short chains of amino acids present in brain as well as non-neural tissues, are primarily known for their role as neurotransmitters[22]. In the central nervous systems of the recently evolved mammals, neuropeptides are regionally distributed being largely localized in those limbic and cortical regions primarily responsible for sensory processing, memory, behavior and mood[10]. As such, neuropeptides are candidates for the biochemical mediators of these events. It is becoming clear that these compounds, far from acting solely within the nervous system, are localized throughout the brain and body, and have pleiotropic effects serving as transmitters, growth hormones, and signals for many body systems. These peptides and their receptors have been extensively conserved structurally and are widely distributed across phyla[23,24] where they presumably also function as components in a network for intercellular communication. The presence of varied, distinct neuropeptide receptors on macrophages and other immune system cells, coupled with reports of neuropeptide synthesis by immune cells, suggests that immune cells are in communication with, potentially, themselves as well as other neuropeptide secreting and responding cells. Neuropeptides and their receptors thus join the nervous system, glands, and immune system in a network of information exchange which exists throughout the body, as well as the brain. We have called this a "psychoimmunoendocrine" network and the purpose of such a network may be to prioritize the body's defense and repair mechanisms within the context of the whole internal milieu. Because neuropeptide-rich loci in the central nervous system have been inferred to mediate numerous behavioral and mood states we have proposed that this neuropeptide net may form the biochemical basis for observations that emotional states can significantly alter the course and outcome of biological illnesses previously considered to exist strictly in the somatic realm. By this rationale the same mediators which activate mood states in brain also communicate to other cells involved in healing and homeostatic processes. Although speculative it may well be that a particular mood state is associated, biochemically, with a particular neuropeptide tone. Opiates, for example, clearly mediate a state of intense pleasure, while substance P is associate with pain, and benzodiazepines with anxiety. If mood is associated with release of various neuropeptides then the hypothesis of a psychosomatic network implies that all the cells which participate in the network contribute to creation of a neuropeptide tone (mood) which then is perceived throughout the body. All illness and disease may result in alterations in the neuropeptide tone of the mind/body and such changes may have repercussions for health and well-being.

The physiological correlate of _in vitro_ macrophage chemotaxis by neuropeptides is currently unknown although a localized tissue site is implicated as the source of chemoattractant. Macrophages are, as discussed in the introduction, a very heterogeneous population of cells that subserve important roles in immune activation, as well as healing and cancer defense. Chemoattractants often alter other aspects of macrophage physiology and the effects we report here may not be solely limited to enhancement of migration. With respect to the concept that release of neuropeptides may have impact on health, in addition to the effects mediated through the immune and endocrine systems, to cite one example, it may also have direct effects on establishment or maintenance of certain cancers.

Small cell lung cancer (SCLC), which accounts for 25% of all lung cancer deaths, is a tumor whose cells store and secrete numerous neuropeptides. These cells and their normal, non-cancerous progenitors, are therefore components of the psychoimmunoendocrine network and would be expected to be under its tonic influence. Indeed, a most exciting recent paper documents that the characteristic neuropeptide secreted by these cells, the peptide bombesin[25], is also a potent growth factor for these cells[26]. Antibodies to bombesin inhibited cell growth in vitro and tumor formation in vivo. Other work we have been involved in suggests that these cells are derived from macrophages[19] and shows that both macrophages and SCLC tumor cells will chemotax to bombesin[6] and other neuropeptides (Fig. 6)[6]. Neuropeptides released in the brain, as well as the body, due to cognitive, emotional, or other stimuli, may there by have effects on tumor and/or macrophage growth and tissue localization. These observations may be relevant to the metastatic process per se in that cells which have dissociated from the primary tumor mass invade secondary sites by following gradients of neuropeptide signals[6]. Disseminated neoplastic diseases, such as SCLC, breast, or hemopoietic cancers, may, to some extent, develop as a result of dysfunctions in the neuropeptide network which then modifies the course and progression of disease.

One additional prediction of this formulation is that the network and its composite cells can be accessed via any of its members. Thus, to continue with the model for SCLC, an approach which seeks to linearly interrupt the flow of information to the tumor by blocking the action of one peptide or growth factor, such as bombesin, does not accommodate the possibility that, at least on the organismal level, other neuropeptide signals acting directly, or relayed through other cells, may also have effects on tumor growth or the general state of well-being. An understanding of these principles may prove essential to the ultimate goal, which is to re-establish growth homeostasis and health throughout the individual.

REFERENCES

1. E. Schiffmann and J. I. Gallin, Biochemistry of phagocyte chemotaxis, Curr. Topics in Cell Reg. 15:203 (1979).

2. V. H. Perry, D. A. Hume and S. Gordon, Immunohistochemical localization of macrohages and microglia in the adult and developing mouse brain, Neuroscience 15:313 (1985).

3. S. M. Wahl and L. M. Wahl, Modulation of fibroblast growth and function by monokines and lymphokines, Lymphokines 2:179 (1981).

4. D. Van Epps and L. Saland, β-endorphin and met-enkephalin stimulate human peripheral blood mononuclear cell chemotaxis, J. Immunology 132:3046 (1984).

5. M. R. Ruff, S. M. Wahl, S. Mergenhagen and C. B. Pert, Opiate receptor-mediated chemotaxis of human monocytes, Neuropeptides (Europe) 5:363 (1985).

6. M. R. Ruff, E. Schiffmann, V. Terranova and C. B. Pert, Neuropeptides are chemoattractants for human macrophages and tumor cells: a mechanism for metastasis, Clinical Immunol. Immunopath., in press.

7. M. R. Ruff, S. M. Wahl and C. B. Pert, Substance P receptor-mediated chemotaxis of human monocytes, Peptides, in press.

8. M. R. Ruff, C. B. Pert, R. J. Weber, L. M. Wahl, S. M. Wahl and S. M. Paul, Benzodiazepine receptor-mediated chemotaxis for human monocytes, Science 229:1281 (1985).

9. J. D. Levine, R. Clark, M. Devor, C. Helms, M. A. Moskowitz and A. I. Basbaum, Intraneuronal substance P contributes to the severity of experimental arthritis, Science 226:547 (1984).

10. D. G. Payan, J. D. Levine, E. J. Goetzl, Modulation of immunity and hypersensitivity by sensory neuropeptides, J. Immunol. 132:1601 (1984).

11. C. B. Pert, M. R. Ruff, R. J. Weber and M. Herkenham, Neuropeptides and their receptors: a psychosomatic network, J. Immunol. 135:820S (1985).

12. S. J. Paterson, L. E. Robson and H. W. Kosterlitz, Classification of opioid receptors, Br. Med. Bull. 39:31 (1983).

13. M. M. Chang, S. E. Leeman and H. D. Niall, Amino-acid sequence of substance P, Nature (N.B.) 232:86 (1971).

14. M. A. Cascieri and T. Liang, Characterization of the substance P receptor in rat brain cortex membranes and the inhibition of radioligand binding by guanine nucleotides, J. Biol. Chem. 258:5158 (1983).

15. R. B. Rothman, M. Herkenham, C. B. Pert, T. Liang and M. A. Cascieri, Visualization of rat brain receptors for the neuropeptide, substance P, Brain Res. 309:47 (1984).

16. D. G. Payan, D. R. Brewster and E. J. Goetzl, Stereospecific receptors for substance P on cultured human IM-9 lymphocytes, J. Immunol. 133:3260 (1984).

17. S. Garattini, E. Mussini, L. O. Randall, "The Benzodiazepines," Raven, New York (1973).

18. P. Ferrero, A. Guidotti, B. Conti-Tronconi and E. Costa, A brain octadecaneuropeptide generated by tryptic digestion of DBI (diazepam binding inhibitor) functions as a proconflict ligand of benzodiazepine recognition sites, Neuropharmacology 23:1359 (1984).

19. M. R. Ruff and C. B. Pert, Small cell carcinoma of the lung: macrophage-specific antigens suggest hemopoietic stem cell origin, Science 255:1034 (1984).

20. C. B. Pert and M. Herkenham, From receptors to brain circuitry, in: "Biochemistry of Taste and Olfaction," R. Cagan, ed., Academic Press, New York (1981).

21. S. Aswanikumar, B. A. Corcoran, E. Schiffmann, A. R. Day, R. J. Freer, H. J. Showell, E. L. Becker and C. B. Pert, Demonstration of a receptor on rabbit neutrophils for chemotactic peptides, Biochem. Biophys. Res. Comm. 74:81 (1977).

22. D. Krieger, Brain peptides: What, where, why?, Science 222:975 (1983).

23. D. LeRoith, J. Shiloach and J. Roth, Is there an earlier phylo-genetic precursor that is common to both the nervous and endocrine systems?, Peptides 3:211 (1982).

24. D. LeRoith, A. S. Liotta, J. Roth, J. Shiloach, M. E. Lewis, C. B. Pert and D. T. Krieger, Corticotropin and β-endorphin-like materials are native to unicellular organisms, Proc. Natl. Acad. Sci. USA 79:2086 (1982).

25. T. W. Moody, C. B. Pert, A. F. Gazdar, D. N. Carney and J. D. Minna, High levels of intracellular bombesin characterize human small cell lung carcinoma, Science 214:1246 (1981).

26. F. Cuttitta, D. Carney, J. Mulshine, T. Moody, J. Fedorko, A. Fischler and J. Minna, Bombesin-like peptides can function as autocrine growth factors in human small cell lung cancer, Nature 316:823 (1985).

METHIONINE ENKEPHALIN:

IMMUNOMODULATOR IN NORMAL VOLUNTEERS (IN VIVO)

N.P. Plotnikoff*, G.C. Miller**, S. Solomon**, R.E. Faith*,
L. Edwards***, and A.J. Murgo*

Departments of Pharmacology* and Medicine***
School of Medicine
Oral Roberts University and Immuno-Diagnostics Lab**
Tulsa, Oklahoma

INTRODUCTION

The enkephalin, methionine enkephalin (met-enkephalin) was originally discovered to be one of the endogenous ligands for morphine receptors (Hughes et al., 1975; Simontov and Snyder, 1976). However, Plotnikoff et al., (1976) discovered anti-depressant, anti-anxiety, and anti-convulsant effects of the enkephalins, identifying a much broader spectrum of pharmacological effects than originally anticipated.

Earlier studies by several researchers have identified enkephalin receptors on human T-cells, granulocytes, complement, platelets and B cells (Wybran et al., 1979; Lopker et al., 1980; Schweigerer et al., 1982; Hazum et al., 1979). Plotnikoff et al., (1982, 1983) explored the possibility that methionine enkephalin might have an immunomodulatory role. Other investigators studied similar effects with the endorphins (Blalock and Smith, 1980; Gilman et al., 1982; Mathews et al., 1983). In mice, Plotnikoff and Miller (1983) identified enhanced lymphocyte blastogenesis with phytohemagglutinin and also increased size of thymus (Plotnikoff et al., 1985). In rats, Plotnikoff et al., 1984 showed similar effects on the thymus gland.

Studies in humans (in vitro) identified enchanced active T-cell rosettes and NK cell activity in normal volunteers as well as cancer patients (Faith et al., 1984).

The present study is an evaluation of the in vivo effects of methionine enkephalin on levels and activities of T-cells and NK cells in human volunteers.

PATIENTS AND METHODS

Male subjects age 21-39 were recruited and informed consent forms signed. They had complete abstinence from all drugs, including alcohol and tobacco at least three weeks prior to the study. All subjects were within twenty percent of ideal body weight and free of acute and chronic cardiovascular, renal, metabolic and neurological diseases. Those subjects satisfying admission criteria were admitted to the hospital the evening prior to the study, given the drug infusion in the morning of the second day, and discharged on the third day.

Volunteer	One microgram/kg		Ten micrograms/kg		Fifty micrograms/kg	
	#1	#2	#3	#4	#5	#6
Baselines	17/200	31/200	30/200	34/200	33/200	6/200
2 Hours	29/200	77/200	85/200	77/200	82/200	14/200
	(71%↑)	(148%↑)	(183%↑)	(126%↑)	(148%↑)	(133%↑)
24 Hours	26/200	17/200	61/200	43/200	15/200	44/200
	(53%↑)	(45%↓)	(103%↑)	(26%↑)	(54%↓)	(633%↑)

$p < 0.05$ - t-test paired difference ($\frac{10 \text{ volunteers}}{12 \text{ samples}}$)

significant positive increase over controls

METHIONINE ENKEPHALIN FORMATION

A sterile solution of met-enkephalin was prepared. Met-enkephalin (Sigma-Aldrich Chem. Co., St. Louis) was dissolved in sterile saline and filter sterilized by the City of Faith pharmacy. Met-enkephalin has the following characteristics: M.W. 574, water soluble and amino acid sequence Tyr-Gly-Gly-Phe-Met-OH. It was dissolved in 60 ml. of saline at a concentration sufficient to infuse at 2 ml/minute for thirty minutes to give a delivered dose of one, ten, or fifty micrograms/kilogram body weight.

IMMUNOLOGIC TESTS

TOTAL AND ACTIVE T LYMPHOCYTE ROSETTE DETERMINATION

Peripheral blood was collected by antecubital venipuncture, diluted with RPMI 1640 medium, layered over a Ficoll-Paque gradient and centrifuged for thirty minutes at 400 x g. The mononuclear band was collected, washed twice, and resuspended in RPMI 1640. Total E rosettes were quantitated by mixing one million lymphocytes with sheep red blood cells in RPMI supplemented with 10% fetal calf serum at 4°C overnight. The cells were gently resuspended and the rosettes quantified. The active T-cells were determined by mixing 0.1 ml volume of 1×10^7 cells/ml and an equal volume of fetal calf serum and incubated at 37°C for 60 minutes. Sheep red blood cells (2×10^7) were added, the cell suspension centrifuged at 200 x g for five minutes, gently resuspended, and rosette forming cells quantitated with a hemocytometer.

NK (NATURAL-KILLER) CELLS

Target cells (K562) were adjusted to 2×10^6 cells in 0.2 ml RPMI 1640 and labeled with $Na^{51}CrO_4$ (1mCi) for 45 minutes at 37°C in 5% Co2. The cells were washed twice, resuspended in 2 ml RPMI 1640, and adjusted to 5×10^4 cells/ml.

The effector cells were collected on Ficoll-Paque gradients as described above. The cells were collected, washed and adjusted to 5×10^6 cells/ml and three serial three fold dilutions were made.

Equal volume of effector cells and target cells were added to wells in microtiter plates. The cell mixtures were incubated at 37°C in 5% CO_2 for four hours. One-tenth milliliter supernatant was harvested from each well, and quantified in a liquid scintillation counter. The killing capability of the NK cells was calculated as follows:

$$\text{NK ratio} = 1 - \frac{\text{Experimental counts} - \text{SR}}{\text{Total counts} - \text{SR}} \times 1000$$

where SR = spontaneous release of ^{51}Cr.

RESULTS

ACTIVE T-CELL ROSETTES

Significant increases in the levels of active T-cell rosettes were observed in all six volunteers at all dose levels (1, 10, and 50µg/kg). The range of increases were 26% to 633% over control levels (Table 1).

TABLE 2: TOTAL T-CELL ROSETTES

	One microgram/kg		Ten micrograms/kg		Fifty micrograms/kg	
Volunteer	#1	#2	#3	#4	#5	#6
Baseline	100/200	116/200	62/200	113/200	95/200	110/200
2 Hours	106/200 (6%↑)	124/200 (4%↑)	123/200 (98%↑)	117/200 (4%↑)	128/200 (35%↑)	102/200 (7%↑)
24 Hours	108/200 (8%↑)	110/200 (3%↑)	113/200 (82%↑)	123/200 (9%↑)	117/200 (23%↑)	134/200 (21%↑)

Statistically significant difference from controls

$p<0.05$ – $\frac{10 \text{ volunteers}}{12 \text{ samples}}$ showing positive increase over controls

TOTAL T-CELL ROSETTES

Only a slight increase in total T-cell rosettes was seen in five of the volunteers. However, volunteer #3 demonstrated a very marked increase of 98% and 82% over control levels, (Table 2). A significant increase in 10/12 (5/6 at 2 hours and 5/6 at 24 hours) volunteer samples was obtained with ranges of 4% to 35%.

NK CELL ACTIVITY

11:1 Effector/Target Cell Ratio

Two hours after infusion, volunteers 1 and 5 had increases of 15% and 72% respectively at doses of 1 and 50µg/kg while the other four had decreases of 33%, 59%, and 10%. Volunteer #6 demonstrated no change.

Three of the volunteers administered doses of 1, 10, and 50µg/kg were found to have significant increases in NK activity, 24 hours after infusion. This increase of activity was 30%, 33% and 128% over control levels. Three of the volunteers at doses of 1, 10 and 50µg/kg showed decreases (2%, 39% and 66%) (Table 3).

Similar changes were seen at effector to target cell ratios of 33:1 and 100:1 (Tables 4&5). Overall analyses of all samples indicated that 16/36 showed a positive increase (average 28.2% over controls) ($p<0.05$). At the same time 20/60 samples showed a significant decrease (average 25.3%).

33:1 Effector/Target Cell Ratio

Two hours after infusion of met-enkephalin, at doses of 1 and 10µg/kg, four volunteers showed a slight decrease (6% to 30%). Two volunteers (50µg/kg) showed increases of 19% and 61%.

Twenty-four hours after infusion, three volunteers at doses of 1 and 50µg/kg had increases of 17%, 28% and 106%. Three volunteers (1 and 10µg/kg) had decreases of 16%, 34% and 56%.

TABLE 3: NK CELL ACTIVITY
11:1 Effector/Target Cell Ratio

Volunteer	One microgram/kg		Ten micrograms/kg		Fifty micrograms/kg	
	#1	#2	#3	#4	#5	#6
Baseline	20.4%	14.3%	32.08%	18.6%	17.48%	7%
2 Hours	23.5%	9.6%	13.27%	16.8%	30.13%	7%
	(15%↑)*	(33%↓)	(59%↓)	(10%↓)	(72%↑)*	(0%)
24 Hours	26.6%	8.7%	11.06%	24.8%	17.06%	16%
	(13%↑)*	(39%↓)	(66%↓)	(33%↑)	(2%↓)	(128%↑)*

Significant difference from controls   Overall Analyses (11:1, 33:1, 100:1)
  5/12 positive increase $p < 0.05$ 16/36 samples positive increase
  7/12 negative decrease n.s.   (average 28.2%) $p < 0.05$
                                        20/36 samples negative decrease
                                         (average 25.3%) $p < 0.05$

TABLE 4: NK CELL ACTIVITY
33:1 Effector/Target Cell Ratio

Volunteer	One microgram/kg		Ten micrograms/kg		Fifty micrograms/kg	
	#1	#2	#3	#4	#5	#6
Baseline	39.1%	31.4%	51.0%	37.7%	34.5%	16%
2 Hours	35.9%	22.1%	39.0%	35.5%	55.6%	19%
	(8%↓)	(30%↓)	(24%↓)	(6%↓)	(61%↑)*	(19%↑)*
24 Hours	50.1%	20.7%	22.6%	31.8%	40.2%	33%
	(28%↑)	(34%↓)	(56%↓)	(16%↓)	(17%↑)	(106%↑)*

Significant difference from controls   Overall Analyses (11:1, 33:1, 100:1)
  5/12 positive increase $p < 0.05$ 16/36 samples positive increase
  7/12 negative decrease $p < 0.05$ $p < 0.05$
                                         20/36 samples negative decrease
                                         $p < 0.05$

100:1 Effector/Target Cell Ratio

Two hours after infusion, met-enkephalin at all doses showed a slight increase in three volunteers (0.4%, 2% and 7%) and three volunteers (0.04%, 2% and 7%) and three volunteers showed a slight decrease (11%, 17% and 7%).

Twenty-four hours after infusion, three volunteers showed an increase (10%, 5% and 127%) and three showed a decrease (25%, 35% and 17%).

DISCUSSION

The present in vivo study of met-enkephalin at doses of 1, 10 and 50µg/kg confirms and extends our original in vivo studies (Plotnikoff et al.,

1981, 1982, 1983). In fact the minute doses of met-enkephalin employed (1, 10 and 50 μg/kg) corresponds to 10^{-5} mg/ml blood which was a high dose range of out in vitro studies. Marked activity on T-cells and NK cells was seen at concentrations of 10^{-6} to 10^{-14} mg/ml blood.

TABLE 5: NK CELL ACTIVITY
100: 1 Effector/Target Cell Ratio

Volunteer	One microgram/kg #1	#2	Ten micrograms/kg #3	#4	Fifty micrograms/kg #5	#6
Baseline	58.8%	58.8%	70.9%	57.8%	58.3%	30%
2 Hours	59.8% (2%↑)*	48.9% (17%↓)	62.9% (11%↓)	58.1% (0.4%↑)*	68.6% (18%↑)*	28% (7%↓)
24 Hours	64.9% (10%↑)*	44.2% (25%↓)	46.3% (35%↓)	48.3% (17%↓)	61.5% (5%↑)*	68% (127%↑)*

Statistical difference from controls   Overall Analyses
   6/12 positive increase n.s.   16/36 positive increase p<0.05
   6/12 negative decrease n.s.   20/36 negative decrease p<0.05

Previous in vitro studies have shown that volunteers with low NK cell baseline values had significant increases of NK activity with met-enkephalin treatment. Low baseline conditions appear to be most sensitive to the stimulant effects of met-enkephalin in elevating NK cell activity have less response following enkephalin treatment (Faith et al., 1984). Similar effects on NK cell activity have been reported with the interferons (Lotzova et al., 1983).

Such increases in active T-cell rosettes as well as NK cells may have implications in the immunomodulatory control of infectious and neoplastic diseases, (Wybran and Fudenberg, 1973; Herberman, 1982). Certainly the elevations of blood levels of enkephalin as well as NK cell activity in times of stress have been now documented by several researchers (Udenfriend and Kilpatrick, 1983, Gilman et al., 1982; Hanbauer et al., 1982; Viveros et al., 1980; Farrell et al., 1982). It is possible that the enkephalins have a reciprocal relationship with the steroid hormones in modulating immune function in times of stress (Riley, 1981; Ader, 1982; Besedovsky et al., 1983).

It is hoped that the administration of met-enkephalin to patients with infections as well as cancerous tumor growth will be found useful in modulating the immune system, as measured by its restorative effects on T-cells and NK cells.

REFERENCES

Ader R., 1982, in: "Psychoneuroimmunology", Academic Press, New York.
Besedovsky, H. O., del Rey, A. E., and Sorkin, E., 1983, What do the immune system and brain know about each other? Immunol. Today, 4:342.
Blalock, J. E., and Smith, E. M., 1980, Human leukocyte interferon: structural and biological relatedness to adrenocorticotropic hormone and endorphins, Proc. Nat'l. Acad. Sci., 77:5972.
Faith, R. E., Liang, H. J., Murgo, A. J., and Plotnikoff, N. P., 1984, Neuroimmunomodulation with enkephalins: enhancement of human natural killer (NK) cell activity in vitro, Clin. Immunol. Immunopathol., 31:412.
Farrell, P. A., Getes, W. K., Maksud, M. G., and Morgan, W. P., 1982, Increases in plasma beta-endorphin/beta-lipotropin immunoreactivity after treadmill running in humans, J. Appl. Physiol., 52:1245.

Gilman, S. C., Schwartz, J. M., Milner, R. J., Bloom, F. E., and Feldman, J. D., 1982, Beta-endorphin enhances lymphocyte proliferative responses, Proc. Nat'l. Acad. Sci., 79: 4226.

Hanbauer, J., Kelly, G. D., Saiani, L., and Yang, H. Y. T., 1982, Met-enkephalin like peptides of adrenal medulla: release by nerve stimulation and functional implications, Peptides, 3: 469.

Hazum, E., Chang, K. J., and Cuatrecasas, P., 1979, Specific non-opiate receptors for beta-endorphins, Science, 205: 1033.

Herberman, R. B., 1982, in: "NK Cells And Other Natural Effector Cells", Academic Press, New York.

Hughes, I., Smith, T. W., Kosterlitz, H. W., Fotergill, L. A., Morhan, B. A., and Morriss, H. T., 1975, Identification of two related pentapeptides from the brain with potent opiate agonist activity, Nature, 258: 577.

Laszlo, J., Muang, A. T., Brenchman, W. D., Jeffs, C., Koren, H., Cianciolo, G., Metzgar, R., Cashdollar, W., Cox, E., Buckley III, C. E., Tso, C. Y., and Lucas, V. S., 1983, Phase I study of pharmacological and immunological effects of human lymphoid blasts interferons given to patients with cancer, J. Cancer Research, 43: 4458.

Lopker, A., Abood, L. G., Hoss, W., and Lionetti, F. J., 1980, Stereo-selective muscarinic, acetylcholine and opiate receptors in human phagocytic leukocytes, Biochem. Pharmacol., 29: 1361.

Lotzova, E., 1983, Function of natural killer cells in various biological phenomena, Surv. Synth. Path. Res., 2:41.

Mathews, P. M., Froelich, C. J., Sibbitt, Jr., W. L., and Bankhurst, A. D., 1983, Enhancement of natural cytotoxicity of beta-endorphin, J. Immunol., 130: 1658.

Miller, G. C., Murgo, A. J., and Plotnikoff, N. P., 1984, Enkephalins-Enhancement of active T-cells rosettes from normal volunteers, Clin. Immunol. and Immunopathol., 31: 132.

Plotnikoff, N. P., 1982, The central nervous system control of the immune-system-Enkephalins: Anti-tumor activities, Psychopharm. Bulletin, 18: 148.

Plotnikoff, N. P., Kastin, A. J., Coy, D. H., Christensen, C. W., Schally, A. V., and Spirtes, M. A., 1976, Neuropharmacological actions of enkephalin after systemic administration, Life Science, 19: 1283.

Plotnikoff, N. P., and Miller, G. C., 1983, Enkephalins as immunomodulators, Int. J. Immunopharmac., 5: 437

Plotnikoff, N. P., and Murgo, A. J., Faith, R. E., 1984, Neuroimmuno-modulation with enkephalins: Effects on thymus and spleen weights in mice, Clinical Immunology and Immunopathology, 32: 52.

Plotnikoff, N. P., Murgo, A. J., Miller, G. C., Corder, C. N., and Faith, R. E., 1985, Enkephalins: immunomodulators, Fed. Proc. 44: 118.

Prange, A. J. Jr., Wilson, J. C., Zara, P. P., Alltop, L. B., and Breese, G. R., 1972, Effects of thyrotropin-releasing hormone in depression, The Lancet, 2: 999.

Riley, V., 1981, Psychoneuroendocrine influences on immunocompetence and neoplasia, Science, 212: 1100.

Robbins, D. S., Donnan, G. G., Fudenberg, H. H., and Strelkauskas, A. J., 1981, Functional subsets of human T cells defined by 'active' rosette formation, Cell. Immunol., 59: 205.

Rossier, J., Dean, D. M., Livett, B. G., and Udenfriend, S., 1981, Enkephalin congeners and precursors are synthesized and released by primary cultures of adrenal chromaffin cells, Life Sci., 28: 781.

Schweigerer, L., Bhakdi, S., and Teschemacher, H., 1982, Specific non-opiate binding sites for human beta-endorphin on the terminal complex of human complement, Nature, 296: 572.

Simantov, R., and Snyder, S., 1976, Morphine-like peptides in mammalian brain: isolation, structure elucidation, and interactions with the opiate receptor, Proc. Nat'l Acad. Sci., 73: 2515.

Targan, S., Britvan, L., and Dorey, F., 1981, Activation of human NKCC by moderate exercise: increased frequency of NK cells with enhanced capability of effector-target lytic interactions, Clin. Exp. Immunol., 45: 352.

Udenfriend, S., and Kirkpatrick, D. L. 1983, Biochemistry of the enkephalins and enkephalin-containing peptides, Arch. Biochem. Biophys., 221: 309.

Vaught, J. L., and Takemori, A. E., 1979, Differential effects of leucine and methionine enkephalin on morphine-induced analgesia, acute tolerance and dependence, J. Pharmacol. Exp. Ther., 208: 86.

Viveros, O. H., Diliberto, E. J., Hazum, E., and Chang, K. J., 1980, Enkephalins as possible adrenomedullary hormones: storage, secretion, and regulation of synthesis, Adv. Biochem. Psychopharmacol., 22: 191.

Wybran, J., Appelboom, T., Famaey, J. P., Govaerts, A., 1979, Suggestive evidence for receptors for morphine and methionine-enkephalin on normal human blood T lymphocytes, J. Immunol., 123: 1068.

Wybran, J., and Fudenberg, H. H., 1973, Thymus-derived rosette-forming cells in various human disease states: cancer, lymphoma, bacterial and viral infections and other diseases, J. Clin. Invest., 52: 1026.

Wybran, J., Appelboom, T., Famaey, J. P., and Goverts, A., 1980, in: "International Symposium on New Trends in Human Immunology and Cancer Immunotherapy", B. Serrou and C. Rosenfeld, ed., Doin Press, Paris.

ACKNOWLDEGEMENTS

These studies were generously supported by a grant from TNI Pharmaceuticals, Inc., Tulsa, Oklahoma and Travenol Laboratories, Morton Grove, Illinois.

METHIONINE ENKEPHALIN: CLINICAL PHARMACOLOGY

N.P. Plotnikoff, S. Solomon, J.L. Valentine, M. Fesen, R.E.
Faith, L. Edwards, R. Richter, A.J. Murgo, and G.C. Miller*
Departments of Pharmacology and Medicine
School of Medicine
Oral Roberts University
Immuno-Diagnostics Laboratory*
Tulsa, OK 74171

INTRODUCTION

Earlier studies indicated that methionine enkephalin infusions (1,000 micrograms) in normal volunteers induced facial flushing, general vaso-dilation and noisy stomach (borborgymi). Blood pressure and pulse rate were normal in all experiments. Plasma levels of pancreatic polypeptide, somatostatin, T_3 and T_4, TSH, FSH, PRL, ACTH, and GH were unchanged. However, there was some reduction of LH (Rolandi et al., 1980, Goldstein et al., 1981). The present study is an evaluation of the effects of methionine enkephalin (over a broad dose range) on all of the vital signs as well as measurements of blood level.

PATIENTS AND METHODS

Twelve male subjects age 21-39 years were recruited for these studies and given appropriate informed consent documents approved by Oral Roberts University Institutional Review Board. They also provided a signed statement of complete abstinence from drugs, including alcohol and tobacco, at least three weeks prior to the study. All subjects were within 20% of ideal body weight and free of acute and chronic cardiovascular, renal, metabolic and neurological diseases. Those subjects satisfying admission criteria were admitted to the hospital the evening prior to the study, given the drug infusion in the morning of the second day and discharged on the third day.

LABORATORY/PHYSICAL EXAMINATION--PREHOSPITALIZATION CLINIC

A routine physical examination was done which included medical and social history, habits, medications and comprehensive physical examination. The examination included supine and erect heart rate, blood pressure, and examination of occult blood.

LABORATORY (CERTIFIED CLINICAL LABORATORY)

The laboratory work-up included: 12 lead electrocardiograms, chest x-rays, PA and lateral. A standard blood chemistry profile (SMAC 26) was done which routinely includes sodium, potassium, chloride, carbonate, glucose, BUN, creatinine, calcium, osmolality, phosphate, total protein, albumin, globulin, total bilirubin, SGOT, AST, ALK., phosphatase, LDH, cholesterol, triglyceride, uric acid and iron. Also included in the lab-

407

oratory testing were serum amylase, VDRL, ANA, HbSAg, clinical blood count (CBC), which includes WBC, RBC, Hg., HCT., Diff., platelet and RBC indices. Urinalysis was also done including pH, Sp. Gr., protein and microscopic. All patients had to have normal data for No. 1 and 2 before entering the hospital phase of the study.

METHIONINE ENKEPHALIN FORMULATION

An investigational new drug (IND) sterile solution of methionine enkephalin was prepared at 10 mg. per ml. Methionine enkephalin (Sigma-Aldrich Chem. Co., St. Louis, Mo.) was dissolved in sterile saline (0.9 gm NaCl per 100 ml) and passed through a 0.22 micron millipore filter. Sigma-Aldrich Chem. Co. provided the Master file for the FDA. The ultra-filtration through the millipore filter was done in the City of Faith Hospital pharmacy. Methionine enkephalin has the following characteristics: M.W. 574, water soluble, Amino acid sequence Tyr-Gly-Gly Phe-Met-OH. It was dissolved in 60 ml NS (0.9 gm NaCl per 100 ml) at a concentration sufficient to infuse at 2 ml per minute for 30 minutes to give a total delivered dose of 1, 10, 50, 100, 150 and 200 micrograms per kilogram body weight.

HOSPITALIZATION

Patients were admitted to the hospital at approximately 1600 on Day 1. A brief physical examination was done and recorded in their chart, and the consent form was signed. The protocol was as follows: Day 1, the patients were admitted, daily body weight taken. Breakfast on Day 2 was a clear liquid diet; thereafter, a regular diet was served. Activity was restricted to room. No visitors were allowed. Supine, standing heart rate and blood pressure were taken at 0800, 1400, 2000 and other times as indicated. Day 2 at 0800: a No. 18 gauge intracath was placed in the antecubital vein with open NS, 1 L. EKG leads and blood pressure cuff were attached. Baseline EKG, supine, erect blood pressure and heart rate were recorded.

SPECIAL PRECAUTIONS

Seizure precautions were taken from 0800 Day 2 to discharge. Usual cardiovascular emergency precautions were taken, including the availability of Naloxone injectibles. Patients used bed pans and urinals for voiding on Day 2 from 0830 to 1200 so that the patient would remain supine.

BEHAVIORAL TEST

100 mm. Mood Line Test. Clinical behavioral mood states were determined by the use of 100 mm Line Test. In this test, a 100 mm line was drawn on a sheet of plain paper and one end was identified "as well as I could be", the other end "as depressed as I could be". The patient marked where he/she stood at the moment of testing. The score, the length in millimeters from the "well" end of the line, was based on the premise that length is analagous to the severity of depression (Prange et al., 1972).

RIA-METHIONINE ENKEPHALIN METHODS

The Immuno Nuclear radioimmunoassay (Immuno Nuclear Corp., Minn.) for methionine enkephalin employs simultaneous addition of sample, rabbit anti-met-enkephalin antibody, and ^{125}I met-enkephalin, followed by an overnight incubation at $4°C$. Phase separation is accomplished by the addition of an equal volume of saturated ammonium sulfate in the presence of carrier gamma globulin. Met-enkephalin is extracted from plasma on ODS-silica, eluted, dried, and reconstituted for assay. Standard were prepared from 1-2000 ng/ml.

PROLACTIN DETERMINATION

The [^{125}I] Prolactin RIA kit by Diagnostic Products Corp., Los Angelos, CA was used for prolactin determinations. This kit requires no preliminary sample extraction. Furthermore, the calibration curve prepared in the presence of serum proteins has a range equivalent to circulating prolactin of 5-200 ng/ml.

RESULTS

Cardiovascular, Respiratory and Temperature Parameters

No significant changes in any parameter measured were recorded. Only transient increases or decreases were seen in heart rate and blood pressure. Representative findings are illustrated in Tables 1-6, showing effects of 1, 10, 50, 100, 150 and 200 micrograms/kg.

TABLE 1
VOLUNTEER #3
MET-ENKEPHALIN (0.001 mg/kg)

11/20/83	BLOOD PRESSURE Supine/Erect		HEART RATE(S/E)	RESP. RATE	TEMPERATURE (^{0}F)
0800	110/80	110/80	52/60	12	98
0830	110/80	110/80	56/60	12	98
0855	110/80	110/80	52/60	12	98
0900	ENKEPHALIN INFUSION				
0910	110/80		55	12	98
0920	110/80		55	12	98
0930	110/80		50	12	98
1000	110/80		54	10	98
1100	110/80	120/80	56/62	12	98
1300	110/80	110/80	55/58	12	98
1600	110/80	110/80	55/58	12	98
11/21/83					
0855	110/80	120/80	54/60	12	98

TABLE 2
VOLUNTEER #1
MET-ENKEPHALIN (0.010 mg/kg)

11/12/83	BLOOD PRESSURE		HEART RATE(S/E)	RESP. RATE	TEMPERATURE (^{0}F)
0800	100/70		44/45	12	98
0855	100/70		50/52	13	98.8
0900	ENKEPHALIN INFUSION				
0910	100/70		60	14	98.8
0920	100/70		60	12	98.8
0930	100/70		60	12	98.8
1000	110/70		64	12	98.8
1100	100/70		60	14	98.6
1300	100/70	100/70	45/60	12	98.4
1600	100/70	100/70	44/56	13	98.4
11/13/83					
0855	100/70	100/70	45/60	12	98.4

TABLE 3
VOLUNTEER #5
MET-ENKEPHALIN (0.050 mg/kg)

	BLOOD PRESSURE Supine/Erect		HEART RATE(S/E)	RESP. RATE	TEMPERATURE (^{o}F)
12/19/83					
0800	110/70	110/70	71/80	12	97.6
0855	110/70	110/70	68/76	12	97.6
0900	MET-ENKEPHALIN INFUSION				
0910	110/70		75	11	97.8
0920	110/70		81	12	97.4
0930	110/70		68	12	97.6
1000	110/70		65	11	97.6
1100	110/70	100/70	68/90	12	97.6
1300	110/70	100/70	64/90	12	98
1600	110/70	110/70	74/88	12	98
12/20/83					
0855	110/70	110/70	68/76	12	97

TABLE 4
VOLUNTEER #7
MET-ENKEPHALIN (0.100 mg/kg)

	BLOOD PRESSURE Supine		HEART RATE(S/E)	RESP. RATE	TEMPERATURE (^{o}F)
2/5/84					
0800	130/80		60/74	14	97.6
0855	120/80		57/64	12	98
0900	MET-ENKEPHALIN INFUSION				
0910	120/80		56	12	98
0920	120/80		54	12	98
0930	120/80		54	13	98
1000	120/80		63	12	98
1100	120/80		54/64	14	98
1300	120/80		64/72	14	98
1600	120/80		72/76	13	98
2/6/84					
0855	120/80		70/76	14	97.4

TABLE 5
VOLUNTEER #9
MET-ENKEPHALIN (0.150 mg/kg)

	BLOOD PRESSURE Supine		HEART RATE(S/E)	RESP. RATE	TEMPERATURE (^{o}F)
3/11/84					
0800	120/80		62/76	14	97.4
0855	120/80		76/80	13	98.2
0900	MET-ENKEPHALIN INFUSION				
0910	120/80		90	13	98
0920	120/80		81	12	98
0930	120/80		73	12	98
1000	120/80		74/102	14	98
1100	120/80		87/100	12	98
1300	120/80		74/80	13	98
1600	120/80		76/80	12	98
3/12/84					
0855	120/80		72/80	13	98

TABLE 6 - VOLUNTEER #11

MET-ENKEPHALIN (01.200 mg/kg)

	BLOOD PRESSURE	HEART RATE(S/E)	RESP. RATE	TEMPERATURE (^{o}F)
6/17/84				
0800	120/80	80/94	12	97.2
0855	120/80	74/76	12	97.2
0900	MET-ENKEPHALIN INFUSION			
0910	120/80	76	13	97.2
0920	120/80	88	14	97.2
0930	120/80	81	12	97.2
1000	120/80	71	12	97.4
1100	120/80	75/78	13	98
1200	120/80	70/74	14	98
1300	120/80	68/76	13	98
1600	120/80	70/74	12	98
6/18/84				
0830	120/80	61/68	12	97

TABLE 7 - HEART RATE

Maximum Increase Over Baseline Control-8:55 a.m.	Peak Time Increase	Maximum % Increase Over Baseline
#1 50 - 64 =	10:00 a.m.	28%
#2 70 - 76 =	10:00 a.m.	9%
#3 52 - 56 =	11:00 a.m.	8%
#4 60 - 74 =	10:00 a.m.	23%
#5 68 - 81 =	9:20 a.m.	19%
#6 76 - 82 =	9:30 a.m.	8%
#7 57 - 72 =	4:00 p.m.	26%
#8 70 - 76 =	9:30 a.m.	9%
#9 76 - 90 =	9:10 a.m.	18%
#10 55 - 62 =	10:00 a.m.	12%
#11 74 - 88 =	9:20 a.m.	19%
#12 66 - 75 =	9:30 a.m.	14%

8/12   10% Increase

7/8 a.m.   1/8 p.m.

Heart Rate

Eight subjects exhibited an increase in heart rate following the infusion of methionine enkephalin. However, no dose response was apparent and the increase in heart rate may have been due to anxiety(Table 7).

100 mm Test

Eight subjects indicated a shift to the "sad scale". (6/8)- Six of the eight subjects indicated this shift in the morning following infusion suggesting "sedation." Three subjects appeared to have transient mystagmus (attributabel to "sedative" effect).

TABLE 8
MET-ENKEPHALIN
100 mm LINE TEST

Maximum Change Over Controls 8:55 a.m.		Post-Infusion Peak Time	%Decrease Over Controls
#1	59mm – 38 =	10:00 a.m.	36%
#2	46mm – 44 =	9:30 a.m.	4%
#3	37mm – 28 =	10:00 a.m.	24%
#4	29mm – 26 =	10:00 a.m.	10%
#5	42mm – 30 =	4:00 p.m.	28%
#6	5.5mm – 3.0 =	4:00 p.m.	45%
#7	26mm – 26 =	11:00 p.m.	0%
#8	37mm – 12 =	4:00 p.m.	67%
#9	50mm – 17 =	1:00 p.m.	66%
#10	33mm – 21 =	4:00 p.m.	36%
#11	34mm – 24 =	1:00 p.m.	29%
#12	39mm – 31 =	4:00 p.m.	21%

$\frac{10}{12}$ 10% Decrease $p < 0.05$ Paired Difference Analyses

$\frac{3}{10}$ a.m. $\frac{7}{10}$ p.m.

TABLE 9
MET-ENKEPHALIN
100 mm LINE TEST

Maximum Change Over Controls 8:55 a.m.		Peak Time	%Increase Over Controls
#1	59 – no increase		0%
#2	46 – 50 =	11:00 a.m.	8%
#3	37 – 41 =	9:30 a.m.	10%
#4	29 – 38 =	4:00 p.m.	24%
#5	42 – 53 =	10:00 a.m.	26%
#6	5.5 – 17.0 =	1:00 p.m.	209%
#7	26 – 29 =	10:00 a.m.	11%
#8	37 – 61 =	11:00 a.m.	64%
#9	50 – no increase		0%
#10	33 – 38 =	9:30 a.m.	13%
#11	34 – 37 =	9:30 a.m.	8%
#12	39 – 54 =	10:00 a.m.	38%

8/12 10 % Increase $p < 0.05$ Paired Difference Analyses

6/8 a.m. 2/8 p.m.

Ten subjects indicated a shift to the "happy side of the scale". (7/10)-
Seven of the ten subjects reported a shift to the "happy side of the scale"
in the afternoon. See Table 9.

Prolactin

No significant alteration in plasma prolactin levels were observed over
the course of the study except for two subjects who showed an increase in
blood levels of prolactin after recieving a dose of ten micrograms/kilogram.

Blood Levels-Methionine Enkephalin

The pre-infusion levels of methionine enkephalin were quite high. This
was probably due to the stress of pre-infusion procedures(indwelling catheter,
EKG, as well as anticipation of the infusion). Volunteers maintained high
levels throughout the study.

Levels elevated above baseline were seen in volunteers administered 50
micrograms/kilogram, 100 micrograms/kilogram, 150 micrograms/kilogram, and
200 micrograms/kilogram. No apparent dose response was seen due to
administered methionine enkephalin.

TABLE 10:PROLACTIN BLOOD LEVELS(ng/ml)

DOSE	1 microgram/kg		10 micrograms/kg		50 micrograms/kg
Volunteer Number	1	2	3	4	5
0855 Day One	a	4.9	10.6	3.1	20.1
0910	0.2	3.8	7.7	3.3	2.6
0920	1.2	4.4	6.5	8.5	22.3
0930	0.9	2.1	10.6	29.1	14.0
1000	a	0.8	15.3	16.9	12.4
1100	a	6.4	25.1	42.4	9.4
0855 Day Two	0.3	6.3	14.3	24.0	18.7

[a]Below level of detection for the assay

TABLE 11: BLOOD LEVELS–MET ENKEPHALIN (pg/ml)

DOSE	1 microgram/kg	10 micrograms/kg	50 micrograms/kg
0855 Day One	763.5	377.9	130.3
0910	618.1	216.4	221.1
0920	557.2	162.6	179.9
0930	540.0	140.3	218.2
1000	706.7	138.8	860.9
1600	890.2	--	240.8
0855 Day Two	608.9	--	--

TABLE 12: BLOOD LEVELS–MET ENKEPHALIN (pg/ml)

DOSE	100 micrograms/kg	150 micrograms/kg	200 micrograms/kg
Control 0855	157.1	652.7	1315.4
0910	--	735.9	660.7
0920	252.4	759.6	1679.3
0930	196.4	1311.9	779.9
1000	--	785.8	264.5
1600	180.6	664.4	269.2
0855 Day Two	115.5	559.2	237.0

SIDE EFFECTS

No consistent changes or any dose response were observed.

Initial facial flushing following infusion; sedation, "stomach noises", skin tingling, were reported similar to other human enkephalin studies (Table 13).

SMAC 26 and Urinalysis

No consistent changes or dose response changes were observed.

The principal side effects observed were vaso-flushing(5/12) and gastro-intestinal disturbances(4/12). See Table 13.

414

TABLE 13: MET-ENKEPHALIN - PHASE I SUMMARY (12 Volunteers)

Side Effects	Frequency

Flushing

Warm feeling during infusion	1 (50 µg/kg)
Tingling and flushing scalp	1 (150 µg/kg)
Burning sensation -- head	1 (200 µg/kg)
Flushing face	1 (150 µg/kg)
(hands-head chest-body)	1 (200 µg/kg)
	TOTAL...5/12

Gastro-Intestinal

Crampy abdominal pain	1 (200 µg/kg)
Increased bowel sounds	1 (150 µg/kg)
Intra-umbilical abdominal cramps	1 (150 µg/kg)
Slightly nauseated	1 (100 µg/kg)
	TOTAL...4/12

Headache	2/12 (1 & 10 µg/kg)
Euphoric and light-headed	1/12 (1 µg/kg)
Angry for a couple of minutes	1/12 (50 µg/kg)
Drowsy-sleeping	1/12 (200 µg/kg)

DISCUSSION

The present study demonstrates that methionine enkephalin can be administered safely to humans over a wide dose range. No significant alterations in vital signs were observed. Biphasic behavioral changes were recorded on the 100 mm line test ("sedated" effects following the infusion in the morning and a "stimulant" effect in the afternoon). Only slight effects were seen in elevating prolactin levels (two volunteers). Blood levels of methionine enkephalin recorded were highly variable and appeared to be independent of any dose response relation. The side effects recorded were minimal and consisted predominantly of "vaso-dilation-flushing" (5/12) and gastro-intestinal effects (4/12). In general these effects were transient and seen at high doses.

In the earlier study reported by Golstein et al. (1981) methionine enkephalin at a dose of 1000 µg induced side effects of facial flushing, vasodilation and borborgymi, while blood pressure and pulse rate were normal. Hormone levels remained unchanged.

Other clinical studies with derivatives of methionine enkephalin indicated that various degrees of analgesia were observed because of stability as well as more side effects. Drowsiness, sensation of heaviness in extremeties, burning at injection site, and nasal congestion were the side effects reported (Calimlin et al., 1982).

FK 33-824, another enkephalin derivative apparently resulted in a larger rate of side effects in man; oppression of chest, red eyes, whole body flushing, as well as a flare reaction with intradermal injection (Von Grafferied et al., 1978). In addition, FK 33-834 increased PRL and GH and reduced cortisol (del Pozo et al., 1980).

The present study supports and extends the original findings by Golstein et al., (1981) that methionine enkephalin can be administered safely to man over a wide range.

The blood levels of methionine enkephalin observed would support the findings of Roda et al. (this volume) that there is protective binding to plasma proteins resulting in sustained blood levels. Also the difference in side effects compared to the synthetic derivatives suggest that methionine enkephalin may have great receptor specificity in the delta family of receptors.

REFERENCES

Calimlin, J. F., Sriwatanakul, K., Mardell, W. M., Lasagna, L., and Cox C., 1982, Analgesic efficacy of parenteral met-enkephamide acetate in treatment of post-operative pain (LY 127623), The Lancet, 1(2):1374.

del Pozo, E., Kleinstein, J., Brun del Re R., Derrer F., and Martin-Perez, J., 1980, Failure of oxytocin and lysine-vasopressin to stimulate prolactin release in humans, Horm. Metab. Res., 12:26.

Golstein, J., Cantraine, F., Copinschi, G., L'Hermite, M., Pipeleers, D., Robyn, C., Velkeniens, B., and Vanhaelst, L., 1981, Effects of enkephalin infusion on hormonal levels in man: Inhibition of the episodic secretion of LH by methionine enkephalin, IRCS Med. Sci., 9:218.

Plotnikoff, N. P., Murgo, A. J., Miller, G. C., Corder, C. N., and Faith, R. E., 1985, Enkephalins: Immunomodulators, Fed. Proc., 44:118.

Prange, A. J. Jr., Wilson, J. C., Zara, P. P., Alltop, L. B., and Breese, G. R., 1972, Effects of thyrotropin-releasing hormone in depression, The Lancet, 2(1):999.

Rolandi, E., Pescatore, D., Milesi, G. M., Gilberti, C., Sannia, A., and Barreca, T., 1980, Evaluation of LH, FSH, TSH, PRL, and GH secretion in patients suffering from prostatic neoplasms, Acta Endocrinol. (Copenh), 95:23

Von Graffenried, B., Del Pozo, E., Roubicek, J., Krebs, E., Poldinger, W., Burmeister, P., and Kerp, L., 1978, The effects of the synthetic enkephalin analogue FK 33-824 in man, Nature, 272:729.

METHIONINE ENKEPHALIN: T-CELL ENHANCEMENT IN NORMAL VOLUNTEERS (IN VIVO)

N.P. Plotnikoff, G.C. Miller*, S. Solomon
R.E. Faith, L. Edwards, and A.J. Murgo

Departments of Pharmocology and Medicine
Oral Roberts University, School of Medicine
Immuno-Diagnostics Laboratory*
Tulsa, Oklahoma 74171

INTRODUCTION

Earlier studies by our group indicated that methionine enkephalin enhanced PHA induced lymphocyte proliferation in mice, active rosette forming cells and NK cells in the cells of normal volunteer and cancer patients,(Plotnikoff et. al.,1985). More recently, several groups have reported that methionine enkephalin stimulates macrophage function as well as chemotaxis(Foris, 1984;Weber, 1984). Finally several groups have reported increased lymphokine production by methionine enkephalin(Brown, et al.,1985;Youkilis et al.,1985).

The present study demonstrates that methionine enkephalin increases circulating lymphocyte numbers, exhibited by increased numbers of various T-lymphocyte subpopulations, and enhances lymphoproliferation of PBL's stimulated with PHA.

METHODS

PATIENTS

Seven normal volunteers (males were studied clinically and immuno-logically prior to and following methionine enkephalin treatment.

METHIONINE ENKEPHALIN

Methionine enkephalin(Sigma-Aldrich Chem. Co., St. Louis, MO) was dissolved in sterile saline and filter sterilized by the hospital pharmacy. It was dissolved in 60 ml of saline at a concentration sufficient to infuse at 2 ml per minute for 30 minutes to give a total delivered dose of 10 to 25 micrograms per kilogram per body weight.

CELL PREPARATIONS

Heparinized peripheral blood was collected, incubated with 25 microliters of a 1:100 dilution of latex bead preparation/10^6 cells for 30 minutes at 37C, diluted with phosphate buffered saline(PBS), layered over a Ficoll-Paque(Pharmacia) gradient and centrifuged for 30 minutes at 400 x g. The mononuclear cell band was collected, washed twice with PBS, resuspended in RPMI 1640 and quantified.

ACTIVE T-CELLS

An equal volume of 1×10^6 lymphocytes and heat inactivated fetal calf serum was incubated at 37°C for 60 minutes. The fetal calf serum had been absorbed against both sheep and human AB erythrocytes. The lymphocytes were then gently mixed with an equal volume of sheep red blood cells (SRBC) at 4×10^7/ ml suspended in saline, centrifuged at 200x g at 4°C for 5 minutes gently resuspended and rosettes quantified using a hemacytometer. An active rosette forming cell is defined as a lymphocyte which has bound three or more SRBC.

T LYMPHOCYTES AND T SUBSETS

10^6 cells in 50 microliters PBS with 0.1% sodium azide was incubated for 30 minutes at 4°C with monoclonal antibodies (MoAb-s(10 micrograms/ml)). The cells were washed twice, incubated with FITC labeled goat anti-mouse serum at 4° for 30 minutes, washed twice again with PBS with sodium azide and gently resuspended in 1 drop of PBS with the sodium azide and quantified under a Nikon epi-illumination fluorescent microscope. Three hundred cells were counted: the monoclonal antibodies utilized were OKT 3, OKT 4, OKT 8, and OKT 11 (Ortho Pharmaceu., N.J.)

LYMPHOCYTE PROLIFERATION ASSAY

Lymphocyte proliferation, stimulated by Phytohemagglutinin (PHA), pokeweed mitogen (PWM), concanavalin A (con A) and Staphylcoccal Protein A was performed in triplicate. The mitogens, in varying concentrations, were plated with 1×10^5 cells per well in 96 microculture plates and were incubated for 96 hours. Sixteen hours before harvesting, 1 microCurie of ^{3}H thymidine (2 Ci/mmole; Amersham, Arlington Heights, Bethseda, MD) suction-filter apparatus and the activity of tritium bound to acid insoluble material was quantified in a liquid scintillation spectrometer.

NATURAL KILLER (NK) CELL ASSAY

K562 target cells, adjusted to 2×10^6 cells in 0.2 ml RPMI 1640, were labeled with $Na^{51}CrO_4$ (1mCi) for 45 minutes at 37°C in 5% CO_2. The cells were washed twice, resuspended in 2 ml RPMI 1640 and adjusted to 5×10^4 cells per ml. Peripheral blood lymphocytes were collected on a Ficoll-Paque gradient, washed twice and adjusted to 5×10^6 cells/ml and 3 serial 3 fold dilutions made. An equal volume of effector cells and target cells were added to wells in microtiter plates. These cell mixtures were incubated at 37°C in 5% CO_2 for 4 hours. A 0.1 ml aliquot was collected from each of the wells and quantified. The killing capabilities of the NK cells was calculated as follows:

$$NK \text{ ratio} = 1 - \frac{\text{Experimental counts } -SR}{\text{Total counts } - SR} \times 100$$

where SR = spontaneous release of ^{51}Cr.

INTERLEUKIN 2 RECEPTOR

Lymphocytes collected from a Ficoll-Paque gradient were incubated with Phytohemagglutinin for 96 hours, the cell harvested, washed twice and incubated with anti-human IL-2 receptor (Becton-Dickinson, Mtn. View, Calif.) for 30 minutes at 4°C. The cells were washed twice in PBS with sodium azide, incubated with FITC goat anti-mouse antibody, washed twice with PBS, resuspended in 1 drop of PBS with sodium azide and examined under the fluorescent microscope. Three hundred cells were counted.

RESULTS

TOTAL LYMPHOCYTES - There was a significant increase in numbers of circulating lymphocytes two hours after infusion in six volunteers (Table 1).

B LYMPHOCYTES - At two hours, there was a slight decrease in three
volunteers. At 24 hours there was a significant increase in five subjects
(Table 1).

ACTIVE ROSETTE FORMING CELLS - Significant increases of E rosettes were
found at both the 2 hour(six subjects) and 24 hour period(seven subjects)
(Table 1).

T-LYMPHOCYTES (OKT 11) - Significant increases in number of OKT 11 cells
were seen at both 2 hours in six volunteers and 24 hours in all seven
volunteers(Table II).

T-HELPER LYMPHOCYTES (OKT 4)- Six subjects recieving methionine enkephalin
showed a significant increase in OKT 4 labeled cells 2 hours after infusion.
All seven subjects had a significant increase at 24 hours(Table II).

T-SUPPRESSOR LYMPHOCYTES (OKT 8)- Five subjects exhibited an increase in
OKT 8 labeled cells 2 and 24 hours after infusion. Two subjects had a slight
decrease. There was no significant alteration of the ratio OKT 4 and OKT 8
labeled cells in those subjects at baseline and 1.6 at 2 and 24 hours
(Table II).

ACTIVE T-LYMPHOCYTES (ROSETTES) - Significant increases in number of rosettes
was seen in seven subjects at 2 hours and in six subjects at 24 hours
(Table II).

BLASTOGENESIS ConA - Significant increases in proliferative rates were seen
at 2 hours in six subjects (Table III).

BLASTOGENESIS ConA - Four subjects were found to have significant increases
at 24 hours while three subjects had significant decreases (Table III).

BLASTOGENESIS-POKEWEED - Five subjects were found to have a significant
increase at 2 hours (Table III).

BLASTOGENESIS-STAPH A - No significant changes were observed in four subjects
studied(Table III).

NK CELL ASSAY - At 2 hours, five of the volunteers were recorded to have
a significant decrease in NK activity at effector to target ratios of 100:1
and 11:1. At 24 hours, six volunteers registered a significant decrease at
a ratio of 100:1 while four subjects expressed a decrease at a ratio of
11:1 (Table IV).

NK CELLS (LEU 7) - No significant changes recorded in the four subjects
studied (Table IV).

DISCUSSION

The present study in normal volunteers demonstrates that methionine enkephalin
significantly elevates numbers of lymphocytes, active rosette forming cells,
and T lymphocyte subsets. In addition there is a significant increase in PHA
and ConA stimulated blastogenesis in some but not all individuals. Earlier
studies indicated that in vitro , methionine enkephalin increased numbers of
rosette forming cells in normal volunteer cells(Plotnikoff et al.,1985). In
this regard, significant increases in T lymphocyte subsets have now been

TABLE I - LYMPHOCYTES FROM VOLUNTEERS
ADMINISTERED METHIONINE ENKEPHALIN

Lymphocytes

0 hours	2 hours	24 hours
1864±90	2375±185* (6/7 +)	--
0 hours 1739±129		2212±223 (7/7 +)

B Lymphocytes

0 hours	2 hours	24 hours
212±25 (4/7 +)	295±27 (4/7 +)	--
247±33 (3/7 +)	225±40* (4/7 +)	--
226±24 (5/7 +)		*323±39 (5/7 +)

T Lymphocytes (OKT 11 Rosettes)

0 hours	2 hours	24 hours
1004±74 (6/7 +)	1495±133* (6/7 +)	
972±70 (7/7 +)		1184±215* (7/7 +)

* Significant difference from controls $p < 0.05$ paired difference analysis

TABLE II - T LYMPHOCYTES FROM VOLUNTEERS

ADMINISTERED METHIONINE ENKEPHALIN

T Lymphocytes (OKT 11)

0 hours	2 hours	24 hours
1353±108 (6/7 +)	1791±138* (6/7 +)	
1282±115 (7/7 +)		1774±171* (7/7 +)

T Helper Lymphocytes (OKT 4)

0 hours	2 hours	24 hours
719±89 (6/7 +)	983±55* (6/7 +)	
690±81 (7/7 +)		979±110* (7/7 +)

T Supressor Lymphocytes (OKT 8)

0 hours	2 hours	24 hours
419±39 (5/7 +)	635±89* (5/7 +)	
374±82 (5/7 +)		632±163* (5/7 +)
Ratio 1.7	Ratio 1.6	Ratio 1.6

Active T Lymphocytes

0 hours	2 hours	24 hours
31±6 (7/7 +)	66±13* (7/7 +)	
34±6 (6/7 +)		87±17* (6/7 +)

* Significant difference from controls p<0.05 paired difference analysis

421

TABLE III—BLASTOGENESIS FROM VOLUNTEERS ADMINISTERED METHIONINE ENKEPHALIN

Blastogenesis PHA

0 hours	2 hours	24 hours
219±77 (6/7 +)	468±130* (6/7 +)	
246±88 (5/7 +)		357±81 (5/7 +)

Blastogenesis ConA

0 hours	2 hours	24 hours
173±54 (4/7 +)	238±87 (4/7 +)	
211±69 (4/7 +)		375±50* (4/7 +)
192±15 (3/7 −)		136±24* (3/7 −)

Blastogenesis —Pokeweed

0 hours	2 hours	24 hours
33±10 (5/7 +)	53±16 * (5/7 +)	
37±10 (5/7 +)		63±11 (5/7 +)

Blastogenesis-Staph A

0 hours	2 hours	24 hours
12±7 ($\frac{2}{4}$ + $\frac{2}{4}$ −)	15±11 ($\frac{2}{4}$ + $\frac{2}{4}$ −)	
11±7 ($\frac{2}{4}$ + $\frac{2}{4}$ −)		13±8 ($\frac{2}{4}$ + $\frac{2}{4}$ −)

*Significant difference from controls $p < 0.05$

found in a patient with Kaposis' sarcoma(AIDS) as well as a lung cancer patient(Plotnikoff et al.,1985). Therefore, it may be of great interest to expand the clinical studies into patients with T-cell deficiencies. However, in the present study no significant increase in NK cell activity was observed in contrast to earlier in vitro studies, perhaps because of high baseline control levels. The highly significant increase in T lymphocytes and T-cell subsets and PHA induced blastogenesis is supported by our earlier findings that methionine enkephalin may be stimulating in the maturation of T-cells in the thymus gland. This effect on T-cells is separate from other natural hormone immunomodulators such as interferons, and interleukins(Einhorn et al.,1983).

TABLE IV - NK CELLS FROM VOLUNTEERS
ADMINISTERED METHIONINE ENKEPHALIN

NK CELL ASSAY

100:1 Effector/Target Ratio

0 hours	2 hours	24 hours
54+ 6 (5/7 -)	51+6* (5/7 -)	
56+4 (6/7 -)		47+4* (6/7 -)

33:1 Ratio

27+6 (4/7 +)	29+5 (4/7 +)	
37+3 (3/7 -)	35+2 (3/7 -)	
34+4 (6/7 -)		29+4 (6/7 -)

11:1 Ratio

| 20+2 (5/7 -) | 15+3* (5/7 -) | |
| 19+4 (4/7 -) | | 16+4* (4/7 -) |

NK CELLS(LEU 7)

0 hours	2 hours	24 hours
252+68 ($\frac{2}{4}$ + $\frac{2}{4}$ -)	374+95	
297+66 ($\frac{2}{4}$ + $\frac{2}{4}$ -)		288+86

* Significant difference from controls p less than 0.05

REFERENCES

Brown, S. L. and Van Epps, E. E., 1985, Beta endorphin (BE), met-enkephalin (ME), and corticotrophin (ACTH) modulate the production of gamma interferon (INF) in vitro, Fed. Proc., 44:949.

Einhorn, S., Blomgren, H., Stander, H., and Troye, M., 1983, Activity following treatment with Interferon In Vivo, in: "Mediation of Cellular Immunity in Cancer by Immune Modifiers", M. A. Chirigos, ed., Raven Press, New York.

DeMaeyer, G., Galasso, G., and Schellenkens, H., eds. 1983, in: "The biology of the interferon system", 347-352, Elsevier/North Holland Biomedical Press, Amsterdam.

Foris, G., Medgyesi, G. A., Gyimesi, E., and Hauck, M., 1984, Met-enkephalin: induced alterations of macrophage functions, Mol. Immun., 21:747.

Plotnikoff, N. P., Murgo, A. J., Miller, G. C., Corder, C. N., and Faith, R. E., 1985, Enkephalins: Immunomodulators, Fed. Proc. 44:118.

Plotnikoff, N. P., Miller, G. C., Wybran, J., and Nimeh, N. F., April 10, 1985, Methionine enkephalin T-cell enhancement in Kaposis' sarcoma, Serono Symposium, Copley Plaza Hotel, Boston, Recent Advances in Primary and Acquired Immunodeficiencies (in Press).

Weber, R. J., and Pert, C. B., 1984, Opiatergic modulation of the immune system, in: "Central and Peripheral Endorphins: Basic and Clinical Aspects", E. E. Muller and A. R. Genezzani, eds., Raven Press, New York.

Youkilis, E., Chapman, J., Woods, E., and Plotnikoff, N., 1985, In Vivo immunostimulation and increased in vitro production of interleukin 1 (IL-1) activity by met-enkephalin, Int. J. Immunopharm., 7:79.

METHIONINE ENKEPHALIN: ENHANCEMENT OF T-CELLS IN

PATIENTS WITH KAPOSIS'SARCOMA, AIDS, AND LUNG CANCER

N.P. Plotnikoff[*], J. Wybran[**], N.F. Nimeh[***], and G.C. Miller[****]

Departments of Pharmacology[*] and Medicine [***]
Oral Roberts University School of Medicine,
Immuno-Diagnostics Laboratory, Inc. [****]
Tulsa, Oklahoma; Hospital Erasme, Universite Libre de
Bruxelles, Brussels, Belgium [**]

INTRODUCTION

The enkephalins were originally described as endogenous opiate peptides modulating perception of pain (1). Other behavioral functions for the peptides were identified including anti-depressant and anti-anxiety actions (2).

More recently we reported that the enkephalins were immunomodulators, resulting in very significant activation of the T-cells in mice and men (3,4,5,6,7,8). Based on the latter studies we started a series of in vivo studies in normal volunteers as well as cancer patients.

Patient one, age 27, was admitted to our hospital with swollen lymph nodes, fever, and suspected Kaposis'sarcoma and Pneumocystitis. Initially he was placed on Pentamidine therapy for suspected Pneumocystis carinii pneumonia. After the initial treatments with Pentamidine, the patient was placed on methionine enkephalin treatment. The schedule employed was daily infusion the first week for five days and twice a week thereafter. The dose employed was ten micrograms per kilogram prepared in a normal saline solution and infused over a thirty minute time course. Twenty four hours after infusion, blood samples were withdrawn and analyzed for T-cells (E rosettes), OKT 3 T lymphocytes, mature thymocytes, OKT 11 T lymphocytes-early development stage thymocytes, T helper cells (OKT 4), T suppressor cells (OKT 8), blastogenesis or mitogen stimulated proliferation, phytohem-agglutinin (T helper cell mitogen), concanavalin A (a T helper and T suppressor cell mitogen), pokeweed (a T dependent B cell mitogen), and Staph A (a B cell mitogen). NK cell assay (natural killer cells) was conducted against the K-562 tumor cell line labeled with ^{51}Cr (7).

This patient received infusions of methionine enkephalin (10 micrograms per kilogram) each day of the first week (five days, Monday thru Friday). Blood samples were taken each day before infusion of methionine enkephalin. The data in Table 1 indicates that absolute number of T helper cells increased (57 to 94/mm^3) and the absolute number of suppressor cells (OKT 8) decreased from 382 to 264 per mm^3 on the fifth day. There was a slight increase in OKT 3 and OKT 11 cells. The T helper/T suppressor ratio rose from 0.149 to 0.354. The total lymphocyte count dropped from 516 on day 1 to 368 on day 4 and rose again to 550 on day 5. Active T-cells rose significantly from 201 on day 1 to 396/mm^3 on day 5.

No methionine enkephalin was infused on day 6 or day 7. Day 8 blood samples were withdrawn followed by methionine enkephalin infusion (dose of 25 micrograms per kilogram) corresponding to one-half of the first week total dose. The T-cells were still elevated on day 8 compared to day 5. T helper cells were 119 compared to 94; T suppressor cells increased to 409 from 264; OKT 3 increased from 341 to 491/mm^3; and OKT 11 increased from 429 on day 5 to 558 on day 8. The active T-cells increased to 565/mm^3 on day 8 compared to 396/mm^3 on day 5. Futhermore, the total lymphocytes increased to 774/mm^3 on day 8 compared to 550/mm^3 on day 5. The NK cell assay on day 8 was slightly decreased compared to day 1 values.

On day 11 blood samples were taken once again followed by methionine enkephalin infusion. All of the T-cell subsets increased except active T-cells. The total lymphocyte count diminished slightly.

The patient was discharged from the hospital with signs of subjective improvement. Of great interest was that the original lesion of the sarcoma including biopsy hole, was crusting and healing. Lymph nodes in the axillary and groin area were palpably smaller.

AIDS PATIENT STUDY BY DR. J. WYBRAN (BRUSSELS, BELGIUM)

Patient 2

Methionine enkephalin was given to a 26 year old male caucasian AIDS patient from Zaire, Africa whose clinical manifestations included resected cerebral lymphoma and opportunistic infections (Candida albicans and Mycobacterium bovis). Methionine enkephalin (UCB, Brussels) was administered at a dose of 20 micrograms/kilogram in saline perfusion over a period of 30 minutes. Lymphocyte population were studied using monoclonal antibodies (Ortho, Raritan, New Jersey and Becton-Dickinson, Mtn. View, California). After incubation with the monoclonal antibodies, the cells were further incubated with goat anti-mouse coupled particles of colloidal gold (Janssen Life Science Products, Beerse, Belgium) and the smears were put in a silver developer and counter-stained with May-Grunwald-Giemsa (9). This smear method allows morphology and is about twenty times more sensitive than immunofluorescence.

RESULTS

Lymphocytes	Before	After 2 hours	After 24 hours
OKT 3	30 %	26 %	27 %
OKT 10	45 %	53 %	49 %
OKT 11	31 %	34 %	31 %

Blood T-cells increased in number slightly as judged by the OKT 10 and OKT 11 antisera. Of special interest is the increase in OKT 10 which is similar to in vitro data obtained by incubating human lymphocytes with methionine enkephalin (10).

LUNG CANCER PATIENTS (W.A.)

Patient 3

This woman was found refractory to chemotherapy and had a positive X-ray diagnosis of lung cancer. The dose schedule was the same as our Kaposis' sarcoma patient (10 micrograms/kilogram per day the first week and 25 micrograms per kilogram two to three times a week thereafter).

Patient 1	Day	1	2	3	4	5	8	11
ASSAYS	Rx Conc	10 μg/K/da	10 μg/K/da	10 μg/K/da	10 μg/K/da	10 μg/K/da	25 μg/K/2x wk	25 μg/K/2x wk
WBC		4300/mm^3	2600/mm^3	2300/mm^3	2300/mm^3	2500/mm^3	3100/mm^3	2950/mm^3
Lymphocytes		516/mm^3	442/mm^3	391/mm^3	368/mm^3	550/mm^3	774/mm^3	738/mm^3
Active T cells								
Percent		39%	83%	79%	72%	72%	76%	26%
Absolute		201/mm^3	367/mm^3	309/mm^3	265/mm^3	396/mm^3	565/mm^3	192/mm^3
T LYMPHOCYTES & SUBSETS								
T lymphocytes (OKT 3)								
Percent		60%	80%	82%	82%	62%	66%	76%
Absolute		310/mm^3	354/mm^3	321/mm^3	302/mm^3	341/mm^3	491/mm^3	561/mm^3
T lymphocytes (OKT 11)								
Percent		79%	88%	80%	80%	78%	75%	81%
Absolute		408/mm^3	389/mm^3	313/mm^3	294/mm^3	429/mm^3	558/mm^3	598/mm^3
T lymphocytes (OKT 4)								
Percent		11%	13%	14%	17%	17%	16%	17%
Absolute		57/mm^3	58/mm^3	55/mm^3	63/mm^3	94/mm^3	119/mm^3	125/mm^3
T lymphocytes (OKT 8)								
Percent		74%	63%	53%	53%	48%	55%	61%
Absolute		382/mm^3	278/mm^3	207/mm^3	195/mm^3	264/mm^3	409/mm^3	450/mm^3
T helper/T suppressor ratio		0.149	0.209	0.264	0.321	0.354	0.291	0.278
BLASTOGENESIS								
Phytohemagglutinin		20X	---	---	---	---	134X	---
Concanavalin A		11X	---	---	---	---	49X	---
Pokeweed		12X	---	---	---	---	18X	---
Staph A		1X	---	---	---	---	3X	---
Interleukin 2 Receptor		14%	---	---	---	---	48%	---
NK cell Assay								
100:1		26%	---	---	---	---	16%	17%
33:1		11%	---	---	---	---	8%	---
11:1		5%	---	---	---	---	3%	---
Slope of killing		0.237	---	---	---	---	0.156	---

DAYS

ASSAYS	1	2	3	4	5	8	11	15	18	22	25	29	32	36
Lymphocytes(per mm³)	1360	1088	1952	1488	2002	2040	1908	1716	1974	N.D.	N.D.	1830	3159	1452
Active T-cells Percent	52%	54%	34%	43%	23%	58%	30%	40%	16%	36%	74%	40%	23%	52%
Absolute(per mm³)	707	578	664	639	460	1183	572	686	316	685	N.D.	732	727	755
T LYMPHOCYTES & SUBSETS														
T lymphocytes (OKT 3) Percent	64%	–	–	–	–	47%	–	–	–	–	–	67%	–	–
Absolute (per mm³)	870	–	–	–	–	959	–	–	–	–	–	985	–	–
T lymphocytes (OKT 11) Percent	77%	–	–	–	–	50%	–	–	–	–	–	74%	–	–
Absolute(per mm³)	1047	–	–	–	–	1020	–	–	–	–	–	1088	–	–
T lymphocytes (OKT 4) Percent	36%	–	–	–	–	28%	–	–	–	–	–	44%	–	–
Absolute(per mm³)	489	–	–	–	–	571	–	–	–	–	–	647	–	–
T suppressor cells (OKT 8) Percent	20%	–	–	–	–	17%	–	–	–	–	–	22%	–	–
Absolute(per mm³)	272	–	–	–	–	347	–	–	–	–	–	323	–	–
T helper/suppressor Ratio	1.8	–	–	–	–	1.65	–	–	–	–	–	2.0	–	–
BLASTOGENESIS														
Phytohemagglutinin	723X	–	–	–	–	432X	–	–	–	–	–	864X	–	–
Concanavalin A	704X	–	–	–	–	576X	–	–	–	–	–	711X	–	–
Pokeweed	83X	–	–	–	–	78X	–	–	–	–	–	73X	–	–
Staph A	21X	–	–	–	–	84X	–	–	–	–	–	44X	–	–
Interleukin-2 Receptor	52%	–	–	–	–	60%	–	–	–	–	–	80%	–	–
NK Cell Assay 100:1	50%	–	–	–	–	28%	–	–	–	–	–	30.6%	–	–
33:1	23%	–	–	–	–	11%	–	–	–	–	–	19.3%	–	–
11:1	11%	–	–	–	–	6%	–	–	–	–	–	8.8%	–	–
Slope of killing	.4369	–	–	–	–	0.2515	–	–	–	–	–	.227	–	–

The accompanying table illustrates the finding that OKT 3, OKT 4, OKT 8, increase significantly over the 29 days. The degree of blastogenesis with phytohemagglutinin also increased. However, one of the most striking increases was seen in the percent of interleukin-2 receptors. A slight decrease in NK cell activity was observed. Finally, there was a significant increase in the absolute lymphocyte count.

DISCUSSION

The patient with Kaposis' sarcoma was diagnosed as an AIDS patient on the basis of defective T helper cell levels compared to T suppressor cell levels. Seligmann et al. have indicated that AIDS is characterized by a decreased OKT 4 lymphocyte subset (11).

The present study with methionine enkephalin is based on our earlier findings that methionine enkephalin stimulates PHA-induced blastogenesis (a T helper cell antigen) in mice and also markedly stimulates OKT 4 (T helper cell) production in normal volunteers (Plotnikoff et al.). Similar elevation of T helper cells by methionine enkephalin was seen in the present AIDS patient with Kaposis' sarcoma. In addition there is a marked elevation of interleukin-2 receptors to 48% of the lymphocytes compared to 14% on day one. In addition, the primary sarcoma lesion appears to be healing. Similar findings on T-cell subsets were seen both in the AIDS patient studied by J. Wybran as well as the lung cancer patient studied by our group.

REFERENCES

1. J. Hughes, T. W. Smith, H. W. Kosterlitz, Z. A. Fothergill, B. A. Morgan, and H. T. Morris, Identification of two related pentapeptides from the brain with potent opiate agonist activity, Nature, 258:577 (1975).
2. N. P. Plotnikoff, A. J. Kastin, D. H. Coy, C. W. Christensen, S. V. Schally, and M. A. Spirtes, Neuropharmacological action of enkephalins after systemic administration, Life Science, 19:1283 (1976).
3. N. P. Plotnikoff and G. C. Miller, Enkephalins as immunomodulators, Int. J. Immunopharm., 5:437 (1983).
4. N. P. Plotnikoff, A. J. Murgo, and R. E. Faith, Neuroimmunomodulation with enkephalins: Effects on thymus and spleen weights in mice, Clin. Immunol. Immunopathol., 26:446 (1983).
5. G. C. Miller, A. J. Murgo, and N. P. Plotnikoff, Enkephalins: Enhancement of active T-cell rosettes from lymphoma patients, Clin. Immunol. Immunopathol., 26:446 (1983).
6. G. C. Miller, A. J. Murgo, and N. P. Plotnikoff, Enkephalins: Enhancement of active T-cell rosettes from normal volunteers, Clin. Immunol. Immunopathol., 31:132 (1984).
7. R. E. Faith, H. J. Liang, A. J. Murgo, and N. P. Plotnikoff, Neuroimmodulation with enkephalins: Enhancement of human natural killer (NK) cell activity in vitro, Clin. Immunol. Immunopathol., 31:412 (1984).
8. J. Wybran, Enkephalins and endorphins as modifiers of the immune system: Present and future, Fed. Proc., 44:92 (1985).
9. F. Romasco, J. Rosenberg, and J. Wybran, An immunogold silver staining method for the light microscopical analysis of blood lymphocyte subsets with monoclonal antibodies, Amer. J. Clin. Pathol., (in press).
10. J. Wybran and L. Schandene (in preparation).
11. M. Seligmann, L. Chess, J. L. Fahey, A. A. Fauci, P. Lachmann, J. L'Age-Stehr, J. Ngu, A. J. Pinching, F. S. Rosen, T. J. Spira, and J. Wybran, AIDS: An immunologic re-evaluation, N. Eng. J. Med., 311:1286 (1984).

Robert E. Faith[a], Anthony J. Murgo[b], and Nicholas P.
Plotnikoff[c]

[a]University of Houston, Houston, TX; [b]West Virginia
University Medical Center, Morgantown, WV; [c]Oral Roberts
University School of Medicine, Tulsa, OK

When immunology was a new science the immune system and immune response were viewed in rather simple terms. The immune system was viewed to
be rather autonomous in function and to be a primairly internally regulated
system. This view was supported by the fact that various elements of the
immune system are capable of functioning in in vitro systems and by the
natural antibody selection theory (1). As our knowledge of immunity and the
immune system has increased it has become increasingly clear that the immune system is quite complex, both in its make up and its functions.

In the early 1960's it was demonstrated that there is a division of
labor in the immune response and that lymphocytes could be divided into
thymus-derived lymphocytes (T-cells) and bursal or bursal-equivalent derived lymphocytes (B-cells). Subsequent studies have shown that the two
divisions are further subdivided with each having several functionally
different subpopulations of cells. The two divisions have been shown to
interact in various ways providing both help and suppression.

As the complexity of the immune system has become increasingly clearer
it has also become apparent that the immune system interacts with other
bodily systems, especially the endocrine system and the central nervous
system. In fact, it has recently been suggested that perhaps the immune
system should be viewed as an internal sensory organ recognizing non-
cognitive stimuli such as bacteria, viruses, antigens, etc and relaying
information to the neuroendocrine system by lymphocyte derived hormones (2).

The recurrent theme in this volume is that there exists an intimate
interrelationship between the immune, endocrine and central nervous systems.
Indications of this interrelationship discussed in this volume are briefly
reviewed here. An early indication of the interaction of the endocrine
and immune systems was provided by the now well known effects of adrenal
glucocorticosteroids on immune function. Other, more recent findings include the observation that the estrogens suppress immune functions, primarily through interactions with thymic epithelial cells. In contrast,
androgens have been shown to be immunoenhancing. Thyroxine has been shown
to increase phagocytic activity and the inhibition of thyroid activity to
suppress immune responses.

The endogenous opioid peptides, which have now been shown to be produced and stored in and secreted by the adrenals, as well as the central

nervous system, now appear to play a role in regulation of immune function. These peptides are apparently protected from hydrolysis by enzymes in circulation which allows for half-lives sufficiently long for the peptides to be physiologically active. Lymphocytes, monocytes, granulocytes and mast cells have been shown to have receptors for the opioid peptides. The enkephalins and beta-endorphin have been shown to modulate a number of immune functions in vitro, generally enhancing T cell functions and natural killer (NK) cell activity. These peptides also modulate the functions of neutrophils and macrophages. It appears that these peptides may be shown to be critically involved in the regulation of immnue responses.

In addition to the effects of the neuropeptides on immune function there are other manifestations of central nervous system effects on immune function. Undoubtedly some of these central nervous system effects will be observed to be mediated via the neuropeptides while others will be shown to be mediated in other ways. It has now been demonstrated that stress may or may not induce suppression of immune response depending upon whether the stressed individual is able to "cope" with his stress or not. Indeed some forms of stress actually appear to be healthful while other forms of stress can lead to disease conditions. Other interactions of the central nervous system with the immune system include the observations that depressive illness may lead to abnormalities in immune regulation and in neuroendocrine regulation. Physical lesioning of various areas in the hypothalmus lead to modulation of immune responses. Lesions in some areas lead to suppression while lesions in other areas lead to enhancement. One of the most intriguing observations is that immune responses can be conditioned in a Pavlovian manner just as other physiological responses.

The interaction of the central nervous and endocrine systems with the immune system is not a one way street. There is a growing body of evidence that the cells of the immune system produce molecules which allow communication with the other two systems. It has now been well documented that lymphocytes produce active neuropeptide hormones (ACTH, endorphins, etc.) and also produce thyrotropin, vasoactive intestinal peptide and somatostatin. Further evidence for feedback regulation from the immune system to the central nervous system is provided by the observation that there are receptors for lymphokines in the central nervous system and lymphokines such as interleukin-1 and interleukin-2 may directly influence pituitary fuction.

Other observations of interest are those which show endogenous opioid levels to be increased both by exercise and trauma. These observations lead to speculation that the increased levels of enkephalins/endorphins may be a partial explanation as to why well conditioned individuals are apparently healthier and more resistant to disease than sedentary individuals. Perhaps the increased levels of endogenous opioids enhance immune function in well conditioned individuals leading to increased resistance to disease. By the same token increased levels of endogenous opioids following trauma would function to enhance the body's ability to resist infection at the site of the injury as well as provide an endogenous source of analgesia.

We feel that further investigation will show the enkephalins/endorphins to be significant endogenous regulators of immune function. As such we feel they will become important tools for immunotherapy of various disease states, especially certain immunodeficiency states and neoplastic disease. Indeed the final chapters of this volume provide the initial observations indicating that this is the case.

REFERENCES

1. N. K. Jerne, 1955, The natural selection theory of antibody formation. Proc. Natl. Acad. Sci. (U.S.A.), 41: 849.
2. J. E. Blalock, 1984, The immune system as a sensory organ. J. Immunol., 132: 1067.

CONTRIBUTORS

INDEX